Improve International

MANUAL OF SMALL ANIMAL DIAGNOSTIC IMAGING

Improve
Veterinary Education

First published 2024

Published by
Improve International Ltd.
Alexandra House, Whittingham Drive
Wroughton, Swindon,
Wiltshire SN4 0QJ
United Kingdom

Tel: +44 (0) 1 793 759 159
https://improveinternational.com/uk/

Important note
Veterinary medicine is an ever-changing science, so the contents of this publication, especially recommendations concerning diagnostic and therapeutic procedures, can only give an account of the knowledge at the time of publication. While utmost care has been taken to ensure that all specifications regarding drug selection and dosage and treatment options are accurate, readers are urged to review the product information sheet and any relevant material supplied by the manufacturer, and, in case of doubt, to consult a specialist. From both an editorial and public interest perspective, the publisher welcomes notification of possible inconsistencies. The ultimate responsibility for any diagnostic or therapeutic application lies with the reader.

A catalogue record for this book is available from the British Library.

ISBN: 978-1-913352-17-2

Copywriter: Clare Farrar
Illustrator: Elaine Leggett
Photos by the authors unless otherwise indicated.

Inclusion in this publication of the logo, advertising or commercial name of any company other than Improve International does not imply that it has participated in the elaboration, writing or revision of the content. This inclusion does not signify the endorsement of the owner or editors or collaborators of said brands, products, or services.

Any comments regarding this publication will be considered to improve future editions.

Please contact us via email:

info.es@improveinternational.com

Or via our website:

https://www.improveinternational.com

The erratum and other updates will be published on the following website:

https://publication.improveinternational.com

Authors

Amalia Agut Giménez

DVM PhD Dipl. ECVDI
Amalia obtained her DVM and PhD in veterinary medicine from the University of Zaragoza, and is a diplomate of the European College of Veterinary Diagnostic Imaging (ECVDI). She is currently lecturer in Radiology of the Department of Small Animal Surgery and Medicine and Head of the Diagnostic Imaging Service at the Clinical Veterinary Hospital at the University of Murcia. She has completed several short stays at various centres in universities in the United Kingdom, in addition to the University of Sydney (Australia). She has been a member of the Board of the ECVDI and is Associate Director of the International Veterinary Radiology Association. She has presented papers, lectures and seminars at national and international congresses and published articles in both national and international journals as well as authoring and co-authoring books on small animal diagnostic imaging.

Pablo Amengual Batle

DVM, Dipl. ECVN
Pablo completed his veterinary degree at the Autonomous University of Barcelona in 2012, followed by an internship in small animal medicine and surgery. After working in general practice for six months he moved to the United Kingdom where he spent six months with the Department of Neurology and Neurosurgery at the University of Edinburgh and subsequently completed a second internship at the same university. In 2016 Pablo started a residency in neurology and neurosurgery at the University of Glasgow and in 2019 he returned to the University of Edinburgh as lecturer in neurology. In 2020 he became a diplomate of the European College of Veterinary Neurology. Since 2020 he has worked in multiple hospitals in the United Kingdom and is currently Head of Neurology at Hospital Puchol.

Agustina Ansón Fernández

DVM, PhD, Dipl. ECVDI
Agustina completed her veterinary degree at the University of Murcia in 2007 and after working in private practice for two years subsequently completed a master's degree in diagnostic imaging techniques in 2010 and an internship in diagnostic imaging in 2011, both at the University of Murcia in 2010. From 2011 to 2014 Agustina completed a residency in diagnostic imaging becoming a European diplomate (ECVDI) and obtained her PhD at the same university in 2016. She has received numerous prizes including best oral presentation at the International Congress of Veterinary Radiology in Turkey (2012) and best poster (Rhodes prize) at the International Congress of Veterinary Radiology in Australia (2015). She was an associate lecturer at the University of Vienna (Austria) from 2014 to 2019 and since 2019 has been as lecturer at Tufts University (Boston, USA), during which time she has also worked in teleradiology. She has also spent time visiting various European and American universities, including Glasgow, Dublin, and North Carolina amongst others. Agustina has also authored multiple publications in both national and international journals, in addition to presenting scientific communications and talks both nationally and internationally.

Abby Caine

MA VetMB, Dipl. ECVDI, CertVDI
Abby graduated from Cambridge Veterinary School in 2001. During five years in a busy small animal practice, she developed an interest in radiology and ultrasound, and gained the RCVS Certificate in Veterinary Diagnostic Imaging. She returned to Cambridge in 2006 to undertake a Residency in Diagnostic Imaging, was awarded the European Diploma in Veterinary Diagnostic Imaging in 2009, and since then has worked as an imaging specialist at Dick White Referrals (DWR), a multidisciplinary referral hospital managed by specialists situated in the east of England.

She is an active member of the British and Irish Division of the European Association of Veterinary Diagnostic Imaging and has been a member of the Board of the European College of Veterinary Diagnostic Imaging. Abby is interested in all aspects of imaging, in particular MRI, trauma imaging and musculoskeletal ultrasound. She has published numerous articles and book chapters in the diagnostic imaging field. She has been responsible for the supervision of a large number of diagnostic imaging residents due to the prestigious DWR resident programme and enjoys teaching students and general practitioners to perform ultrasound.

Vicente Esteve Bernet

DVM
Vicente obtained his degree in veterinary medicine from the Cardenal Herrera University-CEU, Valencia in 2011. He then completed a rotating internship at the Veterinary Teaching Hospital at the same university. He subsequently worked as an associate lecturer at the Cardenal Herrera University-CEU. He has spent time with the diagnostic imaging departments

in both national and international hospitals, such as the Small Animal Teaching Hospital of the University of Liverpool. He currently works as a lecturer at the Cardenal Herrera University-CEU Valencia in the Department of Animal Medicine and Surgery where he fulfills his academic and research role within the diagnostic imaging service.

M. Josefa Fernández del Palacio

PhD, Dipl. ECVIM-CA
M. Josefa Fernández del Palacio is a lecturer at the Department of Medicine and Animal Surgery of the University of Murcia and Head of the Cardiorespiratory Service of the Veterinary Hospital of the University of Murcia. She holds a diploma in Cardiology from the European College of Veterinary Internal Medicine (Dipl. ECVIM-CA [Cardiology]). She has published numerous articles and book chapters on cardiology in both national and international journals. Her fields of interest are cardiology and nephrology.

Patricia Laborda Vidal

DVM, MSc, PhD, Dipl. ECVDI
Patricia obtained her degree in veterinary medicine from the Cardenal Herrera University-CEU (Valencia). In 2005, she completed an internship at the LMU University Hospital in Munich, Germany. In 2006 she obtained an FPI scholarship to undertake her PhD at the Institute of Animal Science and Technology of the Polytechnic University of Valencia, defending her master's thesis in 2007 and her PhD in 2011. From 2010-2012, she worked as an associate professor of Diagnostic Imaging at the Cardenal Herrera University-CEU. In 2012 she moved to the UK to complete a residency in diagnostic imaging at the Small Animal Teaching Hospital of the University of Liverpool (2012-2015), becoming a European diplomate in diagnostic imaging in 2017. Between 2016 and 2018 she worked as a lecturer and head of the Diagnostic Imaging service at the Catholic University of Valencia. Since 2018 she has been working as a lecturer of Diagnostic Imaging at the Cardenal Herrera University-CEU. During recent years she has pursued her research interest in the clinical use of computerised axial tomography (CT) for the study of cardiac pathologies.

Panagiotis (Pete) Mantis

DVM, Dipl. ECVDI, FHEA
European Specialist in Diagnostic Imaging in Veterinary Medicine. RCVS-Recognised Specialist in Diagnostic Imaging in Veterinary Medicine. Honorary Associate Professor, University of Nottingham. Pete graduated in 1994 from the Faculty of Veterinary Medicine at the Aristotle University of Thessaloniki, in Greece. He completed an internship in diagnostic imaging at the Royal Veterinary College, later working in veterinary clinics and referral hospitals in London. He spent a year at the Swedish Agricultural University in Uppsala and in 2000 moved to the Royal Veterinary College where he became a senior lecturer in radiology. In 2017 he joined DWR (Dick White Referrals) and in 2019 became head of diagnostic imaging. Pete is a European and RCVS specialist in diagnostic imaging in veterinary medicine and a distinguished member of the Higher Education Academy in addition to being an author, speaker and regular CPD (continuing education) tutor in radiology, ultrasound, computed tomography, and magnetic resonance imaging in small animals.

Miriam Martínez Garrido

DVM, Dipl. ECVDI
Miriam is a diplomate of the European College of Diagnostic Imaging (ECVDI) and accredited in diagnostic imaging by the Spanish Association of Small Animal Veterinary Specialists (AVEPA). She graduated in veterinary medicine from the University of Murcia in 2010. Subsequently, she completed a rotating internship at VRCC Veterinary Referrals in Essex (UK), and an internship in diagnostic imaging at the veterinary teaching hospital at the University of Murcia and the continued to complete a residency in diagnostic imaging (ECVDI) from 2015 to 2018, during which she spent several months at the Universities of Dublin and Glasgow. In addition to a stay at Tufts University (Boston, USA). In February 2019, she obtained her diploma from the European College of Diagnostic Imaging (Dipl. ECVDI). Between 2018 and 2020 she worked in a referral hospital in England (Southfields Veterinary Specialists), as head of the diagnostic imaging service. In February 2020 she founded the company ProtonVet Veterinary Radiology and is currently director. She currently provides a teleradiology service at ProtonVetVeterinary Radiology and with Vet Oracle, in combination with the completion of her PhD at the University of Murcia.

Raquel Salgüero Fernández

DVM MA Dipl. ECVDI MRCVS EBVS European and RCVS Specialist in Diagnostic Imaging
Raquel holds a diploma from the European College of Diagnostic Imaging and is also a RCVS specialist. She is also accredited in diagnostic imaging by the Spanish Association of Small Animal Veterinary Specialists (AVEPA). She graduated from the Complutense University of Madrid in 2006, after which she worked in general practice in Spain and England for 4 years.

From 2010 and 2011 she completed two rotating internships in referral hospitals, VRCC Veterinary Referrals and at the Queen's Veterinary School Hospital at the University of Cambridge, in England, while pursuing a master's degree in education.

Raquel began her residency in diagnostic imaging in 2012 at the University of Cambridge under the supervision of Michael Herrtage, obtaining her diploma from the European College of Veterinary Diagnostic Imaging in 2015. After graduating, she worked as a radiographer at several referral hospitals in England and at Davies Veterinary Specialists for two years before returning to Spain in 2017. After which she was the head of the diagnostic imaging service at a referral hospital in Madrid for 4 years and is currently the head at the Veterios Referral Hospital in Madrid, an associate lecturer at the Complutense University and a telediagnostics consultant nationally and internationally.

Raquel has authored multiple publications, participated in courses and has been a speaker both nationally and internationally. She has experience in all imaging modalities, with special interest in neuroimaging, thoracic and abdominal ultrasound, as well as CT angiography.

Xavier Sánchez Salguero

DVM, MSc, PhD, GPCert CT
Xavier obtained his degree in veterinary medicine from the UAB (2006). Going on to obtain his master's degree (2008) and Doctorate in veterinary medicine from the same university (specialization in radiology, Cum Laude mention, 2012). He authored the book "Manual práctico de radiología torácica en pequeños animales" (Servet, 2018) and is co-author of the books "Diagnóstico ecográfico en pediatría de pequeños animales" (Servet, 2017) and "Manual clínico de diagnóstico por imagen en pequeños animales" (Improve International, 2021). He has also authored national and international scientific publications. He has presented oral communications at international congresses (ACVIM, ECVIM) and been a speaker at dozens of online courses (Vettv, Grupo Asís, Cursovet, Colvet, Ebbenhe, Vetformación) and postgraduate courses in diagnostic imaging (Improve Veterinary Education, Ifevet, Vetmedia, Neo Animalia, Capacitación Veterinaria, VetCam Specialists, UEM, UCV, CEU, UCAM). He has developed educational material for web resources and has been director of diagnostic imaging monographs in the Journal Internal Medicine of Small Animals. He has also collaborated as a radiologist with numerous veterinary clinics.

He is currently an assistant lecturer in Diagnostic Imaging and Domestic Animals Health and Clinic at the University of Lleida and is responsible for the diagnostic imaging service at the same university. He is part of the radiology and CT team at Vetoclock and is also a co-owner of Cursovet and a member of AVEPA's GEDI (in the process of accreditation) and EAVDI.

Marta Soler Laguía

DVM, PhD, CertVDI
Marta graduated in veterinary medicine from the University of Murcia, where she later obtained her PhD. She then went on to obtain an RCVS certificate in diagnostic imaging and subsequently completed a residency in diagnostic imaging at the Faculty of Veterinary Medicine of the University of Murcia becoming a diplomate and undertaking stays at various veterinary faculties such as Dublin, Glasgow and Cambridge and at private referral centres such as Davies Veterinary Specialists (UK) and San Marco (Italy).

She has authored numerous publications in national and international journals, as well as book chapters. She currently works as a lecturer at the Faculty of Veterinary Medicine of the University of Murcia where she teaches in the subject of diagnostic imaging and undertakes clinical work in the diagnostic imaging service of the Clinical Veterinary Hospital of the University of Murcia.

Contents

Diagnostic Imaging Techniques

Abdominal Imaging

Thoracic Imaging

Musculoskeletal Imaging

Diagnostic Imaging Techniques

Physical Principles in Radiology. Digital Radiology. Radiological Interpretation. Contrast Media and Techniques

Miriam Martínez Garrido

Principles of Physics in Radiology

X-rays were discovered by Wilhelm Conrad Roentgen in 1895 and are a type of **electromagnetic radiation** just like visible light or gamma rays. They are produced by electrons interacting outside the nucleus.

Electromagnetic radiation is a combination of electric and magnetic fields that travel together, oscillating in orthogonal planes in the form of waves, which propagate at the speed of light. Electromagnetic radiation is characterised by its wavelength, frequency and energy.

Speed (m/s) =
frequency (waves per second)/wavelength (m)

Since velocity is constant (the speed of light), frequency and wavelength are inversely proportional

The different types of electromagnetic radiation have a wide range of wavelengths, frequencies and energies that make up the spectrum of electromagnetic radiation.

Electromagnetic radiation is quantified into particles called **photons**. The energy of photons is directly proportional to the frequency of the radiation. Radio waves are formed from low-energy photons, whereas X-rays are formed from high energy photons.

When electromagnetic radiation has enough energy to expel electrons from an atom, it is called **ionising radiation**. Radio waves or microwaves cannot ionise atoms, whereas ultraviolet light and X-rays are examples of ionising radiation.

X-ray Formation and the X-ray Tube

In radiology, X-ray formation occurs in the controlled environment of an X-ray tube.

The X-ray tube contains the cathode (negative electrode), which consists of a filament, and the positively charged anode, inside a glass envelope in a vacuum system. The X-ray tube allows the acceleration of electrons from their source in the filament to the metal target at the anode, where X-rays are produced (Fig. 1).

- **The cathode** (**negative electrode**) is formed by the filament (spirally wound tungsten wire) and a focusing cup in which the filament is located.

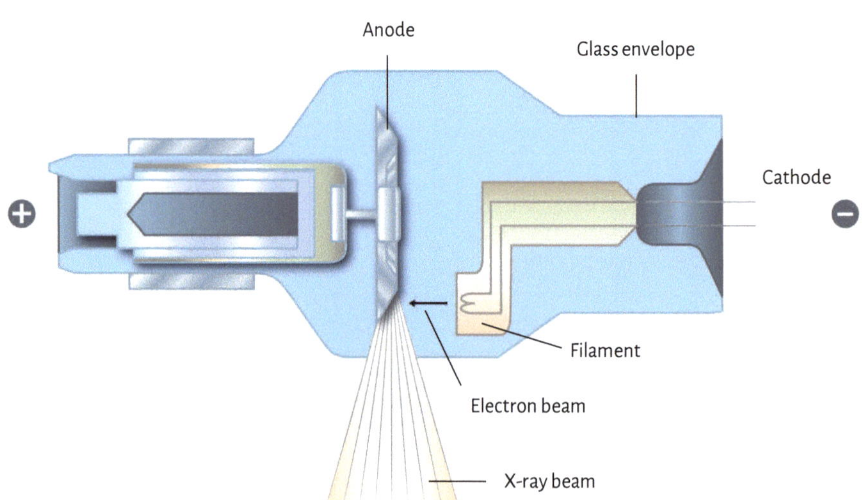

Figure 1. X-ray tube.

To generate a negatively charged electron cloud at the cathode, an electric current is needed, which passes along the filament, raising its temperature. The number of electrons in the cloud is directly proportional to the amount of electrical current passing through the filament, measured in milliamperes (mA), which is selected on the control panel of the X-ray machine.

The electrons produced in the filament are accelerated towards the anode, applying a voltage differential between the two electrodes. As the electrons are negatively charged, they are attracted to the anode, which is positively charged. When they collide with the anode, part of the energy from the electrons is transformed into X-rays. The energy of the X-rays produced depends on the energy of the electrons hitting the metal of the anode, which is determined by the voltage difference between the cathode and the anode and is controlled by the kilovoltage peak (kVp). Increasing the kVp on the control panel increases the voltage difference between the filament and the anode, meaning that the electrons accelerate at higher speeds and have a higher kinetic energy when they hit the anode. Higher-energy electrons can produce higher-energy X-rays.

- **The anode** (**positive electrode**) contains the focal point, the area where electrons collide and X-rays are produced. This is made of **tungsten**.

  The process of X-ray production is very inefficient and about 99% of the energy of the electrons hitting the anode is converted into heat, not X-rays. Therefore, it is necessary for the anode to be made of a material with a very high melting point (3422 °C) so that it is not damaged when subjected to high temperatures. In addition, tungsten has a high atomic number (74), which increases the efficiency of X-ray production.

  The anode can be either stationary or rotary. Stationary (fixed) anodes consist of a tungsten focal point coupled to a copper block. These are often used in portable X-ray machines.

  Rotary anodes consist of a tungsten disc and a molybdenum shaft, and are designed to rotate and thus increase the surface area with which the approaching electrons collide, preventing damage to a single area, as would occur if the electrons continuously hit the same region of a stationary anode. In addition, they have a greater ability to dissipate heat.

X-rays are produced by two mechanisms when electrons collide with the focal point on the anode: collision interactions and radiative interactions.

- **Collision interactions** occur when the approaching electron hits an orbital electron and ejects it from the atom. The energy required to eject an orbital electron is specific to the atom and the shell in which the orbital electron resides, and this is called "**binding energy**". The vacancy that is generated is filled with another electron from the atom, and in this process "characteristic X-rays" are generated. Their energy is characteristic of the atom, the shell from which the electron is expelled and the electron source that fills the vacancy of the atom's shell. The X-rays created by collision interactions represent only a small fraction of the total number of X-rays produced in a diagnostic X-ray tube (Fig. 2).
- In a **radiative interaction**, the approaching electron passes close to the nucleus of the tungsten atom, attracted by the opposite charge. Tungsten has a high positive charge due to the presence of 74 positively charged protons in its nucleus. Therefore, the electron is strongly attracted to the nucleus, which causes the electron to brake and release energy in the form of X-rays.

  The X-rays generated by a radiative interaction are called ***bremsstrahlung*** (**braking radiation**) and have a broad spectrum of energies. Braking radiation is determined by the distance between the incident electron and the nucleus. The closer the electron moves to the nucleus, the more it is attracted, the more its trajectory curves, the more it slows down, the more energy it loses and, consequently, the more energy it produces. Most approaching electrons experience multiple braking interactions, and thus a single electron can produce multiple braking beams. When the electron undergoes a direct impact with the nucleus, this results in a virtually complete loss of its energy, and the greatest amount of X-ray energy is produced (Fig. 3).

Both collision and radiative interaction processes contribute to the total energy spectrum of an X-ray beam, but most X-rays originate from radiative processes.

The highest-energy X-rays in the spectrum have an energy in kiloelectron volts (keV) equal to the kVp that was set on the control panel. The number of X-ray photons in the spectrum with energy equal to the kVp is very small. Additional X-rays that come from collision interactions have specific energies and thus create peaks at specific points on the curve of the spectrum (Fig. 4).

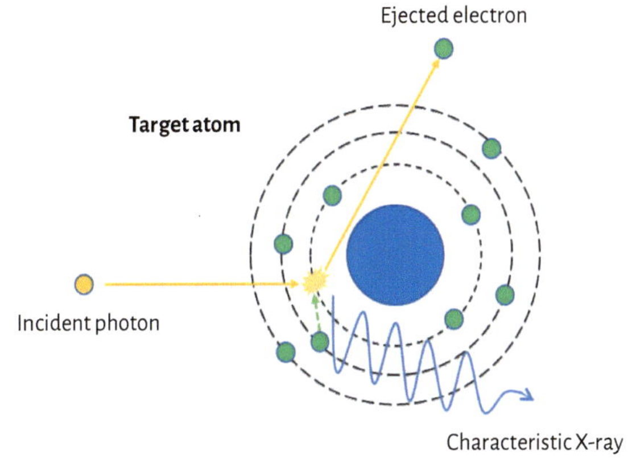

Figure 2. Collision interactions.

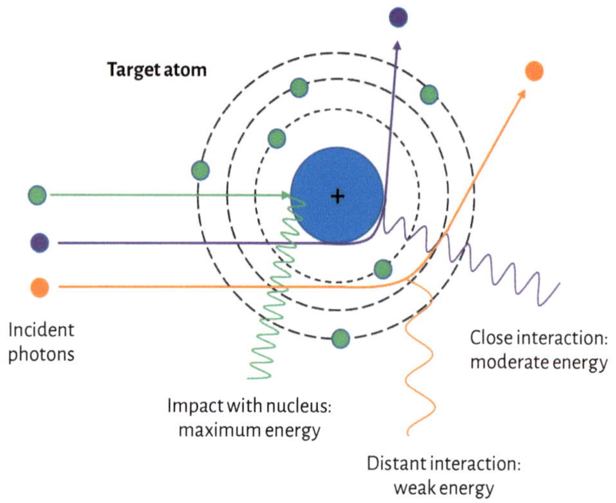

Figure 3. Radiative interactions.

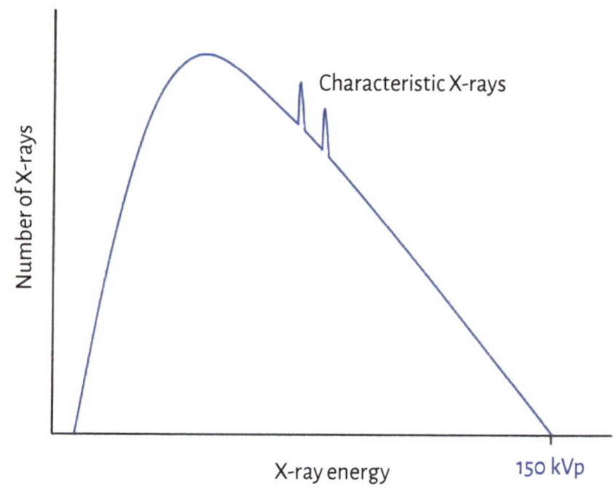

Figure 4. X-ray spectrum.

Properties of X-rays

X-rays are part of the electromagnetic spectrum. Electromagnetic radiation has no mass, is unaffected by electromagnetic fields and has a constant velocity in a given medium.

Some of the properties of X-rays include:

- no charge
- no mass
- travel at the speed of light
- invisible
- not affected by electromagnetic fields
- produce fluorescence when they pass through some substances
- pass through matter. When the X-ray beam strikes the matter there are three possibilities: one part will be absorbed, another part will disperse, and another part will penetrate the matter. The penetration capacity of X-rays depends on the kilovoltage (kV) of the beam and the density and atomic number of the matter
- ability to ionise matter. X-rays have enough energy per photon to cause the ejection of electrons from atoms and, therefore, cause the ionisation of these atoms and certain molecules.

Interaction of Radiation with Matter

In order to understand how an X-ray is produced, it is necessary to understand how photons interact with matter.

Photons can interact with matter in five different ways: **coherent scattering**, **photoelectric effect**, **Compton effect**, **pair production** and **photodisintegration**. Pair production and photodisintegration are not relevant in radiology and will not be discussed here.

Coherent Scattering

This occurs when a low-energy X-ray photon interacts with an object and the photon's direction changes, but the object does not absorb the photon and the photon's energy does not change. Of the fraction of X-rays that a patient receives, the number that undergo coherent scattering represents a very small proportion, approximately 5%. Therefore, this type of scattering is not of much relevance in radiological diagnostics. It is not useful in the production of the X-ray; in fact, it is disadvantageous as it degrades the image quality, or the photons may end up interacting with personnel and increasing their exposure levels.

Photoelectric Effect

This is the most important type of radiation interaction in X-ray production, as it is responsible for the formation of an image. In a photoelectric interaction, the X-rays striking the patient are completely absorbed and thus there are no scattered X-rays.

The X-ray photon encounters an electron from an inner shell of an atom in the tissue and transfers all its energy to it, and the original photon disappears. The secondary electron acquires all the energy from the photon in the form of kinetic energy, and this is sufficient to detach it from its atom and turn it into a projectile (photoelectron). The photoelectron can then

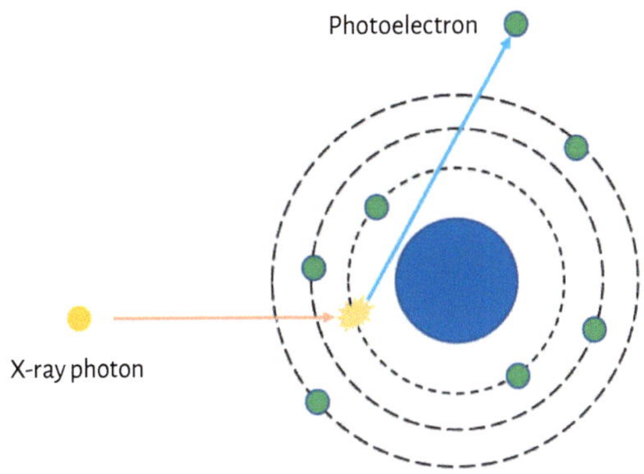

Figure 5. Photoelectric effect.

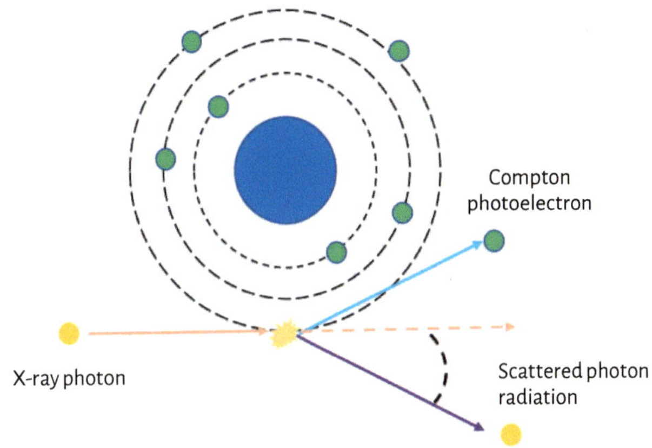

Figure 6. Compton effect.

produce multiple ionisations in the tissue but will eventually be absorbed by the patient (Fig. 5).

Then, electrons from the outermost layers take the vacant position of the photoelectron, and the excess energy is emitted in the form of characteristic X-rays. However, characteristic X-rays produced in tissue have very little energy and are absorbed locally.

Complete absorption of approaching X-rays leads to reduced exposure of the imaging film or plate below that part of the patient. This phenomenon occurs primarily in the absorption of low-energy X-rays and is reduced the lower the atomic number of the tissue is.

Compton Effect

The high-energy photon collides with an electron in the peripheral shell of a tissue atom. The electron acquires only part of the photon's energy and detaches from the atom (this is termed a Compton electron). The rest of the energy is carried away by the original photon, which is deflected with a lower energy and produces scattered radiation (Fig. 6).

All significant scattered radiation in diagnostic radiology results from the Compton effect. Normally, about one-third of all incident energy in a patient is projected outside the patient as scattered radiation. This scattered radiation can impinge on the image detector, causing degradation of image quality (less contrast).

In summary, only the photoelectric effect and the Compton effect are important in radiological diagnosis. The energy of the X-rays and the atomic number of the irradiated tissue will determine the relative proportion of the Compton or photoelectric effect.

With good radiographic technique, the X-ray beams contain energy in which the photoelectric effect predominates. This maximises the differential absorption of X-rays between tissues and so the image contrast. Photon scattering that occurs with the Compton effect is disadvantageous because scattered photons are radiation safety considerations for personnel, and also because they degrade image quality.

Obtaining a Radiographic Image

The radiographic image is generated by the difference in absorption of X-rays by the patient. To obtain a quality radiographic image, a number of practical and technical aspects must be taken into account.

Patient Preparation and Positioning

When carrying out a radiographic study, the patient should be prepared and correctly positioned; these factors are of great importance when it comes to ensuring that the radiographic image is of adequate quality for its subsequent interpretation.

In terms of the **patient's preparation**, it is important that the area or region to be radiographed is clean and the hair is dry. It is also important that radiopaque objects such as collars or harnesses are removed, to avoid the presence of artefacts that degrade the quality of the image.

Correct positioning of the patient while the radiograph is obtained is a fundamental factor in correct radiological interpretation. To ensure correct positioning, aids such as mattresses and other pieces of radiolucent foam, sandbags, ropes or positioners can be used. Use of these aids ensures that the patient is comfortable and reduces patient mobility, but also helps to reduce or prevent rotation of the different anatomical regions.

In many cases it is necessary to immobilise of the patient through the use of **sedation or general anaesthesia**. Immobilisation can have several advantages, such as limiting X-ray exposure of staff holding the patient and the number of radiographic projections needed, and reducing the stress or discomfort to which the patient is subjected.

Exposure Factors

When performing a radiograph, milliamperage and time (mAs) and kilovoltage (kV) are the two exposure factors that determine the quantity and quality, respectively, of the X-ray beam.

Quality and **quantity** are the two terms used to express the characteristics of the X-ray beam. The quality of the X-ray beam refers to its penetrating power and is related to the average energy of the beam. Quantity refers to the number of photons in the beam.

Milliamperage and Time (mAs)

The electric current that heats the filament is measured in milliamperes (mA). The selected milliamperage determines the number of X-rays produced. Thus, when the milliamperage is increased, the number of electrons that are formed at the cathode increases and, consequently, the number of interactions between the electrons and the anode, and therefore the number of X-rays, will increase. The total amount of X-rays produced during an exposure depends on the exposure time. Thus, there is a direct relationship between mA and exposure time (s) = mAs.

The mAs controls the amount of radiation and the dose to which the patient is exposed.

Kilovoltage (kV)

The kinetic energy of the electrons when they reach the anode is proportional to the potential difference between the anode and the cathode (kV).

The kV controls the quality and therefore the penetration power of the X-ray beam. A beam of X-rays of the highest quality is the one with the highest energy.

The kV also controls the contrast of the image. Thus, a low kV produces high-contrast images (e.g. in the limbs or abdomen), whereas a high kV produces a low-contrast image (mainly used in the thorax), because with a high kV there is greater potential for radiation scattering to occur.

In veterinary medicine, the equation known as "Santes' rule" is widely used when estimating kVp and generating exposure factor tables:

2 × X cm
(thickness of the region to be radiographed)
+ 30 for the abdomen, 40 for bone structures or 50 for the thorax
= X kVp

This is why it is important to use a ruler to measure the anatomical region of interest and to be able to select the parameters used on the X-ray machine.

Use of the Collimator and Grid

To reduce the effects of scattered radiation, the collimator and grid are used.

- The **collimator** (or **diaphragm**) is used to control the size of the primary X-ray beam. This is located below the window of the X-ray tube, where the primary beam of generated rays exits, and consists of lead sheets that regulate the size of the beam. In addition, it has a light that is projected on to the table and shows the size of the chosen beam of rays.
  Collimation regulates the area of the patient that is exposed to the primary beam of X-rays, resulting in decreased patient exposure, decreased radiation scattering and improved image quality.
- The **grid** is a rectangular structure made up of a series of thin sheets of lead and aluminium placed alternately, with a set distance between them. It should be placed between the patient and the X-ray film. There are several types of grid depending on their mobility (fixed or mobile, which have a movement mechanism during exposure preventing the lines from appearing in the radiographic image).
  The grid is responsible for absorbing the scattered radiation that is generated by the interaction of the radiation with the patient before it reaches the radiographic film, but it also absorbs part of the primary beam of X-rays. Therefore, when using the grid it is necessary to increase the parameters used, to compensate for this radiation loss. Normally, grids are used when the structures to be radiographed exceed a certain thickness (>15 cm for the thorax and >10 cm for the abdomen and bone, e.g. head, spine, extremities).

Distances

Distances are another factor that must be taken into account.

Film-focus Distance (FFD)

FFD is the distance between the X-ray tube and the chassis. As the distance between the X-ray tube and the film increases, the intensity (amount) of the X-rays decreases. Therefore, maintaining a constant distance is important. In veterinary medicine, the distances established are 100 cm for all regions except for the thorax, where the distance used is 120–150 cm.

It is important to bear in mind that if this distance is greatly reduced, magnification can be created.

Object-to-film Distance (OFD)

The OFD is the distance between the region to be radiographed and the chassis. It is important to keep this distance to the minimum possible, to minimise the magnification and distortion that occur as this distance increases.

- **Magnification** occurs when the area being radiographed is too far from the chassis and, therefore, in the image produced the size of the area is larger than in reality. There will always be some degree of magnification, but this increases as the distance between the object and the film increases, so ideally it should be minimised as much as possible (Fig. 7).
- **Distortion** is caused when the magnification of a region is uneven, as a result of one part of the patient being closer to the X-ray tube than another. This means that the shape of the radiographic image is different from that of the anatomical feature that has been radiographed. To avoid this, the patient should be placed as close to and parallel to the chassis or the X-ray table as possible, and at a 90° angle to the X-ray beam. It is normal to have a certain degree of distortion in some regions, and the radiologist should be familiar with these; however, if the distortion is extreme, the images are confusing and difficult to interpret (Fig. 7).

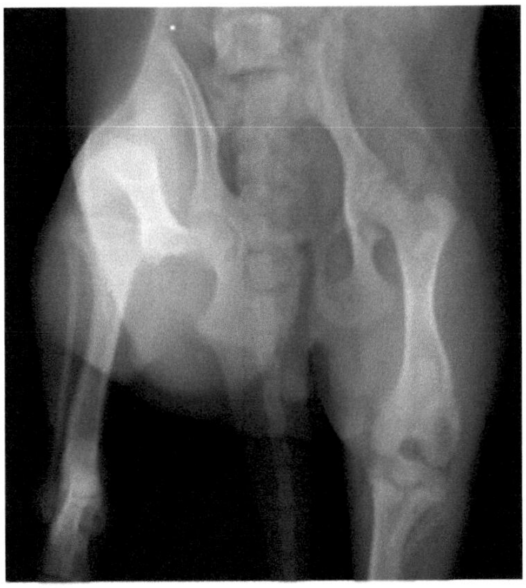

Figure 7. Effect of magnification and distortion. Ventrodorsal radiograph of a dog's hips. The left hindlimb can be seen to be well positioned, with a minimum object-to-film distance and parallel to the chassis, presenting a normal radiographic appearance. The right limb is flexed (poorly positioned), causing magnification of the knee and distortion of the femur.

Factors Affecting Contrast and Resolution

Contrast

Contrast is the difference between two radiographic opacities. On a radiograph, different structures can be distinguished when a structure has a different contrast from the structures around it.

The radiographic contrast depends on several factors: it is affected by the thickness, the physical density and the atomic number of the structures to be radiographed, and by the energy of the X-ray beam.

Patient Contrast

This depends directly on the physical density and atomic number of the tissues being radiographed, and their thickness.

Radiographic Technique

The contrast is affected by the X-ray beam energy (kVp) that is applied when taking the radiograph.

The ability of X-rays to penetrate tissue depends on their energy. Thus, if a very high kVp is used, the X-rays will have a very high penetration power and the radiograph will be overexposed (very dark), whereas if the kVp is very low it will be underexposed (very white) because the X-rays cannot penetrate matter.

The kVp must be combined with the mAs to obtain an image with adequate contrast. If low kVp and high mAs are used, the contrast in the X-ray will be maximised, which is useful when imaging the abdominal cavity, where the patient's inherent contrast is low and, therefore, this technique helps increase the contrast and visualisation of different organs. Conversely, if a high kVp and a low mAs are used, the absorption differences of the X-rays will be similar, and the radiograph will have less contrast. This technique is useful in regions such as the thorax, where the inherent contrast is high, to avoid too much contrast on the radiograph (Fig. 8).

Scattered Radiation

Scattered radiation causes a reduction in radiographic contrast, as it causes darkening of the image. This can be prevented by the use of the collimator and grid to reduce the amount of scattered radiation.

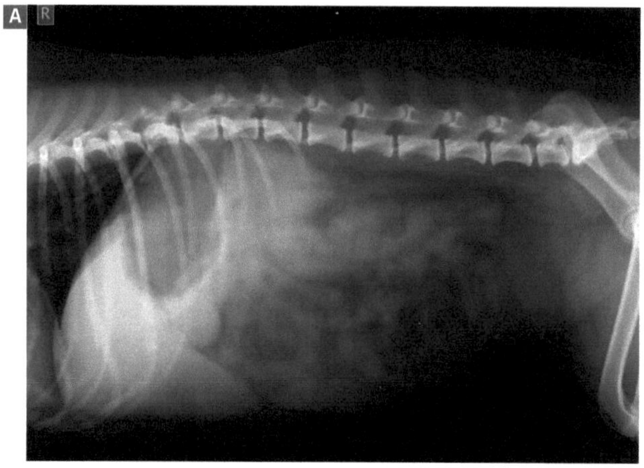

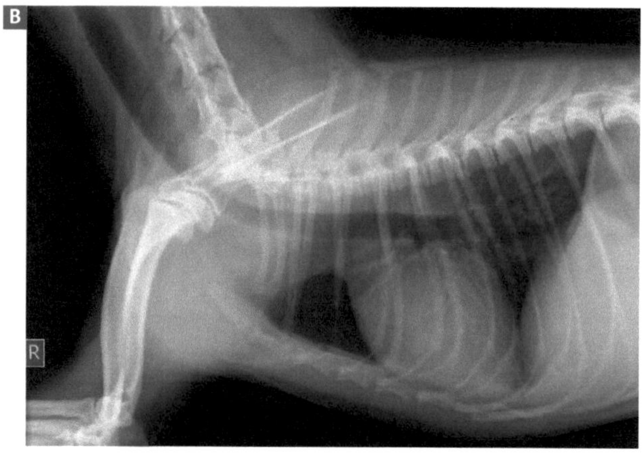

Figure 8. A. Radiograph of a dog's abdomen obtained with a high-contrast technique (low kVp and high mAs). **B**. Thoracic radiograph obtained with a low-contrast technique (high kVp and low mAs).

Resolution

Resolution is the ability to distinguish between small structures that are located near each other, and to differentiate sharp edges in the image.

Resolution depends on several factors.

- **Movement**. Patient movement generates blurring, preventing sharp detail in the image. Patient movement is a significant factor in veterinary medicine, so short exposure times are often used to minimise the effect of movement (Fig. 9). In addition, sedation or general anaesthesia is fundamental to avoid the movement of the patients.
- **Reinforcing screens**. The use of reinforcing screens means that lower mAs values can be used to create a radiographic image with good resolution. Reinforcing screens convert X-rays into visible light and thus increase the efficiency of radiograph production.
- **Use of grids**. Exposure of the radiographic film to scattered radiation causes blackening of the film and, therefore, also affects the resolution. The grid reduces the levels of scattered radiation and thereby improves the resolution of the image.
- **Focal point**. The focal point is the area of the anode where the electron beam impinges. It can be of varying sizes. A small focal point improves the detail of the image. By contrast, a larger focal point causes the margins of the structures to be less sharp, as a "halo" called a penumbra is generated that surrounds the image and makes it less detailed. It should also be noted that this effect becomes more evident with a greater distance between the object and the film.

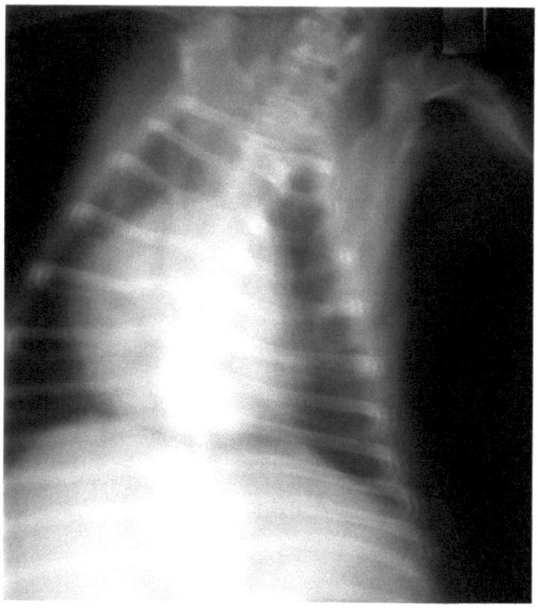

Figure 9. Thoracic radiograph of a dog. Patient movement has generated blur, meaning that the radiograph is not of diagnostic quality.

Digital Radiography

The term digital radiography is used to refer to radiography in which images are obtained directly in digital format without having previously passed through a radiographic film plate. To do this, a digital device that is responsible for recording the distribution of X-rays transmitted through the patient is used.

This involves the following steps.

1. Image generation: electronic measurement of the transmission of X-rays through the patient.
2. Processing and archiving: conversion of the electronic measurement into a digital file.
3. Visualisation of the digital file on a computer monitor.

Digital radiography can be divided into **computed radiography** (CR) and **direct digital radiography** (DDR). Both types use a conventional X-ray machine, with an X-ray table and grid.

Computed Radiography (CR)

In CR systems, the digital device is a chassis containing a photostimulable detector – a plate with a layer of photostimulable phosphors (Fig. 10).

Once irradiated, the photostimulable phosphor plate held in the chassis contains the latent image. The chassis is placed in a reader, which removes the plate from the chassis and scans it with a red-light laser.

This light provides the appropriate excitation for the phosphor to emit the energy it accumulated during irradiation with X-rays, in the form of visible-light photons (photostimulable luminescence process). The light produced is collected by an optical system and directed to a photomultiplier tube. This converts the light into an analogue electrical signal and subsequently passes through an analogue-to-digital converter, to obtain the digital image.

It takes approximately 60–90 seconds to obtain the image from the plate. Then, the photostimulable plate is reintroduced into the chassis, which is ejected from the reader and can be reused.

Direct Digital Radiography (DDR)

In DDR, the digital detector is a rigid image plate or chip (without a chassis) that captures the incident X-rays from the patient and produces a digital image that is sent directly to a computer for interpretation, eliminating the need for a chassis reader as used in CR.

There are two main types of DDR systems.

- **Flat panel detector** (**FPD**)**-based systems**. FPDs are rigid image plates that have a similar appearance to the chassis used in the conventional screen-film system. They can be direct or indirect conversion detectors.
  - Silicon detector or indirect detector. These detectors use a two-phase process to convert X-rays into electrical signals. The X-rays are absorbed and an intensifying screen transforms the X-rays into photons of visible light; these are then detected by the detector, which transforms them into electrical energy.
  - Selenium detector or direct detector. This type of detector directly converts X-ray photons into electrical charge.

Figure 10. Open CR chassis showing the photostimulable detector.

  Both systems convert the X-ray photons that have interacted in the detection zone of a pixel into an electrical charge stored in the matrix element corresponding to that pixel.
- **Systems based on charge-coupled device** (**CCD**) **sensors**. A CCD sensor is a device that captures the images in modern digital cameras and video recorders. There is an intensifier plate in front of and in contact with the active face of the CCD, which acts as a photonic converter: for each X-ray photon that interacts with the intensifier plate, it emits a significant number of light photons. The CCD sensor collects the emitted light and converts it into electrical charge. The process can be carried out with a high throughput rate given its good optical coupling.
  In human medicine, this method is reserved for when the areas being radiographed are small (e.g. dental radiograph or mammogram). In veterinary medicine, the areas that are radiographed are larger and this system is less widely used, as it generates lower-quality images (on larger surfaces) compared with CR and FPD-based systems.

Image Processing and Viewing

Regardless of the type of digital device used, the electronic data obtained are processed by a computer before the image is created and displayed. The aim of the processing is to convert the raw image data into a quality radiographic image, which can subsequently be evaluated in a viewing station.

The image is converted into DICOM (digital imaging and communications in medicine) format, which contains the image and information about it such as the date and time of image acquisition, patient data, the place/institution where the image was taken and other parameters. These images can be viewed and evaluated in a DICOM image viewer.

Subsequently, certain image parameters (e.g. adjusting the window level, zoom, etc.) can be adjusted in the DICOM viewer to enable an appropriate radiological interpretation to be performed.

Artefacts in Digital Radiography

Several specific artefacts can arise in digital radiography as a result of factors such as system error or improper radiographic technique.

- **Underexposure (quantum mottle)**: when a digital radiographic image is underexposed, it acquires a granular appearance. This granular appearance is caused by noise in the image, because some of the image pixels do not provide any information, resulting in dark dots (Fig. 11). This artefact occurs when the mAs is deficient and an insufficient number of X-rays are produced. By increasing the mAs and adjusting the kVp, the noise level in the image is reduced and its quality improved.
- **Overexposure:** when a radiograph is overexposed, the detector becomes saturated. The computer assigns a maximum value (black) to pixels that are saturated. This means that some parts of the radiograph are absent (black) and anatomical structures cannot be evaluated, even if the window level is modified (Fig. 12). These areas usually correspond to areas of lower radiographic density. One of the main factors contributing to overexposure is a high kVp.

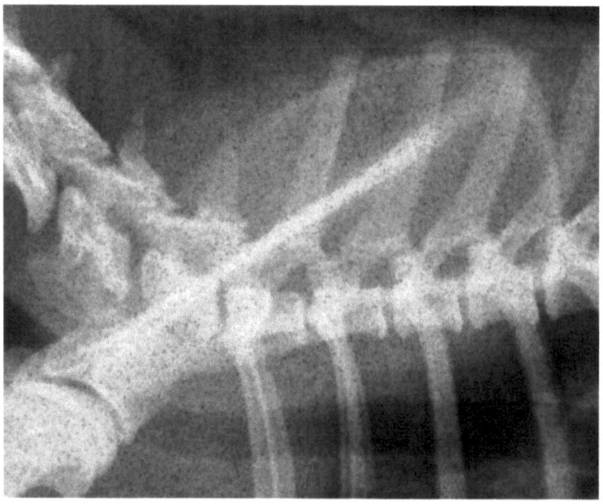

Figure 11. Underexposed radiograph of the cervicothoracic spine showing dark stippling.

- **Edge enhancement** (*Uberschwinger*): excessive application of the edge enhancement algorithm can result in the appearance of an artefact between structures that have very different radiographic densities, for example, between metal and bone or metal and soft tissue. A clear example of this artefact is the appearance of a radiolucent halo around metal implants, which could be misinterpreted as a sign of mobility or implant rejection (Fig. 13). However, it is important to be aware that, when it is an artefact, this halo will appear with a uniform thickness and surrounding the entire metal implant.

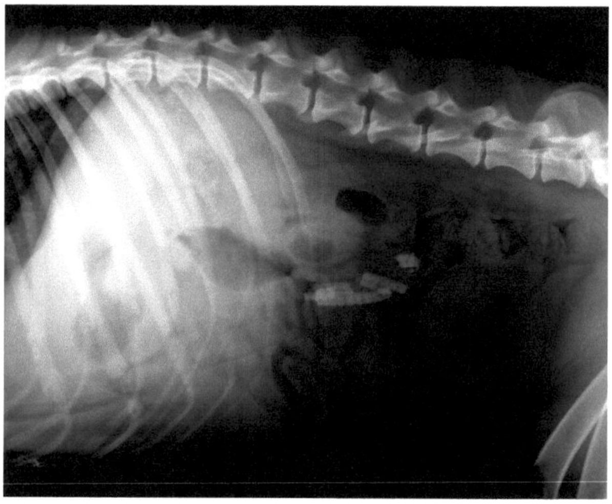

Figure 12. Overexposed abdominal radiograph in which the ventrocaudal aspect appears dark and cannot be evaluated.

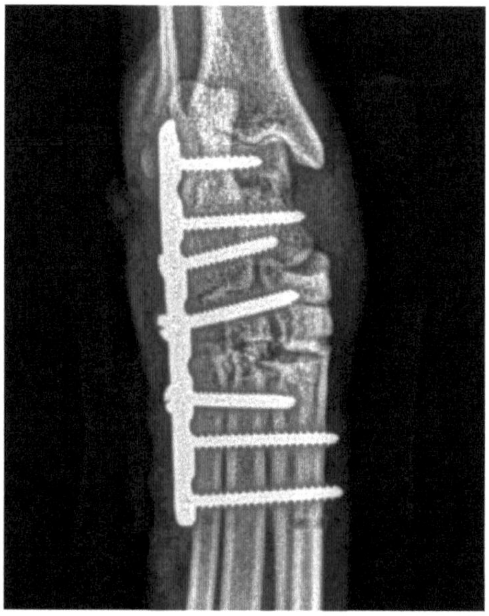

Figure 13. Radiograph of a tarsus showing the edge enhancement artefact, with a radiolucent halo surrounding the entire metallic implant.

- **Moiré artefact**: the use of a static grid, or low-frequency grids, can cause an artefact in which alternating light and dark lines appear in the radiographic image (Moiré effect) (Fig. 14). This occurs when the spaces between the grid sheets coincide with the direction and frequency of the reading lines of the laser light beam in the CR system. Rotating the grid 90° or using a grid that does not coincide with the reading lines solves this problem. Anti-scatter grids (Potter-Bucky grids), which perform a quick movement at the time of X-ray exposure, do not cause this problem.
- **Ghost image** (partial erasure): once the image data captured in the photostimulable phosphor detector have been sent to the computer system of the CR, the reader device erases the detector. If this deletion is incomplete, then when the detector is used to capture the following radiograph part of the silhouette of the previous radiographic image can be seen superimposed, which is called a ghosting artefact (ghost image). This usually occurs when very high exposure values have been used in the first radiographic study.
- **Scattered/stored radiation**: image plates are highly sensitive to radiation. If the CR chassis is exposed to ambient radiation or scattered radiation, this causes image deterioration when the chassis is next used. Therefore, the chassis should be stored and kept away from the area where radiography is performed, and be exposed to radiation only at the time when a radiograph is obtained.
  To avoid the appearance of this type of artefact, if a chassis has been exposed to radiation previously, it must be erased (by passing it through the CR reader) before using it to take another radiograph.
- **Upside down chassis**: if the chassis is placed upside down when performing a radiograph, the construction pattern of the chassis can appear superimposed on the image, generating various artefact patterns.
- **Double exposure**: if two consecutive radiographs are performed using the same chassis, the images will appear superimposed.

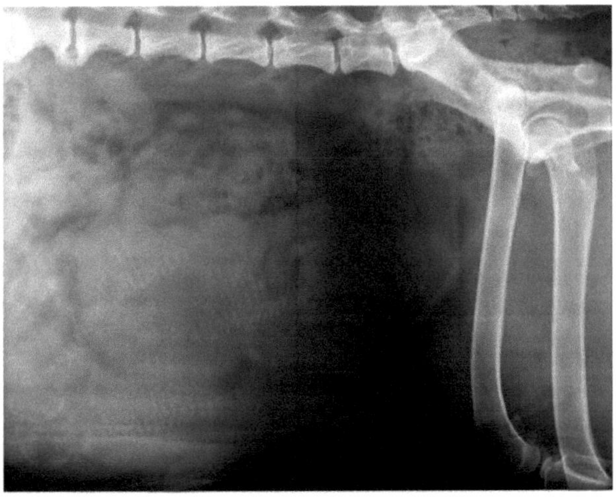

Figure 14. Radiograph of the caudal abdomen, performed with a static grid, generating the Moiré artefact.

Radiological Interpretation. Radiographic Image Evaluation

Definition of Radiography and Radiological Opacities

A radiograph is a two-dimensional image produced from a three-dimensional object (the patient) showing the distribution of X-rays passing through the patient.

The radiograph is produced because X-rays penetrate and interact with matter (the patient). Some of that radiation is absorbed to varying degrees depending on the nature of the different tissues, and a radiation pattern is created that reaches the detector to create a radiographic image. This consists of a black-and-white image with an intermediate grey scale, with shadows or opacities that are familiar and can be recognised.

Radiographic opacity is the degree of blackening of the radiograph caused by the X-rays; it depends on the atomic number (Z), density and thickness of the tissue. The denser a tissue is, the more radiation it will absorb and the less radiation passes through it (Table 1).

Table 1. Density and atomic number of structures that usually appear on a radiograph.

Structure	Density (g/cm^3)	Effective atomic number (Z)
Lung (similar to air)	0.3	7.5
Fat	0.9	6.5
Water	1.0	7.5
Soft tissue	1.04	7.5
Bone	1.7	12
Lead (similar to other metals)	8.7	82

Thus, the black areas of the image represent tissues or other material (e.g. air) where radiation passes through the patient and impinges on the detector, whereas white areas in the image represent areas where radiation is absorbed by the patient and only a few X-rays impinge on the detector (e.g. bone). Between these two extremes there is an intermediate grey scale, in proportion to the number of X-rays that pass through the patient and reach the detector.

Therefore, depending on the patient's absorption of radiation, there are **five radiological opacities** (from lowest to highest) that can routinely be found in a radiographed patient (Fig. 15).

1. **Gas or air**: the most radiolucent material visible on a radiograph.
2. **Fat**: more radiolucent than soft tissue and serves as a contrast for visualisation of soft tissues that are surrounded by fat, especially in the abdomen.
3. **Soft tissue or liquid**: fluid and soft tissue have the same opacity, so fluid-filled organs such as the urinary bladder and parenchymal organs such as the liver have the same opacity.
4. **Bone or mineral**: bone has the highest physiological opacity seen on a radiograph. There are normal variations in the radiopacity of bone, between different types of bones and between different parts of a bone (e.g. cortical bone and bone marrow have different opacities).
5. **Metal:** this is the most radiopaque material. Examples seen on radiographs include contrast media and metallic foreign bodies.

Although these are the only five opacities that can be observed, as mentioned previously the radiographic opacity depends on the thickness of structures. Therefore, it should be taken into account that thick structures will be more opaque than thinner structures, and therefore their opacity is relative. Thus, very thick fatty opacified structures may have an opacity similar to or greater than thinner soft-tissue opacified structures, although in reality the fatty tissue has less radiopacity than the soft tissue.

In addition, when talking about radiological opacity, the term **radiolucent** or **radiotransparent** is used for structures that absorb little radiation so that the number of photons that reach the film is high, which means that black is observed on the radiograph (e.g. air), and **radiopaque** for structures that absorb a lot of radiation and therefore appear white (e.g. metal).

Geometry of the Radiographic Image

As a radiograph is a two-dimensional image of a three-dimensional structure (the patient), the appearance of the structures on the radiograph is affected by several factors that must be taken into consideration when interpreting the radiograph.

- **Loss of depth perception**: in order to evaluate the three dimensions on a radiograph, at least two orthogonal projections are necessary to correctly evaluate a region. These should be performed with a 90° angle between them (e.g. lateral and ventrodorsal projections of the abdomen or thorax).
- **Structure overlap**: in radiography there is a marked overlap of structures. However, being familiar with many of them means they are easily recognisable. Nevertheless,

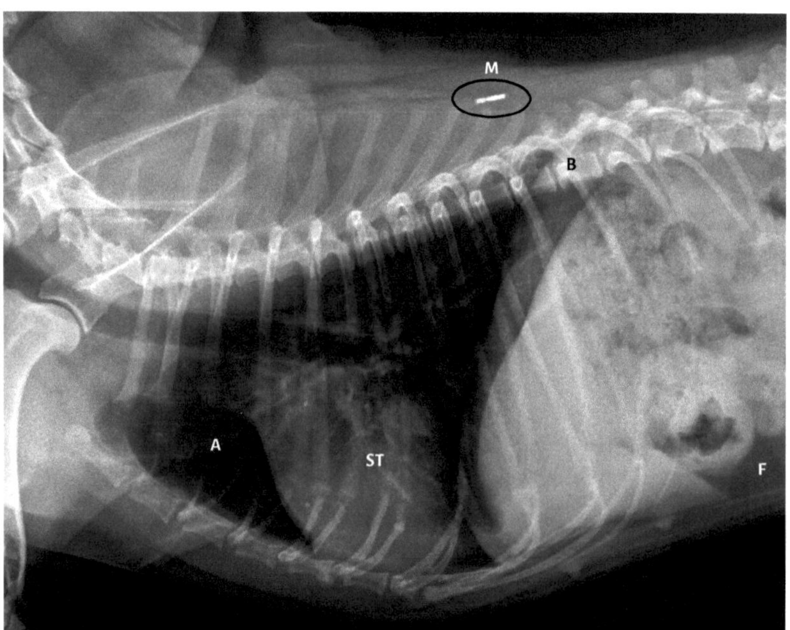

Figure 15. Thoracic radiograph showing the five radiological opacities. A: air, F: fat, ST: soft tissue, B: bone, M: metal.

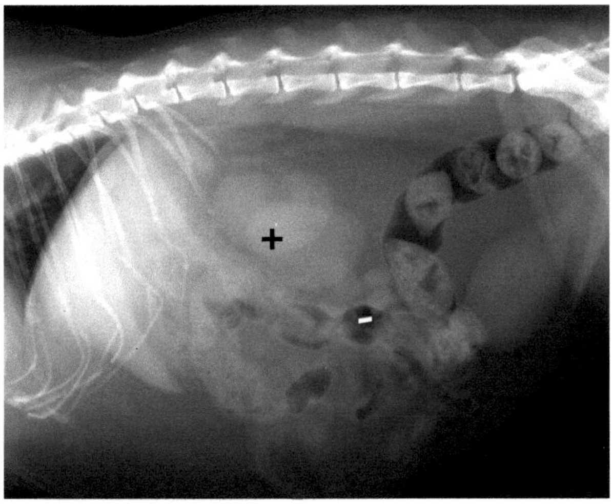

Figure 16. Radiograph of a cat's abdomen. Positive summation sign created by the overlap of both kidneys (+) and negative summation sign (-) created by the overlap of two intestinal loops.

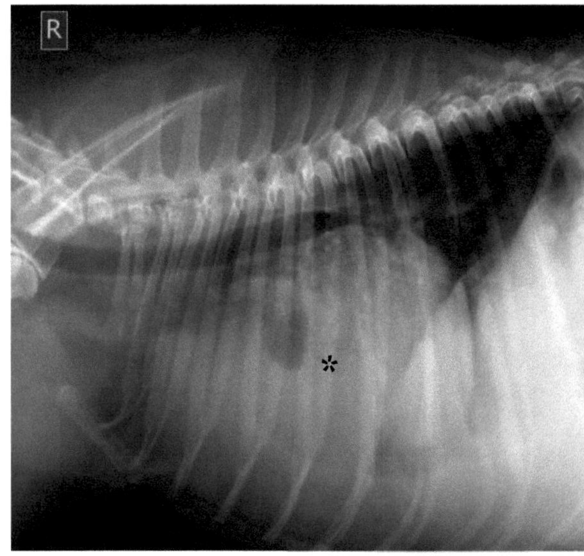

Figure 17. Thoracic radiograph. A cranioventral mediastinal mass is causing a silhouette sign with the cardiac silhouette; the consequence is that the edges of both structures cannot be clearly identified (*).

sometimes, the use of two projections is essential to be able to distinguish them (e.g. the presence of a nipple superimposed on the pulmonary parenchyma, which could be misinterpreted as a pulmonary nodule if two orthogonal projections were not available).

- **Summation sign**: this occurs when two structures with similar radiopacity do not lie in the same plane or are contiguous but are superimposed on a radiographic projection. Owing to superimposition, the opacity of the two structures adds up, creating a more radiopaque region when the opacities that add up are soft tissue or bone (positive summation sign), or a more radiolucent region when two gas-containing regions are added together (negative summation sign) (Fig. 16).
- **Silhouette sign**: this occurs when two structures have the same radiopacity and are adjoining or in contact. This means that there is no contrast between the two structures and the margins between them cannot be distinguished (Fig. 17).
- **Magnification and distortion** (explained in the previous section on obtaining a radiographic image): these factors should be taken into account because they can create unfamiliar images and lead to incorrect interpretation. To avoid magnification, the area to be radiographed should be as close as possible to the chassis; to avoid distortion, the patient should be parallel to the chassis and perpendicular to the X-ray beam.

Radiographic Projections

Radiographic projections are named based on the direction of the primary X-ray beam as it passes through the patient, naming the entry point first and then the exit point. All types of projections in any region of the body are named based on the same principle. Thus, if the patient is placed in sternal recumbency to perform a thoracic radiograph, a **dorsoventral (DV) projection** is obtained.

Laterolateral projections are abbreviated and are simply called lateral; in the case of the thorax and abdomen, the recumbency in which the patient is positioned (**right** or **left lateral**) is added.

It is important that standard projections are always performed by positioning the patient appropriately; this enables familiar radiographs to be obtained and facilitates their interpretation.

Radiological Interpretation

Examination of radiographs must be carried out **systematically**.

- Studies should always be evaluated in a suitable environment, in a **dark room** with dim lighting.
- At the very least a **negatoscope** or a computer screen for interpretation should be available.
- At least **two orthogonal projections** (as described above) should be available, except in exceptional cases where this is not possible.
- **Placement of the radiographs**: the radiographs should be oriented on the negatoscope/screen in a standard way. This is important to ensure familiarity with the image

and easier detection of alterations (Fig. 18). Incorrect positioning of the radiograph can lead to errors in interpretation. The following placements are recommended:

- lateral projections: the cranial or rostral aspect of the patient to the left and the dorsal or proximal aspect of the patient at the top
- ventrodorsal (VD) or dorsoventral (DV) projections: the left of the animal to the right of the observer and the cranial aspect at the top
- craniocaudal (CrCd) or dorsopalmar/dorsoplantar projections of the limbs: the proximal area of the patient is placed at the top. Although it is not determined where the lateral or medial aspect of the patient should be oriented, it is advisable that the lateral aspect of the limb be oriented to the left of the observer.

– **Systematic evaluation** must be performed, examining all structures visible on the radiograph.

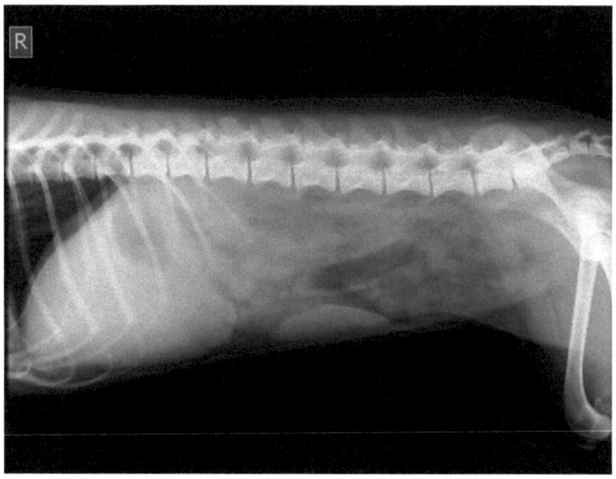

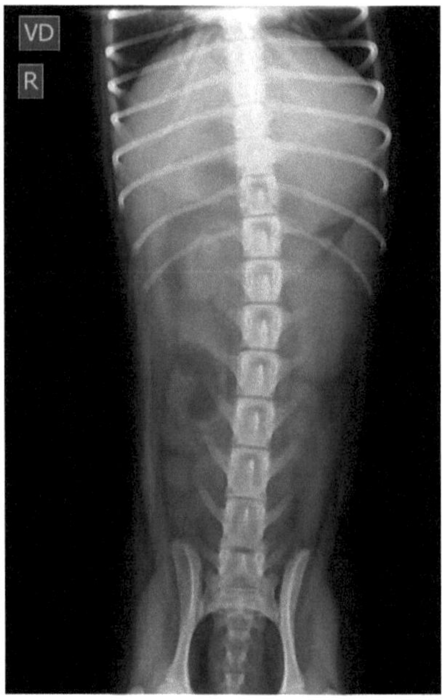

Figure 18. Lateral and ventrodorsal (VD) radiographs of the abdomen, showing correct positioning. The lateral projection has the cranial aspect (Cr) to the left, and on the VD projection the patient's right (R) is to the observer's left.

Radiological Report

There are two ways to interpret a radiograph: either with or without knowledge of the clinical signs or history of the patient. Interpretation without knowledge of the clinical signs of the patient favours a more objective evaluation, whereas being aware of the clinical signs can be critical in helping to determine whether the findings can justify the patient's symptomatology.

The radiological report must be structured and concise. It should contain the following.

- **Patient information**: species, breed, age (radiologically immature or mature), sex and body condition (thin, normal or obese).
- **Region and projections**.
- **Examination of radiographic technique**: evaluation of the technical quality should be mentioned when it might affect interpretation (e.g. in the case of improper positioning, collimation, incorrect centring or exposure factors, presence of artefacts, or missing or incorrect marking of the radiograph).
- **Radiological description**: it is very important that all radiographs are analysed. This must be done systematically by evaluating all the structures, either starting from the periphery and then from the inside, or by organs or systems. To describe radiographs, Roentgen's five radiographic signs (**location, size, shape/margins, number** and **opacity**) should be used, and all projections should be described together. To be able to determine whether there are any abnormalities, familiarity with the normal radiographic appearance is important.
- **Radiological diagnosis**: a summary list of abnormal findings.
- **Differential diagnoses**: a list of possible diagnoses that may be compatible with the findings, always in order from highest to lowest probability and taking into account the signalment, the patient's history and other available information (e.g. test abnormalities).
- **Recommendations/comments**: other diagnostic means that may be recommended to try to reach a definitive diagnosis are described (ultrasonography, computed tomography [CT], magnetic resonance imaging [MRI], cytology/biopsy, etc.).

Contrast Media and Techniques

Radiological contrast studies can be of great help in the diagnosis of certain diseases, as they improve the diagnostic capacity of radiography. In a simple (plain) radiograph, certain structures do not show enough contrast to differentiate them from each other; contrast media make differentiation possible because they increase the visibility of certain organs.

Thus, contrast media may be indicated:

- to identify certain structures
- to obtain information about the wall of certain organs
- to evaluate the function of some organs.

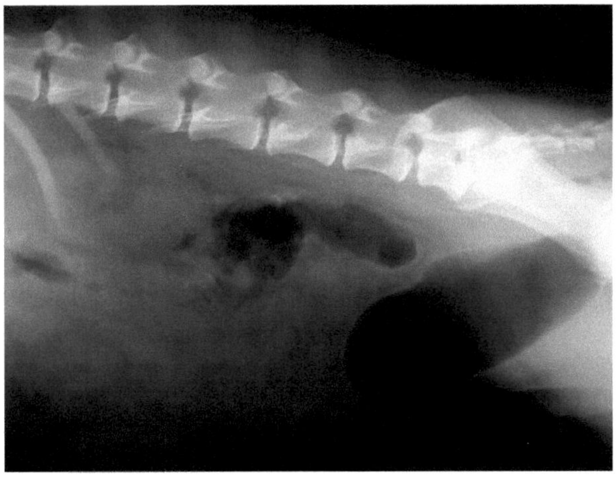

Figure 19. Lateral radiograph of the abdomen after performing a pneumocystogram. Negative contrast (radiolucent) is visible inside the bladder.

Contrast Media

Contrast media can be classified according to their opacity, their chemical content and whether they are ionic or nonionic.

- **Negative (radiolucent) contrast media** (Fig. 19) are based on gases (air, oxygen, carbon dioxide) filling a cavity or hollow organ. The most commonly used is air, although the others are safer as there is a lower risk of air embolism.
- **Positive (radiopaque) contrast media** (Fig. 20) contain elements with a high atomic number (e.g. barium, iodine) to opacify tissues that have a low radiographic contrast in the body. Owing to their high atomic number and density, they absorb X-rays in large quantities and have a metallic opacity. Types of positive contrast include:
  - **barium sulfate**: a water-insoluble barium salt, which can be found in several different formulations (e.g. powder, liquid, paste). It is used exclusively in the gastrointestinal tract, although it is contraindicated when oesophageal or gastrointestinal perforation is suspected because granulomatous reactions can be generated;
  - **iodinated contrast media**: water-soluble contrast media that are excreted via the kidney, so a possible complication is acute renal failure. Therefore, it is important to know if the patient has any renal abnormality or is dehydrated before using these contrast media. These are divided into ionic and nonionic.
    - **Ionic**: can be used for urinary, gastrointestinal or vascular contrast studies, depending on the type. This group consists of high-osmolarity contrast media such as sodium meglumine diatrizoate (e.g. Urografin® or Gastrografin®), or other compounds with lower osmolarity, such as sodium meglumine ioxaglate (Hexabrix®). High-osmolarity compounds are contraindicated for gastrointestinal use in dehydrated patients.
    - **Nonionic**: compounds with a low osmolarity that is close to the osmolarity of the blood. They have similar applications to ionic compounds, although some can also be administered intrathecally (for myelography). They cause fewer adverse effects than ionic contrast media, due to the lack of ions and the reduction of hypertonicity and chemical toxicity. This group contains contrast media such as iohexol (Omnipaque®), suitable for myelography, iopamidol (Niopam®) and iopramide (Ultravist®).

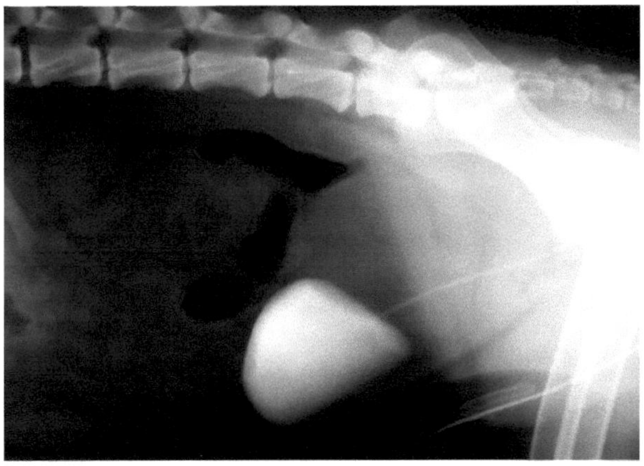

Figure 20. Lateral abdominal radiograph of a dog with a mass in the caudal abdomen. A positive cystogram has been performed and radiopaque contrast is observed inside the bladder; a urinary catheter can also be seen.

Contrast Techniques

This section will focus on contrast techniques for the gastrointestinal and urinary systems.

General Considerations

Radiographic contrast studies require good preparation and systematic execution. Before performing a contrast study, the following aspects must be taken into account.

1. Familiarity with the contrast technique to be performed and with the anatomy of the region to be studied, as well as knowledge of the possible complications that might arise and the contraindications of the contrast medium to be used.
2. The patient should be prepared correctly (some studies require fasting or prior administration of enemas).
3. Preparation of all the material that is to be used during the procedure.
4. Plain radiographs (orthogonal projections) should be performed prior to starting the contrast study. This enables:
   - determination of the appropriate exposure parameters before administering contrast;
   - evaluation of the plain radiographs first, as these can also provide information that is later masked by contrast; and
   - ensuring proper preparation of the patient (e.g. confirming that they have undergone the necessary period of fasting, or that there are no stools in the intestine that may affect the technique).

Other aspects to consider include the sampling of urine for analysis (when necessary) prior to the administration of contrast into the urinary system, as tests may be affected if there is contrast in the urine (e.g. inhibiting bacterial growth or altering density). When performing gastrointestinal studies, it should be taken into account that barium produces a marked artefact (acoustic shadow) on ultrasonography, so this should be performed before the contrast study.

Gastrointestinal System Contrast Techniques

Oesophagogram

- Indications: an oesophagogram is indicated to investigate causes of regurgitation or retching, cases of dysphagia, or when oesophageal abnormalities such as stenosis, foreign bodies (Fig. 21), perforations, megaoesophagus or diverticula, oesophageal masses or alterations in motility are suspected. However, oesophageal motility is best assessed with fluoroscopy, where swallowing of contrast can be observed in real time.
- Patient preparation: 6 hours of fasting.
- Technique
  - Contrast: barium preparations 45–85% m/v. Normally 15–30 ml in dogs depending on size; 5–7 ml in cats. A liquid phase should be performed, followed by a solid phase performed by mixing the contrast with food. In cases where oesophageal perforation is suspected, the use of barium is contraindicated if water-soluble iodinated contrast media can be used (10–15 ml in dogs; 5–10 ml in cats). Nonionic contrast media may be preferable as they are safer in

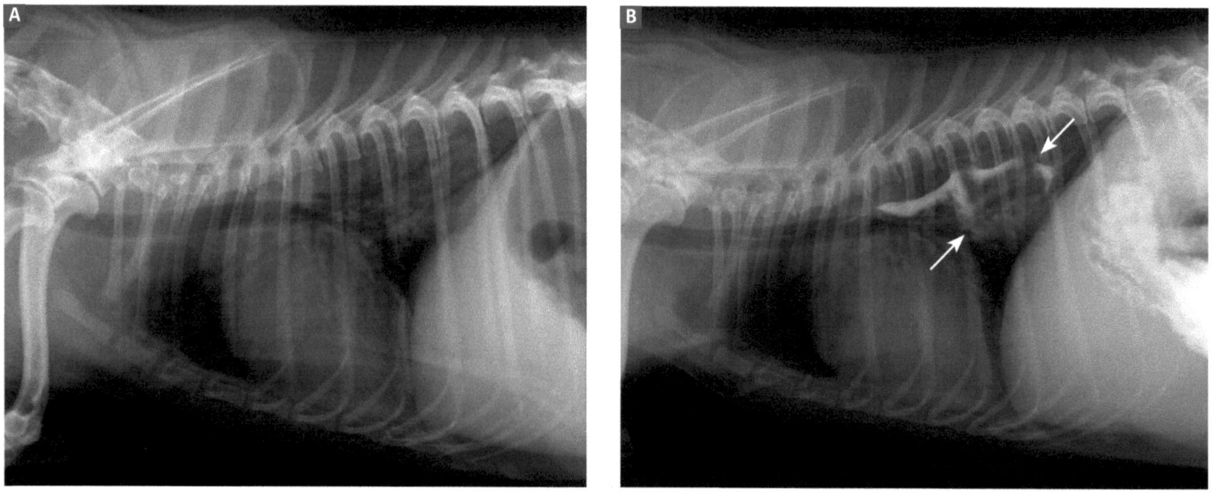

Figure 21. Lateral thoracic radiographs of a dog with retching. **A.** Plain radiograph: an increase in opacity is observed in the caudodorsal region of the thorax, overlapping with the location of the oesophagus. **B.** Oesophagogram: an accumulation of contrast in the caudal portion of the oesophagus, surrounding a radiolucent rectangular structure that corresponds with a foreign body (arrows), can be seen.

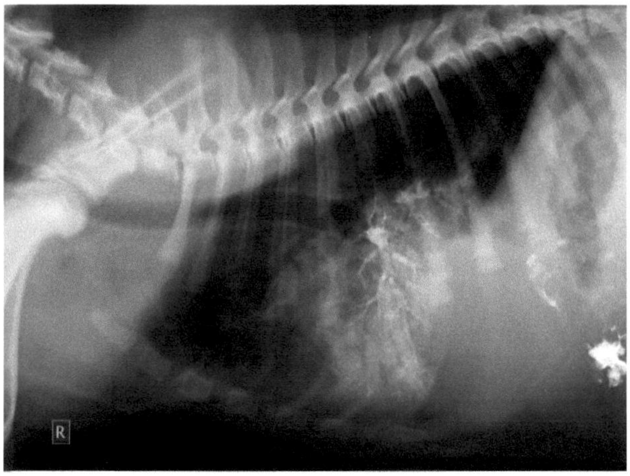

Figure 22. Lateral thoracic radiograph of a dog that has had an oesophagogram and aspirated some of the contrast. Contrast is observed filling the bronchial tree of the right middle and caudal lung lobes.

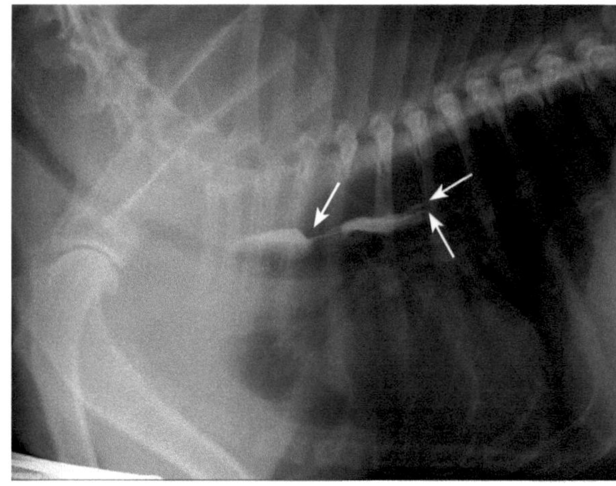

Figure 23. Lateral thoracic radiograph of a dog showing a normal oesophagogram. A small amount of contrast (which corresponds to a bolus) and longitudinal lines of contrast debris accumulated in the oesophageal mucosa (arrows) can be seen.

the event of aspiration, as ionic contrast media can cause pulmonary oedema due to their osmolarity.

- Lateral radiographs of the neck and thorax, and a somewhat oblique orthogonal DV projection so that the oesophagus is not overlapping the spine, should be performed.
- Complications: utmost care must be taken to avoid contrast aspiration (Fig. 22). If aspirated, barium can be removed by coughing or ciliary movements, and at other times it is phagocytosed and observed in the lung or lymph nodes some time after being aspirated. In some cases, it can cause pneumonia or granulomatous reactions.
- Radiological findings: contrast should pass through the oesophagus and not be retained. In dogs, parallel longitudinal lines (which correspond to the folds of the mucosa) can be observed (Fig. 23). In cats, longitudinal lines are seen in the proximal portion, and a "herringbone" pattern is seen in the distal portion because the mucosal folds are transverse or oblique.

Gastrointestinal Transit

- Indications: used to evaluate gastrointestinal transit time, the presence of masses or foreign bodies that are causing obstruction, or to determine the location of the digestive system, and in patients that present with vomiting or diarrhoea. This technique, although still used, has been largely replaced by other techniques such as ultrasonography and endoscopy.
- Patient preparation: fasting for 24 hours.
- Technique
  - Contrast: liquid barium preparation (dogs <20 kg: 8–12 ml/kg; dogs >20 kg: 5–7 ml/kg; cats: 12–20 ml/kg). In cases of suspected gastrointestinal perforation or if subsequent surgery or endoscopy is planned, its use should be avoided. Alternatively, iodinated contrast at a concentration of 240–300 mg iodine (I)/kg (ionic: 3–5 ml/kg; nonionic: 10 ml/kg) can be used. Agents that are hypertonic are not recommended in cases of hypovolaemia or in severely debilitated patients. Contrast should be administered by means of a gastric tube.
  - Immediately after administering the contrast, right and left lateral, VD and DV projections should be performed. Following this, lateral and VD radiographs should be performed at 15, 30 and 60 minutes, and then every hour until the contrast is in the colon. It is important that the time after contrast administration is noted on the radiographs. If any anomalies are observed, projections should be repeated immediately to rule out peristaltic movements. Further radiographs should be taken at 24 hours after administration to make sure there is no contrast left in the stomach or small intestine.
  - Complications: incorrect tube placement and contrast aspiration.
  - Radiological findings: normal gastric emptying occurs 30–120 minutes after contrast administration, and small intestinal transit is 30–120 minutes, with emptying between 180 and 300 minutes (approximately 5 hours). It should be taken into account that these times are variable and are affected by several factors, so their usefulness for evaluating gastric emptying is limited. However, the stomach should be empty by the time contrast reaches the colon (Fig. 24). In the stomach, contrast delimits the gastric folds. The intestinal mucosa should be smooth and uniform. In dogs, at the level of the descending duodenum pseudo-ulcers can be seen at its

antimesenteric border, such as indentations filled with contrast that correspond to Peyer's patches. In cats, the normal appearance of the descending duodenum is a "pearl necklace" pattern, due to peristalsis.

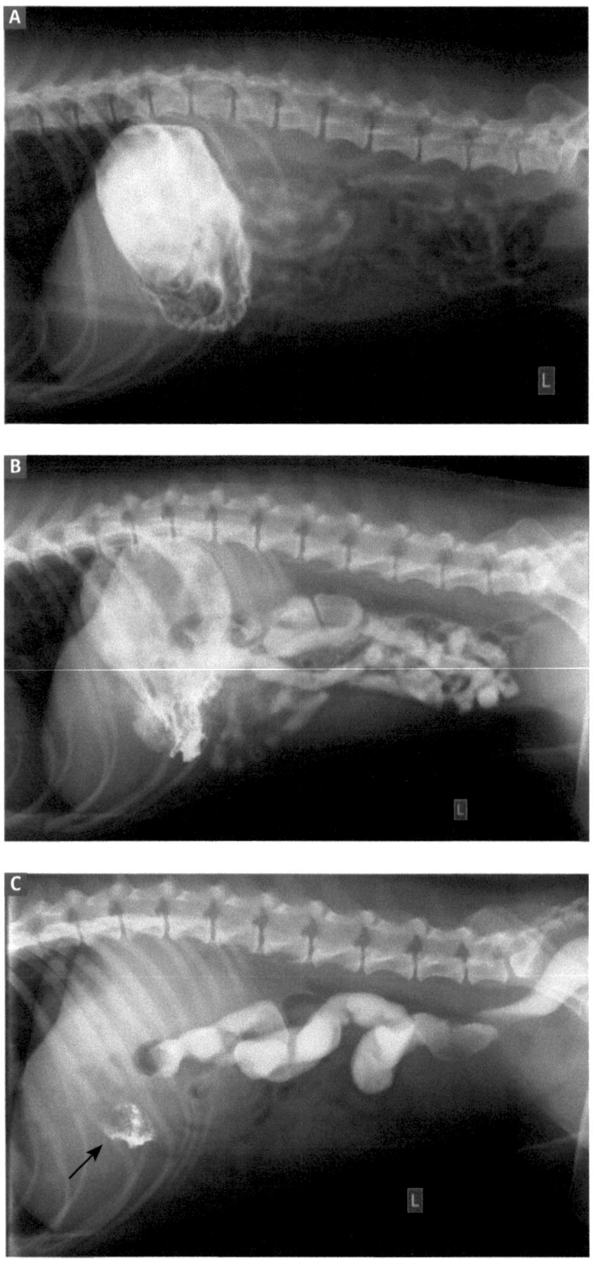

Figure 24. Left lateral radiographs of the abdomen of a dog with chronic vomiting, showing intestinal transit. **A** and **B** show immediate and 1 hour postcontrast radiographs with a normal contrast distribution along the gastrointestinal tract. **C.** Radiograph at 12 hours after contrast administration; the contrast can be seen in the colon. Part of the contrast can be seen in the pyloric antrum surrounding a structure with an irregular shape compatible with a gastric foreign body (black arrow).

Barium Enema and Pneumocolonography

- Indications: used to evaluate the colon in cases of masses or stenosis, or in cases of intrapelvic masses, or to locate the position of the colon when it is empty and differentiate it from the small intestine.
- Patient preparation: the same as for a gastrointestinal transit study, together with enemas to empty the colon. The patient should be anaesthetised.
- Technique
  - Contrast: the study can be performed with positive contrast with a barium solution (20 m/v) at a dose of 10–15 ml/kg in dogs and 7–10 ml/kg in cats. In other cases, a double contrast study can be performed, introducing air (11 ml/kg in dogs and 7–11 ml/kg in cats) after introducing the barium and when part of it has been drained. As in other techniques, barium is contraindicated in cases where perforation is suspected. Sometimes only air can be administered (pneumocolonography) (Fig. 25). The contrast is administered with a Foley balloon catheter to seal the anus so that there are no leaks. The contrast must be warmed at room temperature, and it should be administered slowly, taking a radiograph to check the degree of distension that is being achieved.
  - Lateral and VD projections should be performed when the appropriate degree of distension is achieved.
  - Complications: colon perforation can be caused by overdistension.
  - Radiological findings: the normal mucosa can be evaluated, and this should be smooth.

Urinary System Contrast Techniques

Excretory Urography

- Indications: helps with evaluation of the kidneys and ureters, allowing evaluation of their size, shape and position in cases of urinary incontinence, haematuria, pyuria, etc. This technique is being replaced by CT, which allows observation of the same organs without overlap of structures, thus avoiding the need to perform multiple radiographic projections.
- Patient preparation: 24 hours of fasting and enemas to make sure there is no food content or stools in the gastrointestinal tract. Performed under general anaesthesia.
- Technique
  - Contrast: an ionic or nonionic iodinated contrast should be used (the latter is preferable, especially in patients with kidney problems) at a dose of 600 mg I/kg. However, these types of contrast are contraindicated in cases of anuria, severe dehydration or when it is known that the patient has sensitivity or allergy to iodinated contrast media. The contrast should be administered as an intravenous bolus using a catheter

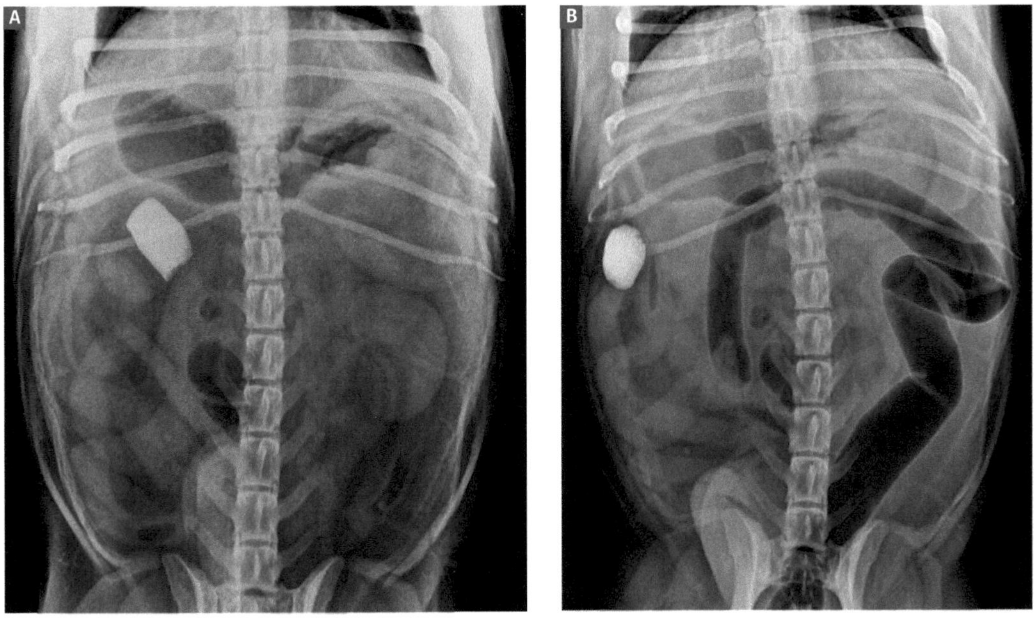

Figure 25. Ventrodorsal radiographs of the abdomen of a dog with vomiting. **A**. Plain radiograph in which a foreign body is observed in the right cranial abdomen (location unclear). **B**. A pneumocolonogram is performed to determine the location of the colon and reveals that the foreign body is located in the small intestine.

with the largest possible bore. Administration of fluid therapy from the beginning of anaesthesia is advisable, and the contrast should be warmed before administration. A negative cystogram can be performed before injecting the positive contrast to more easily assess the ureterovesical junction and ureters.

- A VD projection should be performed immediately after administering the contrast and then at 1, 5, 20 and 30 minutes. Slightly oblique lateral projections should be taken at 5, 10 and 20 minutes after administering the contrast to evaluate the ureters.
- Complications: less likely if nonionic iodinated compounds are used.
- Radiological findings (Fig. 26): this technique has two main phases. The first is the **nephrogram** phase, in which the renal parenchyma is homogeneously opacified within seconds after administering contrast, up to 5 minutes. Subsequently, the contrast is filtered by the kidney with urine and the **pyelogram** phase occurs, in which the renal pelvis and diverticula are opacified, between 2 and 5 minutes post injection. Finally, the contrast starts to be excreted through the ureters at between 5 and 10 minutes post injection, and reaches the bladder. Normally, contrast in the ureters can be seen in segments with filling defects due to peristalsis.

Cystography

- Indications: this technique is used to evaluate the bladder in patients with urinary problems (dysuria, haematuria, urine retention or incontinence) or post trauma to evaluate bladder integrity. There are three types of cystography depending on the contrast used: **positive cystography** is indicated to evaluate the position of the bladder and the integrity of its wall; **negative cystography** can also help locate the position of the bladder, and is used as a complementary technique to excretory urography to evaluate the ureterovesical junction; **double contrast cystography** is used to evaluate the bladder wall, and is a technique rarely used nowadays.
- Patient preparation: the same as for excretory urography.
- Technique: the bladder should be catheterised and emptied completely (with a urinary catheter in male patients and a Foley catheter in females) before contrast is introduced. In general, to avoid overdistension, and regardless of the type of contrast, the contrast is administered gradually while palpating the bladder, controlling the degree of distension, since the dose is variable.
- Negative contrast cystography: the bladder is inflated with air using a syringe and a three-way adapter tap, at a dose of 5 ml/kg in dogs. Once the bladder is full, the catheter can be partially removed to evaluate the bladder neck. This technique is contraindicated in suspected cases of severe cystitis or haematuria, as a gas embolism may occur.
  - Positive cystography: ionic or nonionic iodinated contrast (the latter is preferable, especially when there is a suspicion of severe cystitis because it is less irritating) are used, at a dose of 5 ml/kg in dogs and 2–5 ml/kg in cats, with a concentration of 150 mg I/kg. If the urethra needs to be evaluated at the same

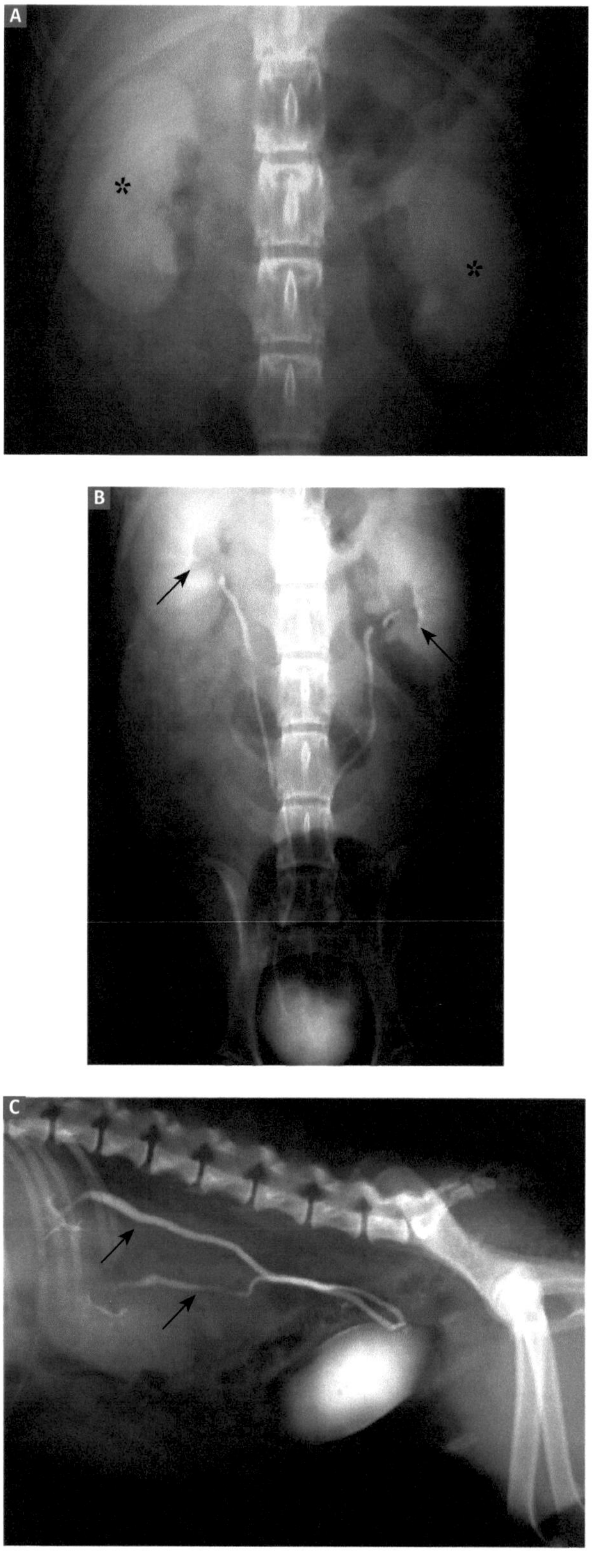

Figure 26. Ventrodorsal and lateral radiographs of the abdomen showing normal excretory urography. **A**. Radiograph at 30 seconds post contrast administration showing the nephrogram phase, with opacification of the kidneys (*). **B**. Radiograph at 5 minutes post contrast showing the pyelogram phase, with opacification of the renal pelvis (arrows). **C**. Radiograph at 10 minutes post contrast showing both ureters filled with contrast (arrows) with a normal ureterovesical junction, and contrast in the bladder.

time, the tip of the catheter should be placed in the penile urethra in males or in the vaginal vestibule in females.

- Double contrast cystography: pneumocystography should be performed, and then lower doses of iodinated contrast (13 ml/kg in dogs and 0.5–1 ml/kg in cats at a concentration of 300 mg I/kg) introduced. The patient should then be moved and the bladder massaged carefully to distribute all the contrast across the bladder mucosa.

– Complications: iatrogenic trauma to the bladder or urethra, or a urinary tract infection secondary to catheterisation, can be caused. In cases where air is introduced; a gas embolism can be caused.
– Lateral and VD projections should be performed.
– Radiological findings
  - Negative cystography (Fig. 27): distended bladder with air opacity and a thin, smooth and homogeneous wall.
  - Positive cystography: distended bladder containing contrast, with a smooth surface, no filling defects in the wall or lumen, and no loss of contrast.
  - Double contrast cystography: the thickness of the bladder wall can be evaluated; it should be thin, smooth and homogeneous. Contrast should be visible in the centre of the bladder, surrounded by gas.

Retrograde Urethrography

– Indications: in patients with abnormal urination (stranguria, haematuria, dysuria), where obstruction or rupture of the urethra is suspected, or the presence of vaginal masses.

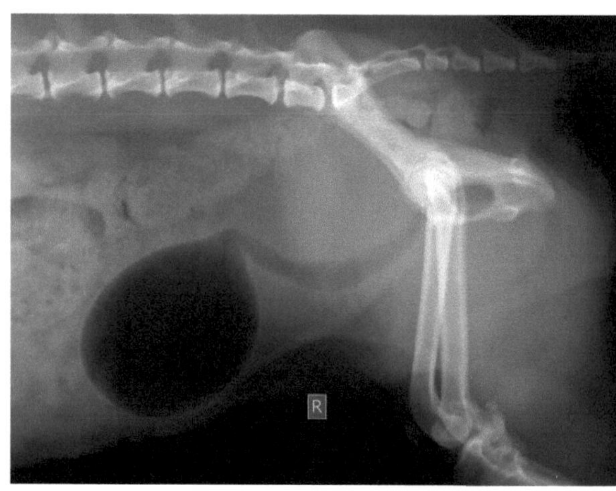

Figure 27. Lateral radiograph of the abdomen showing a mass in the caudal abdomen. A negative cystogram has been performed to determine the location of the bladder and urethra; the bladder and urethra can be seen distended with air and ventrally displaced by the mass.

- Patient preparation: the same as for excretory urography.
- Technique: the patient should always be catheterised and all urine emptied from the bladder before proceeding.
  - Males (retrograde urethrography): the catheter should be introduced into the penile urethra and the sheath/penis sealed with atraumatic forceps. The catheter must be filled with contrast before it is inserted, to avoid the introduction of air bubbles.
  - Female (retrograde vaginourethrography): a Foley catheter is placed in the vulvar region, the balloon is filled with air in the vestible, and the vulva is sealed with atraumatic forceps. As with males, the catheter must be filed with contrast previously in order to avoid the introduction of gas within the urethra.
- Contrast: ionic or nonionic iodinated contrast should be used as in other urinary techniques. In males, contrast is used at a dose of 10–20 ml in dogs and 5–10 ml in cats. In females, the dose is 1 ml/kg (10–30 ml in bitches depending on size, and 5–10 ml in cats). In both sexes, the contrast should be diluted to a concentration of 150 mg I/ml by mixing it with saline.
- A lateral projection with the limbs slightly extended forward to avoid overlap with the urethra should be performed when the contrast injection is finishing. This is the most useful projection, although an orthogonal projection (VD) can also be performed and in many cases it will also provide information.
- Complications: rupture of the urethra or vagina.
- Radiological findings (Fig. 28)
  - Males: the normal urethra appears as a column of homogeneous contrast with smooth margins. In some cases, there may be reflux in the prostatic ducts at the level of the prostatic urethra.
  - Females: contrast fills the vagina homogeneously and then fills the urethra and bladder by reflux. Both the vagina and urethra should have smooth, homogeneous walls without filling defects.

Bibliography

- Agut, A., Soler, M. (2014) Producción de los rayos X: obtención de la imagen radiológica. In: Agut, A., et al. (eds). *Diagnóstico por Imagen en Pequeños Animales.* Multimédica Ediciones Veterinarias, pp. 1-12.
- Agut, A., Sánchez-Valverde, M.A. (1992) *Radiodiagnóstico de Pequeños Animales.* Interamericana McGraw-Hill.
- Ayers, S. (2012) *Small Animal Radiographic Techniques and Positioning.* 1st ed. Wiley-Blackwell.
- Bushberg, J.T., et al. (2012) *The Essential Physics of Medical Imaging.* 3rd ed. Lippincott Williams & Wilkins.
- Carrera, I. (2014) Captura de la imagen a través de la digitalización de la radiografía. Imagen digital. In: Agut, A., et al. (eds). *Diagnóstico por Imagen en Pequeños Animales.* Multimédica Ediciones Veterinarias, pp. 23-33.
- Corzo, N. (2014) Técnicas de contraste radiológico. In: Agut A., et al. (eds). *Diagnóstico por Imagen en Pequeños Animales.* Multimédica Ediciones Veterinarias, pp. 43-61.
- Huda, W. (2016) *Review of Radiologic Physics.* 4th ed. Wolters Kluwer.
- Muhlbauer, M.C., Kneller, S.K. (2013) *Radiography of the Dog and Cat: Guide to Making and Interpreting Radiographs.* 1st ed. Wiley-Blackwell.
- Shetty, C.M., et al. (2011) Computed radiography image artifacts revisited. *Am J Roentgenol*, 196, pp. W37–W47.
- Soler, M., Agut, A. (2014) Evaluación de la imagen radiológica. Calidad de la imagen radiológica. Contraste. Resolución. Geometría. In: Agut, A., et al. (eds). *Diagnóstico por Imagen en Pequeños Animales.* Multimédica Ediciones Veterinarias, pp. 13-22.
- Thrall, D.E. (2018) *Textbook of Veterinary Diagnostic Radiology.* 7th ed. Elsevier.

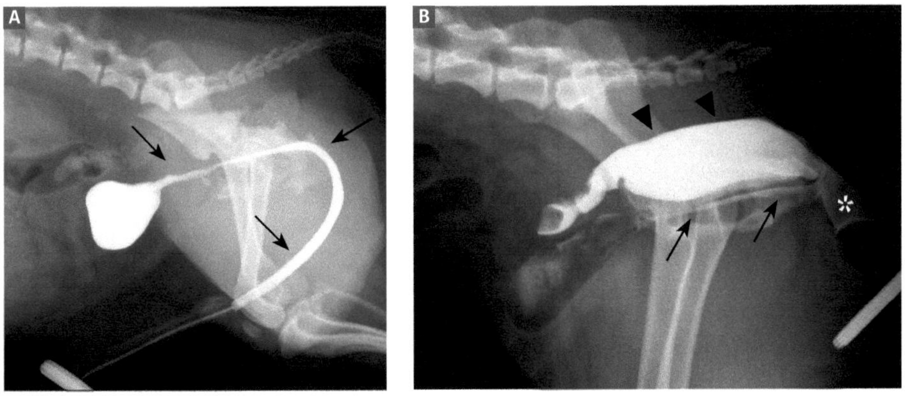

Figure 28. A. Lateral abdominal radiograph of a polytraumatised dog with multiple hip fractures. A urethrogram is being performed to assess the integrity of the urethra; note the homogeneous appearance of the normal urethra (arrows). **B**. Normal retrograde vaginourethrography, showing homogeneously distributed contrast in the vestibule (*), vagina (arrowheads) and urethra (arrows).

Physical Principles of Ultrasonography. Principles of Interpretation. Artefacts

Amalia Agut Giménez

Introduction

Ultrasonography is a diagnostic imaging technique that uses the reflection of **ultrasound waves** to form an echographic image. This chapter covers the following topics:

- formation of the ultrasound image
- ultrasound image interpretation
- artefacts.

Definition of Ultrasound

Ultrasound waves are sound waves with a frequency greater than 20 000 Hz, which makes them inaudible to humans. Sound is mechanical energy that propagates in a medium through compression and rarefaction of the particles composing the medium.

Sound waves are defined by different characteristics and properties.

- **Frequency** (*f*) is the number of waves that are repeated per unit of time, expressed in cycles per second or hertz (Hz: 1 Hz = 1 cycle/s, 1 MHz = 1000 Hz).
- **Wavelength** (λ) is the distance travelled in a cycle, expressed in metres.
- **Velocity** (v) is the product of frequency and wavelength, expressed in metres/second. The speed of sound depends on the characteristics of the medium through which the wave propagates. In soft tissues, the speed of sound is considered practically constant at 1540 m/s.
- **Amplitude**: sound waves cause particle displacement and variation in the local pressure of the propagation medium (Coltera, 2010).

Ultrasound Formation

Ultrasound waves are formed in the **transducer**, which is a component of the ultrasound equipment (ultrasound scanner) and is made up of crystals with a piezoelectric effect.

Piezoelectricity is the electrical charge that accumulates in certain solid materials, such as crystals and some ceramics, in response to the application of mechanical stress, resulting in brief bursts of mechanical energy in the form of ultrasound.

Piezoelectric crystals (which can be natural quartz or synthetic ceramic materials such as lead zirconate titanate [PZT]) have the ability to transform electrical energy into mechanical energy and vice versa.

Thus, the transducer emits ultrasound pulses. Each pulse is a mechanical vibration that is characterised by its direction of propagation, speed, frequency and length, and returns to the transducer in the form of an echo. The pulse–echo principle is the basis of ultrasound image formation (Coltera, 2010).

Formation and Visualisation of the Ultrasound Image

Acoustic Impedance

The ultrasound image is formed when ultrasound waves travel through tissues and are then reflected when they meet tissues with different acoustic impedances.

The **acoustic impedance** of a tissue depends on its elasticity and physical density (Table 1). Depending on the difference in acoustic impedance between tissues, the reflected echoes are more or less bright. Depending on the mode used, the image is formed as a map of dots of varying brightness (B mode; see Methods of Ultrasound Image Visualisation, below). When the ultrasound beam impinges perpendicularly on the tissue (specular scattering), the echo that is reflected is brighter; when it is not perpendicular, refraction of the echoes occurs (diffuse scattering) (Kossoff, 2000).

Interaction of Ultrasound with Tissue

There are five basic interactions of ultrasound with tissues: **reflection**, **refraction**, **scattering**, **absorption**, and **attenuation**.

- The **reflection** of echoes occurs at the interface between two tissues that have different acoustic impedances. When two adjacent tissues have very different acoustic

Table 1. Acoustic impedance values of tissues.

Tissue	Density (g/cm²)	Velocity (m/s)	Acoustic impedance (Z) (10^6 kg/m²)
Air	0.0013	331	0.004
Fat	0.97	1470	1.42
Water	0.998	1492	1.49
Blood	1.06	1570	1.63
Muscle	1.04	1568	1.63
Bone	1.7	3600	6.12

impedances, the incident ultrasound beam is reflected almost entirely. This occurs between air and soft tissue, between soft tissue and bone, and between air and bone. However, when the tissues have similar acoustic impedances, for example, soft tissue next to soft tissue, a smaller proportion of the incident beam is reflected. Thus, the difference in acoustic impedance between the tissues determines the proportion of the beam that is reflected towards the transducer in the form of an ultrasound echo to form the ultrasound image and the proportion that remains to be transmitted through the interface of the different tissues to produce images of deeper structures.

- **Refraction** is the change in the direction of ultrasound when it does not strike perpendicularly against an interface of tissues where the speed of sound is different. The angle of refraction is determined by the changes in the speed of sound that occurs at the interface.
- **Scattering** or **diffusion** of ultrasound in different directions occurs when small particles within tissues produce a reflection or refraction of ultrasound, which can be specular or diffuse. This is what causes an echotexture pattern in a given organ. This scattering phenomenon increases with high-frequency transducers, which enables the echotexture of an organ to be observed in greater detail.
- **Absorption** is the process in which acoustic energy is converted into heat energy, in which case ultrasound is lost and cannot be recovered.
- **Attenuation** is the loss of acoustic or ultrasound energy as the beam travels deep through tissues. The attenuation coefficient (expressed in decibels [dB]/cm) is the relative loss of intensity of the ultrasound beam per centimetre of depth travelled. The attenuation coefficient is 0.5 (dB/cm)/MHz frequency of the transducer, which implies that there is greater attenuation when using high-frequency transducers compared with low-frequency ones. This means that high-frequency transducers have better resolution (shorter wavelength) but poorer tissue penetration (Novellas and Espada, 2014).

Methods of Ultrasound Image Visualisation

There are three ways that ultrasound images can be visualised, two of which (B mode and M mode) are used widely clinically.

- **A mode** (amplitude). A mode or amplitude mode is the least often used, but it is especially useful for ophthalmological examinations. The amplitude of the echoes is represented as peaks on a vertical baseline, at the top of which the transducer would be located. The depth of the different echoes is represented along the line, with the deepest echoes located furthest from the transducer.
- **B mode** (brightness). B mode or brightness mode represents the echoes as dots, so that the brightness or grey scale is proportional to their amplitude, and the position corresponds to the depth at which they have originated. Currently, B mode is used in real time, where a moving image in shades of grey is viewed.
- **M mode** (movement). M mode or movement mode uses B mode information to represent echoes from a moving organ, such as the myocardium and heart valves, with the transducer and ultrasound beam in a fixed position relative to the patient. Information from the echoes of a single ultrasound beam passing through a moving structure is acquired and plotted as a function of time, with the depth of the structure on the vertical axis (beam direction) and time on the horizontal axis. M mode allows measurements of cardiac walls and chambers to be made and the motility of cardiac valves and walls to be quantitatively analysed over time (Fischetti and Scott, 2007).

Ultrasound Equipment

Transducers

(Nyland et al., 2002).

The transducer is a fundamental part of the ultrasound apparatus. It is made up of crystals with a piezoelectric effect. Types of transducer include:

a. **mechanical transducers**: these have one or more crystals that rotate or oscillate over a sector. The image on the screen is sector-shaped with a truncated tip. They are more fragile than electronic transducers and are no longer used;
b. **electronic transducers** (Fig. 1): these are formed by groups of crystals organised in an orderly manner (array) and stimulated together. The arrangement of the crystals defines the type of electronic transducer, its application and the appearance of the image on the monitor.

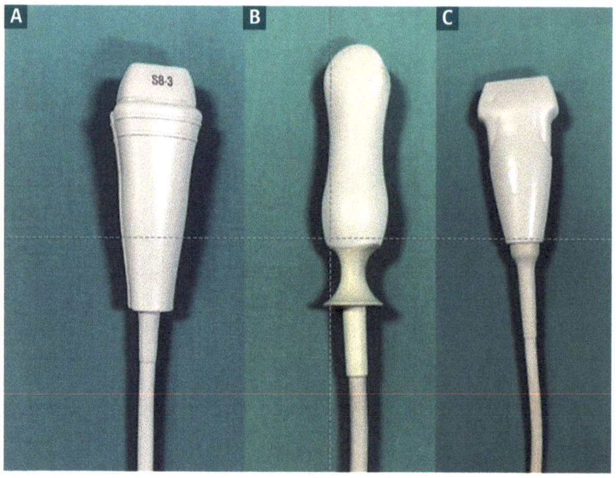

Figure 1. Types of electronic transducers. **A**. Sectoral. **B**. Semiconvex. **C**. Linear.

Both broadband and multifrequency transducers, which cover several frequencies, are currently available.

- **Convex or semiconvex transducers**: the crystals are arranged in a convex shape. The ultrasound beam consequently acquires a fan shape with a greater scanning amplitude, but without artefact in the near field and with a small contact surface. They are used for abdominal and musculoskeletal ultrasonography.
- **Linear transducers**: the crystals are arranged to form a linear contact surface. The image is rectangular with no artefact in the near field. The main drawback is the large contact surface. They are used for abdominal and musculoskeletal ultrasonography.
- **Sectoral transducers** (**phased array**): these have a row of flat crystals. A sectoral field of view is produced, and the beam can be directed in different directions and focused at various levels. They provide a triangular or fan-shaped image with a small echo emission base, with a wider field of view at greater depth. They are used in echocardiography.

In addition to the arrangement of the crystals, the transducers also differ in their frequency; frequencies from 2 MHz to 18 MHz are currently available on the market. The choice of frequency depends on the depth of the structure to be examined: for surface structures high-frequency transducers should be used, whereas for deep structures a lower frequency should be used.

Settings

(Nyland et al, 2002).

The control panel allows the operator to maximise the quality of the image. It is important that the settings are constantly adjusted throughout the ultrasound examination for optimal image quality.

There are some settings that are predetermined depending on the type of examination (preset) and others that are constantly changed while an ultrasound examination is being performed. Among them the following are covered in this chapter: overall gain, time gain compensation (TGC), power, focal point, beam size and depth.

Gain: this amplifies returning echoes. If the gain is increased, the image obtained is whiter over its whole depth. This increases both the useful information signal and the artefactual noise. Excessive gain produces proportionately more noise than useful information, but too low a gain can result in the loss of useful information.

TGC: echoes that come from deeper structures are subject to more attenuation than those that come from surface structures. This difference in attenuation is observed as darker images for deeper structures and brighter images (less attenuated echoes) for surface structures. To compensate for this effect and to be able to obtain a more homogeneous echogenicity throughout the depth of the image, the gain of the echoes coming from deeper structures can be selectively increased.

Power: this is the amplitude of the ultrasound waves that are produced. It is usually determined in the presets of the equipment and is not usually modified. It is advisable to work with the minimum possible power that produces a good image.

Focal points: these are represented in the form of an arrowhead or dots on one side of the image. A focal point is the area where the best lateral resolution is obtained, therefore, it should be placed in the area of interest. With currently available equipment there can be several focal points, and they can be moved to the area of interest.

Beam size: if the beam size is decreased, the lateral resolution is increased (Fig. 2).

Depth: when an organ is evaluated, it must be included completely in the image, so the depth must be adapted according to each organ being studied, to ensure that it is observed in its entirety.

Image Quality

Areas of the Ultrasound Image

The ultrasound beam is not linear but convergent on a point called the focal point, and divergent beyond this point, with a certain thickness in each of the three dimensions.

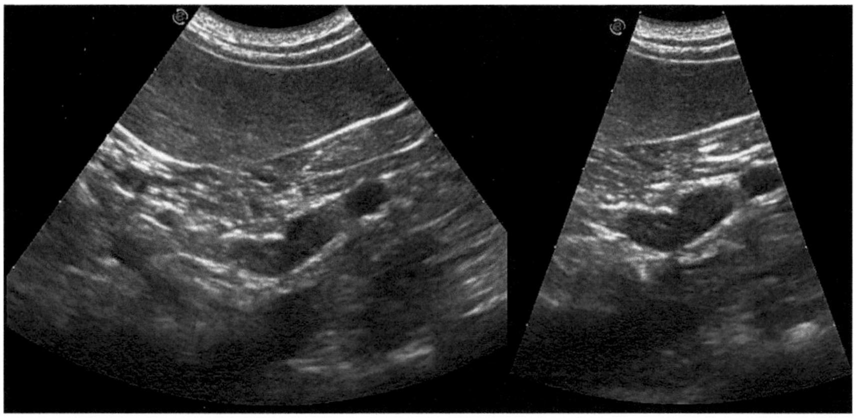

Figure 2. Beam size. The smaller the size, the better the lateral resolution of the image.

Ultrasound images have three areas:

- **near field**: the closest area, the interface between the skin surface and the transducer
- **focal zone**: the area where the beam is narrowest and has the best resolution. It is the area marked with a small triangle or point on the right of the image
- **far field**: includes the deepest area from the focal zone. In this area, the beam begins to widen and its resolution decreases.

Resolution

Resolution is the ability of an ultrasound machine to represent two points or interfaces that are very close together as different echoes. The resolution depends on several factors, such as the frequency of the transducer, the length of the ultrasound pulse, the size of the beam and the resolution of the screen. Some of these factors can be modified but others cannot.

In ultrasonography, there is differentiation between axial, lateral and elevational resolution.

- **Axial resolution** is the ability to differentiate two very close points or interfaces in the direction of the ultrasound beam. The axial resolution is inversely related to the wavelength: if the distance between the two points is less than the wavelength, the ultrasound equipment will not be able to identify the echoes from them separately and will classify them as a single echo. Thus, the axial resolution depends on the frequency of the transducer, and a higher frequency will provide a better axial resolution.
- **Lateral resolution** is the ability to distinguish two points in the direction perpendicular to the axis of the ultrasound beam. It depends on the beam width and the frequency. As the ultrasound beam does not have the same width as the depth changes, the lateral resolution also varies with depth, and is optimal in the focal zone where the beam is narrowest. The ultrasound beam is narrower with higher frequencies; therefore, the lateral resolution will be better when high frequencies are used.

Image Orientation

Orientation of the ultrasound image is important to perform a systematic interpretation.

In an abdominal ultrasonographic examination, the patient is normally placed in dorsal recumbency and to the right of the operator, with the head oriented in the direction where the ultrasound machine is and away from the operator. The animal can also be placed in right or left lateral recumbency, to evaluate the nondependent area.

For each organ, sections defined by a plane whose orientation corresponds to the propagation of ultrasound should be obtained. Thus, there are **transverse** sections, which cross the patient perpendicularly to the spine; **longitudinal/sagittal** plane sections, which are parallel to the spine and can be directed cranially or caudally, right or left; and **dorsal** sections, which are viewed using a right or left lateral approach, parallel to the spine.

The orientation on the monitor is as follows: the top of the monitor represents the part of the transducer that is in contact with the skin, which in the case of an abdominal examination will be the ventral part of the abdomen. In the sagittal and dorsal planes, cranial is to the left of the image on the monitor (Fig. 3). In the transverse plane, the right of the animal is the left of the image on the monitor (Fig. 4).

The orientation of the image on the screen depends on the orientation of the transducer. Each transducer has a mark (e.g. a light or a dot) that corresponds to a dot or image of the logo of the company that manufactured the equipment.

When imaging the abdomen, the transducer mark is placed towards the skull for the sagittal and dorsal planes, and towards the operator for the transverse plane. The indicator mark on the monitor is located to the left of the image for abdominal ultrasonography and to the right for echocardiography.

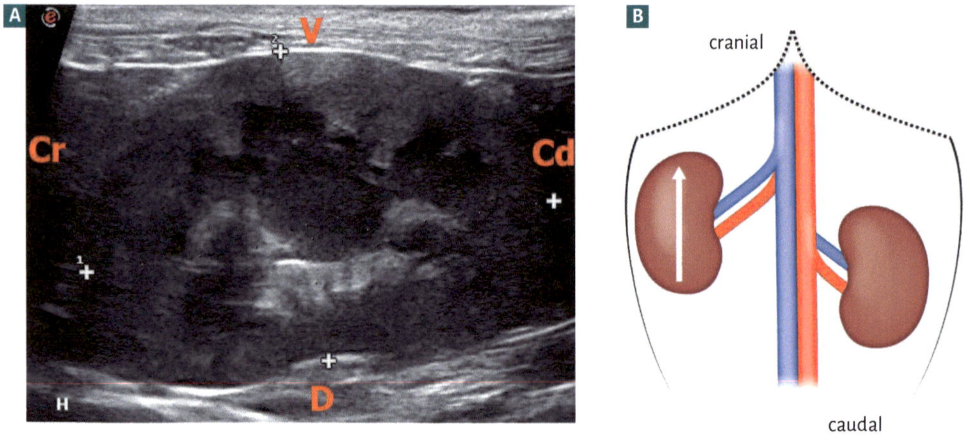

Figure 3. Orientation of the image on the screen in the longitudinal (sagittal) plane. **A**. The position of the transducer is observed with the arrowhead oriented towards the skull, corresponding to the brand reference icon on the screen. **B**. Representation of the ultrasound image in the longitudinal plane obtained according to the position of the transducer in A.

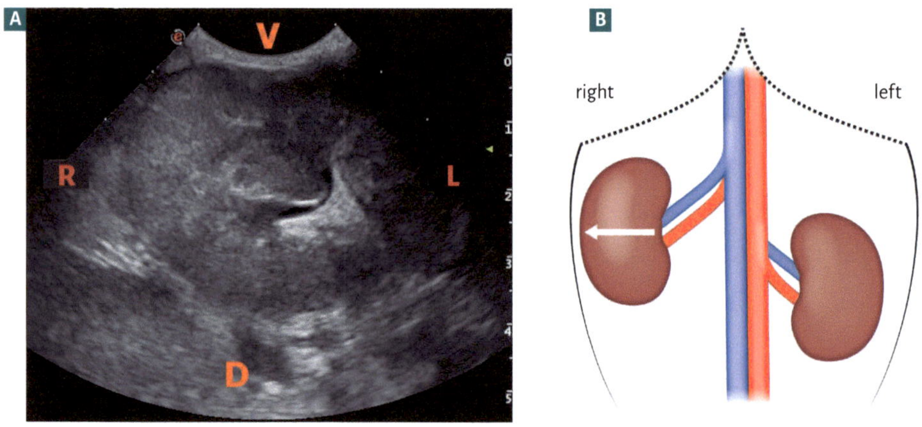

Figure 4. Orientation of the image on the screen in the transverse plane. **A**. The position of the probe is observed with the arrowhead oriented to the right, corresponding to the brand reference icon on the screen. **B**. Representation of the ultrasound image in the transverse plane obtained according to the position of the transducer in A.

If the transducer is placed on the right or the left side, with the animal positioned in lateral recumbency, the upper part of the monitor will be right or left depending on the approach; in sagittal sections, cranial will be located to the left of the monitor, and in transverse sections, dorsal will be located to the left of the monitor (Novellas and Espada, 2014).

Interpretation of the Ultrasound Image and Terminology

The appearance of the ultrasound image depends on numerous factors, such as the structural characteristics of the tissue, the characteristics of the transducer and the adjustment of the gain.

Liquids transmit the ultrasound waves perfectly and appear on the screen as areas devoid of echoes; however, for liquids with high cellularity there may be echoes in suspension.

Soft tissues are observed on the screen with a grainy texture and are displayed in different shades of grey depending on their echogenicity (Box 1).

Fatty tissues are very echogenic; however, fat in certain areas of the body, such as subcutaneous fat in obese animals, has a lower echogenicity. Structural fat can be more echogenic than stored fat because structural fat contains connective tissue, which is very echogenic.

Osseous tissue has a very high acoustic impedance. The difference between the acoustic impedance of bone and soft tissue causes most of the echoes to be reflected, which means that no image can be seen beyond bone. The same happens with air, with artefacts observed beyond images of air and osseous tissue.

The terminology used to describe the appearance of ultrasound images is related to the intensity of the echoes from the tissues (brightness), the attenuation and the echotexture of the organ.

The terminology used to describe the appearance of ultrasound images is as follows.

Box 1. Tissue echogenicity in increasing order

- urine, bile
- renal medulla
- muscle
- renal cortex
- liver
- stored fat
- spleen
- prostate
- renal sinus
- structural fat and vessel walls
- bone, gas and interorgan interface.

- **Anechoic**: area without echo or free of echo. It is black and represents liquid, which easily transmits ultrasound waves without attenuation.
- **Hypoechogenic**: area of low intensity, with few echoes. These areas are observed as different shades of grey and correspond to soft tissues.
- **Hyperechogenic**: high intensity area, with many echoes. These areas are observed in different shades from light grey to white. They correspond to fat, connective tissue, air or minerals.

Because soft tissues all appear as different shades of grey, a comparison of echogenicity is made, using the following terminology:

- **iso:** equal to the surroundings
- **hypo:** less than the surroundings
- **hyper**: greater than the surroundings.

An organ can present a different echotexture depending on the size of the grain (small, medium, large), and can be homogeneous or heterogeneous (Novellas, and Espada, 2014).

Artefacts

(Novellas and Espada, 2014; Penninck, 2002).

Artefacts are anomalies that appear in an image and alter or falsify reality and can be misleading. All imaging modalities feature artefacts that are unique to a particular system. In ultrasound images, some artefacts can facilitate diagnosis. Thus, artefacts in ultrasonography can be classified into two categories, **useful** and **unuseful** (Box 2). Useful artefacts give information regarding the physical properties of the tissue being imaged, whereas unuseful artefacts complicate image interpretation and generally do not give any clinically relevant information.

Box 2. Artefact types

Useful artefacts:

- enhancement effect
- reverberation (comet tail)
- acoustic shadow.

Unuseful artefacts

- split image (refraction)
- mirror image
- propagation speed error
- partial slice thickness (false)
- sidelobe artefact.

Artefacts can also be classified into **attenuation** artefacts (enhancement effect, acoustic shadow and split image [refraction] artefact) according to the physics of ultrasound, or those that are due to **propagation** of the ultrasound beam (sidelobe artefact, partial or false slice thickness, reverberation, comet tail, mirror image and split image).

Enhancement Effect

This effect occurs when the ultrasound beam passes through a structure that does not attenuate ultrasound, such as liquids. It appears as a more echogenic image distally to a structure that does not attenuate ultrasound, for example, the urinary bladder, gallbladder or a cyst (Fig. 5).

Reverberation

This is the result of multiple reflections of the ultrasound beam bouncing between two surfaces or vibrating within a highly reflective surface, typically a gas bubble. It is manifested as a series of parallel hyperechogenic lines (Fig. 6).

Comet Tail

This is a hyperechogenic vertical trace found when the ultrasound beam collides with an air bubble or a mineralised surface. It is a type of reverberation. It can appear when imaging the small intestine, small calculi and small mineralisations.

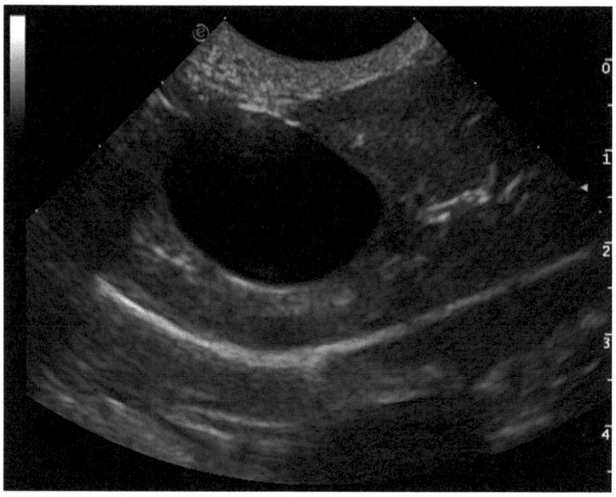

Figure 5. Enhancement artefact. This is formed because there is virtually no attenuation when ultrasound passes through a fluid-filled structure.

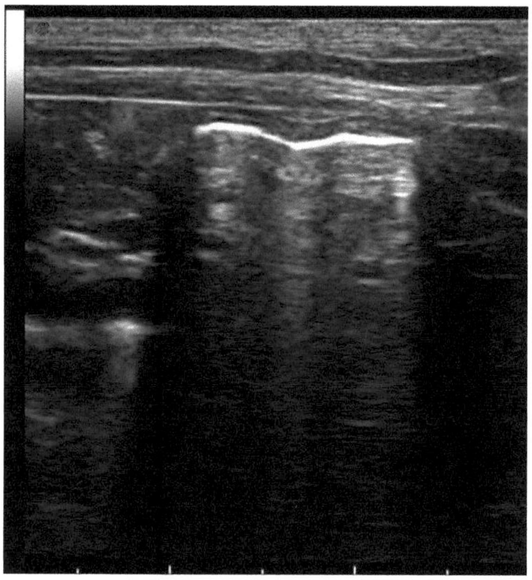

Figure 6. Reverberation artefact. Observed as parallel hyperechogenic lines produced by air.

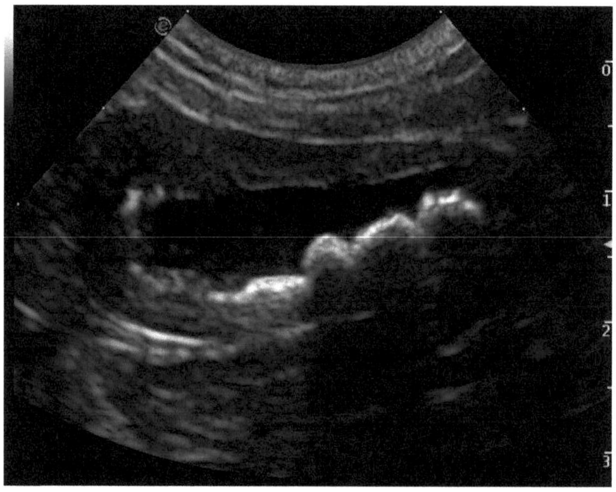

Figure 7. Acoustic shadow artefact. This is visualised as a hyperechogenic structure followed by an anechoic cone. It is produced by structures that almost completely reflect ultrasound, such as bone and minerals.

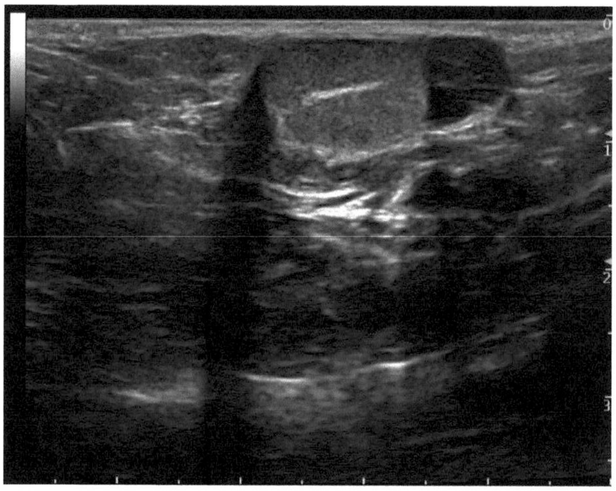

Figure 8. Split image (refraction) artefact. Produced by the refraction of ultrasound when it encounters a rounded structure.

Acoustic Shadow

This is observed as a hypoechoic or anechoic region that is located distally to a hyperechogenic structure due to a high attenuation or reflection of the ultrasound beam. Very few of the initial ultrasound waves pass through the hyperechogenic surface, meaning that very few echoes return from structures located deep to this surface. This artefact is typical of bone or other mineral structures, gas and many nonbiological materials, including some foreign bodies (Fig. 7).

Split Image (Refraction)

This artefact arises due to the slowing of ultrasound through a liquid-filled structure, causing refraction of the ultrasound beam at the tissue–liquid interface. It can also be observed between two tissues when one has a curved surface and there is a difference in the speed of sound between them. The ultrasound beam is refracted in the direction of the tissue with the lower propagation speed, therefore there are no echoes that can return from regions below the rounded margin. It is observed in the margins of rounded structures as a thin line or anechoic conical region (Fig. 8).

Mirror Image

This occurs when the ultrasound beam impinges on a curvilinear structure that acts as a mirror interface. In these types of interfaces, the echoes return directly to the transducer when the incidence is perpendicular, but if it is not, some echoes may return after changing their trajectory and bouncing against another interface that reflects them towards the probe, so they will have a greater delay in returning due to the greater distance travelled.

A physiological example of a structure that generates this artefact is the diaphragm; part of the liver is seen reflected on the other side of the diaphragm when air from the lung is on the other side. It is observed as two symmetrical images separated by a hyperechogenic line (Fig. 9). Typically, the artefact can be removed by changing the position of the transducer.

Propagation Speed Error

The software of the ultrasound machine assumes that ultrasound is transmitted into soft tissues at a constant velocity of 1540 m/s, and uses this velocity and the time it takes for the echoes to return to calculate the depth at which the structures are located. The speed of ultrasound in fat is actually slightly lower (1450 m/s); thus, fat, in addition to slowing down the speed of ultrasound waves, absorbs and reflects them in large quantities. This causes deep areas to appear with few echoes and low amplitude, that is, it produces subsequent attenuation. This causes image distortions to occur.

Partial or False Slice Thickness

The width of the ultrasound beam varies with the design characteristics of the transducer. When a fluid-filled structure and a tissue structure are included in that width at the same time, the echoes returning from that location are a combination of the echoes of the liquid and the surrounding tissues, represented as if the tissue were inside the liquid.

The artefact can be seen as echoes in the bladder, which actually come from the bladder wall or other adjacent tissues (Fig. 10). A sediment-like image can be seen in the gallbladder if part of a liver lobe is also included in the width of the beam. The artefact can be eliminated or reduced by adjusting the beam angle.

Sidelobe Artefact

The ultrasound beam is formed by a primary beam and other small accessory and less-penetrating beams on both sides of the main beam, called side beams or lobes. If a highly reflective structure is in the path of these side beams, the echoes returning from them may be powerful enough to reach the transducer and produce a signal, which will be represented in the image as if it were in the plane of the primary beam.

This can be observed in the bladder due to echoes that come from, for example, the colon. Changing the direction of the transducer or ultrasound beam will alter or remove the artefact.

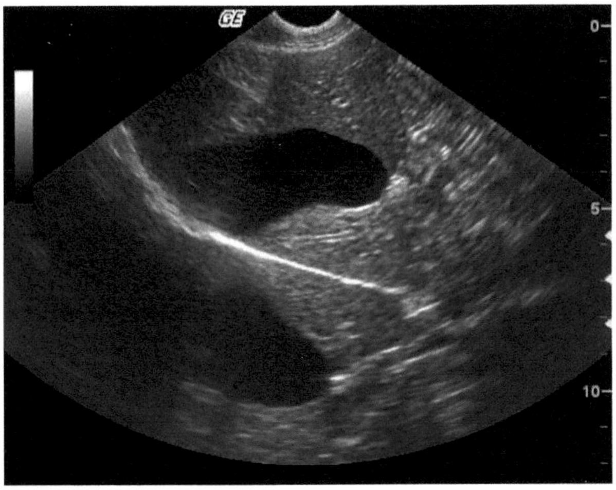

Figure 9. Mirror image artefact. This occurs when ultrasound is reflected at the curved lung–air interface against the diaphragm.

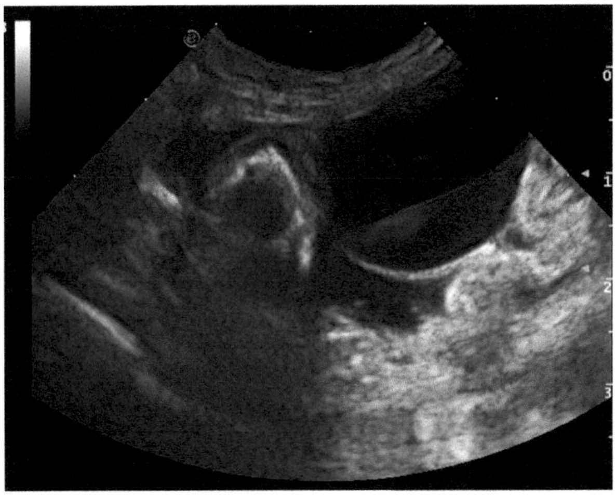

Figure 10. A laminar thickness artefact that looks like sediment, but does not move with the patient's position and disappears when the transducer position is changed.

Advantages and Disadvantages of Ultrasonography

Advantages

Ultrasonography is a technique that:

- is harmless
- is quick
- is sensitive to tissue changes
- allows repeated checks, which are very important for monitoring the evolution of diseases
- can be used to perform ultrasound-guided punctures or biopsies
- allows a dynamic study to be performed
- has easy portability, that is, the equipment is portable and can be moved easily
- is easily accessible in terms of cost.

Disadvantages

Ultrasonography is a nonspecific technique that, most of the time, requires punctures or biopsies to be performed to help reach a definitive diagnosis.

It is operator dependent; knowledge of anatomy is essential, as well as understanding the physical principles of ultrasound imaging and keeping up to date on knowledge of different diseases.

Tissues beyond gas-filled and osseous tissue cannot be visualised by ultrasound imaging. To overcome this drawback, it is necessary to look for acoustic windows (Novellas and Espada, 2014).

Bibliography

- Coltera, M.(2010) Ultrasound physics in a nutshell. *Otolaryngol Clin North Am*, 43, pp. 1149–1159.
- Fischetti, A.J., Scott, R.C. (2007) Basic ultrasound beam formation and instrumentation. *Clin Tech Small Anim Pract*, 22, pp. 90–92.
- Kossoff, G. (2000) Basic physics and imaging characteristics of ultrasound. *World J Surg*, 24, pp. 134–142.
- Mattoon, J.S., Berry, C.R. (2021) Fundamentals of Diagnostic Ultrasound. En: *Small animal Diagnostic ultrasound*. Ed Mattoon JS. Sellon RK. Berry CR. 4th ed Philadelphia: WB Saunders, pp. 1-48
- Novellas, R., Espada, Y. (2014) Diagnóstico ecográfico. Producción y propiedades. Aplicaciones. Principio de interpretación. In: Agut, A., et al. (eds). *Diagnóstico por Imagen en Pequeños Animales*. Multimédica Ediciones Veterinarias, pp. 63-78.

Notes

Doppler Techniques

Abby Caine

This chapter describes the basic Doppler techniques that can be used in abdominal ultrasonography in small animals. These techniques are used to evaluate the great vessels, identify anomalous vessels such as portosystemic shunts, investigate the vascularisation of lesions and assess the velocity of blood flow through vessels such as the portal vein.

The Physics of the Doppler Effect

When imagining a static reflective interface that interacts with an ultrasound beam, the ultrasound wave emitted by the transducer travels to the static interface and is reflected back to the transducer at the same frequency. The Doppler effect is based on the fact that an ultrasound wave that is reflected by a moving object will travel back at a frequency that is different from the frequency that had been emitted. If the object is moving towards the transducer, the frequency of the reflected wave will increase as the wavelength is compressed; for an audible sound, this would be heard as an increase in pitch. Conversely, if the object is moving away from the transducer/listener the wavelength of the reflected wave is increased and the frequency or pitch of the wave decreases (Fig. 1). The difference between the frequencies that are transmitted and received is known as the Doppler effect. During an abdominal ultrasound examination, in an ideal "perfect" situation the only moving object would be the blood in the vessels, so the Doppler signal should be received only from the vessels. In practice, however, things are not perfect, and the movement of the animal, including its breathing, can cause interference.

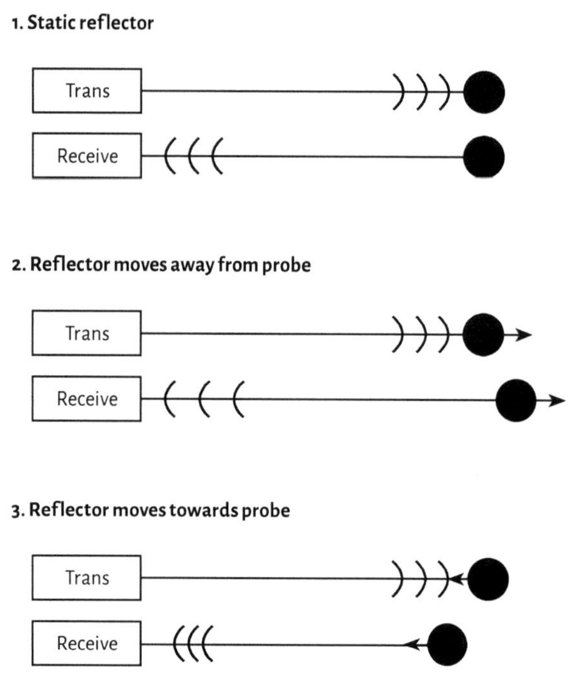

Figure 1. Illustration of the physics of the Doppler effect. 1. The transducer and the reflective object are both static, so the frequency transmitted (Trans) and the frequency received (Receive) are the same. 2. The reflective object is moving away from the transducer, so the received frequency is lower than the frequency transmitted. 3. The reflective object is moving towards the transducer, so the received frequency is higher than the transmitted frequency.

The difference between the frequencies of the emitted and reflected ultrasound waves can be used to calculate the velocity at which the mobile interface is moving and the direction (relative to the transducer) in which it is moving. Accurate calculation of the velocity is dependent on the difference between the angle of the ultrasound beam and the angle of the blood vessel/direction of blood flow, because the Doppler shift in frequency can be used to calculate only the portion of movement towards the transducer. Ideally, the direction of blood flow and the ultrasound beam should be parallel so that the Doppler angle between these two directions is as close as possible to 0°. If it is not possible to align the transducer with the direction of blood flow, as happens frequently in abdominal ultrasonography because the direction of flow in the great vessels is from the head to the feet, then angle correction should be applied or the velocity of the moving blood will be underestimated. To correct the angle, the vessel should be aligned with an angled line superimposed on the sample gate visible on the monitor (Fig. 2). The error in the calculated velocity after angle correction increases with the size of the Doppler angle; as a rule of thumb, the Doppler angle (between the ultrasound beam and the blood flow) should be less than 60° even when angle correction is applied. If the angle is greater than 60°, the calculated velocity is progressively less accurate: at 60° the error is approximately 10%, and at 80° it is 42%. Therefore, to obtain meaningful measurements, the angle between the ultrasound wave and the vessel should not exceed 60°.

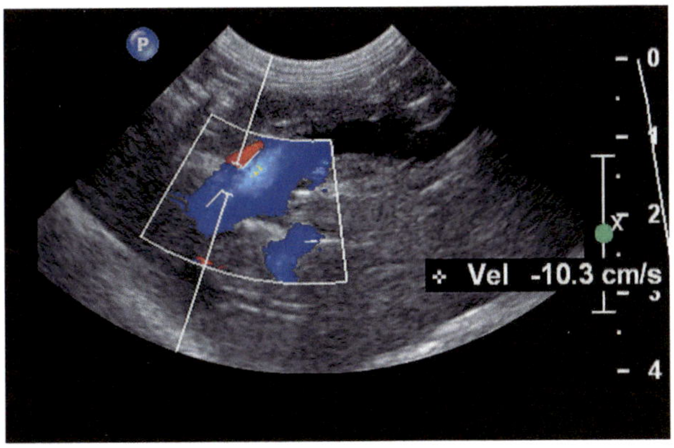

Figure 2. Application of angle correction when measuring the velocity of portal blood flow in the abdomen of a cat.

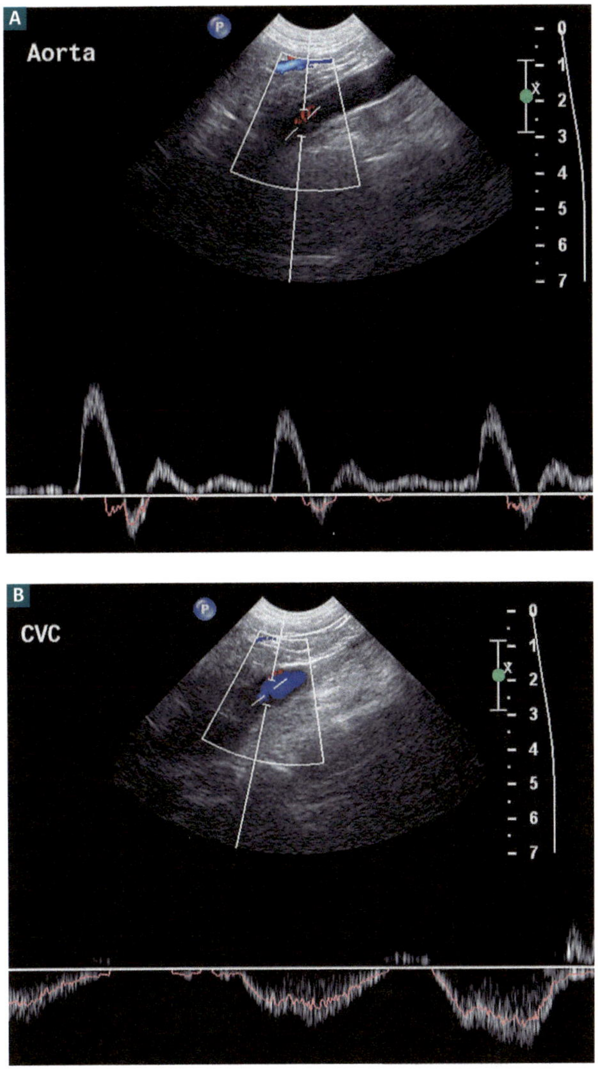

Figure 3. The character of the flow can be used to differentiate between arterial and venous flow. **A**. Aorta showing a "clean" envelope and pulsatile flow typical of large-diameter arteries. **B**. Caudal vena cava (CVC) showing a "dirty" trace due to the variation of velocity in the venous flow.

Information Obtained with Doppler

Visualisation of Doppler Information in Diagnostic Ultrasonography

There are two methods for visualisation of the information obtained from the Doppler effect: a **spectral Doppler** signal, which displays the velocity of the blood over time, and a **colour Doppler** signal that maps the frequency and direction of the blood movement within each pixel of the two-dimensional (2D) image.

In the abdomen, **pulsed-wave** (PW) Doppler, a type of spectral Doppler, is used. In this technique, an ultrasound wave is emitted and the transducer "listens" for the returning echo at a specific time later. The depth of the "gate" selected on the image is the only place where the Doppler signal is acquired and analysed. This technique cannot be used in the case of high-velocity blood flow, for example, in echocardiography of stenotic valvular anomalies, in which the flow velocity can exceed the display capacity of the PW gate, resulting in an artefact called aliasing. PW Doppler is ideal for abdominal vascular imaging because in this location the blood flow velocity should not exceed 1.5–2 m/s (greater velocities typically lead to aliasing). **Continuous-wave** (CW) spectral Doppler, which can measure higher velocities without aliasing artefact, is not necessary for abdominal imaging.

Spectral Doppler information is displayed as a black and white plot on a graph of calculated velocity against time. Blood flow towards the transducer is shown above the baseline, and flow away from the transducer is shown below the baseline. The baseline is the point at which the interface is not moving relative to the probe.

The information from spectral Doppler can be used to calculate, among others, the **direction** of flow (towards or away from the transducer) and the **character** of the flow, which allows arterial and venous flow to be distinguished (Fig. 3). The character of the flow is determined by measuring the difference in pressure between the start and end of the vessel being imaged, and the diameter of the vessel. In large vessels with fast flow, the flow can be described as uniform and laminar across the entire diameter of the vessel. In narrower vessels, it might be described as blunted or parabolic, with a greater range of velocities due to the slower flow adjacent to the vessel walls resulting from frictional forces from the walls.

Turbulent flow, with the blood "swirling" in various directions, can be seen at points where vessels narrow or where the flow passes through an abnormal junction, for example, with a shunt.

In general, arterial flow is pulsatile because it is subject to pressures due to the cardiac cycle. Very large arteries, such as the aorta, have laminar flow and so they demonstrate a "clean" envelope because all the blood in the vessel is moving at the same speed, resulting in a single-line trace indicating the maximum velocity (Fig. 3 A). Smaller arteries still have pulsatile flow, but may have a "dirty" trace because frictional forces reduce the flow velocity at the edges of the vessel. This is displayed as pulsatile flow with the area within the maximum flow profile filled in to varying degrees because there is more than one flow velocity. Arteries that supply a capillary bed that has high resistance, for example, in the extremities, may show a slight flow reversal during diastole. This phenomenon does not occur in arteries that supply low-resistance organs, such as the renal or carotid arteries.

Veins show different Doppler traces because they are under influences other than the cardiac cycle because the blood that flows through them has passed through a capillary bed. Even large-diameter veins do not have a "clean" envelope because they always have a range of flow velocities. The caudal vena cava is subject to different influences because it empties into the heart (and therefore is affected by the cardiac cycle), and also because it passes through the caudal thorax and so is affected by respiratory movements. These influences cause it to have a "dirty" trace with a biphasic maximum velocity (with the cardiac pulsation superimposed on the respiratory pulsation) (Fig. 3 B).

The portal vein is also subject to different influences and has a distinctive appearance when viewed with spectral Doppler. It empties into the capillary bed of the hepatic portal system, which has a constant pressure; therefore, it has a "dirty" trace, since many velocities are present, as described above for venous flow. However, if the portal vein is located within the sample gate during the Doppler study, the maximum velocity is constant (Fig. 4).

Colour Doppler gives a good indication of the presence and direction of blood flow in the vessels included in the sample volume, and provides some qualitative information about the velocity of blood flow, since flow with a higher mean velocity is displayed with greater colour saturation. The information about velocity should be viewed as qualitative rather than quantitative. If a quantitative measure of velocity is required, PW Doppler should be used; this assesses only the mean velocity (not the peak velocity). Using colour Doppler requires the use of multiple pulses per scan line, which will reduce the refresh rate; if this causes a problem with the system, the width of the Doppler sample volume should be reduced.

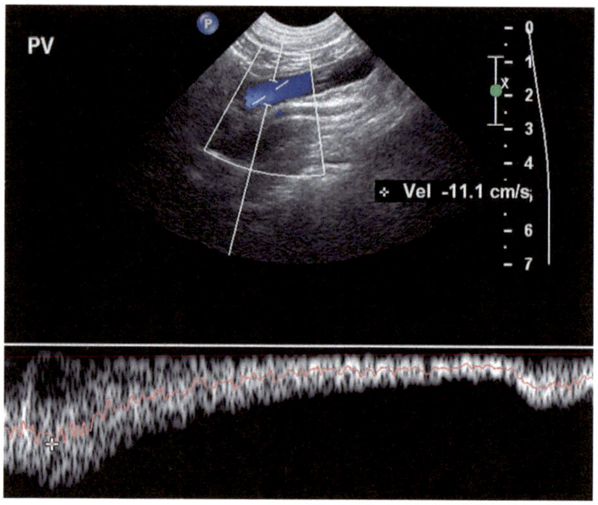

Figure 4. The portal vein has a "dirty" trace because it is venous flow (with many velocities); however, the constant downstream pressure as it empties into the capillary bed of the hepatic portal system leads to the maximum velocity being almost constant, varying only with respiratory movements. Here the mean flow is superimposed on the pulsed wave trace so it can be measured.

In general, large arteries and veins have laminar (uniform colour) flow and are usually visualised following the **Blue Away, Red Towards** (**BART**) directional coding. If the flow is turbulent and nonlaminar, then a mosaic of colour is displayed, with some flow towards and some away from the transducer (this can be displayed as variance, or green, if this setting is selected). Turbulent flow occurs in the case of an abnormal entrance to a vessel (e.g. an anomalous vessel such as a portosystemic shunt) or if the flow passes through a narrowing in the vessel (e.g. due to neoplastic invasion or a thrombus).

Obtaining Accurate Doppler Information

Obtaining a good Doppler signal, and therefore accurate readings, relies on optimising the image quality. To obtain a good-quality spectral Doppler trace, the following steps should be followed.

1. First of all, a good-quality 2D image should be obtained (a poor-quality 2D image will result in an inadequate Doppler signal).
2. Colour Doppler should be used to identify the blood vessels if there is doubt about their anatomy or the direction of blood flow.
3. The transducer should be aligned as closely as possible with the direction of flow in the blood vessel, because differences between the direction of flow and the direction of the ultrasound beam may result in an inaccurate

measurement of flow velocity (remember the rule of thumb of 60°).

4. The sample gate should be placed in the vessel of interest and the gate opened as wide as possible within the vessel, to ensure that all flow velocities are detected.
5. The vessel wall filter should be adjusted so that it is as low as possible (less than 50–60 Hz), to eliminate noise from peripheral blood vessels.
6. The display should be adjusted so that the Doppler waveform fills at least 75% of the Doppler screen and a sweep speed that allows 4–6 full cardiac cycles to be displayed should be used.

It is important to adjust the pulse repetition frequency (PRF) properly to avoid errors in interpreting the information provided by the Doppler signal. The PRF determines how many pulses of ultrasound are emitted by the transducer in a set period of time (usually measured in pulses per second). If the Doppler shift frequency is greater than 50% of the PRF, then these high frequencies will be misinterpreted as lower frequencies – this is aliasing, which leads to the signal being placed on the wrong side of the baseline (for spectral Doppler) or the blood in the centre of the vessel, which is the fastest moving, being displayed as green (if the variance is switched on) or as the colour indicating the opposite direction to that expected in colour Doppler (Fig. 5).

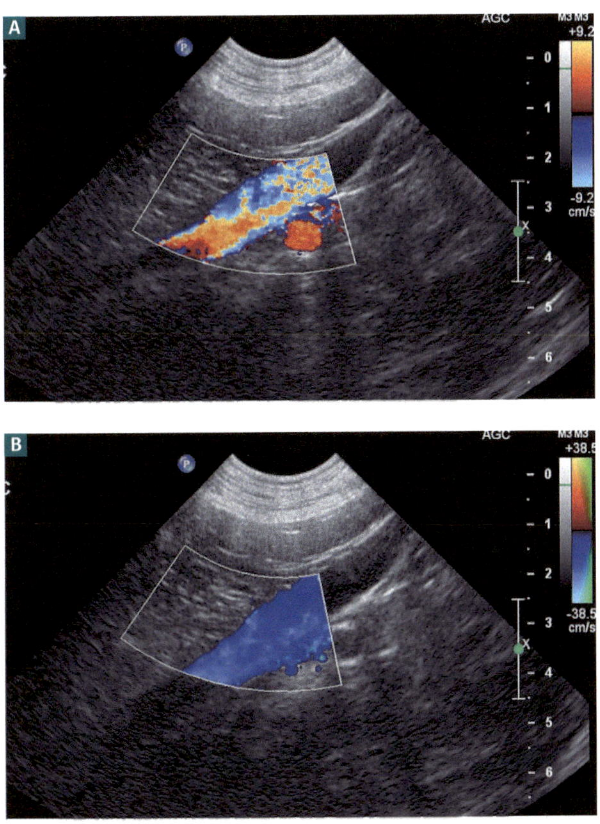

Figure 5. Different appearances of blood flow in colour Doppler. **A**. Flow in the caudal vena cava (CVC) showing aliasing in the faster-flowing central region because the pulse repetition frequency has been set too low. **B**. The same CVC with the settings adjusted to eliminate aliasing, showing uniform flow in blue.

Analysis of Doppler Information

Doppler information can be evaluated in various ways.

1. To determine whether blood flow is present: either in a large vessel (e.g. to look for a thrombus) or in the small vessels within an organ in the case of identifying infarction.
2. To determine the direction of blood flow: this can help to identify the vessel that is being evaluated if the operator is unfamiliar with the anatomy. It also helps in identifying flow reversal, which can occur in cases of severe portal hypertension.
3. To determine the maximum velocity of the blood flow: this can be helpful in cases of portal hypertension, which reduces the velocity of flow towards the liver, and in cases of portosystemic shunting, in which the flow velocity can be increased if the shunt arises from the portal system downstream of the site of measurement.
4. To evaluate the spectral waveform: this qualitative evaluation might be used to distinguish an artery from a vein, or, in the case of evaluating Doppler indices (see section Specific Doppler Indices) can be used to help diagnose a variety of pathologies in the organ into which the vessel being studied empties.

Bibliography

- Lamb, C., Boswood, A. (2005) Doppler ultrasound examination in dogs and cats: The principles. *In Practice*, 27:4:183-189. https://bvajournals.onlinelibrary.wiley.com/doi/abs/10.1136/inpract.27.4.183
- Oglat, A.A. et al. (2018) A review of medical doppler ultrasonography of blood flow in general and especially in common carotid artery. *J Med Ultrasound*, 26(1):3-13. https://www.ncbi.nlm.nih.gov/pmc/articles/PMC6029191/

Computed Tomography

Xavier Sánchez Salguero

Computed tomography (CT) was developed by Godfrey Hounsfield and Allan McLeod Cormack in the 1970s. Both won and shared the Nobel Prize in Physiology or Medicine in 1979. The first veterinary use of CT was approximately 10 years after the introduction of the modality, and it was mainly used for the diagnosis of intracranial pathologies such as nasal and neurological abnormalities. Shortly afterwards, CT was modified for the study of large animals. Since then, the technology behind this advanced imaging technique has progressed considerably. Progress in the design of the detectors has made it possible to increase the speed at which studies are performed and has also enabled the acquisition of high-resolution images. The availability of CT equipment in veterinary centres has grown over the past 20 years: initially there were few available machines, most of which were single-slice equipment, whereas now many veterinary centres have multi-slice CT equipment.

CT is similar to the other conventional imaging modalities used for the diagnosis of a wide range of pathologies that affect the patient's anatomy. However, in many cases it is considered superior to the other modalities because it offers an excellent representation of the anatomy due to the absence of overlapping anatomical structures in the patient or interference caused by gas or the size of the patient, and the ability to examine the patient's body in its entirety. It is important to recognise that in many cases taking samples of the lesions observed by CT is necessary to establish a definitive cytological or histopathological diagnosis.

CT scans are noninvasive, can be performed quickly (often under sedation) and provide a wealth of anatomical information about the patient. In addition, advanced image capture and storage methods allow CT studies to be readily available for review by a specialist who is not necessarily on site. CT, therefore, has become a very useful diagnostic tool for veterinary medicine, helping veterinarians to reach more complete diagnoses, propose more precise interventions and treatments and, especially with the use of three-dimensional (3D) reconstructions, communicate better with owners.

Physical Principles of CT

CT uses the same physical principles as radiology but, unlike the latter, shows a wide range of grey shades in anatomical cross sections of the patient. Unlike in radiology, in CT the X-ray tube rotates around the patient, emitting radiation that crosses the anatomical region of interest. The X-rays are captured by a series of detectors that are responsible for transforming the X-rays into an electrical signal that is transmitted to a computer, which reconstructs the data obtained into a two-dimensional image that represents a cross section of the patient's anatomy.

CT Machine Components

A CT machine consists of the following elements.

- The **gantry** contains the X-ray tube and the detectors, and has a ring shape that allows the patient to be accommodated and advanced through it during the study (Figs. 1 and 2).
  - At the top of the gantry there is a numerical display that shows the position and height of the table, and the inclination of the gantry. Depending on the equipment, the display may show other parameters (Fig. 3).
  - The **collimators**: these are red lasers indicating the x axis (horizontal) and the y axis (vertical) that coincide at the isocentre of the gantry. Their orientation is essential for correct positioning of the patient by focusing the region of interest on the isocentre.
  - The **generator** or power source.
- The **table**, where the patient is positioned and oriented on the z axis of the scanner, allowing the patient to be moved through the gantry.
- The **console** allows patient information to be entered, the exposure parameters to be adjusted and the images to be reconstructed. It is connected to the computer linked to the CT equipment, which allows the scanner to be controlled and is where the images are processed and reconstructed (Fig. 4).

Types of Equipment

CT equipment can be classified according to the arrangement and movement of its components during image acquisition (generation) and according to the number of slices (single-slice or multi-slice).

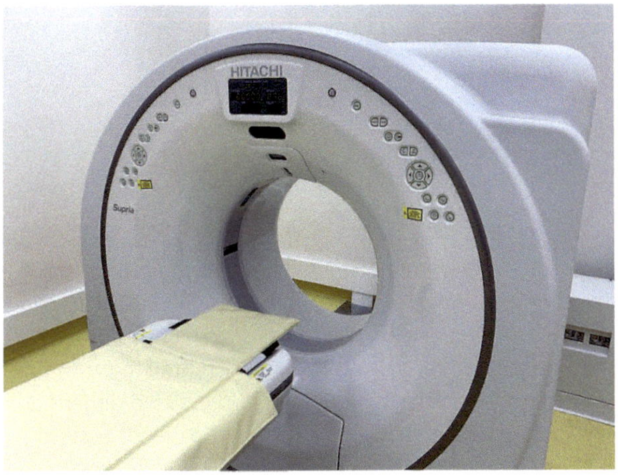

Figure 1. CT equipment. The gantry can be seen with its characteristic ring shape, as well as the table on which the patient will be positioned.

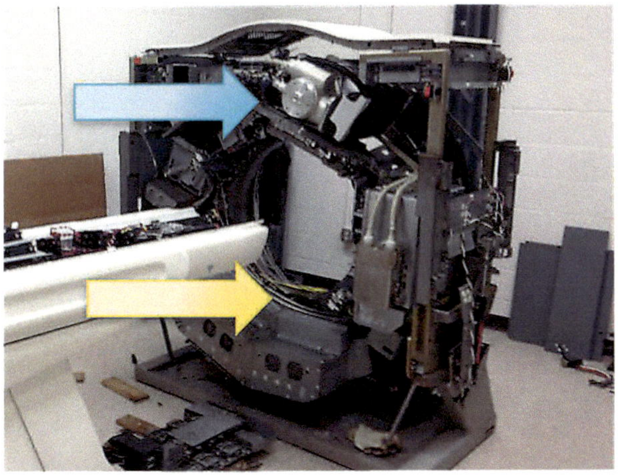

Figure 2. CT equipment where the gantry casing has been removed. The blue arrow points to the X-ray tube and the yellow arrow indicates the detectors (image courtesy of Randi Drees).

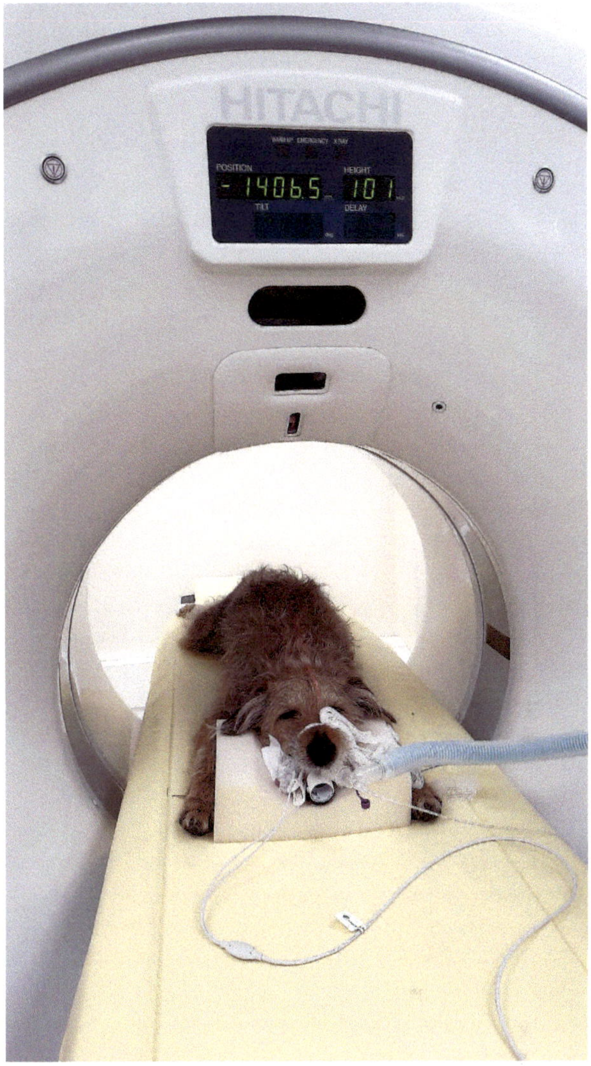

Figure 3. Magnified image showing the gantry with its numerical display, on which the position and height values of the table can be seen. The red laser can also be seen on the z axis .

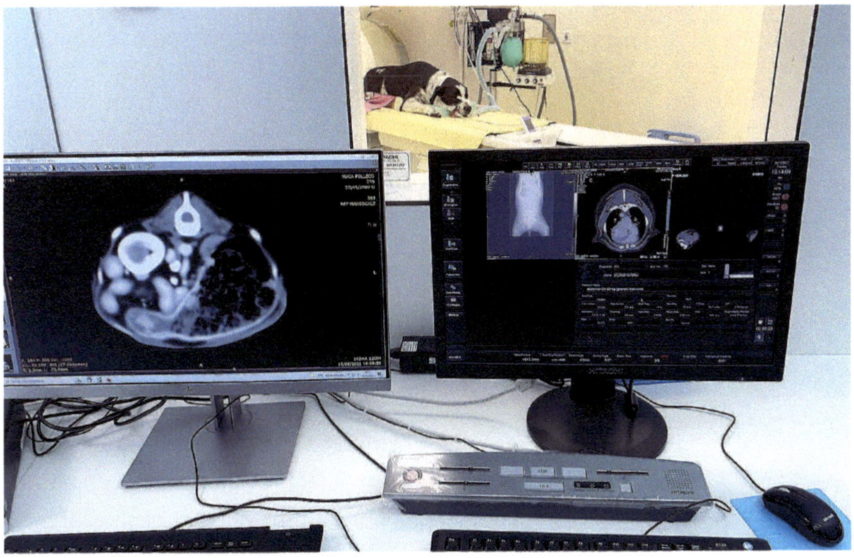

Figure 4. Workstation consisting of the console and a computer for the visualisation and interpretation of the images.

Classification by Generation

First-Generation "Rotation Translation"

In first-generation equipment, both the X-ray tube and the detector move along the patient (translation), allowing different projections to be obtained at a specific angle. Subsequently, there is a rotation movement to obtain another series of images. This process is carried out 180 times. The scan time is approximately 25–30 minutes.

Second-Generation "Rotation Translation"

In second-generation equipment, more detectors are added (up to 30); this perform the same types of movement as first-generation equipment but acquire multiple projections at the same time.

Third-Generation "Rotation Rotation"

In third-generation equipment there is simultaneous synchronised rotation at constant speed of both the X-ray tube and the detectors. Both the number of detectors (from 288 to more than 800) and the angle of the X-ray beam (fan beam) are considerably larger, allowing the entire patient to be scanned. With this equipment, the scanning time is substantially reduced (0.5 seconds), and although these systems initially suffered from ring artefacts (see later in this chapter), technology has now solved this problem.

Fourth-Generation "Rotation Stationary"

Fourth-generation equipment was designed to solve the problem of the ring artefacts presented by third-generation equipment. The number of detectors (more than 2000) that are arranged along the entire gantry (360°) is increased, and they remain stationary while the X-ray tube rotates. They are less commonly used due to the high cost associated with the large number of detectors.

Classification According to the Number of Slices

Single-Slice CT

Single-slice CT has a single row of detectors, which are 1 cm wide, in the x–y plane of the gantry. The slice thickness is controlled by the degree of collimation: a narrower collimation results in a thinner slice whereas a wider collimation results in greater slice thickness. This setting is selected by the user depending on the study requirements. The slice thickness that is set cannot be changed after acquiring the images.

Multi-Slice or Multi-Detector CT

Multi-slice CT machines have multiple rows of detectors (2–320), aligned on the z axis of the gantry, allowing multiple slices to be obtained simultaneously. The number of detectors determines the number of slices that the equipment can acquire simultaneously. The slice thickness is controlled by the detectors used rather than being determined by collimation alone.

With newer machines, the term "channels" is also used; this refers to the connections of the detectors that allow separate signals from multiple rows of detectors to be combined, depending on the requirements of the image.

Currently, most CT equipment used in veterinary medicine is multi-slice (16–64 slices). The availability of more detectors, and their smaller size, allows improved spatial resolution of the acquired images.

Unlike single-slice CT equipment, multi-slice CT allows the thickness to be modified after image acquisition.

Cone Beam CT

In cone beam CT (CBCT), the collimation of the X-ray beam has a cone shape. These devices are widely used in human medicine, especially in dentistry, mammography, angiography, interventional radiology and for radiotherapy. In recent years they have started to be used in veterinary practice.

Image Formation

The radiation emitted by the X-ray tube reaches the detectors, which are responsible for measuring it based on its attenuation and transform it into an electrical signal. The data acquired by the equipment corresponds to a specific location in the X-ray tube.

Each CT image represents a section, or thin slice, of the patient's anatomy, and is composed of an array of small cubic sections known as **voxels** or volume elements. The image is presented on a flat monitor as an array of **pixels** or image elements. Each voxel in the array is associated with an electronic signal that is spatially located in the body and processed by a computer. The variations in intensity of these electronic signals are shown as variations of the brightness of pixels on the monitor. In this way, a voxel associated with higher X-ray attenuation will correspond to a brighter or whiter pixel, whereas tissues or anatomical regions exhibiting lower X-ray attenuation (e.g. air) will appear dark.

Hounsfield Units

CT technology uses the spatial distribution of the linear attenuation coefficient for each pixel. The relative attenuation, or shade of grey of each pixel, is shown in relation to the attenuation of water. Thus, the shade of grey of an individual pixel is relatively independent of the X-ray spectrum used. These CT values are referred to as Hounsfield units (HU) in reference to Godfrey Hounsfield.

On the HU scale, water is assigned the value of 0 as the reference material. Any tissue with a density lower than that of water and, therefore, an attenuation coefficient value lower than water, will have negative values, while tissues with a higher density will have positive values (Table 1).

Except for water and air, these categories are associated with approximate values or ranges. HU can be obtained in a CT study after identifying the anatomical region of interest (Fig. 5).

Table 1. The Hounsfield units of tissues and materials of different composition.

Composition	Hounsfield units (HU)
Bone	700 to 3000 HU
Soft tissue	30 to 50 HU
Cerebrospinal fluid	15 HU
Water	0 HU
Fat	−50 to −100 HU
Lung	−500 to −700 HU
Air	−1000 HU

Image Visualisation

Five different radiopacities can be identified through radiography (see Chapter 1). CT displays up to 4096 shades of grey; although many of them can be displayed on a computer monitor, the human eye is able to detect and differentiate only 30–90 shades of grey.

The user can adjust two parameters, related to the number of grey tones or the HU range shown in the image (window width [WW]) and the central grey tone or midpoint of the range of values shown (window level [WL]) (Fig. 6).

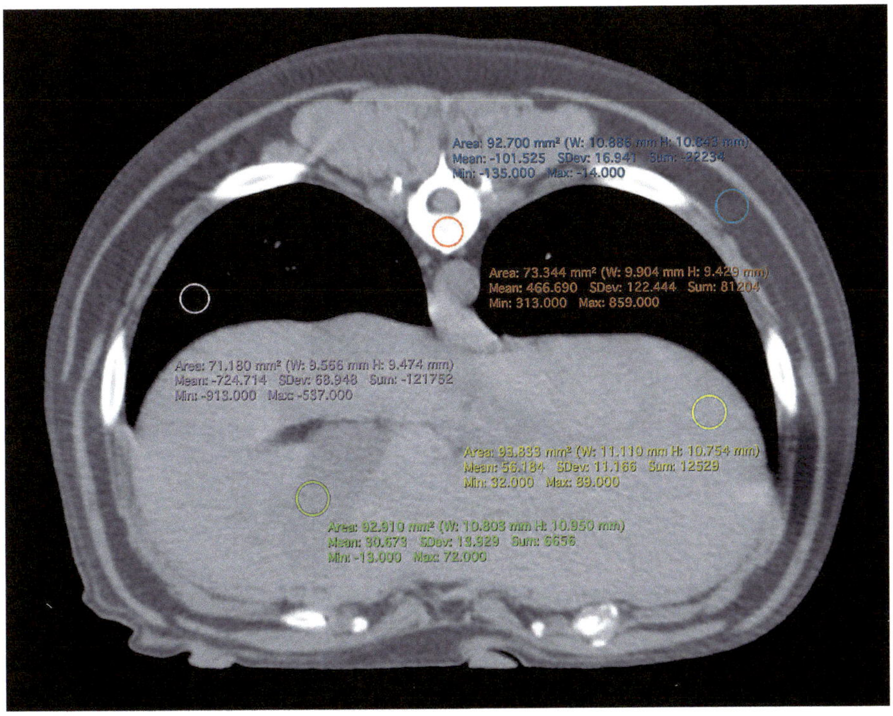

Figure 5. CT image showing the mean HUs of the lung (−725 HU, violet), fat (−102, blue), bile (31, green), liver parenchyma (56, yellow) and a vertebral body (467, orange).

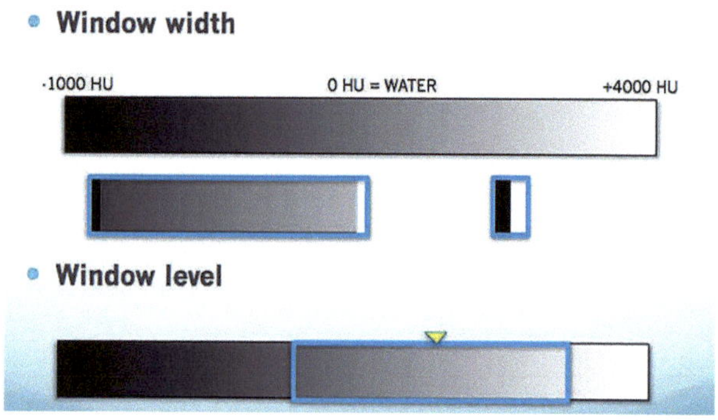

Figure 6. Illustration depicting the concepts of window width and window level (image courtesy of Randi Drees).

The **window level** is usually set to the mid-range for the tissue or organ of interest (e.g. approximately –500 HU if the lungs are to be evaluated).

It is important that the **window width** is correctly adjusted, taking into account that a very wide window width will offer more shades of grey than the human eye can differentiate, whereas a very narrow window width can reduce the shades of grey to exclusively black and white.

Both the window width and the window level are easily modifiable using any CT visualisation software. With a simple movement of the mouse to one side or the other, up or down, both parameters can be modified (Fig. 7).

Depending on the anatomical region, certain window width and level values will be used. In the thoracic cavity, the mediastinum (soft tissue), the bone and the pulmonary parenchyma are assessed. Each of these tissues is best visualised with certain window width and level values (Fig. 8).

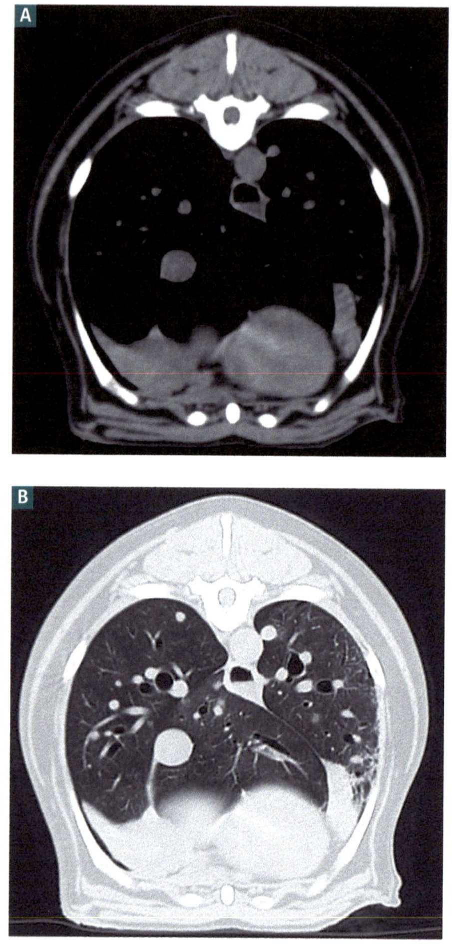

Figure 8. Two visualisations of the same cross section of a canine patient's thorax. **A**. The window width and level values are 350 HU and 40 HU, respectively. **B**. The window width and level values are 1400 HU and –500 HU, respectively. A narrow window width allows soft tissue structures to be assessed, but not the pulmonary parenchyma (A); by expanding the window width the pulmonary parenchyma can be assessed, although soft tissue detail is lost (B).

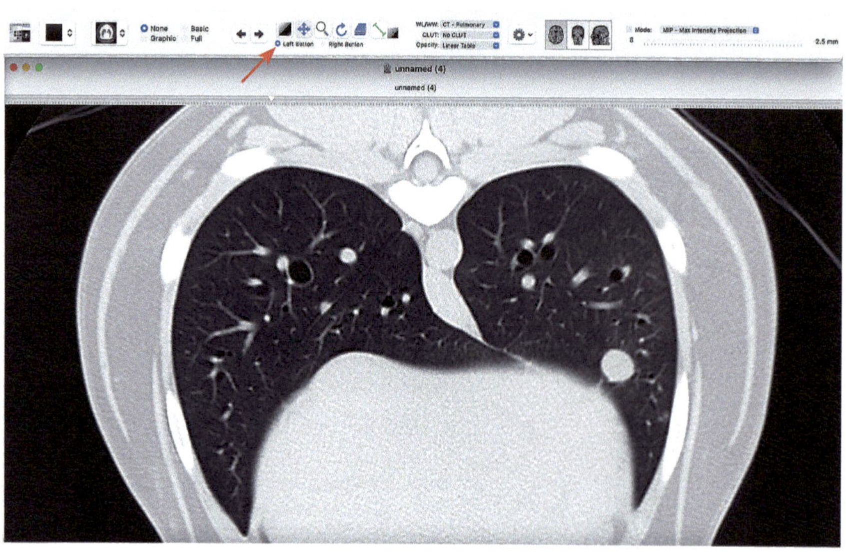

Figure 7. Cross section of a patient's lungs, displayed by software used for visualisation of CT studies. The red arrow indicates the button with which both the window level and window width can be easily modified.

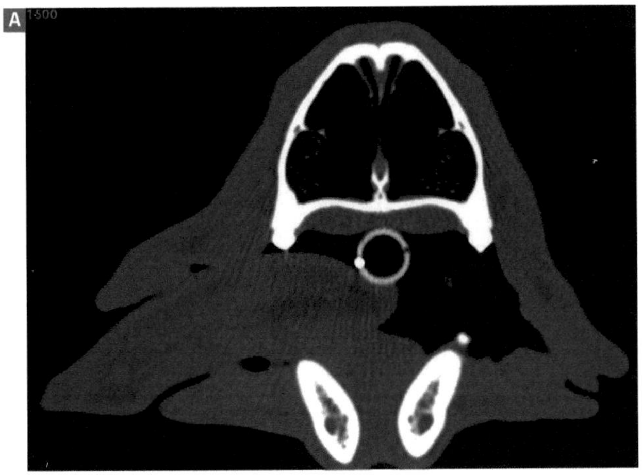

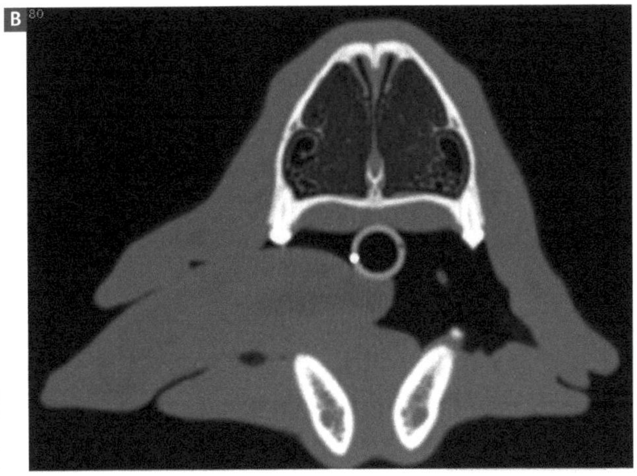

Figure 9. Two visualisations of the same cross section of a dog's nasal cavity. In **A**, the window width and level values are 1500 HU and 300 HU, respectively. The nasal turbinates are not correctly visualised in this image. In **B**, the window width has been extended to 3480 HU. The turbinates can now be observed in detail.

As the thoracic cavity is an anatomical region containing structures of very different densities, the window width should be wide. On the other hand, in the abdominal cavity, where most of the organs have a very similar density (soft tissue), a narrow window width should be used.

In the case of the nasal cavity, if a narrow window width is used the nasal turbinates cannot be correctly visualised; however, by expanding the window width these anatomical structures can be correctly visualised and assessed (Fig. 9).

Normally, the window width and level parameters are preconfigured in both the CT console and the viewers, but they can be adjusted based on individual preferences (Table 2).

For visualisation of the images, a DICOM viewer (e.g. Horos, Osirix, RadiAnt) is usually used. By convention, images are interpreted by placing the right side of the animal to the viewer's left and the left side of the animal to the viewer's right (Fig. 10).

Table 2. Examples of preset window width (WW) and window level (WL) settings for different organs and tissues.

Organ/tissue	WW	WL
Brain	100	50
Bone	1500	300
Abdomen/mediastinum	400	40
Lungs	1500	–500

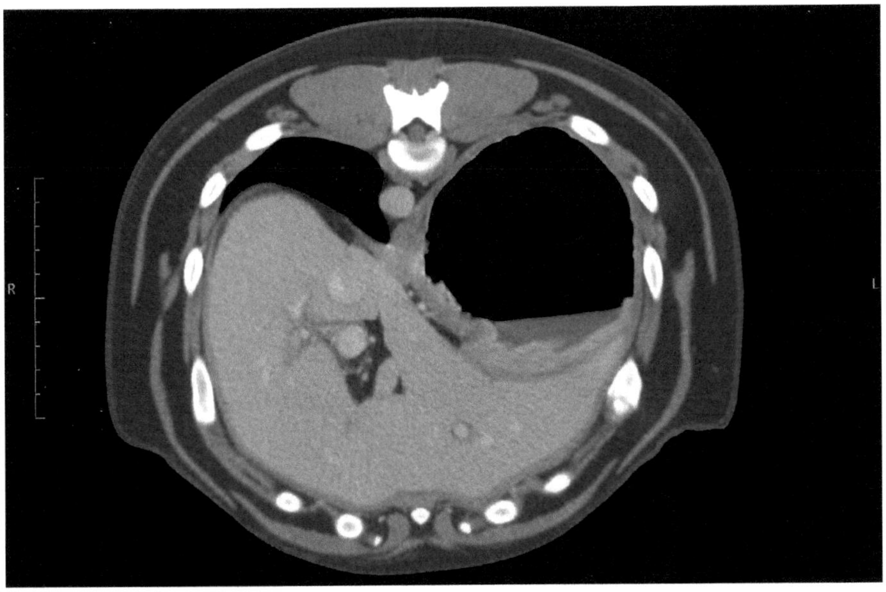

Figure 10. Cross section of a dog's abdomen. The letter L marks the left side of the animal, located to the viewer's right, and the R indicates the right side of the animal, located to the viewer's left.

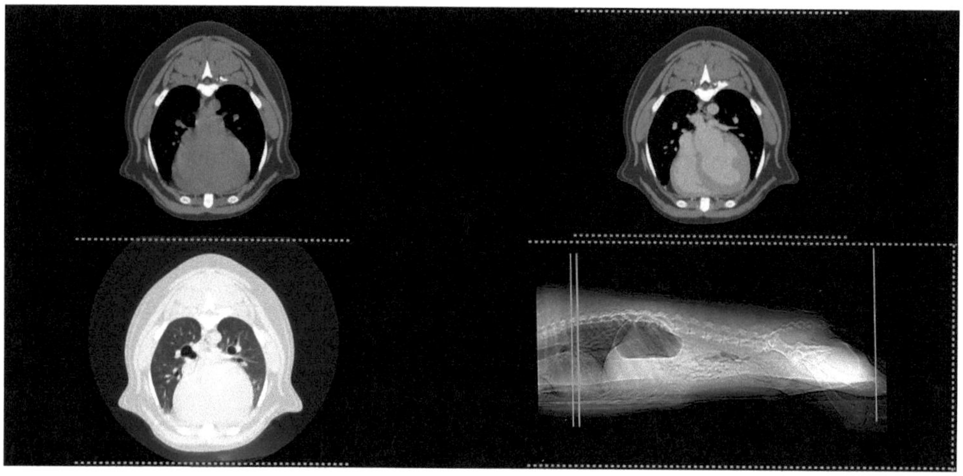

Figure 11. Three visualisations of the same cross section of a dog's thorax (both upper and lower left images). A soft tissue window has been applied without contrast (upper left image) and with contrast (upper right image), and a lung window has been applied (lower left image). The lower right image shows the topogram, in which the orange lines mark the anatomical region selected for the study and the green line indicates the location of the cross section displayed in the other three images.

For interpretation of CT studies, the same cross section is usually displayed at the same time using different windows, in different series (precontrast and postcontrast), often in addition to the topogram to make localisation of the section shown on the screen easier (Fig. 11).

Image Acquisition Parameters

Before starting a CT study, the patient's data should be entered, the anatomical region or regions of interest selected using the preconfigured protocols in the system, and the topogram, scout or locator view acquired. The latter is achieved by moving the patient, positioned on the table, through the gantry where the X-ray tube is active but in a fixed position (0° and 90°); this allows images very similar to ventrodorsal/dorsoventral and lateral radiographs to be obtained, respectively. The topogram (Fig. 12) is useful to verify that the patient is positioned correctly on the CT table.

As with any other imaging technique, performing CT studies that allow high-quality images to be obtained is essential, thus making the most of the equipment's performance. Many parameters can be adjusted on the operator console to achieve this aim. These parameters will have an impact not only on the quality of the study but also on the dose of radiation received by the patient.

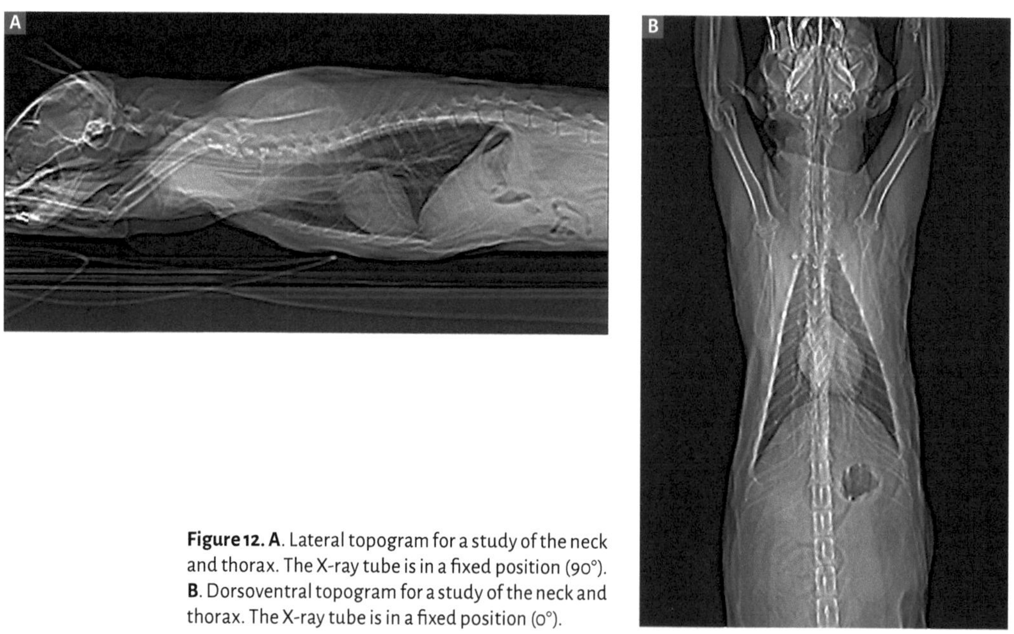

Figure 12. A. Lateral topogram for a study of the neck and thorax. The X-ray tube is in a fixed position (90°). **B.** Dorsoventral topogram for a study of the neck and thorax. The X-ray tube is in a fixed position (0°).

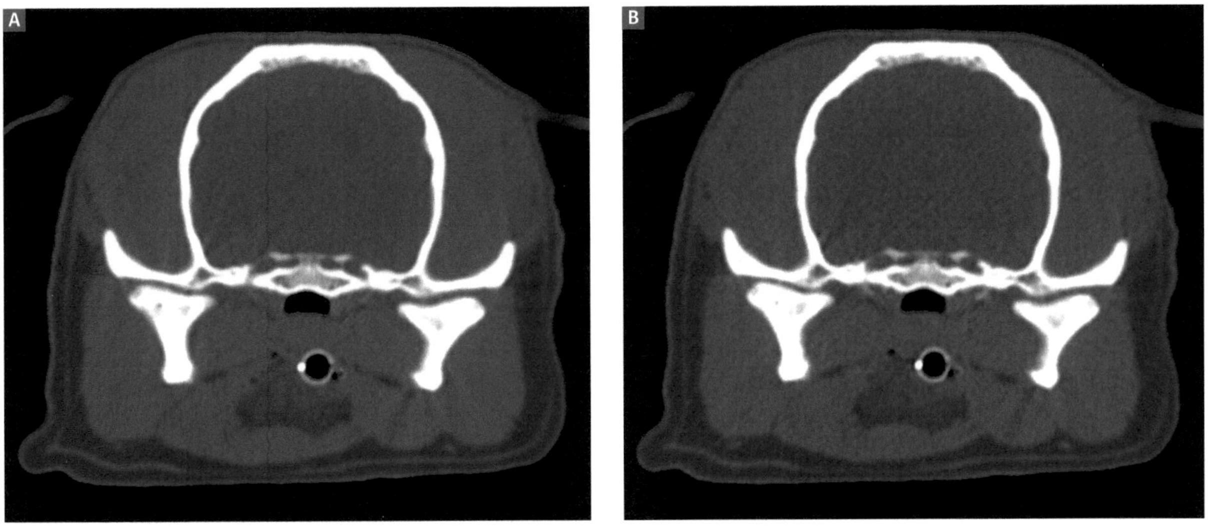

Figure 13. Two visualisations of the same cross section at the level of the temporomandibular joint. Only the mA has been modified: **A**, 200 mA; **B**, 80 mA. The image in B is more grainy due to the smaller number of photons involved in the signal.

Knowledge of the basic tomographic anatomy and the effect caused by the **adjustment of these technical parameters** is essential, both to optimise CT studies and to improve safety when interpreting them.

Kilovoltage (kV)

High kV values are usually used in CT and are limited to a range of 80–140 kV. A value of 120 kV is the most widely used, as it is useful for most CT studies in small animals. Values above 120 kV are indicated in large patients to ensure adequate penetration of the X-rays. To obtain the best possible image quality, milliamperage (mA) values should be selected based on the kV value used. When a high kV is required (140 kV), low mA values should normally be used so, in these cases, maximising the mA at the expense of the kV is recommended.

A low kV affects the image quality in a similar way to a low mA (producing a grainy image with noise) and also generates artefacts due to the inadequate penetration of X-rays.

Tube Current (mA) and mAs

The mA determines the number of electrons colliding with the anode and thus the number of X-ray photons that are generated. The mAs is determined by the tube current per unit time (seconds).

Tube current values are limited to the range of 50–400 mA. The number of photons reaching the detector is directly related to the noise in the image: with a low mA the noise and the grainy appearance of the image increase, resulting in a lower-quality study. A high mA improves the quality of the image (Fig. 13) but also increases the dose of radiation received by the patient; in addition, it will cause heating of the X-ray tube (as will a high kV value).

Depending on the CT equipment and the heating capacity of the X-ray tube, the use of high values for both kV and mA is limited by narrowing the mA range to 100–250 mA in small animals. Many of the current multi-slice CT systems incorporate a dose-modulation system that regulates and adapts the mA based on the density information obtained from the topogram.

X-Ray Tube Rotation Time

Normally, the rotation time of the X-ray tube is adjusted so that it is as short as possible. This parameter is especially important in CT studies of the chest and abdomen due to respiratory movement. In these cases, the rotation time of the X-ray tube is usually in the range of 0.5–1 second. Depending on the CT equipment, this parameter can be adjusted independently or automatically together with the mA.

Slice Thickness

Slice thickness is one of the most important parameters for acquiring good-quality images. The thinner the slice on the z axis, the smaller the voxel depth and the smaller the anatomical region collected in a CT image. Thin slices provide a very detailed picture when combined with the correct mA settings.

In a thick slice, more anatomical information is collected per slice to the detriment of its detail; thus, blurred images are obtained, but without noise. In contrast, thinner sections provide more information and anatomical detail, but with more noise in the image due to the lower number of photons received by the detector. In studies that require thin slices (e.g. of the lung, skull, joints) increasing the mAs to compensate for and reduce this increase in noise is recommended. The image quality of multiplanar reconstructions, as well as 3D reconstructions, is higher in studies where thin slices have been obtained (Figs. 14 and 15).

The drawbacks of acquiring thin slices are the greater difficulty in obtaining images free of motion artefacts, the longer duration of the study and, consequently, the greater radiation dose received by the patient. In the same way as is the case with high kV and mAs values, carrying out studies with very thin slices will cause greater heating of the X-ray tube, so using very thin slices is not always advisable.

Thicknesses of between 1.25 mm and 3 mm are recommended for thoracic and abdominal CT studies, with thinner slice thicknesses reserved for musculoskeletal imaging, for example, of the elbow joint (0.5–1 mm) or the spine.

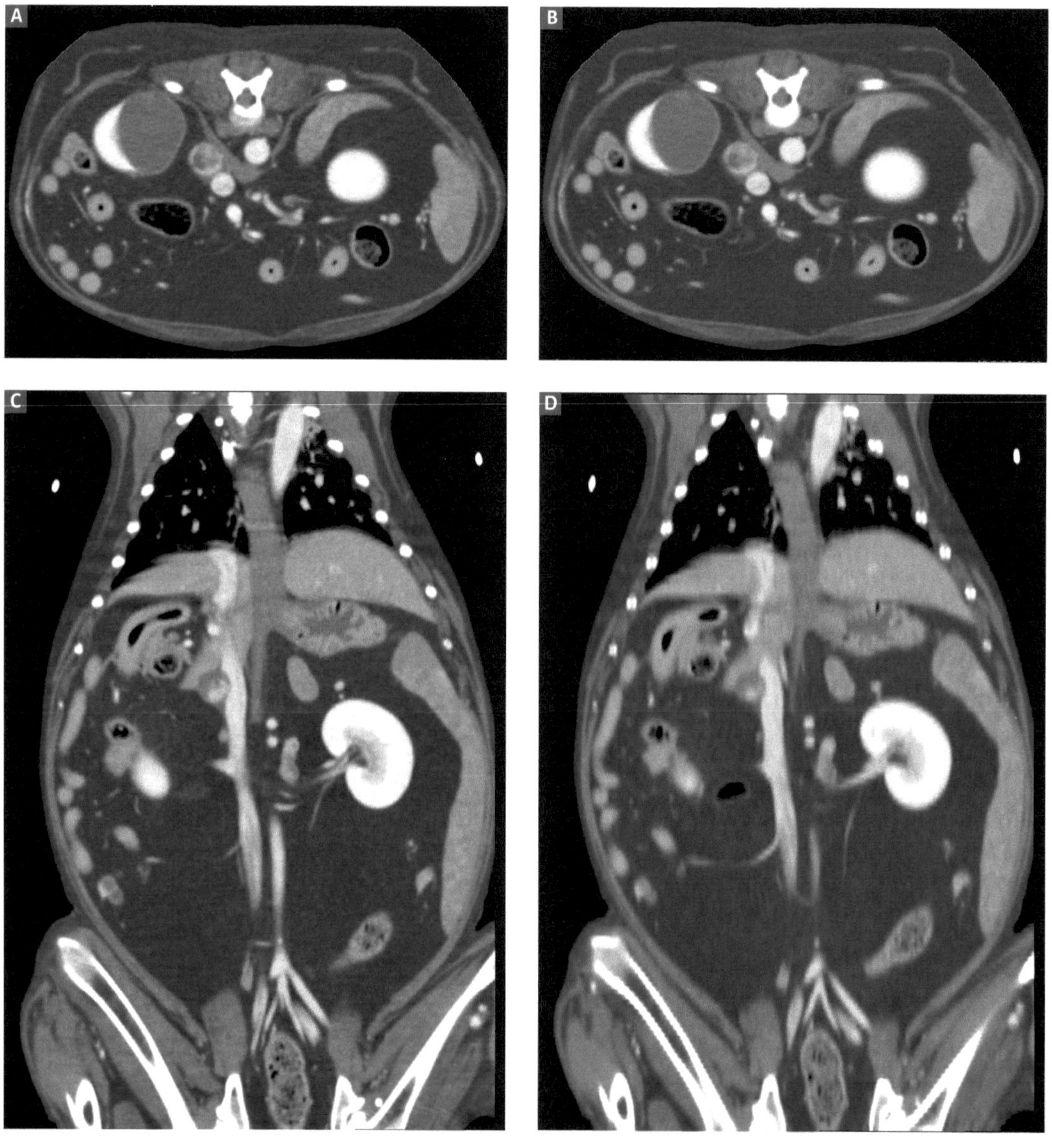

Figure 14. A and **B** show cross sections obtained at slice thicknesses of 1.25 mm (A) and 2.5 mm (B). **C** and **D** correspond to dorsal reconstructions from the cross sections in A and B, respectively. While there is little apparent difference between A and B, greater anatomical detail is evident in C, a reconstruction from the section with the smaller slice thickness (A), compared with D.

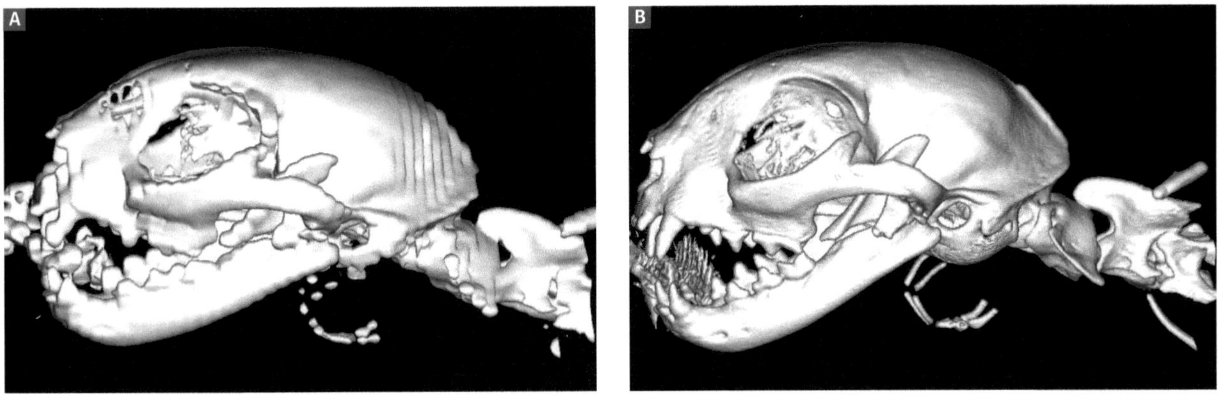

Figure 15. 3D reconstruction of the skull of a cat. **A**. Reconstruction from 1.25 mm slices. **B**. Reconstruction from 0.625 mm slices. Greater resolution and anatomical detail can be observed in B.

Slice Interval

The slice interval represents the interval of space between CT images when scanning in axial mode or reconstruction of the images obtained in helical mode (reconstruction interval). It is often set to the same value as the slice thickness. If the slice interval is less than the slice thickness, overlapping slices will be produced.

Scan Field of View (SFOV)

The SFOV is the central region of the gantry that is available for image acquisition. Normally, it cannot be adjusted by the operator and it is set at the maximum possible value. If any anatomical region of the patient is outside the SFOV, the X-ray beam is attenuated, but the computer is unable to precisely locate this attenuation by generating a white ring at the periphery of the image. This parameter cannot be modified once the CT study has been performed, so it is essential to correctly position the patient within the SFOV, specifically at the isocentre of the gantry, with the help of the lasers (collimators).

Display Field of View (DFOV)

The DFOV is the area of the SFOV from which the image is reconstructed. This adjustment must not exceed the SFOV and must be as small as possible because it has a decisive impact on the quality of the image. A default 512 pixel array is typically used to display the CT image. The size of the DFOV selected determines the size of the pixel. The larger the pixel, the more information it will contain, thus decreasing the definition of the image. Adjusting the DFOV as closely as possible to the anatomical region of interest is recommended and to ensure that no anatomical structures are left outside it. Unlike the SFOV, with most CT equipment the DFOV can be reconstructed retrospectively.

Apart from adjusting the different parameters for acquiring the images, the **acquisition mode** can also be configured.

Axial or Sequential

In an axial or sequential study, the table does not move while the X-ray tube and the imaging detectors rotate around it. For acquisition of the next image, the table moves while the X-ray tube remains inoperative; the table then stops and a new rotation occurs. This mode should be used only in machines with fewer than 8–16 slices, especially in those with a single slice, where a higher image quality is appreciated. When using equipment with 16 or more slices, there is no benefit from obtaining the images in sequential mode.

Helical or Spiral

In helical or spiral studies, the table moves at the same time as the rotation of the X-ray tube and the detectors occurs, producing a spiral (helical) path. This type of study acquires the volumetric information but does not completely obtain the data, which is completed later through mathematical processes. Using this mode of image acquisition decreases the duration of the study. Currently, it is the most commonly used type of study because artefacts associated with patient movement are decreased, resulting in high-quality images.

In this type of study, the **pitch** can be adjusted, which refers to the relationship between the distance travelled by the table during a complete rotation of the X-ray tube and the slice thickness (Fig. 16). This adjustment affects the quality of the image obtained. Pitch values of 1–1.4 are normally recommended with single-slice machines, and values less than 1 are recommended for multi-slice machines. If the value of the pitch is greater than 1, the images obtained will probably be blurred. This adjustment will also affect the study duration and the radiation dose received by the patient. Low pitch values will increase the study duration and consequently the radiation dose.

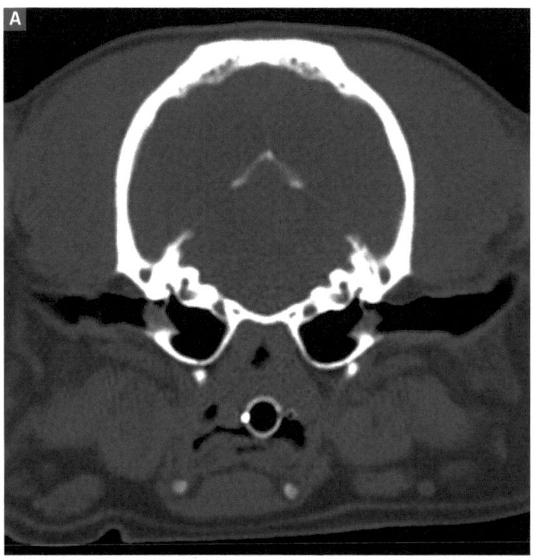

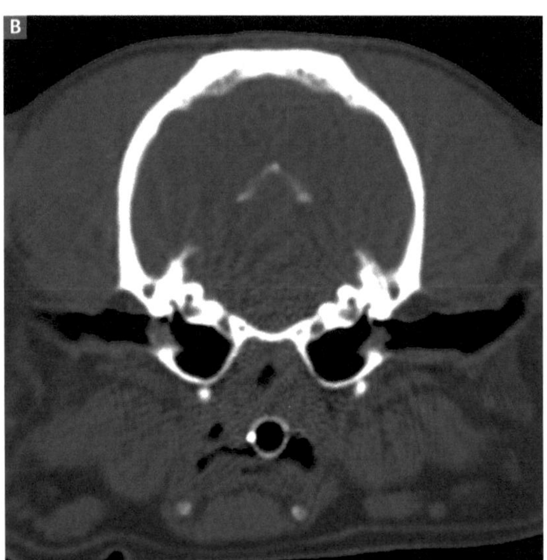

Figure 16. Two visualisations of the same cross section at the level of the middle ear. In both images, the same kV (120) and mA (200) values have been used, and only the pitch has been changed: in **A**, the pitch is 0.5 and in **B** the pitch is 1.56. Higher image quality can be seen in A.

Image Reconstruction

Image reconstruction algorithms are used to calculate the matrix of the image that will be displayed on the screen from the raw data (raw information or primary data) from the detectors. This is achieved by a mathematical process known as **transformation** or the **Fourier transform**.

These **spatial reconstruction algorithms** are described, based on their spatial frequency, as high, medium, and low spatial frequency algorithms.

- **Medium or low spatial frequency algorithms** improve contrast resolution by reducing noise. They allow good differentiation between slightly different shades of grey. They should be used for anatomical regions that have little inherent contrast, such as the abdomen, brain or mediastinum, where a narrow window width is used to compare and differentiate similar shades of grey. They will also be very useful for all postcontrast studies.
- **High spatial frequency algorithms** improve the sharpness of the image but increase the noise. They are used for anatomical regions that have a lot of inherent contrast such as the lungs, bones, or nasal and auditory cavities, in which a wide window width is used in order to increase the range of shades of grey.

These algorithms are applied by the operator via the console at the time of study setup. To acquire an image using a different algorithm, no additional scans are required. Reconstructions can also be generated retrospectively, using different algorithms, as long as the raw data are available in the equipment.

For thoracic CT studies, both high-frequency (bone, lungs) and medium-frequency (soft tissue/mediastinum/lymph nodes in the pre- and postcontrast series) algorithms are recommended. The lungs can be checked using a medium-frequency algorithm, although the pulmonary parenchyma will be slightly more blurred than if a high-frequency algorithm were used, and this may make it difficult to define lesions (Fig. 17).

Sagittal and dorsal multiplanar reconstructions can also be performed in 3D, as well as "virtual endoscopy".

Maximum Intensity Projections (MIPs)

In MIPs, the thin slices are grouped or overlapped into thicker slices. They are especially useful for locating and differentiating pulmonary nodules from the rest of the pulmonary vasculature (Fig. 18).

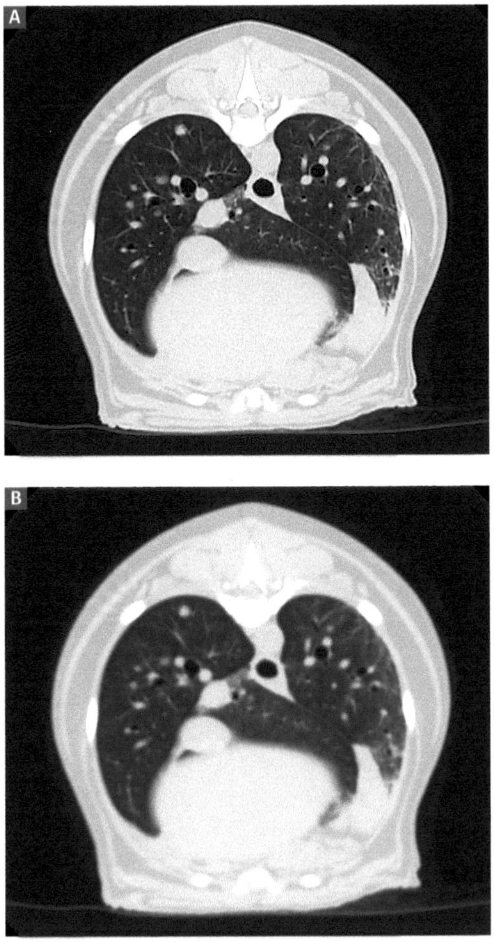

Figure 17. Two visualisations of the same cross section of a dog's thorax. In **A**, a high-frequency algorithm has been used; in **B**, a medium-frequency algorithm has been used. Loss of definition is evident in B, resulting from the lung window having been applied in an algorithm configured for assessment of the mediastinum.

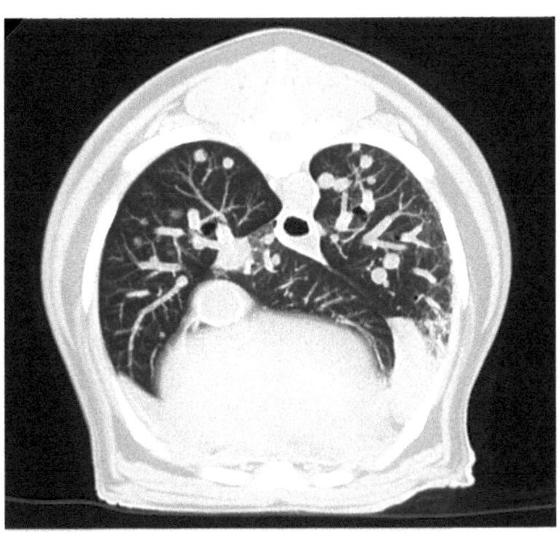

Figure 18. Cross section of a thoracic CT study obtained using 1.25 mm slices. This image shows a slice thickness of 10 mm (MIP), and presents a 3D appearance compared with Fig. 17 (images of the same patient without using MIPs).

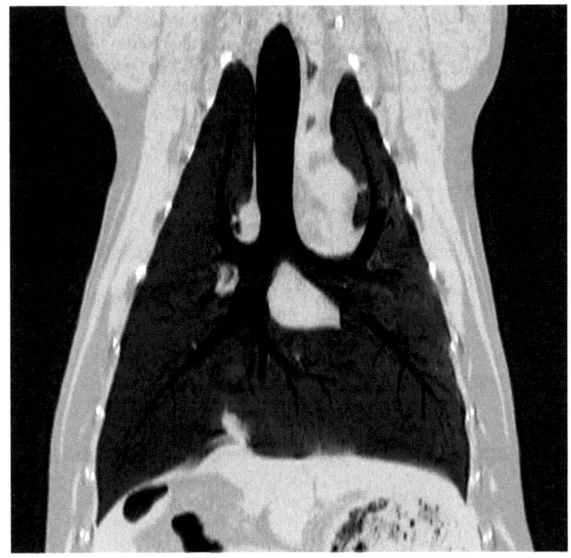

Figure 19. Dorsal reconstruction of a thoracic CT study obtained using 1.25 mm slices. This image shows a slice thickness of 11.7 mm (MiniP), presenting a 3D appearance of the bronchial tree and allowing subtle alterations in lung attenuation to be ruled out.

On some occasions, when a pulmonary nodule is visible in only a single slice due to its small dimensions, it can go unnoticed unless MIPs are used; these projections allow slices to be combined, meaning that the nodule will be present in more images and allowing it to be visualised more readily.

Minimum Intensity Projections (MinIPs)

These projections, like MIPs, also combine slices, but eliminate all radiodense structures. They are very useful for assessing the airways and to detect alterations in the attenuation of the pulmonary parenchyma (Fig. 19). Slight increases in lung attenuation may go unnoticed during the interpretation of the study; these subtle alterations become more evident when using MinIPs.

Contrast Media and Angiography

Intravenous administration of contrast media is part of the routine for CT studies. The iodinated contrast is injected through a catheter placed in a peripheral vein, preferably in the forelimb.

Contrast media are used to improve the ability to observe anatomical details, increase contrast in the parenchyma of different organs (soft tissue) and visualise the blood vessels (angiography).

Contrast Media

Iodinated contrast media can be classified as ionic or nonionic; the latter are recommended due to the lower incidence of side effects when using them. Soft tissue lesions (inflammation, neoplasia) are better identified on contrast studies due to increased contrast accumulation. The recommended dose of contrast is 600–800 mg I/kg and it can be administered manually or with a mechanical injector.

Angiography

Ionic or nonionic iodinated contrast media can be used for angiography. The use of a mechanical injector is essential for faster, better-controlled administration, delivered at the desired time and to obtain an even distribution of the contrast medium. Delivery of contrast via an injector is not painful, but if sedation or anaesthesia is not deep enough, the patient may feel the pressure of the contrast being delivered and move. If an injector is not available, diagnostic-quality angiography studies can be obtained with manual contrast administration so long as the timing of the injection is very well coordinated, the administration is fast and the study is started quickly by leaving the CT room immediately after the injection. In angiography studies in which contrast administration is manual, the exact moments at which contrast is visualised in the different vascular structures cannot be determined (Fig. 20). Therefore, the use of a mechanical injector is essential in some cases.

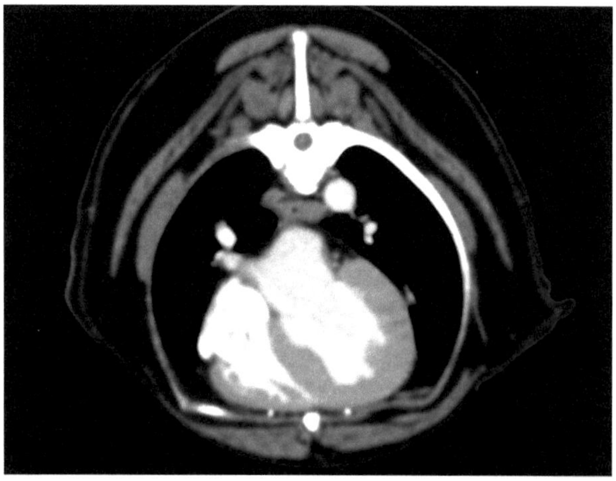

Figure 20. CT study (angiography) at the level of the heart. Higher contrast intensity can be seen on the right side of the heart than in the left atrium and ventricle. Contrast is also visualised in the aorta.

Depending on the anatomical region and the clinical suspicion, the visualisation of some structures is prioritised over others. Many factors contribute to the quality of angiography studies: the technology and speed of the CT apparatus itself, the method of contrast administration and the contrast medium used, and factors related to the patient such as its size and cardiovascular status. These studies require practice, but once integrated into the study protocols they are very useful for detecting vascular pathologies such as portosystemic shunts or anatomical variations.

It is important to avoid movement artefacts caused by the patient's breathing, so carrying out these studies under general anaesthesia and with the induction of apnoea is recommended. It is important to plan these studies well, with a previous precontrast evaluation, and then perform a dynamic CT or bolus test that shows the exact times at which a certain vascular structure is visualised with the greatest possible contrast. Next, the CT study is performed in dual phase, obtaining the arterial phase (from caudal to cranial, from the cranial pole of the left kidney to the most cranial area of the diaphragm) and the portal venous phase (from cranial to caudal, from the most cranial area of the diaphragm to the pelvic cavity). If a three-phase (or triple-phase) angiography study is to be conducted, a flush phase 1 minute after the venous phase should be included.

While the patient is on the CT table, it is important to ensure that the contrast has reached the vascular region of interest and there are no movement artefacts that may hinder or prevent the correct interpretation of the study. In the event that the images are not of sufficient quality due to breathing artefacts or because the contrast is not yet located in the region of interest, the study can be quickly repeated. If the images are obtained too late and there is not enough vascular enhancement, the study and contrast injection can be repeated after waiting the necessary time for the contrast medium to be excreted.

Artefacts

Artefacts are frequent in CT. Unlike the artefacts present in ultrasound imaging, some of which are useful and allow the identification of lesion characteristics (see Chapter 2), in CT they have no use and can significantly degrade the image. An artefact is defined as the appearance of a structure in an image that is not representative of a structure inside the patient's body. In veterinary medicine, most artefacts are very evident due to the anatomical variation between patients and the limited performance of some unsophisticated CT machines. In CT, any discrepancy between the reconstructed values in the image and the true attenuation coefficient of the structure represents an artefact that must be recognised as such, and it is important to know the different ways to avoid or remedy it.

Most artefacts are due to interactions between the patient and the machine; therefore, they are subject to the laws of physics.

Artefacts can be classified according to their appearance (stripes, rings, shadows) and according to their cause (caused by the patient, those based on physics and those generated by the CT equipment).

Patient-Based Artefacts

Patient Movement

Movement of the patient during image acquisition will result in a blurred or distorted image. These artefacts are primarily caused by **respiratory, gastrointestinal, and cardiac movement** (Fig. 21). **Respiratory movement** artefact can be avoided by hyperventilating the patient before the study and, if a CT study of the thorax or abdomen is being performed, scanning from caudal to cranial or from cranial to caudal, respectively, quickly moving away from the diaphragm, which is one of the main causes of this artefact. The image acquisition speed can also be adjusted to decrease respiratory artefact by increasing the pitch or slice thickness, at the cost of decreased resolution and increased partial volume artefact (see below).

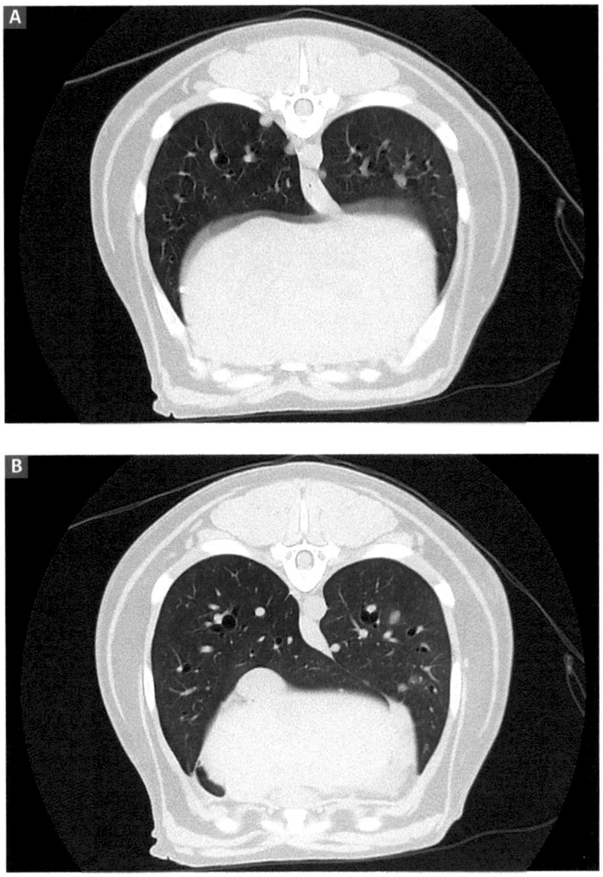

Figure 21. Thoracic CT study with two images of the lung parenchyma of the same patient. In **A**, the section is more caudal, and shows the artefact caused by breathing at the level of both the diaphragm and the bronchi and bronchioles. In **B**, which is much sharper, the section is more cranial; the bronchial branches are better defined and delimited.

Gastrointestinal movements are difficult to control; the speed of image acquisition can be increased or the study of the anatomical region of interest can be repeated if necessary.

To avoid artefacts caused by the **heartbeat**, specific imaging techniques are required.

Metallic Implants

Structures with a density higher than those included in the normal range of the CT equipment cause incomplete attenuations, appearing as black and white stripes or bands. This is the case for contrast media and metal objects such as the animal's identification microchip, surgical implants or gun pellets (Fig. 22). The detector receives a reduced signal or does not receive it, and will not process it properly. To build the image, the CT computer needs information from all angles; since this does not occur in these cases, white or black stripes are generated.

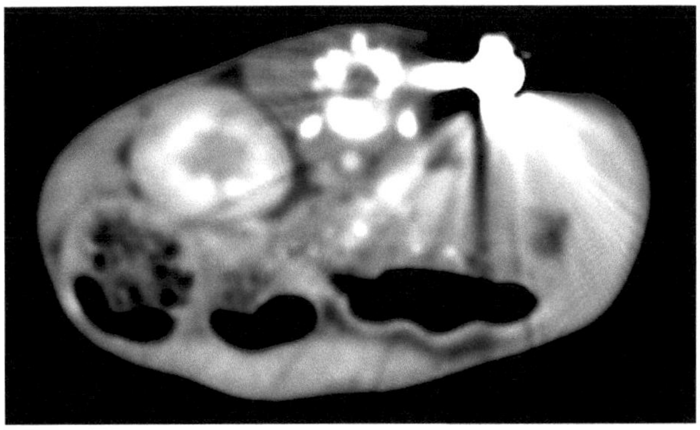

Figure 22. CT image of the abdomen of a cat showing black and white stripes caused by a metal pellet.

To resolve this artefact, the high-density object should not be included in the SFOV if possible, by modifying the patient's position or varying the angle of the gantry to try to scan around the object. Newer CT equipment may have correction algorithms that allow this artefact to be minimised in cases in which it cannot be avoided.

Physics-Based Artefacts

Photon Starvation

This artefact can occur between high-density objects such as temporal bones or hip joints. In these anatomical regions, the artefact, in the form of horizontal stripes, usually appears because the mAs is not high enough to go through them, and so a smaller number of photons is generated. The mAs can be increased or the patient's position modified to avoid this artefact. There are also algorithms for the correction of this artefact, but they are normally designed for human anatomy, meaning that it is difficult to completely avoid in veterinary medicine.

Beam Hardening

This describes the process by which lower-energy X-ray photons are attenuated by high-density objects through which only higher-energy X-rays can penetrate. This can occur in high-density anatomical regions such as the hip; it causes streaks on the image and makes structures behind the high-density object appear radiolucent. It can be corrected using either higher mA and kV values or correction algorithms.

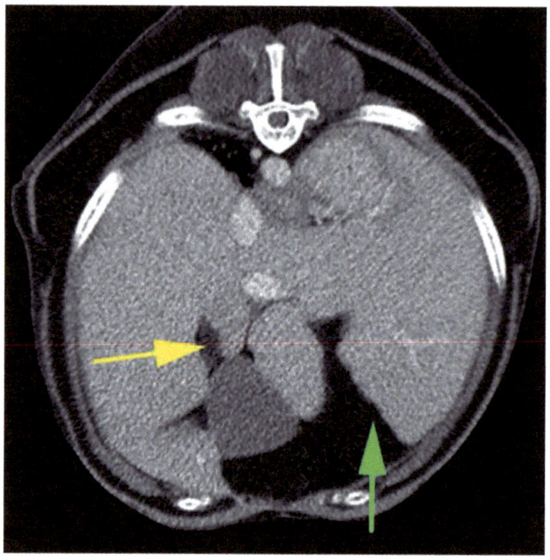

Figure 23. Cross section of the abdomen at the level of the liver, obtained using a single-slice CT scanner (3 mm slice thickness). The yellow arrow points to the peritoneum located between the right lobes of the liver, which appears as a lighter shade of grey compared with the peritoneum adjacent to the left liver lobes (green arrow). This is due to the partial volume artefact present along the curved margins and should not be confused with a focal peritoneal effusion (image courtesy of Randi Drees).

Partial Volume Artefact

This artefact can be thought of as an overlap within the slice. The greater the thickness of the acquired slice, the more anatomy it will contain. The greater the anatomy included in a slice, the less differentiation there will be. This artefact is frequently observed in the margins of organs with curved contours and is difficult to avoid. It appears as blurred margins, and small lesions or anatomical details may be invisible (Fig. 23). This artefact can be resolved by using a smaller slice thickness.

Aliasing

In diagnostic imaging this term refers to imaging artefacts caused by insufficient data collection. Radial stripes are generated from an object with defined or sharp margins due to undersampling. The simplest way to suppress this artefact is by increasing the beam width to filter or remove the high-frequency components.

Stair Step Artefact

This occurs when the interval between slices is too large, giving rise to images where the margins of the structures have staggered morphology. This artefact is resolved by decreasing the interval between slices (in sequential mode) or the reconstruction interval (in helical mode).

Uberschwinger Artefact

Edge enhancement is inherent in high-frequency reconstruction algorithms. It can cause the appearance of a dark halo around high-density structures such as the ribs or internal margins of the vertebral canal. It should not be confused with a pneumothorax or epidural fat as it is an artefact (Fig. 24). It can be recognised as such by its symmetry and location. It can be minimised by using low- or medium-frequency algorithms.

Artefacts Caused by Equipment

Ring Artefact

This artefact occurs in third-generation equipment when one of the elements along the row of detectors is damaged or defective and does not pick up the signal on a regular basis. As the detector moves around the patient, this defect will cause a circular pattern or ring in the image (Fig. 25).

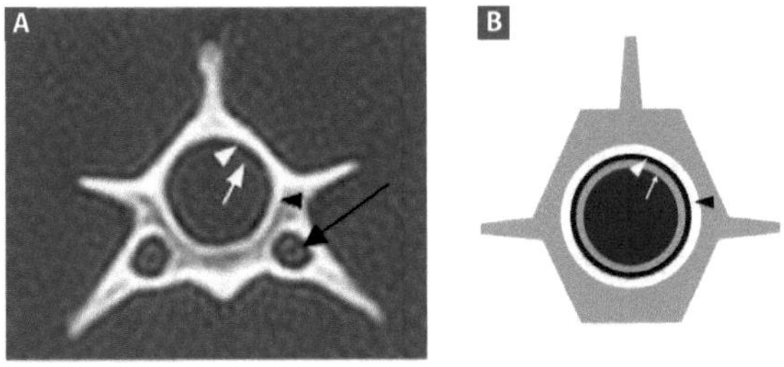

Figure 24. Cross section of a vertebra. **A.** CT image (1 mm slice thickness). **B.** Corresponding illustration. The Uberschwinger artefact can be seen, consisting of a hyperattenuating ring at the periphery of the vertebral canal lumen (white arrow), adjacent to a hypoattenuating ring (white arrowhead) that is bordering the hyperattenuating margin (black arrowhead) of the vertebral canal bone. A similar phenomenon can be seen in the transverse canal (black arrow) (image courtesy of Randi Drees, from Drees et al., 2009).

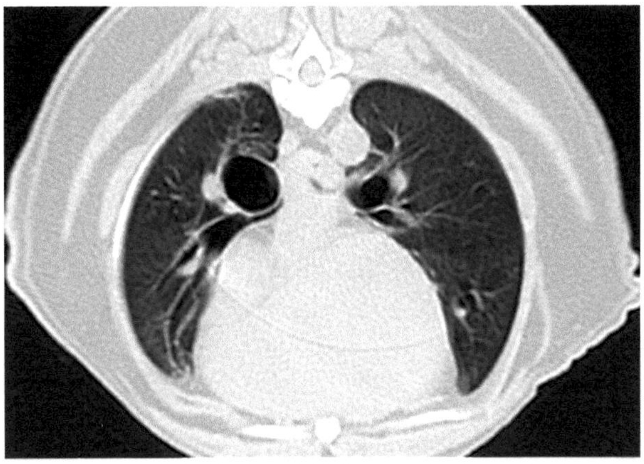

Figure 25. Thoracic CT image, with a lung window, at the level of the right middle bronchus. A line can be seen running through the central part of the heart following a curvilinear path (ring artefact).

The more centrally the damaged detector is located, the smaller the ring will be. This artefact can be resolved by calibrating the equipment (without the patient present) but, if it remains, the machine may require repair by a technician.

Image Quality

Whether an image is of diagnostic quality or not will depend on the spatial and contrast resolution, as well as the noise present in the image.

Contrast Resolution

Contrast resolution is the ability to differentiate structures that appear as different shades of grey due to their different densities. The contrast of the image itself will depend on both the contrast of the screen used to view the image and the subjective contrast. The latter is defined as the difference between the attenuation of a lesion and that of the surrounding tissues. The screen contrast is adjusted by the window width and window level.

Spatial Resolution

Spatial resolution is the ability to distinguish small structures that are close to each other. It depends on the slice thickness, the array size and the reconstruction algorithm. The use of thin slices, bone algorithms and reconstructions with a small DFOV improve the spatial resolution.

Bibliography

- Barrett, J.F., Keat, N. (2004) Artifacts in CT: recognition and avoidance. *RadioGraphics*, 24, pp. 1679–1691.
- Bertolini, G. (ed.) (2017) *Body MDCT in Small Animals: Basic Principles, Technology, and Clinical Applications.* 1st ed. Springer.
- Bushberg, J.T., Seibert, J.A., Leidholdt, E.M., Boone, J.M. (2012) *The Essential Physics of Medical Imaging.* 3rd ed. Lippincott Williams and Wilkins.
- Drees, R., Dennison, S.E., Keuler, N.S., Schwarz, T. (2009) Computed tomographic imaging protocol for the cervical canine and lumbar spine. *Vet Radiol Ultrasound*, 50, pp. 74–79.
- Gavin, P.R., Bagley, R.S. (eds.) (2009) *Practical Small Animal MRI.* 1st ed. Wiley-Blackwell.
- Porat-Mosenco, Y., Schwarz, T., Kass, P.H. (2004) Thick-section reformatting of thinly collimated computed tomography for reduction of skull-base-related artifacts in dogs and horses. *Vet Radiol Ultrasound*, 45, pp. 131–135.
- Schwarz, T., Saunders, J. (eds.) (2011) *Veterinary Computed Tomography.* 1st ed. Wiley-Blackwell.
- Thrall, D.E. (ed.) (2018) *Textbook of Veterinary Diagnostic Radiology.* 7th ed. Elsevier.
- Wisner, E.R., Zwingenberger, A.L. (eds.) (2015) *Atlas of Small Animal CT and MRI.* 1st ed. Wiley-Blackwell.

Basic Principles of Magnetic Resonance Imaging

Pablo Amengual Batle

Physical Principles of Magnetic Resonance Imaging

Magnetic resonance imaging (MRI) is a very complex advanced imaging technique. Put simply, in practice, the steps that are followed are:

1. the patient is placed in the MRI machine, where they are exposed to a very strong magnetic field
2. a radio wave is emitted by the machine
3. when the radio wave finishes, the patient's body sends a signal back that is captured by the machine
4. the computer that is part of the MRI machine reconstructs the information obtained to produce an image.

In order for readers to better understand these steps, this chapter will cover basic concepts of physics first.

Every atom in the body is made up of at least one positively charged proton and one negatively charged electron. A property of protons is that they constantly rotate around their axis, which is known as **spin**. Spin is a vital concept in MRI that must be remembered. Following the principles of physics, every charge that moves (or spins) creates an electric current, which in turn produces a minuscule magnetic field in the case of protons.

When the patient is exposed to MRI, the protons in its body act like tiny magnetic bars and align with the powerful magnetic field produced by the machine. This alignment can occur in two different ways: one where they are in parallel (that is, "facing" the direction of the field) and one where they are antiparallel (with their "back" to the direction of the field). Since parallel protons contain less energy, and are therefore more stable, there will always be a slightly greater number of protons in parallel than in antiparallel.

In addition to rotating on their axis (spinning), protons perform another type of motion called **precession**, which changes the angle of their axis. This movement is described as being similar to that of a spinning top when it loses kinetic energy and goes from rotating completely straight to moving in a circle around its initial axis. The precession frequency can be calculated using the Larmor equation; however, for practical purposes it is not necessary to be familiar with this concept in depth. It is more important to simply remember that the stronger the magnetic field used, the higher the frequency of precession. The result of these processes gives rise to so-called **magnetisation vectors**.

Magnetisation Vectors

Another important physical concept to understand that underlies magnetisation vectors is that two magnetic forces that are in opposite directions cancel each other out. Since there will always be more protons in parallel form than in antiparallel form, as outlined above, this leaves a net magnetic force "facing" the direction of the magnetic field, which is known as **longitudinal magnetisation**. Although the magnetic field of each proton is deflected slightly because its axis is not completely straight (due to precession), these deflections will also cancel each other out. This is because one that is slightly tilted to the right will cancel out another that is tilted to the left, enhancing its longitudinal magnetisation (Fig. 1).

Unfortunately, it is not possible to measure the strength of this magnetic field because it is parallel to and in the same direction as the external magnetic field produced by the MRI machine, and for obvious reasons it is much weaker. Therefore, the direction needs to be varied so that it can be detected, that is, to convert the external field into a transverse field. This is known as **transverse magnetisation**. To do this, a short radio wave known as a **radiofrequency pulse** (RP) is sent to the patient. As a result, the direction of the protons varies. However, for this to happen, the RP must be of the same frequency as the protons. To achieve this, the Larmor equation is used, which allows calculation of the precession frequency of the protons. When both frequencies are aligned, the protons are able to capture energy from the RP in a process called **resonance** (hence the name of this imaging technique). The effect is very interesting. When capturing energy, some protons that were facing the magnetic field will begin to turn away form it, which will create increased cancellation of the longitudinal magnetisation. In addition, although the axis of each proton has a different angulation due to precessional motion, they will also align, which is known as "being in phase". When they are in phase, the cancellation due to precession mentioned previously disappears, enhancing transverse magnetisation. This new magnetisation can be detected by an antenna located in the MRI machine, and is known as **echo** (Figs. 2 and 3).

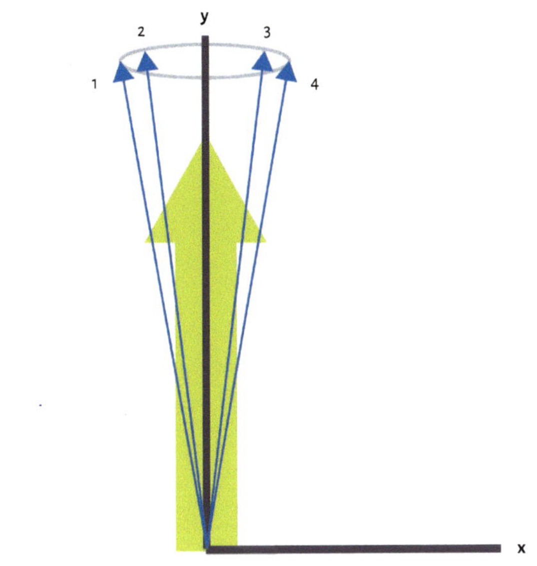

Figure 1. This image illustrates the principle of longitudinal magnetisation. After the parallel and antiparallel protons have cancelled each other out, there are four parallel protons left facing in the direction of the magnetic field (y axis). In addition, the magnetisation of the x axis produced by the precession motion of the protons is cancelled out between the protons (1 by 3 and 2 by 4). The result is a longitudinal magnetisation completely parallel to the external magnetic field (green arrow on the y axis) that is not detectable by MRI.

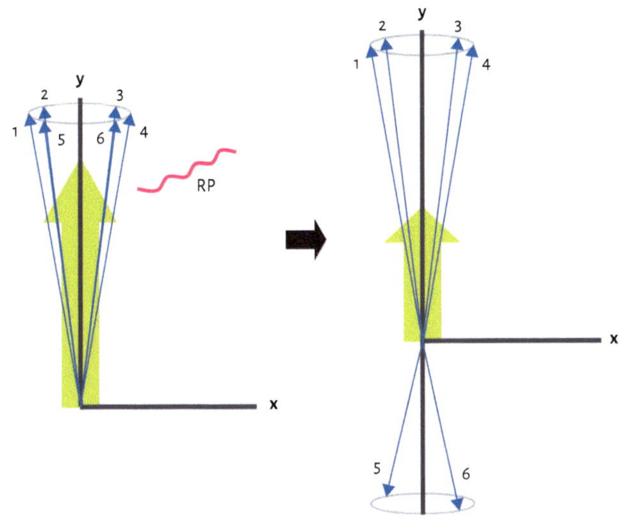

Figure 2. Principle of transverse magnetisation. In this case, by sending a RP, some protons that were parallel (5 and 6) capture energy and become antiparallel. This reduces the longitudinal magnetisation (green arrow on the axis), but this event on its own is not enough to create sufficient transverse magnetisation.

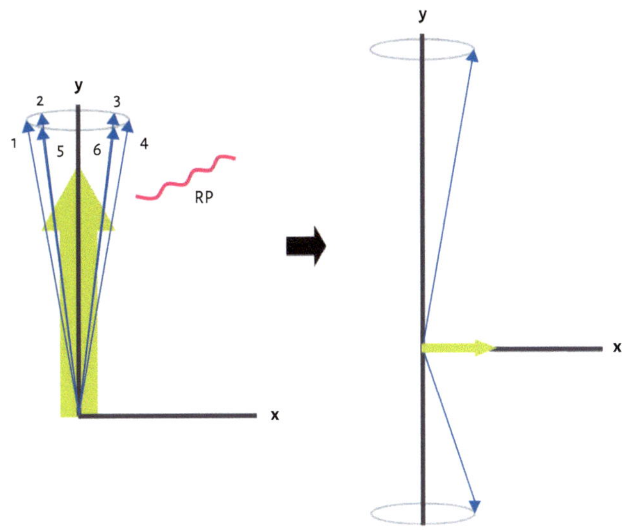

Figure 3. Principle of transverse magnetisation. In this image, in addition to the effect explained in Fig. 2 with the appearance of new antiparallel protons, the protons begin to align and go into phase. In this way, the cancellation seen when the precession movement was free does not occur and this ends up creating a certain amount of transverse magnetisation (green arrow). In this case, since it is not parallel to the external magnetic field, it can be detected by MRI.

Types of Relaxation

Once the RP ceases its activity, the protons return to their natural state through two different types of relaxation.

- **T1 relaxation** (spin-lattice relaxation): this process occurs when, while losing energy, the protons realign with the magnetic field and lose transverse magnetisation; as more of these protons face the magnetic field instead of turning away from it, they cancel themselves out and return to full longitudinal magnetisation.
- **T2 relaxation** (spin-spin relaxation): the in-phase state of the protons is also lost, so they cancel each other out again as their axes have different inclinations. The rate at which the coherence between protons is lost when precessing is produced by two distinct processes. The first process is due to the interferences between the different protons as they spin (they create small magnetic fields that affect other protons). The second process, also known as T2* relaxation, occurs as a result of external alterations, such as the presence of paramagnetic or ferromagnetic materials (iron) or imperfections in the MRI machine. The latter will result in a much faster loss of phase than the former. Fig. 4 illustrates the process of phase loss and the return to longitudinal magnetisation.

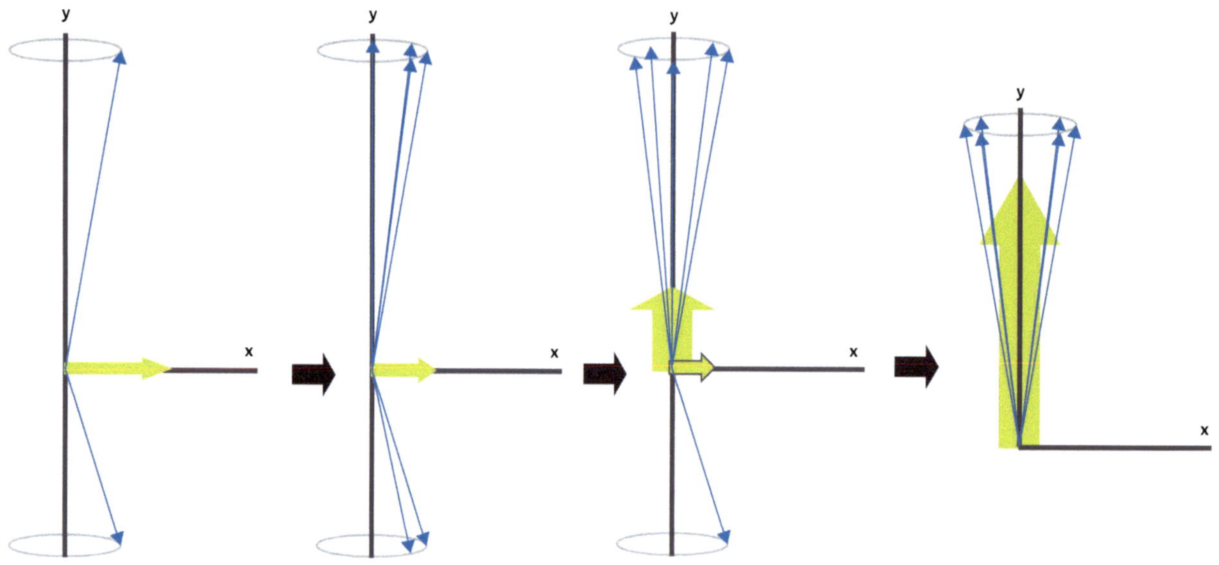

Figure 4. Spin-spin relaxation. Once the RP is no longer being applied, the protons begin to lose phase, in such a way that the transverse magnetisation weakens. In addition, antiparallel protons are placed in parallel to the external magnetic field again and cancel each other out as they cease to be in phase, causing the longitudinal magnetisation to become stronger and the transverse magnetisation to disappear completely.

Despite these definitions, it is difficult to determine the exact moment at which the transverse magnetisation is completely lost and the longitudinal magnetisation is recovered. Therefore, the following definitions can also be used:

- T1 relaxation: the time in which 63% of the longitudinal magnetisation is recovered
- T2 relaxation: the time in which 37% of the transverse magnetisation is lost.

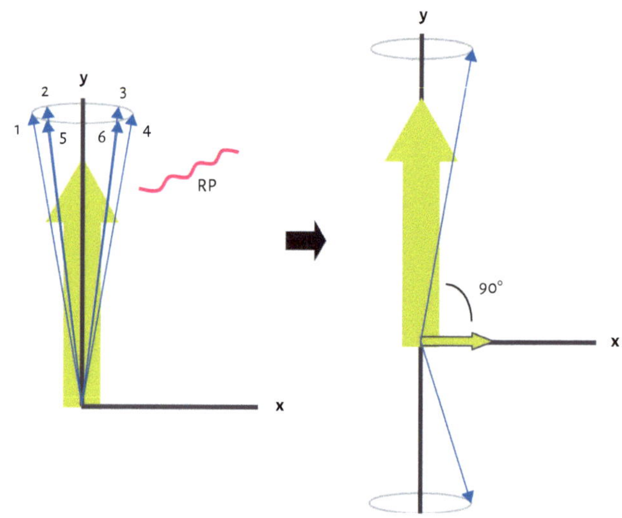

Figure 5. In this image the effect of an RP on magnetisation can be seen. In this case, when the RP is applied, a transverse magnetisation occurs at 90° to the longitudinal magnetisation.

Repetition Time and Echo Time

The different sequences that are used in MRI are created from the use of different RPs. In some cases, this is a 90° RP, whereas in others a 180° RP is used. Other angles are possible, and later in this chapter the usefulness of using RPs will be covered (Fig. 5).

The process of excitation of protons must occur multiple times, since the energy released after a single RP is not enough to be detected by the MRI machine. The time between a 90° RP and the echo is known as **echo time** (**ET**). The time between successive RPs at 90° is known as the **repetition time** (**RT**). These are covered in greater detail later in the chapter in the sections explaining the different types of sequences.

Magnetic Susceptibility

Magnetic susceptibility is a property that all tissues have that depends on their ability to magnetise when exposed to an external magnetic field, as in the case of MRI. This concept is of great importance in MRI, since it is the principle by which artefacts can be produced, some of which are indistinguishable from some types of pathological lesions. These events can occur especially when there are two adjacent tissues with different magnetic susceptibilities. As a consequence, a distortion of the magnetic field occurs. This distortion is much more marked in the presence of paramagnetic or ferromagnetic substances, such as blood-derived products containing iron.

One of the clearest examples is the interface between air and tissue, as can be seen in the sinuses and adjacent tissues. An example of the artefact caused by the difference in magnetic susceptibility at the air–tissue interface is shown in Fig. 6.

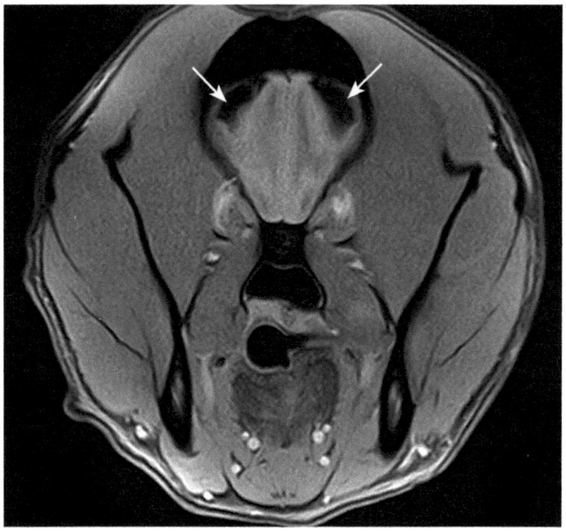

Figure 6. Example of artefact caused by differences in magnetic susceptibility. A loss of signal is observed inside the frontal cortex (white arrows) due to the difference in magnetic susceptibility between the air and other tissues.

Magnetic Resonance Signal

As in the case for most imaging modalities, MRI has its own nomenclature when describing the different observable signals. These signals are divided into three different types and are always compared to a standard reference tissue (e.g. cortical grey matter on MRI of the head and paravertebral musculature on MRI of the spine).

The signal is described as **hyperintense** when it is bright, **hypointense** when it is dark, and **isointense** when it is similar to the signal of the reference tissue.

Magnetic Resonance Sequences

All the concepts introduced above enable better understanding of what the different types of magnetic resonance sequences consist of. Each tissue in the body has different T1 and T2 relaxation characteristics. Once these are understood, they can be used to the operator's advantage to send different RPs and create the images, which will be described later. The most commonly used group of sequences is known as spin echo.

Spin echo (SE) sequences follow an RP pattern characterised by an initial RP of 90° followed by a second 180° pulse exactly halfway between the 90° RP and the echo. This 180° pulse is of great importance as it allows elimination of the effects caused by external interference, blocking the effect of T2* relaxation. Therefore, in this type of sequence only T1 and T2 relaxation will have an effect.

Inversion recovery (IR) sequences, which include FLAIR (fluid-attenuated inversion recovery), with fluid suppression, and STIR (short tau inversion recovery), with fat suppression, are also based on the principles of SE, although extra RPs are applied to suppress the signal of different types of tissues. In these cases, a starting RP of 180° is used, followed by the standard SE sequence. The time between the application of this 180° RP and the 90° RP is known as **inversion time** (IT).

The main tissues that will serve as a reference for this type of sequence are fat and liquid.

T1-Weighted SE Sequences (T1W)

In T1W sequences, the aim is to enhance T1 relaxation differences between tissues by using short RTs, while minimising the effect of T2 relaxation with short ETs. As explained above, each type of tissue has specific magnetic characteristics. Fat has short T1 relaxation times, so in this sequence it will be seen as hyperintense, since a maximum transverse magnetisation will be encountered. However, fluid will appear hypointense with long T1 relaxation times. Soft tissue has intermediate relaxation times, and the intensity varies depending on the specific tissue. Fig. 7 shows the behaviour of fluid and fat protons in the T1W sequence. Fig. 8 shows an example of a T1W cross section in which hyperintense fat can be observed while the fluid is hypointense.

The main use of T1W is for comparison of the images made before and after the administration of contrast. The use of paramagnetic substances (usually gadolinium) shortens the T1 relaxation time of the tissues that take up this contrast, which makes them hyperintense in T1W. Under normal conditions, gadolinium cannot cross the blood–brain barrier, so, unless this barrier is disrupted, lesions inside the brain or spinal cord should not show contrast uptake. Later in the chapter, exceptions to this rule will be covered.

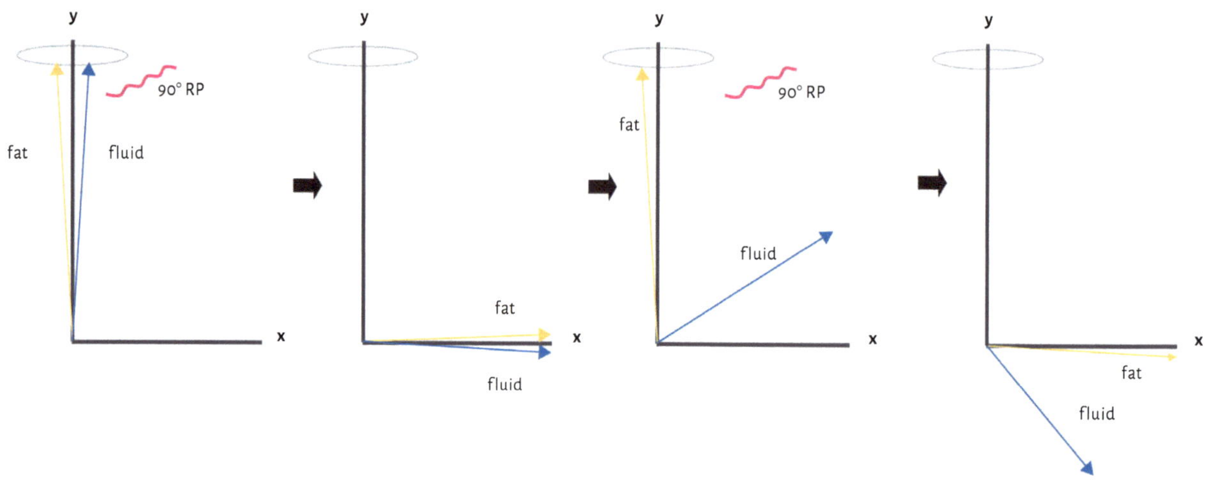

Figure 7. Behaviour of fluid and fat protons in the T1-enhanced SE sequence (T1W). First, a 90° RP is applied in such a way that the protons in the fluid and fat have maximum transverse magnetisation. When emission of the RP ceases, all protons progressively lose transverse magnetisation, mainly due to the T1 relaxation principle. As fat has a shorter T1 relaxation time than fluid, when the second 90° RP is applied, the protons in the fat will be transverse to the magnetic field again (since they are realigned with the external magnetic field), whereas those of the fluid will not. In this way, a hyperintense signal from fat is achieved in T1W, while the fluid appears hypointense.

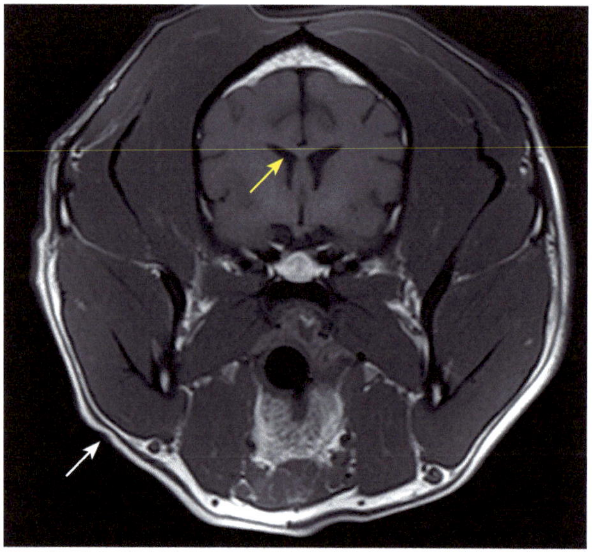

Figure 8. Transverse T1W cross section of the skull of an adult dog at the level of the piriform lobes. In this sequence, hyperintense fat (white arrow) is observed, while cerebrospinal fluid is hypointense (yellow arrow) compared to the cortical grey matter.

It is important to remember that there are certain structures that will take up contrast physiologically, and this helps to determine if the contrast has reached the patient. The most important are:

- the pituitary gland (Fig. 9)
- the choroid plexuses (Fig. 10)
- the trigeminal nerves (Fig. 11).

Historically, with low-field MRIs, this sequence was also used for its anatomical detail, since other sequences did not distinguish grey matter and white matter in such detail. However, current high-field MRIs allow other sequences, such as T2-enhanced SE sequences, to show sufficient anatomical detail.

T2-Weighted SE Sequences (T2W)

In the case of T2W sequences, long ETs are used to maximise the differences in T2 relaxation time between the different tissues. In addition, a long RT is used to minimise the effect of relaxation time in T1. This means that tissues with a short T2 relaxation time (e.g. fat) have lost their transverse magnetisation, in such a way that they appear hypointense, while tissues with long T2 relaxation times (e.g. fluid) still maintain it and appear hyperintense. However, this sequence has been replaced by the so-called fast SE or turbo SE, where additional RPs are applied in such a way that the fat also appears hyperintense. Fig. 12 shows the behaviour of fluid and fat protons in the T2W sequence. Fig. 13 shows an example of a T2W cross section where fat and hyperintense fluid can be observed due to the use of fast SE and turbo SE sequences.

This sequence is the most important when describing pathological lesions. The reason for this is that many of these lesions increase the amount of fluid present (e.g. inflammation, infection, neoplasia, oedema), such that hyperintensity is usually present on T2W compared to normal or reference tissue.

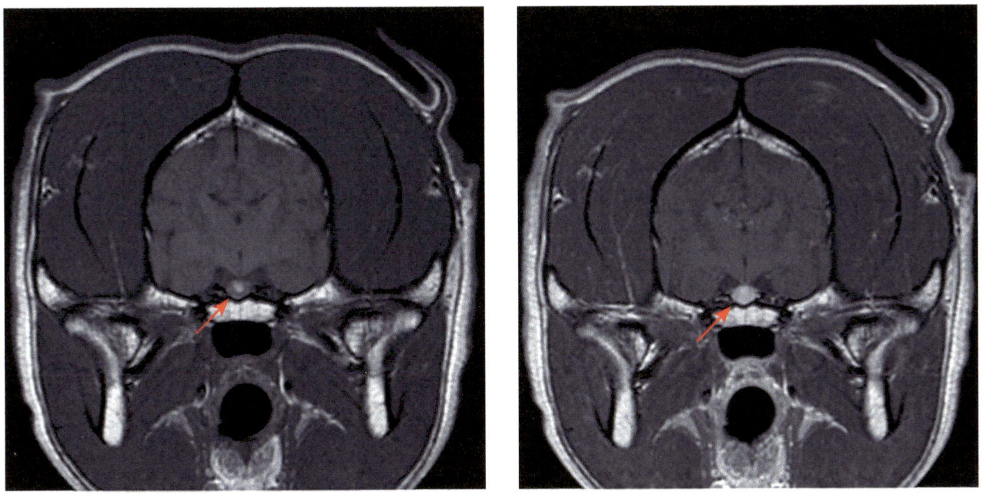

Figure 9. Transverse pre- and postcontrast T1W sequence of the skull of an adult dog at the level of the pituitary gland (red arrow). This image shows how this structure captures contrast physiologically.

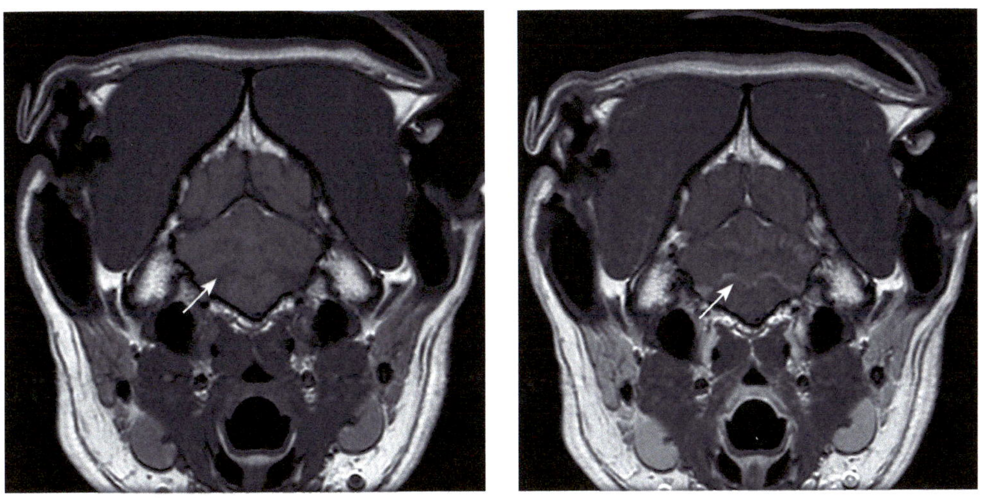

Figure 10. Transverse pre- and postcontrast T1W sequence of the skull of an adult dog at the level of the fourth ventricle with the choroid plexus inside (white arrow). These images show how this structure captures contrast physiologically.

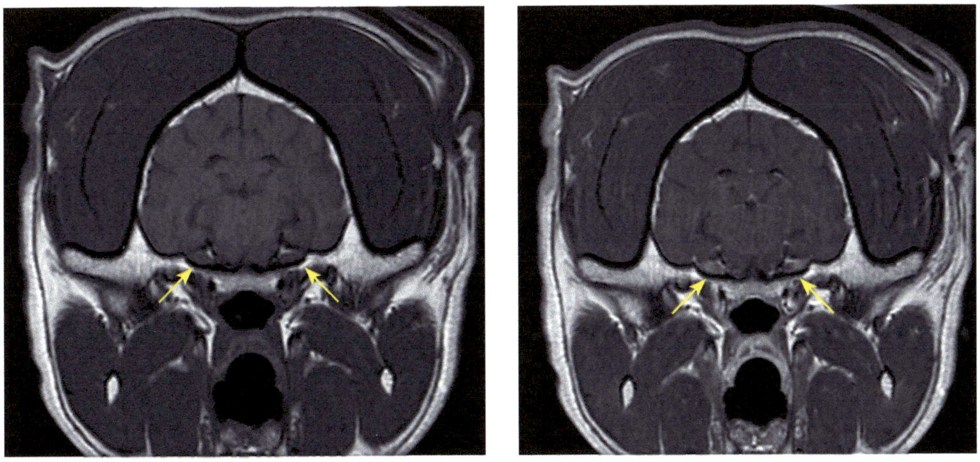

Figure 11. Transverse pre- and postcontrast T1W sequence of the skull of an adult dog at the level of the trigeminal nerve as it exits the pons (yellow arrows). These images show how this structure captures contrast physiologically.

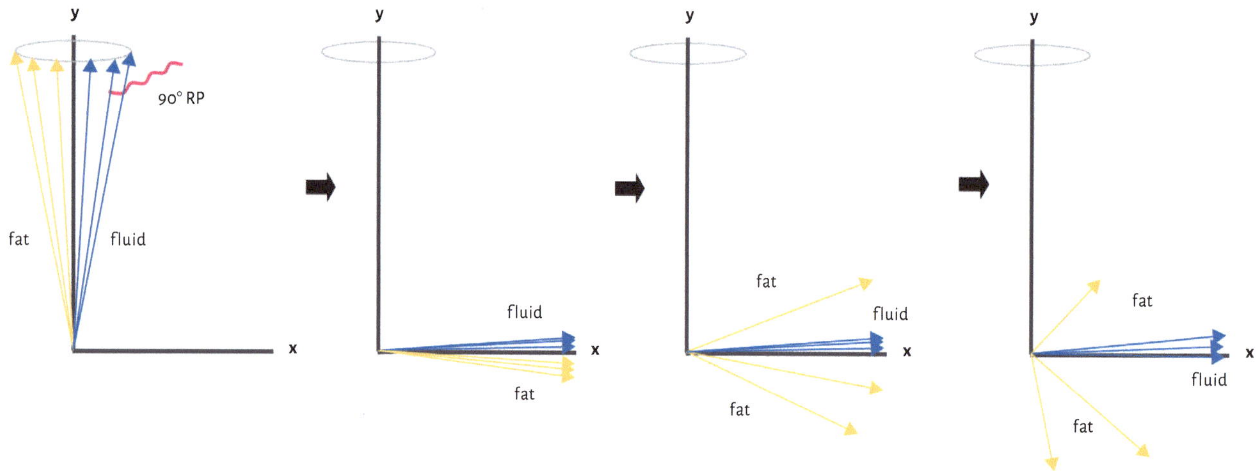

Figure 12. SE sequence enhanced in T2 (T2W). First, a 90° RP is applied in such a way that the protons in the fluid and the fat have maximum transverse magnetisation while they are in phase. When emission of the RP ceases, all protons progressively lose transverse magnetisation, but in this case the phase loss is more important, with dispersion of the protons, due to T2 relaxation. As fluid has a very high T2 relaxation time, it does not lose as much coherence as fat. As it takes a long time to obtain a signal, the fat has already lost its transverse magnetisation, while the fluid still maintains it. This is why in a T2W sequence, the fluid is hyperintense and the fat is hypointense. It should be remembered that fast SE or turbo SE sequences are used, which apply more RPs in such a way that the fat will also be in phase when the signal is captured, so it will also appear hyperintense.

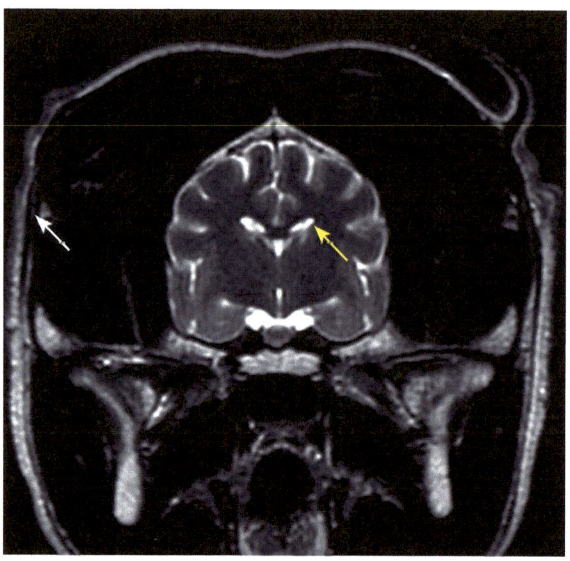

Figure 13. Transverse T2W sequence (turbo SE in this case) of the skull of an adult dog at the level of the piriform lobes. In this image, the hyperintense fat (white arrow) is observed and the cerebrospinal fluid also emits a hyperintense signal (yellow arrow) compared to the cortical grey matter.

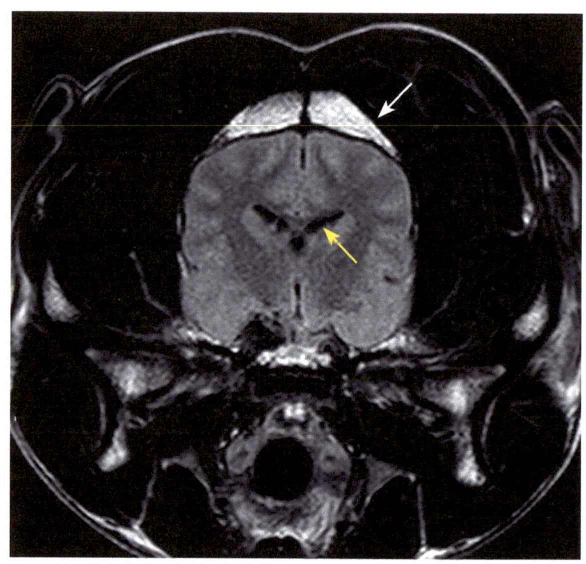

Figure 14. FLAIR cross section of the skull of an adult dog at the level of the caudate nuclei. In this sequence, hyperintense fat (white arrow) is observed, while the cerebrospinal fluid signal is suppressed (yellow arrow), compared to the cortical grey matter. Note that the cerebrospinal fluid signal in FLAIR is more hypointense than in T1W (same as air).

Fluid Suppression Sequences (FLAIR)

FLAIR is an example of an IR sequence. In FLAIR, a long IT is applied in such a way that the signal from the free fluid (fluid with low cellularity and protein content) is suppressed. Unfortunately, this sequence does not allow the suppression of types of fluids with high cellularity, such as blood. Fig. 14 shows an example of a cross section in FLAIR where the hyperintense fat can be seen while the signal from free fluid, such as cerebrospinal fluid, is suppressed. This sequence is used in

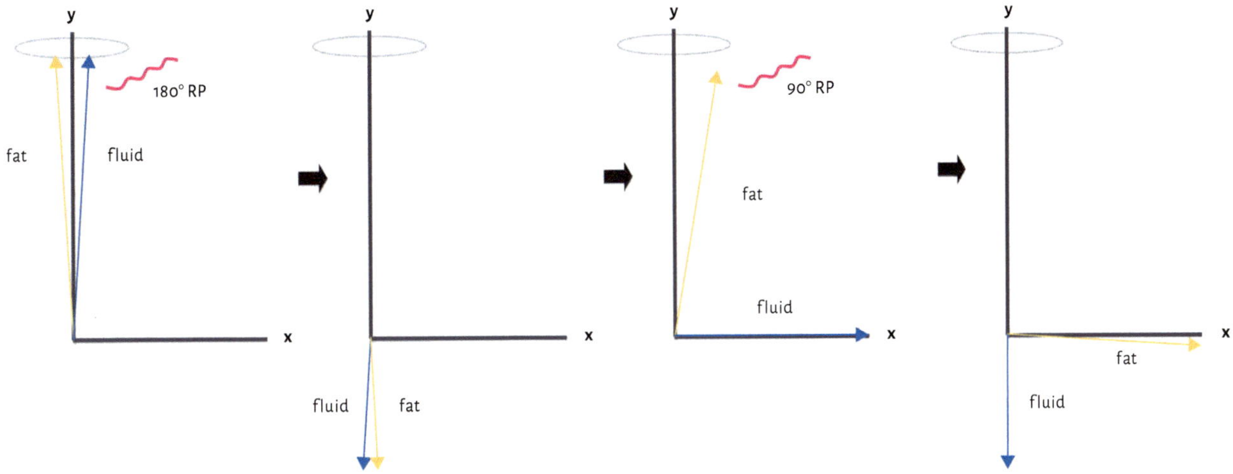

Figure 15. Behaviour of fluid and fat protons in a FLAIR sequence. First, a 180° RP is applied in such a way that the protons in the fluid and the fat are positioned antiparallel to the external magnetic field. Over time, the protons, under the T1 relaxation effect, will return to their parallel position. Fat has a shorter T1 relaxation time, so it will be closer to its longitudinal magnetisation. Fluid, on the other hand, has a longer T1 relaxation time. At the point when the fluid protons are at 90° to the external magnetic field, a RP of 90° is applied. In this way, the fat is transversely magnetised (hyperintense) while the fluid is antiparallel to the magnetic field appearing suppressed in the image.

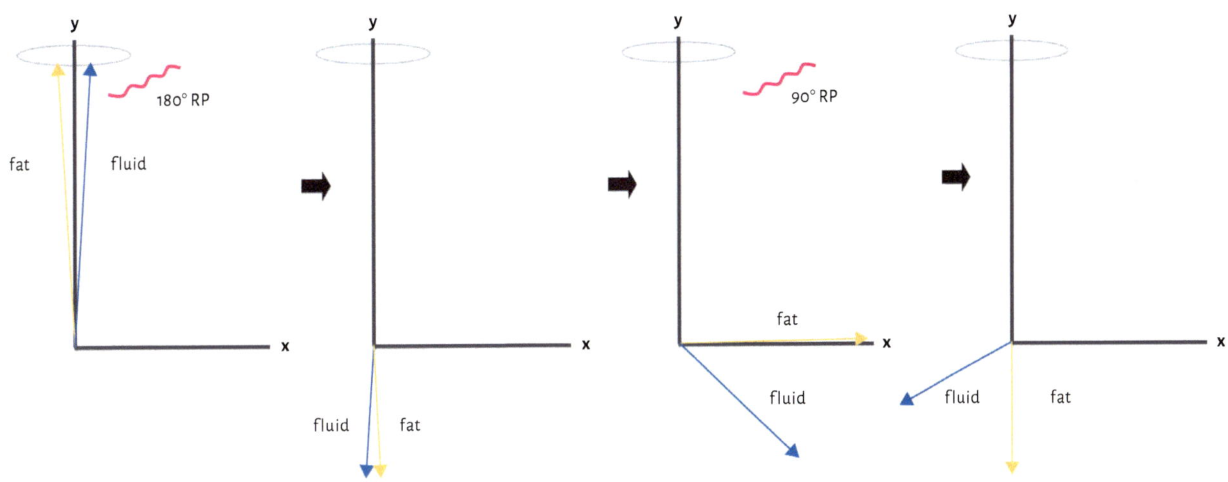

Figure 16. Behaviour of fluid and fat protons in a STIR sequence. First, a 180° RP is applied in such a way that the protons in the fluid and the fat are positioned antiparallel to the external magnetic field. At the point when the protons in the fat are at 90° to the external magnetic field, a 90° RP is applied. In this way, the fluid is transversely magnetised (hyperintense) while the fat is antiparallel to the magnetic field and appears suppressed in the image.

combination with T2W, as it allows a more marked visualisation of lesions that are hyperintense in T2W. In addition, the suppression of free fluid, such as cerebrospinal fluid, helps characterise lesions adjacent to the ventricles, which would otherwise go unnoticed in T2W. Fig. 15 shows the behaviour of fluid and fat protons in FLAIR.

Fat Suppression Sequences (STIR)

STIR is another example of an IR sequence. STIR applies a short IT, so that the fat signal is suppressed. Fig. 16 shows the behaviour of fluid and fat protons in this sequence. Fig. 17 shows an example of a dorsal section in STIR where the hyperintense fluid can be observed whereas the fat signal is suppressed.

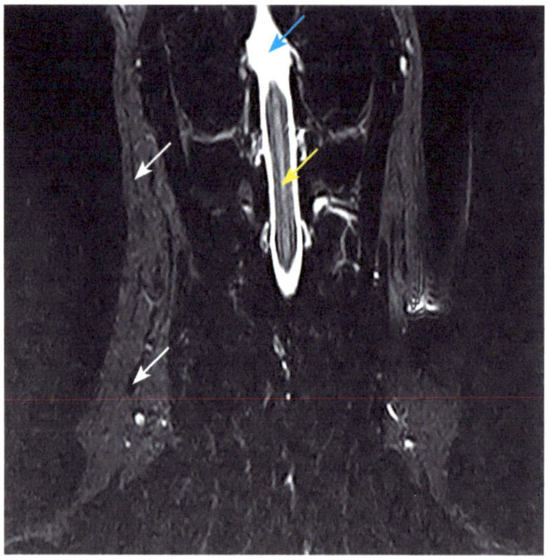

Figure 17. Dorsal section in STIR of the cervical spine of an adult dog. In this sequence, hyperintense cerebrospinal fluid (blue arrow) is observed around the spinal cord (yellow arrow), with the fat signal suppressed (white arrow) compared to the paravertebral musculature. Note that the signal from fat in STIR is similar to that of air, similar to the appearance of fluid in FLAIR.

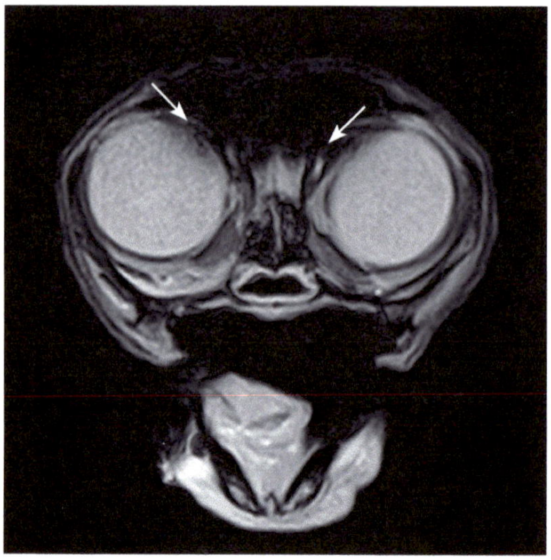

Figure 18. A T2* cross section of the skull of an adult cat at the level of the frontal sinuses. In this sequence, an artefact is observed due to the absence of the 180° RP (susceptibility artefact), which produces a distortion of the image in the form of a shadow (white arrows).

The main practical use of this sequence is for imaging the spine, since it allows hyperintense vertebral lesions to be distinguished from fat in the bone marrow, which also appears hyperintense on T2W.

Gradient Echo Sequences (GE)

These types of sequences show significant differences from the SE and IR sequences. First, they do not use 90° and 180° RP angles, but use smaller angles. In addition, the RTs are lower, meaning that the acquisition time is shorter. In addition, as the 180° RP is not applied, the external interference is not eliminated. The most widely used GE sequence is T2*. Fig. 18 shows an example of a cross section in T2* where air interference can be observed when the 180° RP is not applied.

This sequence is mainly used for the detection of haemorrhagic infarcts or blood byproducts.

Advantages and Disadvantages of MRI

Advantages of MRI

MRI is the modality of choice for the diagnosis of most diseases of the central nervous system and even some of those affecting the peripheral nervous system, such as neuritis and nerve tumours. This imaging modality allows excellent visualisation of the central nervous system and parts of the peripheral nervous system, such as certain spinal or cranial nerves, as well as soft tissues, such as the musculature, glands and lymph nodes, among others.

In addition, MRI allows imaging of the body in multiple planes, which significantly increases the ability to detect lesions and determine their extent.

Disadvantages of MRI

As with the other imaging modalities, MRI is not 100% sensitive or specific either for the detection of lesions or for establishing a diagnosis. One of the clearest examples of this disadvantage is found in the differentiation between a glioma and an ischaemic infarction, which can be very difficult to distinguish on MRI. Although MRI shows the soft tissues in great detail, it is not as useful for the study of bone lesions, unlike computed tomography (CT).

MRI also requires general anaesthesia of the patient, which may be contraindicated in some cases due to either systemic disease (e.g. cardiac, renal, hepatic) or the severity of intracranial lesions (e.g. increased intracranial pressure). In addition, it is an expensive technique and takes significantly longer than other imaging techniques, especially CT.

Artefacts

An artefact can be defined as any feature of an image that does not represent the object as it should. A large number of artefacts are found on MRI. They can be mainly divided into two types:

- patient-associated artefacts
- artefacts associated with image acquisition.

In some cases, artefacts are evident, causing significant image distortion. In others, discrete artefactual lesions may appear difficult to distinguish from an actual lesion. Therefore, being aware of the main types of artefact will help interpret any imaging technique correctly. It is also important to remember that some of these artefacts can be corrected by modifying the imaging parameters.

This section of the chapter will cover some of the most common artefacts and provide some images as examples.

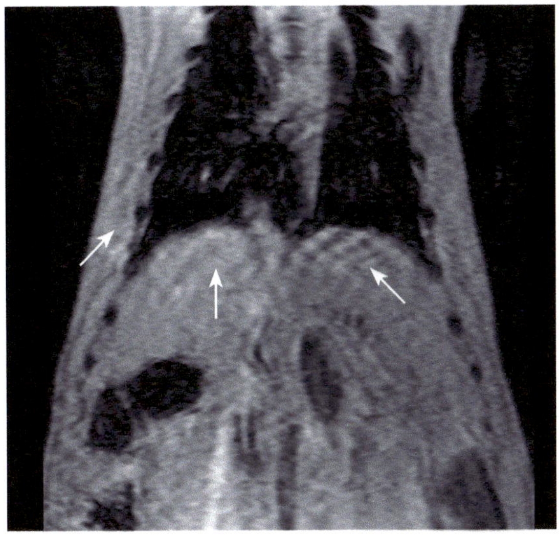

Figure 19. This image shows the locator used by the technician to prescan the region of interest, in this case a dorsal image of the thoracic and cranial abdominal region. These images are very susceptible to artefacts, as can be seen in this case, where lines caused by the movement of the patient's breathing (white arrows) can be seen.

Patient-associated Artefacts

Motion Artefact

Motion artefact is probably one of the most frequently observed artefacts. It occurs when there are (even minimal) movements of the patient during the acquisition of images. It takes a significant time to obtain a single sequence, and patient movement causes the MRI system to misinterpret the exact location of protons. The result is similar to that of a photograph taken when the subject (or camera) is in motion, with a distorted image (Fig. 19).

Fig. 19 shows the locator used by the technician to prescan the region of interest, in this case a dorsal image of the thoracic and cranial abdominal region. These images are very susceptible to artefacts, as can be seen in this case, where lines caused by the movement of the patient's breathing (white arrows) can be seen.

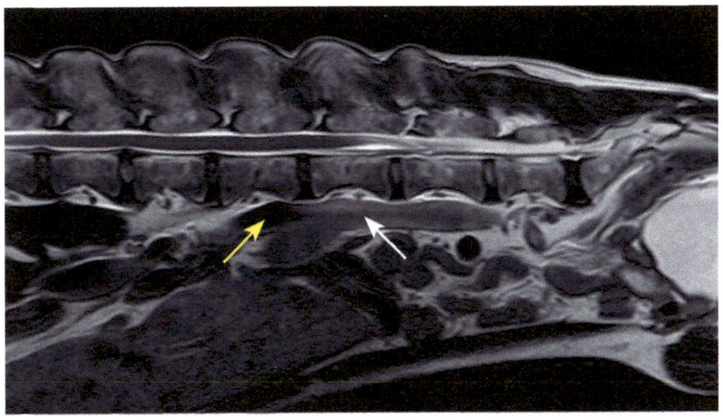

Figure 20. Sagittal T2W sequence of the abdominal cavity of a dog. Blood showing different intensities can be observed inside the caudal vena cava. In some regions it presents a more hyperintense signal (white arrow), whereas in others it appears hypointense (yellow arrow). This is a consequence of blood flow artefacts.

Blood Flow and Cerebrospinal Fluid Artefacts

Collectively, these are another of the most common artefacts. Although there are different types, the best known is caused by blood flow in the so-called **time-of-flight phenomenon**. This occurs due to constant movement of the blood during imaging; the same amount of blood may receive a 90° RP but not a 180° RP, or neither of the two, and the result is usually a loss of signal. In the case of the **entry slice phenomenon** the opposite situation is seen. As the blood is stimulated in each section, it presents an increasingly hyperintense signal compared to the blood in the first section, which presents much less signal (Fig. 20).

The flow of cerebrospinal fluid can produce a similar effect, resulting in a decrease in the signal in T2W (Fig. 21) and partially losing the suppression in FLAIR.

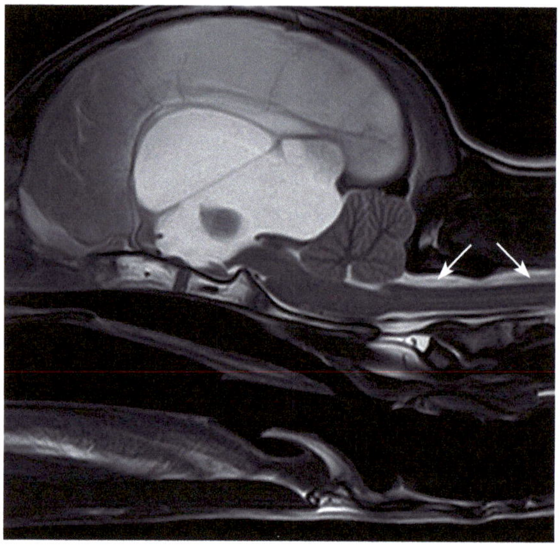

Figure 21. Sagittal T2W sequence from a young dog with severe hydrocephalus. A loss of signal can be observed in the subarachnoid space of the cervical region in the form of a hypointense line (white arrows) as a result of the flow of cerebrospinal fluid.

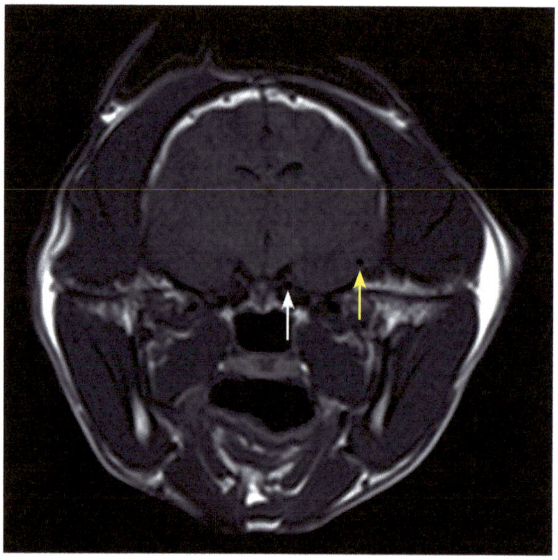

Figure 22. Cross section of a precontrast T1W sequence of the skull of a cat. In this case, the white arrow shows the location of a real vessel, represented as a markedly hypointense rounded structure. The yellow arrow shows a pulsatility artefact, appearing as a vessel similar to the real one but inside the piriform lobe.

Pulsatility Artefact

The pulsatility artefact is produced by the pulsation of vessels of a certain size, creating ghost images (images of structures that are not actually there) arranged in the direction of the phase encoding. They are usually present in only one of the planes, so it is easy to rule out that they are not real lesions (Fig. 22).

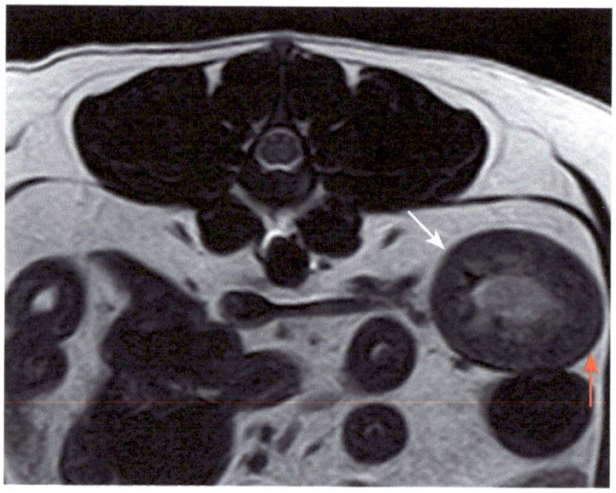

Figure 23. Example of a chemical shift artefact in a transverse T2W sequence at the level of the cranial lumbar region. The kidney in this image presents a hyperintense border (white arrow) while the contralateral border is markedly hypointense (red arrow).

Artefacts Associated with Image Acquisition

Chemical Shift Artefact

Chemical shift artefact occurs in structures where fat and water are in close proximity. It occurs because water and fat have a slight difference in their resonance frequencies, which means that the signal from the fat is not properly recorded. Consequently, a dark line is observed on one side and a bright one on the other side at interfaces between fat and soft tissue (Fig. 23).

Partial Volume Averaging Artefact

In the partial volume averaging artefact, a sum effect of the signals emitted by adjacent tissues is observed, especially when these tissues have very different intensities (e.g. very hyperintense cerebrospinal fluid with hypointense medullary parenchyma). Therefore, the parenchyma may appear more hyperintense than it should, which could lead the viewer to think that there is an intramedullary or intra-axial lesion (Fig. 24).

Susceptibility Artefact

The susceptibility artefact has been discussed in previous sections, where some examples have also been provided. It occurs in areas at the junction between tissues with different magnetic susceptibilities (see Figs. 6 and 18 for examples of this artefact).

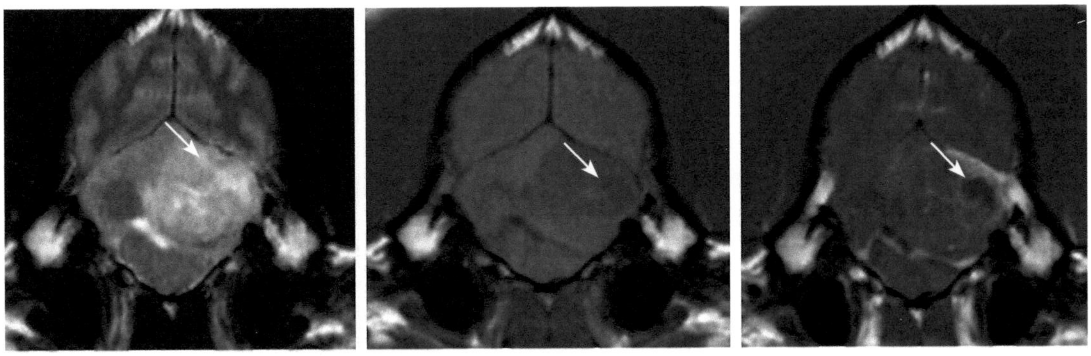

Figure 24. An example of an intra-axial injury primarily affecting the cerebellum, although it also compresses the medulla oblongata dorsally. The lesion is heterogeneous, poorly-defined, and appears hyperintense on T2W (left slice) and hypointense on precontrast T1W (middle slice), and shows poor and mainly peripheral constrast enhancement (right slice). Considering the appearance, it is possible that most of it is oedema surrounding the actual lesion. The presence of a glioblastoma multiforme affecting the left cerebellum was confirmed.

MRI Interpretation

The interpretation of an image produced by MRI, as with all imaging techniques, must be done considering several points. To begin with, and as discussed earlier in the chapter, some diseases can have a very similar appearance (e.g. glioma versus ischaemic infarction), so the age, sex, breed (and species) of the patient should always be taken into account, as well as the presentation and progression of clinical signs. In addition, some changes visible on MRI may be artefacts, as discussed in the previous section, and this possibility must always be kept in mind when assessing an MRI. They may also simply be a normal variant or an incidental lesion that is not related to the patient's current condition.

Having a basic understanding of neuroanatomy is vital in order to evaluate an MRI. It is not the intention of this chapter to provide a detailed description of the structures of the nervous system, so referring to neuroanatomy books for more information is recommended. In addition, observation of all structures, not only those belonging to the nervous system, is extremely important, because in some cases lesions are of extracranial origin.

Establishing a differential diagnosis is vital for effective interpretation of MRI. The use of the mnemonic VITAMIN D (V: vascular; I: inflammatory/infectious; T: traumatic/toxic; A: congenital anomaly; M: metabolic; I: idiopathic; N: neoplasia/nutritional; D: degenerative) helps to ensure that no group of diseases is forgotten.

Lesion Description

As a rule, the description of an MRI study should begin by indicating the region studied (e.g. skull, cervical region, thoracic region, lumbar region, sacral region) and the species in question (dog, cat). It should be noted whether the patient is adult (dentally, when the skull is being studied, or skeletally, in the case of a study of the spine) or immature (in the same way). Then, all the sequences included in the study are indicated, with their respective planes.

Regarding the description of the lesion, the following points should be noted:

1. location
2. distribution and extent of the lesion
3. shape of the lesion
4. size of the lesion
5. signal from the lesion
6. changes associated with the lesion.

Location

After providing the introductory information mentioned above, the location of the lesion must be determined. First, it should be established whether the lesion is inside or outside the central nervous system. To do this, the following nomenclature should be used.

- **Brain**
  - Intra-axial: in this case, the lesion is located within the brain parenchyma. The lesion is surrounded by parenchyma, with little or no contact with external structures. Although these types of lesions do not

have a homogeneous appearance and there are some exceptions, generally they cause expansion of the parenchyma, with displacement or invasion of adjacent structures, and have little or no contrast uptake. Intraventricular lesions, which are located inside the intraventricular system, can be considered intra-axial in some cases. These include cerebrovascular accidents (strokes), some neoplasms such as glioma, or inflammatory processes such as meningoencephalitis of unknown origin (Fig. 24).

- Extra-axial: the lesion originates from outside the brain parenchyma, including the meninges. As the dura mater is attached to the skull and there is no epidural space in the cranial cavity, it is difficult to determine if the lesion is meningeal or originates externally. In general, extra-axial lesions cause compression of the brain parenchyma, displacing it, and have a wide base of contact with the skull and usually show more contrast uptake when they are outside the blood–brain barrier. They include some neoplasms such as meningiomas and histiocytic sarcomas, skull fractures and abscesses (Fig. 25).

– **Spinal cord**

- Extradural: these are lesions that originate from outside the meninges. There are many examples of extradural lesions, such as intervertebral disc extrusions, bone neoplasms, the accumulation of purulent material in the epidural space or empyema. The extradural location is probably the most common with regard to lesions affecting the spinal cord (Fig. 26).
- Intradural/extramedullary: in these cases, the lesion is located in the meninges. The best known lesions in this location are meningiomas, although other processes, such as arachnoid diverticula, are also located here.
- Intramedullary: as in the case of intra-axial lesions, these are located inside the parenchyma. Fibrocartilaginous thromboembolism, glioma and meningomyelitis of unknown origin are some examples of lesions of the spinal cord parenchyma (Fig. 27).

Distribution and Extent of the Lesion

Regarding the distribution and extent of the lesion, the number of lesions present in the case should be described as follows.

- Focal: a single lesion located in a specific region.
- Multifocal: several lesions located in one or more regions.
- Diffuse: a single lesion that extends over several regions or structures.

This also helps determine the most likely aetiology. For example, primary neoplasms of the nervous system usually present as focal lesions, whereas it is common to find several lesions in cases of metastases. A large haemorrhagic lesion may be more suggestive of a traumatic cause, while several haemorrhagic lesions larger than 5 mm could indicate the presence of the heartworm *Angiostrongylus vasorum*.

Another important aspect to remember when assessing the distribution of lesions is their lateralisation and symmetry. The central nervous system is practically bilateral and symmetrical. Some processes are more commonly presented as lateralised (e.g. neoplasms, inflammatory/infectious or vascular processes), whereas others may be bilateral and symmetrical (e.g. metabolic, toxic or neurodegenerative diseases). Although this aspect can help establish the most likely of the differential diagnoses, it should not be forgotten that there are exceptions to this rule (e.g. some vascular damage or inflammatory and infectious processes of the spinal cord can be so extensive that they affect both sides with the same intensity, so there is no obvious lateralisation).

Lesion Shape

The shape and definition of the lesion should be evaluated in detail. Some neoplastic lesions, especially metastases, or abscesses are usually rounded in shape, with well defined edges. This appearance may also apply to territorial ischaemic infarcts (e.g. occlusion of a major artery of the brain, such as the middle cerebral artery) in which the boundary between the affected region and a healthy region vascularised by another artery can be observed clearly. Other processes, such as infection or inflammation, have poorly defined borders and erratic shapes that are difficult to describe.

Lesion Size

The size of the lesion is another aspect that should be considered when describing an MRI study. Although a subjective assessment (e.g. large, extensive, small) can be used when describing the lesion, the use of more objective methods is recommended. For example, whenever possible the lesion should be measured (when it has well defined edges and is focal), or the exact extent of the lesion should be described (e.g. it extends from the right frontal cortex to the right occipital cortex); doing this will give a more reliable idea of the true size of the lesion.

Lesion Signal

The signal from the lesion is probably one of the most vital aspects which should be described. The signal of all pathological changes that can be observed should be described. As previously discussed, T2W and FLAIR are very useful as they are the sequences best able to detect the presence of lesions in the central nervous system.

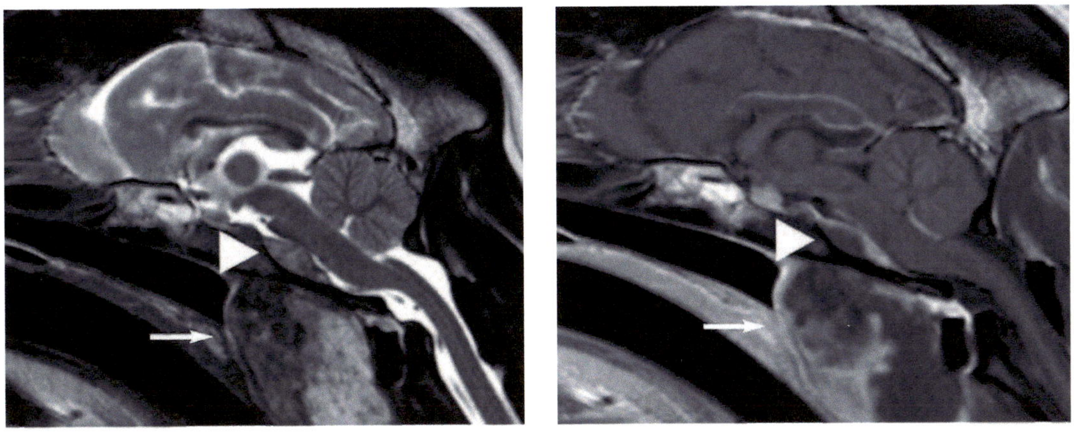

Figure 25. Example of an extra-axial lesion causing compression of the pons (arrowhead) due to a large mass inside the pharynx (white arrow). The first image corresponds to a sagittal T2W section and the second is a postcontrast sagittal T1W section. The lesion can be seen showing heterogeneous contrast uptake, mostly located in the periphery. Histopathology confirmed the presence of a multilobular bone tumour.

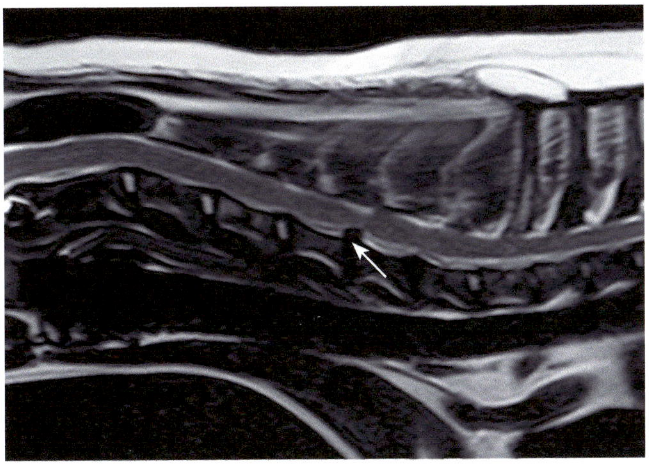

Figure 26. A T2W sagittal section of the spinal cord of an adult dog is shown. Strongly hypointense extradural material compatible with a disc protrusion is observed at the level of the C5–C6 intervertebral space (white arrow). Note the spinal cord compression caused by the herniated disc.

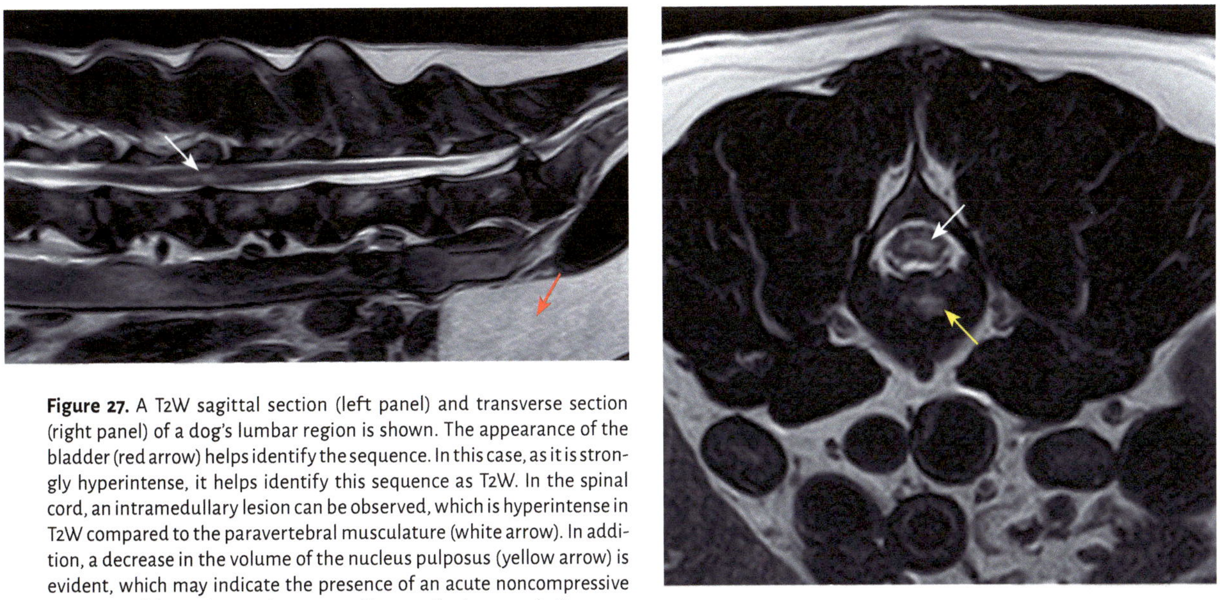

Figure 27. A T2W sagittal section (left panel) and transverse section (right panel) of a dog's lumbar region is shown. The appearance of the bladder (red arrow) helps identify the sequence. In this case, as it is strongly hyperintense, it helps identify this sequence as T2W. In the spinal cord, an intramedullary lesion can be observed, which is hyperintense in T2W compared to the paravertebral musculature (white arrow). In addition, a decrease in the volume of the nucleus pulposus (yellow arrow) is evident, which may indicate the presence of an acute noncompressive extrusion of the nucleus pulposus or a fibrocartilaginous embolism.

Many processes (neoplasia, infection, inflammation, gliosis and oedema) will be hyperintense in both T2W and FLAIR (although this may vary in some specific cases). This is because the increase in cellularity that occurs in the first four processes will also increase the amount of fluid present. In the case of oedema, since it is the presence of excess fluid, it will also appear hyperintense in both sequences, regardless of its location (vasogenic or cytotoxic).

In some cases, the signal from the lesion may not be homogeneous. For example, some neoplasms may contain calcified or haemorrhagic areas, so the periphery of the lesion may show a different intensity from the rest. In such cases where different intensities are found, a heterogeneous signal should be noted.

Changes Associated with the Lesion

In addition to the specific observations regarding the lesions that are present, the effect they have on the parenchyma of the nervous system should also be taken into account.

One of the most characteristic changes is the **mass effect**, which is defined as the displacement of any structure from its physiological position caused by the growth or invasion of, or compression by, one or more lesions. It can be present in many pathological processes, including neoplasms, inflammatory and infectious processes, and cerebrovascular accidents (both ischaemic and haemorrhagic), among others. In some cases, the mass effect will not be caused primarily by the disease itself but by changes secondary to it. For example, many meningiomas and gliomas are associated with large amounts of oedema, which will further increase the volume of the lesion. When describing the mass effect, the main structures affected should be listed, as well as the degree to which they are affected.

Another characteristic associated with the mass effect is displacement of the midline (Fig. 28).

If the intracranial volume reaches a critical level and the mechanisms that control intracranial pressure fail, displacement of large areas of parenchyma or herniation will become evident. There are three **types of herniation**.

- **Cerebellar herniation**: in this case, the cerebellum crosses the foramen magnum and moves towards the cisterna magna.
- **Transtentorial herniation**: the cerebellar tentorium separates the cerebral hemispheres from the cerebellum. In this case, part of the brain parenchyma passes through this structure and compresses the cerebellum.
- **Subfalcine herniation**: the falx cerebri partially separates the cerebral hemispheres along the midline. In this case, part of a hemisphere is displaced medially and compresses the contralateral side.

Fig. 29 shows the two most frequent types of herniation, cerebellar and transtentorial.

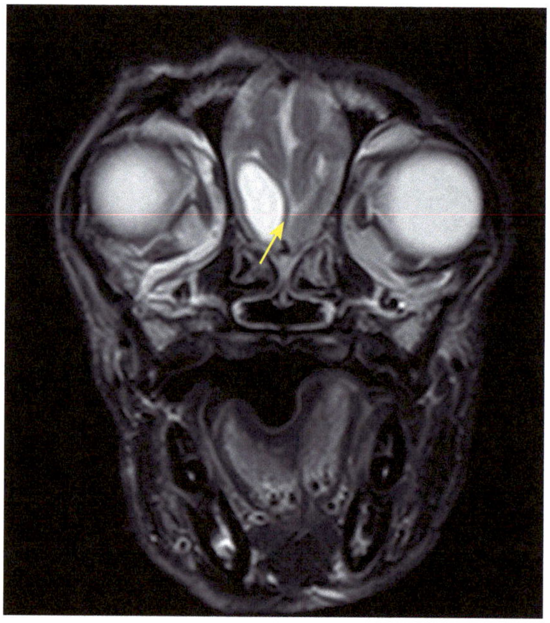

Figure 28. This cross section in T2W shows a cystic lesion in the right frontal region of the right cerebral hemisphere. A slight displacement of the midline to the left side (yellow arrow) can be observed.

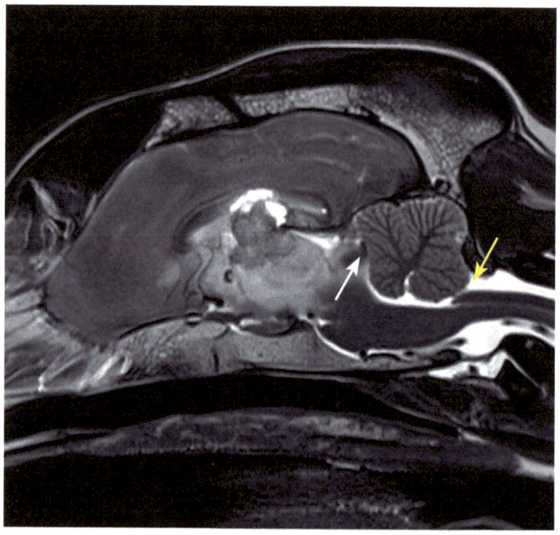

Figure 29. Sagittal T2W section of the head of an adult dog in which a heterogeneous mass is observed in the region of the third ventricle. The intense rostral compression of the cerebellum (white arrow) produced by a transtentorial herniation can be seen. In addition, cerebellar herniation is observed as part of the cerebellum extends caudally into the foramen magnum (yellow arrow).

Description of the Tissue Surrounding the Lesion

Description of the tissue surrounding the lesion should follow the guidelines described above. It is important to always look for small changes that may go unnoticed, such as lesions in the pituitary gland, ventricular system, meninges or bones of the skull/spine. It is also important to pay attention to the cranial and spinal nerves, as the patient's clinical signs could be associated with the peripheral nervous system (Fig. 30).

Assessment of Extracranial Structures or Adjacent Structures of the Spine

Other structures that are of interest in neurology are the tympanic bullae and the inner ear, the masticatory muscles (temporal muscle, masseter muscle, medial pterygoid muscle and the rostral portion of the digastric muscle, all of which are innervated by the mandibular branch of the trigeminal nerve) and the intervertebral discs (which are of utmost importance in neurology, since degenerative diseases of the intervertebral discs are among the most frequent processes in dogs).

It is also important to look at other structures that are not part of the nervous system, such as the salivary glands, lymph nodes and other paravertebral muscles. Abdominal organs can also be scanned for potential lesions, although in most cases abdominal ultrasound imaging or computed tomography is recommended for confirmation. In the case of thoracic structures, it is common for artefacts produced by the heartbeat and inspiratory/expiratory movements to hinder correct visualisation of these organs, so the use of MRI to visualise these structures is not recommended.

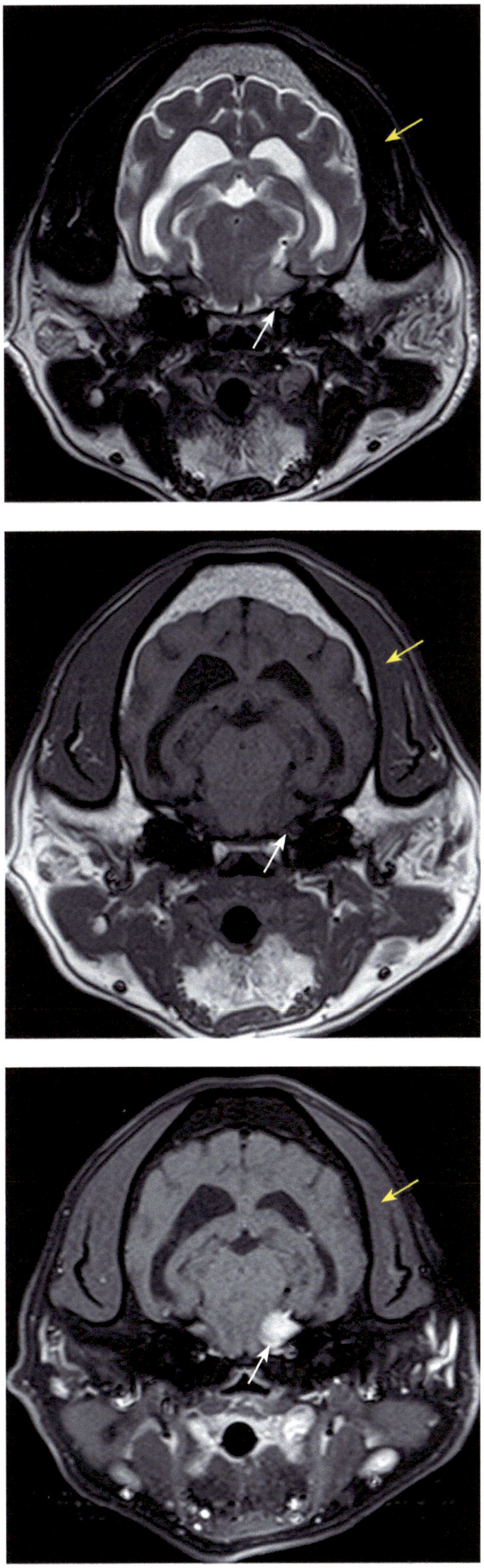

Figure 30. These images show three cross sections in T2W (top panel), T1W precontrast (middle panel) and T1W postcontrast (bottom panel). In these images, an increase in the size of the left trigeminal nerve is observed, which presents an increase in T2W intensity and marked and homogeneous contrast uptake (white arrows). This also produces a degree of mass effect, with medial displacement of the pons. It is important to note the atrophy of the ipsilateral masticatory muscles, especially the temporal muscle (yellow arrow).

Bibliography

- Cervera, V., Mai, W., Vite, C.H., et al. (2011) Comparative magnetic resonance imaging findings between gliomas and presumed cerebrovascular accident in dogs. *Vet Radiol Ultrasound*, 52(1):33–40.
- Havsteen, I., Ohlhues, A., Madsen, K.H., et al. (2017) Are movement artifacts in magnetic resonance imaging a real problem?—A narrative review. *Front Neurol*, 8:232.
- Hecht, S. (2016) Principles and application of magnetic resonance imaging (MRI). In: Dewey CW, da Costa RC. (eds). *Practical Guide to Canine and Feline Neurology*, pp. 87–139. Wiley-Blackwell.
- Lowrie, M., De Risio, L., Dennis, R., et al. (2012) Concurrent medical conditions and long-term outcome in dogs with nontraumatic intracranial hemorrhage. *Vet Radiol Ultrasound*, 53(4):381–388.
- Mai, W. (2018) General principles of magnetic resonance imaging. In: Mai, W. (ed). *Diagnostic MRI in Dogs and Cats*, pp. 3–35. CRC Press.
- Mai, W. (2018) Imaging characteristics in MRI and principal pulse sequences. In: Mai, W. (ed). *Diagnostic MRI in Dogs and Cats*, pp. 36–69. CRC Press.
- McConnell, J.F. (2018) MRI artifacts. In: Mai, W. (ed). *Diagnostic MRI in Dogs and Cats*, pp. 70–87. CRC Press.
- Schenck, J.F. (1996) The role of magnetic susceptibility in magnetic resonance imaging: MRI magnetic compatibility of the first and second kinds. *Med Phys*, 23(6):815–850.
- Schild, H.H. (1990) *MRI Made Easy*. 1st ed. Schering AG.

Notes

Abdominal Imaging

Radiography and Computed Tomography of the Abdomen: Abdominal Cavity, Liver, Spleen

Agustina Ansón Fernández

Introduction

Abdominal radiographs are an essential tool in the small animal clinic and are one of the first modalities of choice for the investigation of most abdominal pathologies. Computed tomography (CT) is also a very useful tool in the assessment of abdominal structures thanks to its excellent resolution, its ability to differentiate soft tissue from fluid and its tomographic nature, which avoids organ overlap.

Abdominal Radiographic Technique

For the study of the abdominal cavity at least two orthogonal projections are always necessary. Standard projections include a **right lateral and a ventrodorsal** (**VD**) **projection**. However, additional projections such as **left lateral or dorsoventral** (**DV**) **projections** are especially useful in studies of the gastrointestinal system and are included in routine protocols at many referral centres. In general, patients do not need a period of fasting or administration of an enema prior to abdominal radiographic studies. However, there are exceptions, for example, when the aim is to rule out small masses or calculi in the urinary system (especially the ureters) or when a contrast study is performed.

It is imperative that the entire abdominal cavity is included in the study. If this is not possible due to the size of the animal, radiographs of the cranial and the caudal abdomen should be obtained. Abdominal radiographs should cover the area from the diaphragmatic dome to the pelvic cavity. This is generally achieved by positioning the cranial aspect of the X-ray beam approximately 5 cm cranial to the xiphoid process of the sternum, and the caudal aspect of the X-ray beam approximately 5 cm caudal to the greater trochanter of the femur (Figs. 1 A and 2 A). Both bony structures are easily palpable in most animals. Sometimes it is also necessary to include the entire pelvic cavity and perineum. In lateral projections (Fig. 1), the hindlimbs should be positioned perpendicular to the lumbar spine. In this way, they do not overlap the caudal abdomen, nor are they overretracted caudally, which would cause compression of the caudal abdomen and subsequent overlapping of structures. Similarly, in VD projections (Fig. 2), the hindlimbs should not be stretched caudally but should be left flexed on both sides of the cavity in a "frog" position.

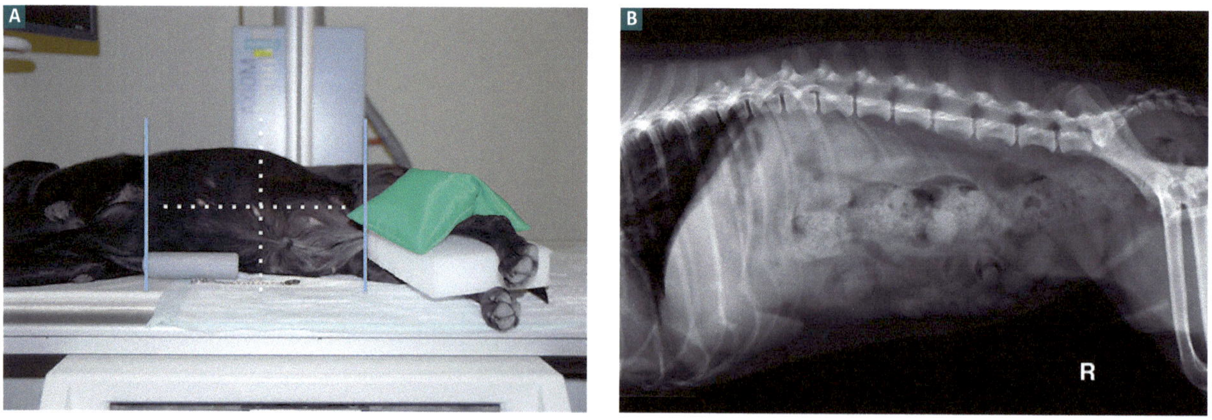

Figure 1. A. Patient positioning and collimation when performing a lateral projection of the abdomen. **B**. Right lateral projection of the abdomen of a dog.

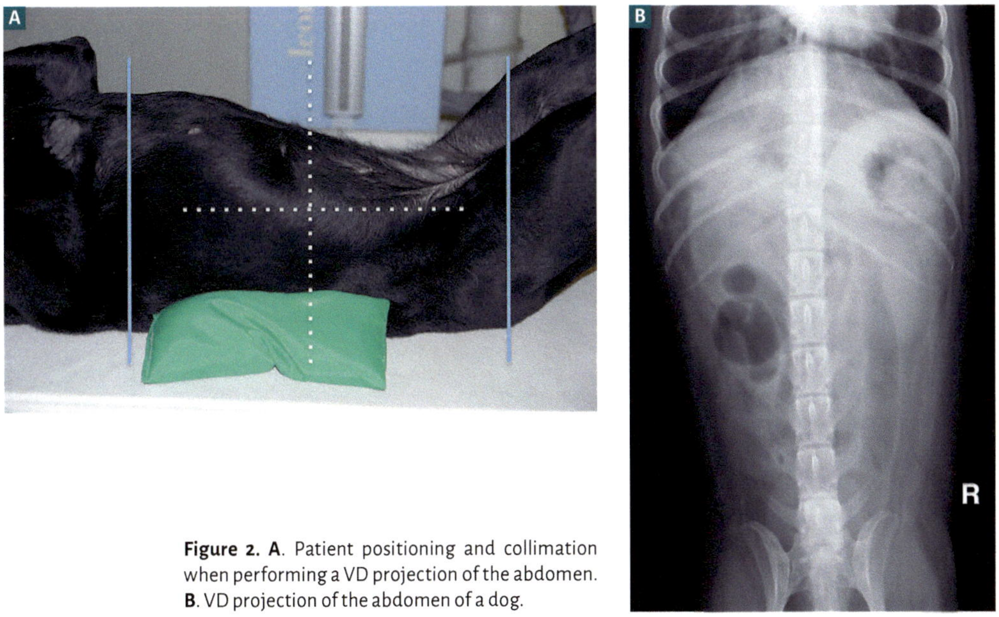

Figure 2. A. Patient positioning and collimation when performing a VD projection of the abdomen. **B**. VD projection of the abdomen of a dog.

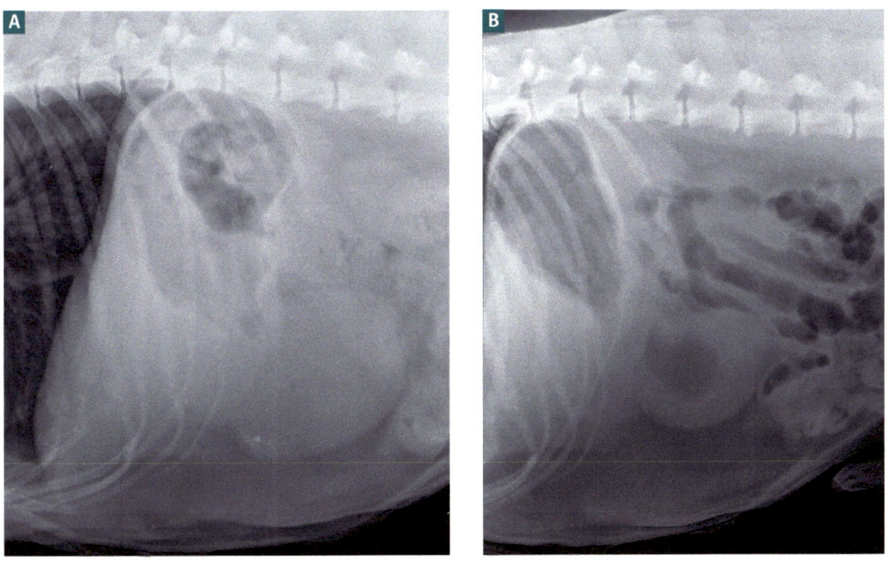

Figure 3. A. Right lateral projection of the cranial abdomen of a dog. The pyloric antrum is visualised as a rounded mass of soft tissue opacity in the cranioventral abdomen, which should not be interpreted as an abdominal (e.g. splenic) mass. **B**. Left lateral projection of the cranial abdomen of the same animal; the pyloric antrum contains gas.

Lateral projections are very helpful when it comes to differentiating gastric contents, because the position of the gas and liquid inside the stomach varies in the different projections. In a right lateral projection, the gas will accumulate in the gastric fundus, as it is the most dorsally located structure, while the liquid accumulates in the pyloric antrum, which is located ventrally, resulting in a rounded structure with the appearance of a mass in the cranioventral abdomen (Fig. 3 A). In contrast, in a left lateral projection, the gas will be located in the pyloric antrum (Fig. 3 B).

The **DV projection** (Fig. 4) of the abdomen is obtained in cases where it is impossible to perform a VD projection. It is also useful for differentiating the gastric contents because, as occurs with lateral projections, the gas and liquid in the stomach change position with the effect of gravity. On a DV projection, the gas will be lodged in the gastric fundus and the fluid will accumulate in the pylorus (Thrall, 2018).

Abdominal radiographs made with the beam horizontal are useful to confirm the presence of free gas. To obtain these, it is necessary to have an X-ray machine that allows rotation by 90° with respect to the vertical axis. A VD radiograph can be made with the beam horizontal and with the animal in left lateral recumbency (Fig. 5). With the animal in this position, free gas accumulates along the right abdominal wall, just below the costal arch. Performing this projection with the animal in right lateral recumbency is not recommended

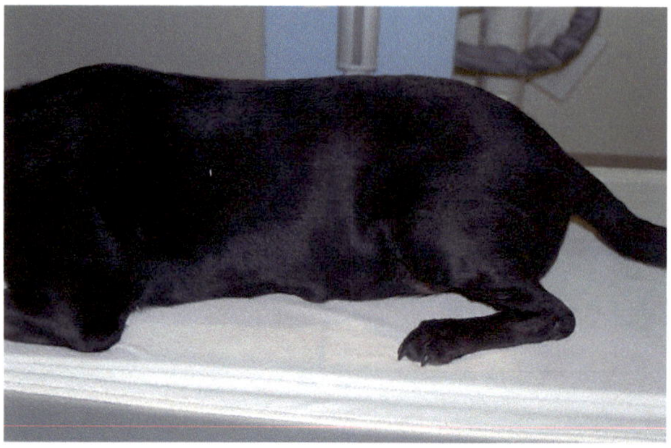

Figure 4. Patient positioning for performing a DV projection of the abdomen. Both hindlimbs should be positioned to the sides of the abdomen and as far away from it as possible to avoid overlap.

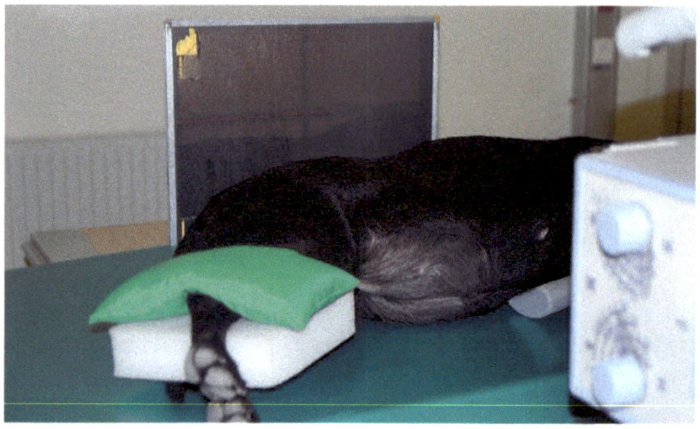

Figure 5. Patient positioning when performing a VD radiograph of the abdomen with the X-ray beam horizontal. The animal is in left lateral recumbency. This position is used to detect small amounts of free gas in the peritoneal space.

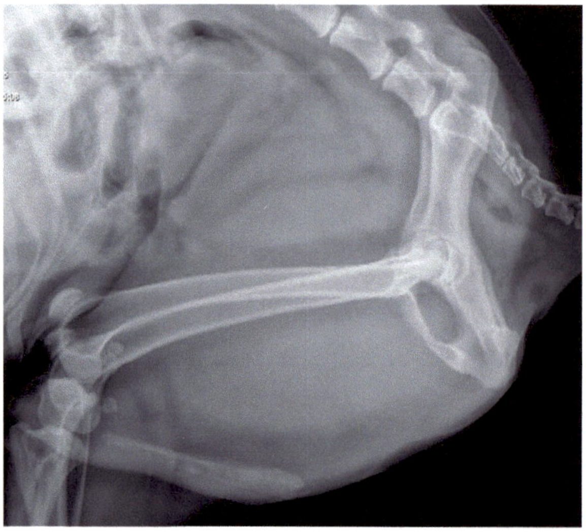

Figure 6. Lateral radiograph of the caudal abdomen with the patient's hindlimbs positioned cranially to allow visualisation of the path of the urethra. Note the calculi at the level of the penile urethra.

because in this position the fundus of the stomach is below the costal arch and, if it contains gas, it could hide or hinder the visualisation of free gas. A left lateral projection can also be performed with the animal in dorsal recumbency. In this position, the free gas will accumulate between the liver, the diaphragm and the ventral abdominal wall, allowing it to be identified (Thrall, 2018). However, a left lateral projection has recently been shown experimentally to be similar to projections obtained with the beam horizontal to diagnose the presence of small amounts of free gas in the abdomen in dogs (Ng et al., 2020).

If the urinary system is to be evaluated in dogs, a radiograph of the caudal abdomen should be performed with the hindlimbs positioned cranially to allow visualisation of both the membranous and penile portions of the urethral pathway (Fig. 6).

Radiographs can be performed with the application of compression, for example, with a wooden spatula, to separate overlapping abdominal structures. This technique is particularly useful when differentiating urinary calculi from small foreign bodies of mineral opacity located in the small or large intestine, which may overlap with the organs of the urinary system (Fig. 7).

When performing abdominal radiography, it is advisable to use a **low kVp and a high mAs**, to obtain an image with few shades of grey and greater contrast between black and white (see Chapter 1). If the abdomen is more than 10 cm thick, the antiscatter grid should be used to avoid scattered radiation (Thrall, 2018).

Once the radiographs have been made, it is important to check that the radiographic technique was correct. To do this, the following points are evaluated:

1. **The mAs is suitable if → the background looks black and grainless.**
2. **The kVp is adequate if → the bony trabeculae of the lumbar vertebrae are visible.**
3. **Collimation is adequate if → the entire abdomen is included, with the X-ray beam centred in the middle of the abdomen.**
4. **There is no rotation.**
5. **There is no movement.**
6. **The hindlimbs do not overlap the abdomen.**
7. **The right and left markers have been included.**
8. **It has been checked that patient preparation was adequate (e.g. fasting, enema) for what needs to be assessed.**

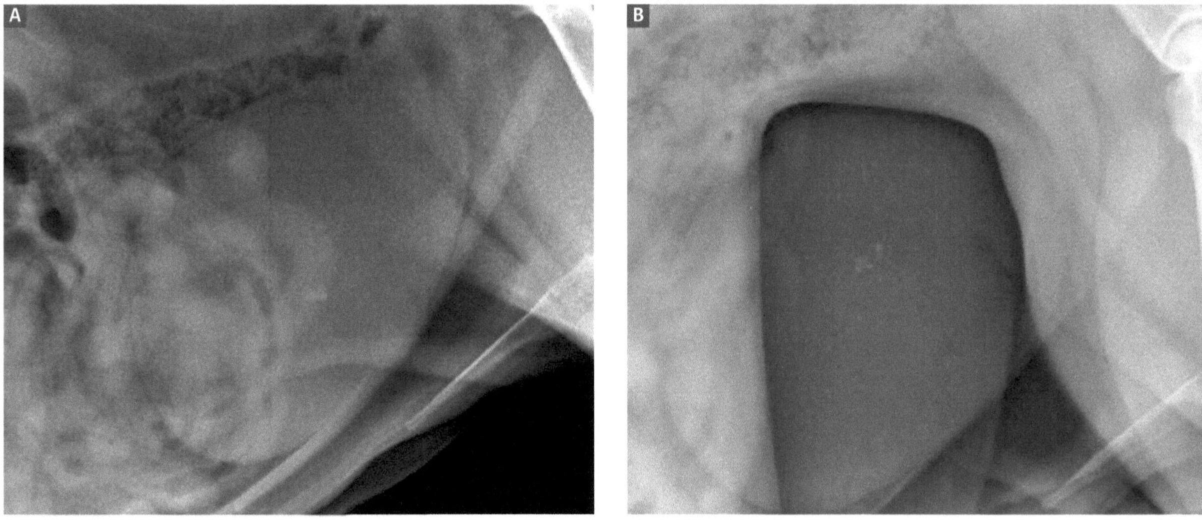

Figure 7. A. Lateral radiograph of the caudal abdomen. A slight irregular mineralisation is observed in the middle aspect of the urinary bladder where several intestinal loops are overlapping. **B**. Lateral radiograph of the caudal abdomen in the same patient obtained while applying compression with a wooden spatula over the urinary bladder to move the overlapping intestinal loops away from the bladder. This image confirms that the mineralisations are urinary calculi.

Computed Tomography of the Abdomen

The main applications of computed tomography (CT) in the abdomen are as follows:

- diagnosis and characterisation of portosystemic shunts (PSS) and other vascular anomalies;
- determination of the origin of abdominal masses, as well as the presence of vascular invasion;
- diagnosis and characterisation of ectopic ureters;
- detection of fistular pathways and abscesses associated with migratory foreign bodies; and
- evaluation of the pelvic cavity and its various pathologies.

To obtain an optimal CT study of the abdomen, it is important to prepare the patient according to the study to be performed. Fasting for at least 12 hours is recommended. Administration of prestudy enemas is necessary in cases where the urinary system is to be evaluated, in particular the ureters and the ureterovesical junction, as well as for studies of the pelvic cavity. General anaesthesia or deep sedation is required in all cases.

For abdominal studies, the animal is positioned in sternal recumbency with the hindlimbs directed caudally. The study begins with a topogram or scout view, which is composed of two orthogonal radiographs of the abdomen obtained by the CT machine, on which the beginning and end of the study should be defined, as well as the borders of the abdominal cavity (Fig. 8). As with abdominal radiographs, the CT scan

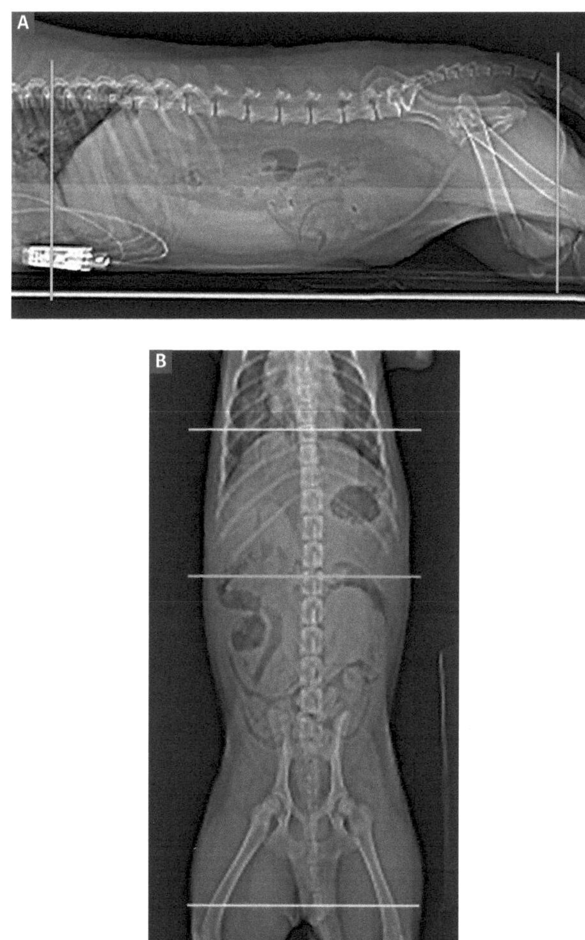

Figure 8. Scout views showing the abdominal cavity boundaries (orange lines) when performing a CT scan. **A**. Lateral view. **B**. DV view.

should include everything from the diaphragmatic dome to the pelvic cavity. The specific technique depends on the organ of interest, but in general a slice thickness of 2–3 mm is recommended in small dogs and cats, and 5–7 mm in large dogs. Images should be processed with both low-frequency (soft tissue or standard) and high-frequency (bone or detail) algorithms (Schwarz and Saunders, 2011).

The use of **intravenous contrast** is essential in abdominal CT studies. For administration of contrast, the catheter should always be placed in the forelimbs, never in the hindlimbs; this is particularly important in vascular studies. A nonionic iodinated contrast medium is used at a dose of 600 mg I/kg, followed by a bolus of physiological saline. The postcontrast series is obtained 60–90 seconds after injection of the contrast medium.

CT **angiography** consists of performing postcontrast series at different times with the aim of enhancing different vascular structures. Angiography can be dual or triple phase depending on the number of phases included in the study:

1. arterial phase
2. portal or venous phase
3. washout phase.

To perform CT angiography correctly, the use of an automatic injector to administer the contrast is essential. The dose used for these studies is 800 mg I/kg. The most widely used techniques to determine the timing of the different vascular phases (arterial and portal) are the use of a bolus test and the bolus tracking technique. The choice of one or the other will depend on the characteristics of the CT machine.

a. The **bolus test technique** consists of the administration of a small bolus of contrast (185 mg I/kg), after which the time it takes for the contrast to reach the aorta and portal vein is measured (Fig. 9). Subsequently, this time is used as a preset during the acquisition of the images in the arterial and portal phases, respectively. The washout phase is obtained 1 minute after the portal phase.
b. The **bolus tracking technique** consists of defining the start time of the vascular study once the contrast has reached a certain concentration in the vessels of interest (aorta and portal vein) (Thierry et al., 2018).

Breathing control is essential when performing a vascular study of the abdomen because the vessels of interest are usually close to the diaphragm and the movement of the diaphragm with respiration may result in a nondiagnostic study. The technique that is normally used for breathing control is hyperventilation of the anaesthetised animal, which causes apnoea for approximately 30–60 seconds, allowing the study to be performed.

Images of the abdomen are visualised using a narrow window for soft tissue assessment —window width (WW): 300–400 Hounsfield units (HU); window level (WL): 40 HU— and a wide window for assessment of mineralised structures (e.g. calculi) and osseous structures, as well as lung tissue included in the study (WW: 1500 HU; WL: 300 HU). Sagittal and dorsal reconstructions are useful for evaluating lesions identified on cross-sectional images.

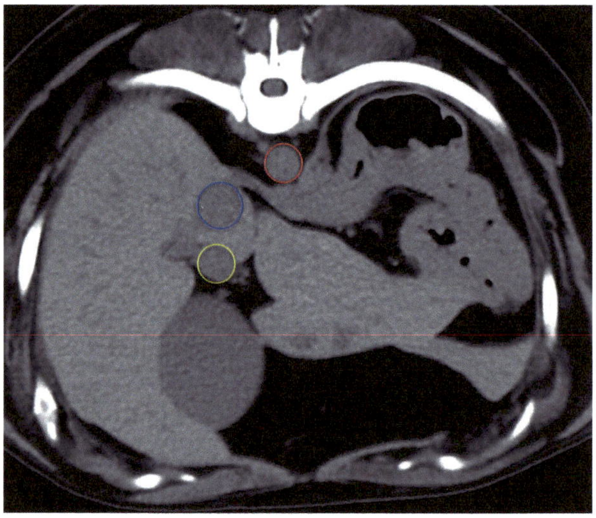

Figure 9. Location of the portal vein (yellow circle), caudal vena cava (blue circle) and aorta (red circle) in a precontrast study at the level of the hepatic hilum.

Abdominal Cavity

All abdominal organs have a similar opacity (soft/liquid tissue), so the way to differentiate them from each other on a radiograph is by the presence of intra-abdominal fat, which has a lower opacity.

The term **good serosal definition** is used when the contrast between the fat and soft tissue of the organs in the abdomen makes the serosal surfaces of the different organs visible (Fig. 10 A). The amount of intra-abdominal fat depends on the patient's age and body condition. If there is not a large amount of intra-abdominal fat, as occurs in very thin or cachectic animals (Fig. 10 B) and in puppies, the differentiation of the serosa from the organs is considerably poorer. In addition, physiologically, puppies have a small amount of free fluid at the peritoneal level and their intra-abdominal fat is brown (unlike the yellow fat in adults), which has a higher water content; together this contributes to poor definition of the serosa (Fig. 10 C). In obese cats (Fig. 10 D), on the other hand, a large amount of fat is deposited in the

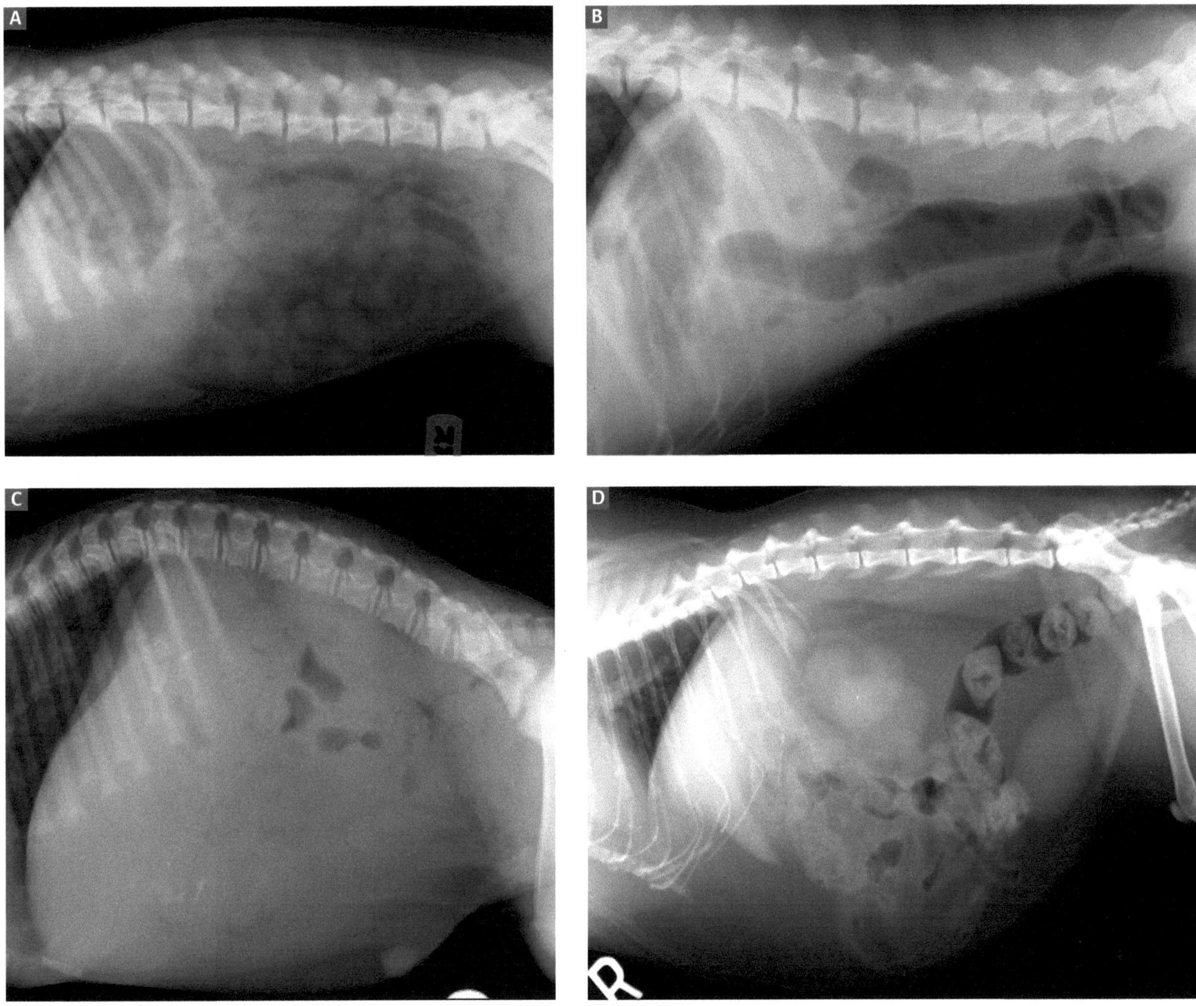

Figure 10. Abdominal radiographs. **A**. A dog with normal serosal definition. **B**. A thin dog. **C**. A puppy. **D**. An obese cat.

falciform ligament (extraperitoneal), the mesentery and the omentum (intraperitoneal), and in the retroperitoneal space, facilitating visualisation of the abdominal organs.However, this large amount of abdominal fat makes it difficult for the loops of the small intestine to move with equal freedom, and they remain "piled up" in the ventral, middle and right areas of the abdomen. The accumulation of fat at the level of the falciform ligament can cause a mass effect in the cranioventral abdomen.

Peritoneal Space

The **peritoneum** is a serosal membrane that is divided into parietal (in contact with the abdominal wall) and visceral (in contact with the organs) parts. Abdominal organs that are surrounded by the visceral peritoneum are considered intraperitoneal and include the liver, gallbladder, spleen, stomach, small intestine, large intestine, pancreas and ovaries. The **peritoneal cavity** is the space between the two layers of the peritoneum.

Loss of Serosal Visualisation or Increased Soft Tissue Opacity

Loss of serosal visualisation is usually accompanied by increased soft tissue opacity of the peritoneal cavity resulting in a loss of intra-abdominal definition and visualisation of the serosal surfaces of the different organs. Differentiation between whether these changes are generalised or localised is important, in addition to whether the increase in opacity is homogeneous or heterogeneous (Table 1).

Table 1. Interpretation algorithm for the loss of visualisation of the serosa in the peritoneal cavity.

	Generalised	Localised
Homogeneous	· Effusion · Puppy · Thin or cachectic animal	· Mass
Heterogeneous	· Mild effusion · Steatitis · Peritonitis · Carcinomatosis	· Mild effusion · Steatitis · Peritonitis · Carcinomatosis · Artefact (e.g. wet hair)

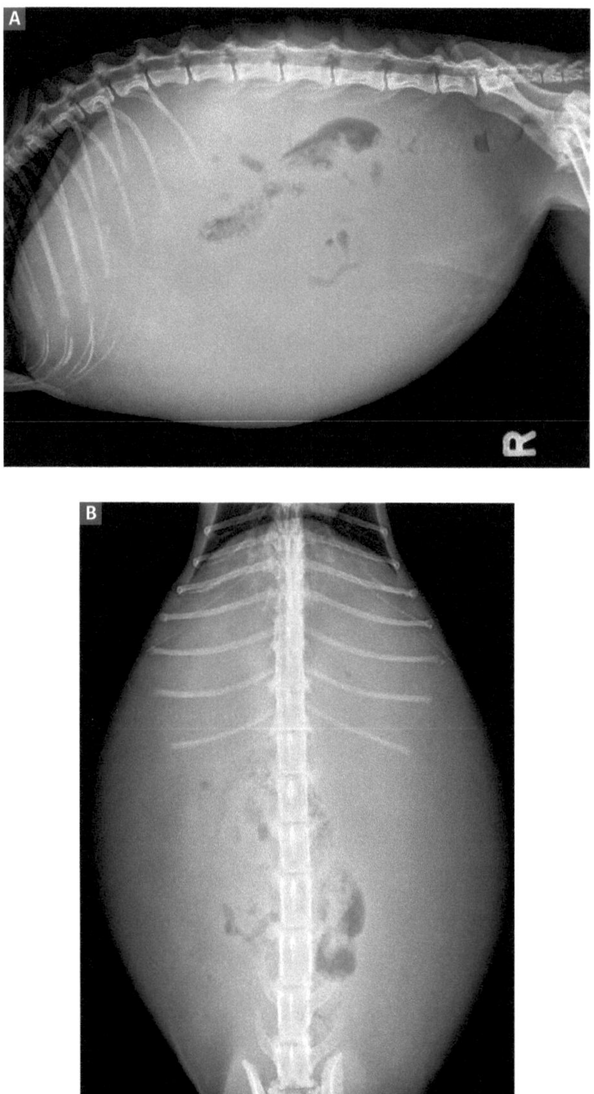

Figure 11. Peritoneal effusion. Lateral (**A**) and VD (**B**) projections of the abdomen of a cat with feline infectious peritonitis. A generalised loss of serosal definition and a homogeneous increase in the opacity of the abdominal cavity are visualised.

The main **causes of loss of serosal visualisation are as follows.**

- The presence of free fluid (**peritoneal effusion**). A large volume of free fluid in the abdominal cavity causes a homogeneous increase in the opacity of the peritoneum, a generalised loss of visualisation of the serous surfaces and abdominal distension (Fig. 11). Sometimes cranial displacement of the diaphragm is also observed. A small amount of free fluid usually causes a localised increase in opacity and a heterogeneous appearance of the peritoneum. However, it must be taken into account that the degree of loss of serosal visualisation will depend not only on the amount of free fluid but also on the ratio of fluid to fat in the abdomen: the greater the amount of fat, the greater the amount of free fluid necessary to cause complete obliteration of the serosa, for example, in obese animals.
- **Steatitis, peritonitis** and **carcinomatosis**. Steatitis refers to inflammation of fat, such as in cases of pancreatitis, which can lead to saponification and fat necrosis. Peritonitis is inflammation of the peritoneum secondary to an infectious cause. Carcinomatosis refers to the presence of metastases of any origin at the peritoneal level. Radiographically, in all cases a focal loss of serosal definition and a heterogeneous increase in peritoneal opacity are observed, similar to that seen with the presence of a small amount of peritoneal effusion, making radiographic differentiation impossible in these cases (Fig. 12). Occasionally, the peritoneum may acquire a miliary nodular appearance.

The distribution of these changes is crucial when establishing possible differential diagnoses. For example, in cases of severe pancreatitis with steatitis of the surrounding fat,

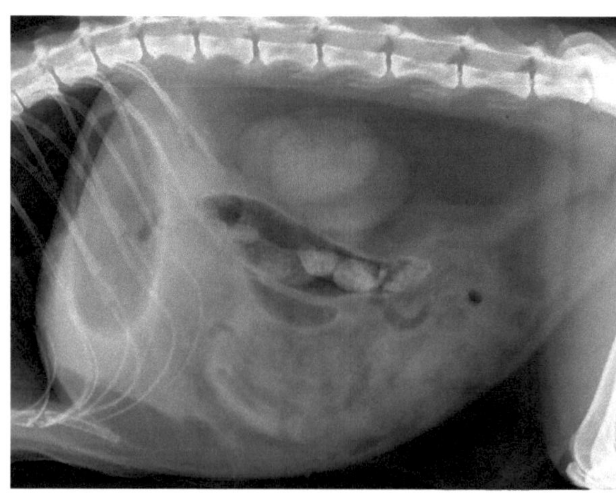

Figure 12. Focal loss of serosal definition and heterogeneous increase in the opacity of the ventral and middle aspects of the peritoneal cavity. Lateral projection of the abdomen of a cat with a ruptured gallbladder.

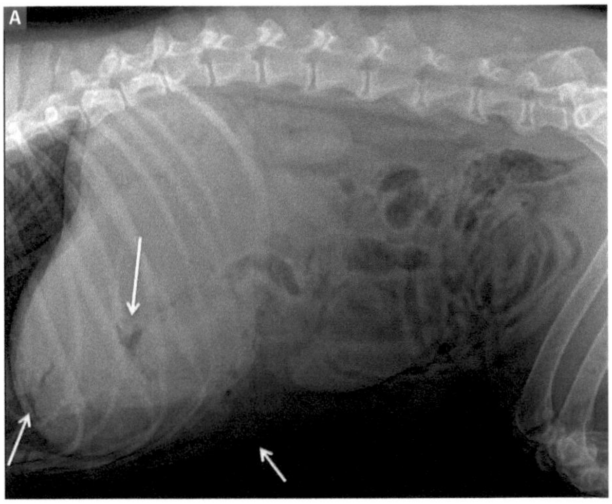

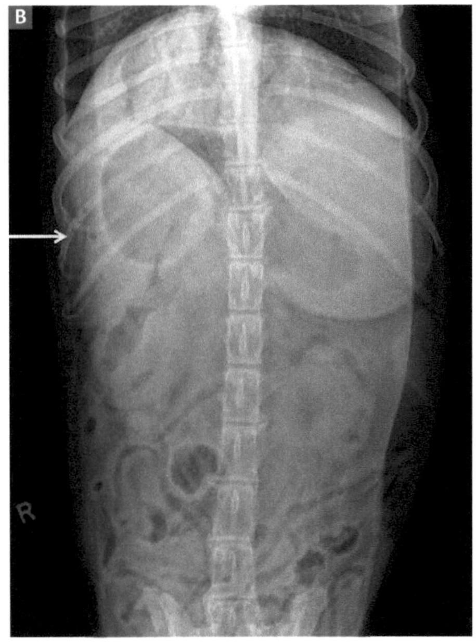

Figure 13. Pneumoperitoneum. Lateral (**A**) and VD (**B**) projections of the abdomen of a dog with intestinal perforation. Irregular areas of gas opacity are observed immediately adjacent to the abdominal wall or in the cranial abdomen between the liver and diaphragm (white arrows).

the changes are usually localised to the right cranial abdomen. A ruptured gallbladder and the presence of biliary peritonitis usually have a similar location. In contrast, in a rupture of the urethra or urinary bladder or prostatitis, changes are localised in the caudal abdomen. It is also important to evaluate whether there is a mass effect, since it may be masked by the presence of free fluid. The intestinal loops are usually floating in the free fluid and are usually located in the central abdomen; by contrast, if there is an abdominal mass in addition to the free fluid, the small intestinal loops are the first to undergo changes in their position.

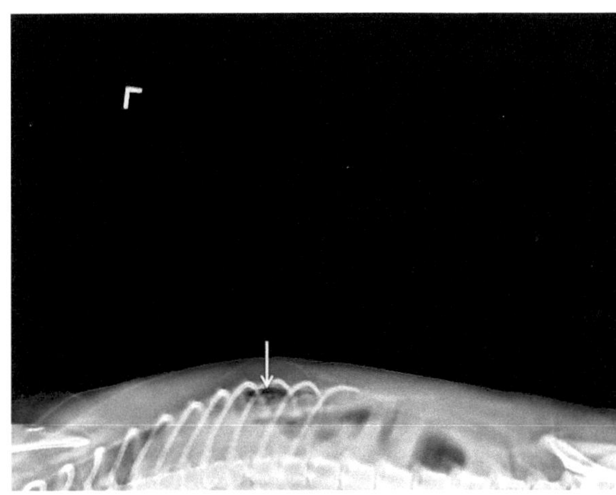

Figure 14. VD projection of the abdomen of a cat with the X-ray beam horizontal and the animal positioned in left lateral recumbency. Note the gas bubble immediately adjacent to the right abdominal wall under the costal arch (arrow).

Gas in the Peritoneal Space (Pneumoperitoneum)

The main causes of pneumoperitoneum are perforation of the digestive tract or abdominal wall, or a recent laparotomy. In the case of the latter, the gas can be visualised radiographically up to 25 days after surgery.

The presence of a large amount of free gas in the peritoneal space causes increased visualisation of the serous surfaces. However, small amounts of peritoneal free gas can be difficult to identify radiographically. Small bubbles of peritoneal free gas can be located in places where the digestive tract would not be expected, such as immediately adjacent to the abdominal wall or in the cranial abdomen, between the liver and the diaphragm (Fig. 13). The morphology of these bubbles can also be useful for their identification: they do not usually have the regular tubular or rounded morphology that is normally seen with gas in the digestive tract. To confirm the presence of pneumoperitoneum, a VD radiograph can be performed with the X-ray beam horizontal and with the animal in left lateral recumbency (Fig. 14), or a left lateral radiograph can be performed with the animal in dorsal recumbency (Frank, 2018).

Mineralisation in the Peritoneal Space

The presence of mineralisation in the abdomen is usually associated with the gastrointestinal, urinary or biliary tract.

Mineralisation of the peritoneum is rare. Where mineralisations in the peritoneum are seen, they are usually dystrophic mineralisations of necrotic mesenteric fat. These are incidental findings with no clinical significance, and they are more frequent in cats than in dogs. Radiographically they appear as mineralised structures which are more radiopaque around the edges than in the centre, with rounded, oval or kidney-shaped morphology (Fig. 15).

Fluid in the Peritoneal Space

CT has a high sensitivity for detecting the presence of free fluid in the peritoneal or retroperitoneal space, and for determining the origin of abdominal bleeding. Measurement of the radiodensity (in HU) of the abdominal fluid allows different types of effusion to be distinguished. Fluids with water-like attenuation, such as bile or urine, have HU values in the range of 0–15 (Fig. 16). Blood causes greater attenuation than these fluids; noncoagulated extravascular blood is usually equivalent to 20–45 HU, while the attenuation of coagulated blood is in the range of 43–70 HU. Tomographic features such as visualisation of a clot, active arterial extravasation or the presence of a triangular area of mesenteric free fluid can help locate the origin of bleeding. Assessment of the presence and location of the "sentinel clot sign" is based on quantification of the HU values of the abdominal fluid to identify which organ is bleeding (Fig. 17). The clot with highest attenuation is located nearest to the bleeding site, whereas the uncoagulated blood with lowest attenuation is located further from the source. Identification of contrast outside the blood vessels when performing a contrast study indicates the presence of active bleeding (Specchi et al., 2017).

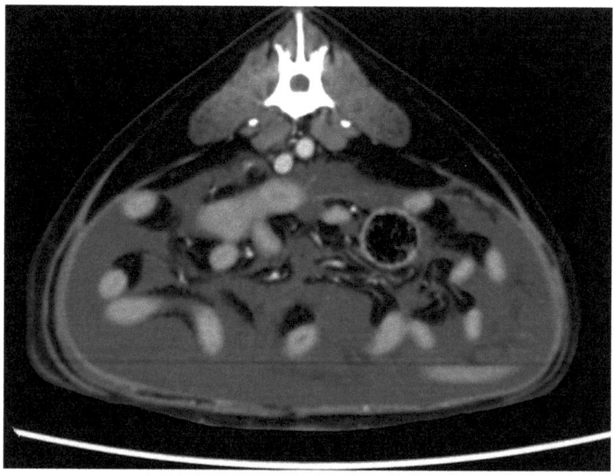

Figure 16. Transverse image of the abdomen of a dog in a soft tissue window (WW: 350 HU, WL: 40 HU) after intravenous contrast administration. A large amount of hypoattenuated free fluid (0–15 HU) is visualised surrounding the intestinal loops and the colon.

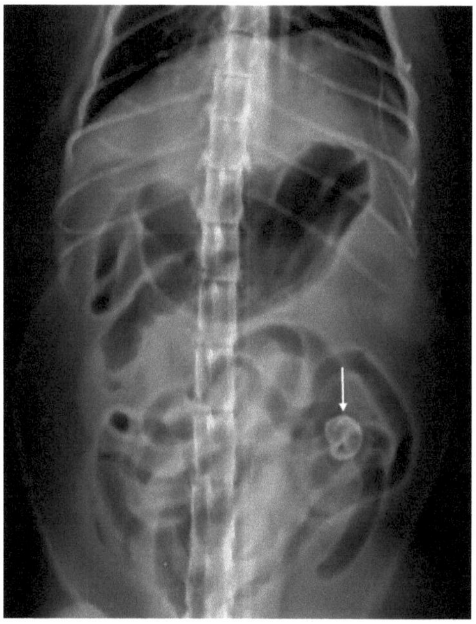

Figure 15. VD projection of the abdomen of a cat. A structure of mineral opacity and kidney-shaped morphology is visualised in the left middle abdomen, compatible with nodular fatty necrosis.

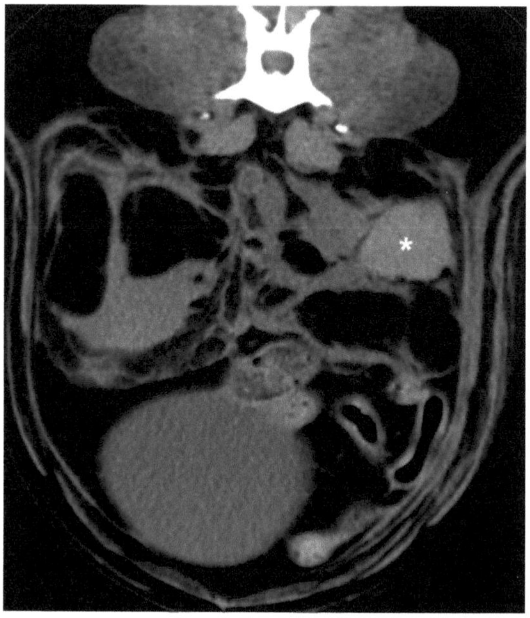

Figure 17. Transverse image of the abdomen of a dog in a soft tissue window (WW: 350 HU, WL: 40 HU). A large amount of free fluid is visualised in the retroperitoneal space. The asterisk indicates the area of greatest attenuation (60 HU), compatible with the signal from the sentinel clot.

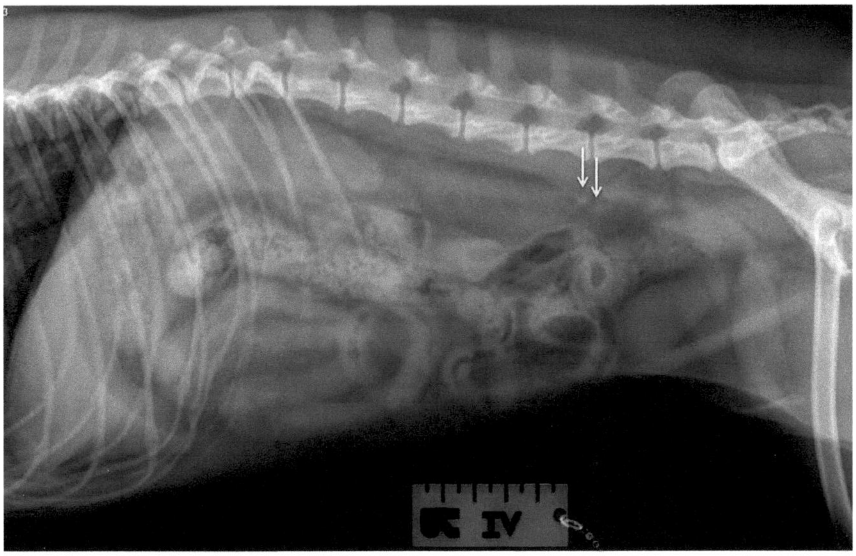

Figure 18. Lateral radiograph showing the deep circumflex iliac arteries and veins in the caudal retroperitoneal space (arrows). Note that the ventral cortex of the L3 and L4 vertebral bodies is slightly less well defined than that of the adjacent vertebrae due to the insertion of the diaphragmatic crura.

Retroperitoneal Space

The retroperitoneum is the space between the dorsal aspect of the parietal peritoneum and the abdominal wall. It extends from the diaphragm to the anus and communicates with the mediastinum and pelvic cavity. The adrenal glands, kidneys, ureters, blood vessels and lymph nodes are located in the retroperitoneum. All of these structures, with the exception of the kidneys, are small in size and not visible radiographically. Occasionally, lateral radiographs may show one or two focal radiopacities in the caudal retroperitoneum that correspond to the deep circumflex iliac arteries and veins (branches of the abdominal aorta and caudal vena cava, respectively), and these should not be misinterpreted as ureteral calculi (Fig. 18) (Thrall and Robertson, 2011). The ventral cortex of the L3 and L4 vertebrae is usually less well defined than that of the adjacent vertebrae, particularly in large dogs, due to the insertion of the diaphragmatic crura. This appearance is normal and should not be confused with aggressive bone injury (Fig. 18) (Thrall and Robertson, 2011). The retroperitoneal space is sometimes difficult to assess using radiography but can be assessed with CT.

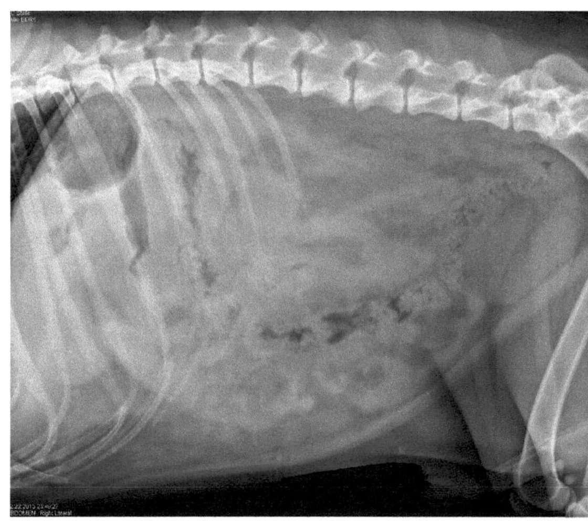

Figure 19. Lateral radiograph showing the appearance of a retroperitoneal effusion. Note the heterogeneous increase in opacity of the retroperitoneal space, with loss of visualisation of the renal silhouettes and the sublumbar musculature.

Loss of Serosal Visualisation and Increased Soft Tissue Opacity

The presence of free fluid in the peritoneum generally causes a heterogeneous image with alternating lines of soft tissue and fat opacity, and loss of visualisation of the renal silhouette and sublumbar musculature. It can also ventrally displace the loops of the small intestine and colon (Fig. 19). The most frequent causes of retroperitoneal effusion (without concurrent peritoneal effusion) are the presence of haemorrhage (e.g. associated with neoplasia or trauma) or urine (due to rupture of the urinary tract). Other causes of increased opacity in the retroperitoneal space include neoplasms (e.g. haemangiosarcoma) and migrating foreign bodies.

Gas in the Retroperitoneal Space (Pneumoretroperitoneum)

The presence of gas in the retroperitoneal space is rare and is usually a consequence of the extension of gas from the mediastinum through the aortic hiatus. Other causes include penetrating wounds, migrating foreign bodies or recent surgery. Gas in the retroperitoneal space can be identified radiographically on lateral projections by the visualisation of structures, such as the abdominal aorta, that would not otherwise be visible.

Mineralisation in the Retroperitoneal Space

Retroperitoneal mineralisation can occur in the adrenal glands, urinary system (nephroliths or ureteroliths) and large vessels. Mineralisation of the adrenal glands is usually bilateral and an incidental finding in cats (Fig. 20), whereas in dogs it may be associated with neoplasia. Aortic wall mineralisation is associated with chronic renal failure, hypervitaminosis D, hyperparathyroidism, hypercalcaemia or (in cats) hypertension.

Abdominal Masses

The radiographic evaluation of abdominal masses on a radiograph is based on the following points.

1. Description of the mass, including the five radiographic signs: opacity, size, morphology, number and edges.
2. Evaluation of the abdominal structures that are displaced by the mass ("mass effect").
3. Location of the mass in the abdomen and knowledge of which organs usually occupy that area.

The mass effect is the change in position of the adjacent structures caused by a mass. In the abdomen, the most mobile organs, such as the loops of the small intestine or the kidneys, are the first to be displaced due to the presence of a mass. To determine the origin of the mass, it is essential to locate the mass in the abdomen and know which organs usually occupy that area. To do this, the abdomen should be divided into quadrants. Thus, in the lateral projection the abdomen should be divided into five areas: cranial, medial, caudal, dorsal and ventral. In the VD projection, the abdomen is divided into cranial, middle, caudal, right and left. Depending on the location of the mass in these quadrants, the possible origin can be established (Agut and Soler, 2014). The organs occupying the different quadrants are shown in Tables 2 A and 2 B. Differential diagnoses of an abdominal mass include neoplasia, abscess, haematoma, cyst and granuloma. In most cases it is not possible to differentiate between these radiographically, however, sometimes, a mass with gas opacity, such as an abscess, or with fatty opacity, such as a lipoma, can be visualised.

CT is a very useful technique for the evaluation of abdominal masses and determination of their origin. It is also considered the technique of choice for the evaluation not only of abdominal masses but of the abdomen in general in large dogs and large breeds (>25 kg), in which radiographic and ultrasonographic evaluation of the abdomen is a challenge (Fields et al., 2012). In addition, it allows the evaluation of adjacent structures and determination of whether there is vascular invasion or the presence of metastasis.

Abdominal Wall

The abdominal wall is formed by the external and internal oblique abdominal muscles and the transverse abdominal muscle.

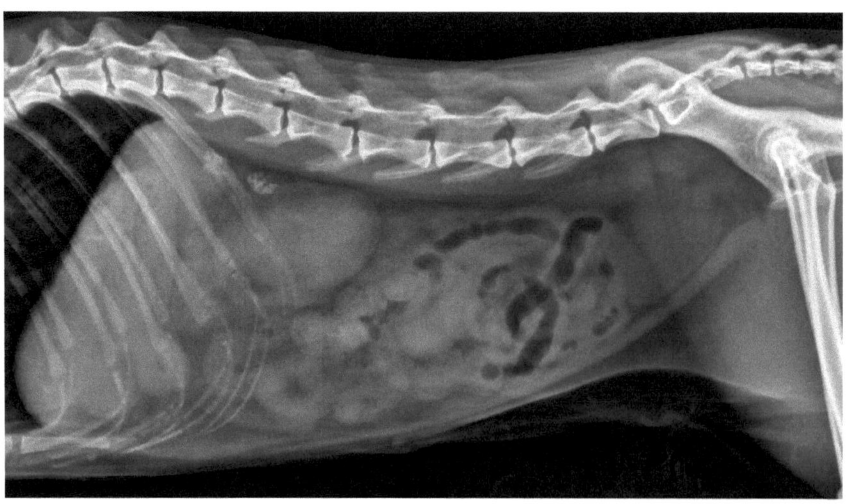

Figure 20. Lateral radiograph of the abdomen of a cat. Two heterogeneous and irregular areas of mineralisation are observed in the dorsocranial aspect of the retroperitoneal space that correspond to mineralisation of the adrenal glands.

Table 2 A. Origin of abdominal masses according to their position on lateral radiographs.

	Generalised	Localised	Caudal
Dorsal	· Liver · Spleen · Kidneys · Adrenal glands · Stomach	· Spleen · Digestive tract · Pancreas · Uterus · Ovaries · Testes · Mesentery · Lymph nodes	· Sublumbar lymph nodes · Colon · Ureters
Ventral	· Liver · Gallbladder · Spleen · Stomach · Pancreas		· Bladder · Uterus · Prostate · Testes

Table 2 B. Origin of abdominal masses according to their position on VD radiographs.

	Cranial	Middle	Caudal
Left	· Liver · Stomach · Head of the spleen · Left kidney · Left adrenal gland	· Spleen · Digestive tract · Pancreas · Uterus · Ovaries · Testes · Mesentery · Lymph nodes	· Sublumbar lymph nodes · Colon · Ureters · Bladder · Uterus · Prostate · Testes
Right	· Liver · Gallbladder · Spleen · Stomach · Duodenum · Pancreas · Right kidney · Right adrenal gland		

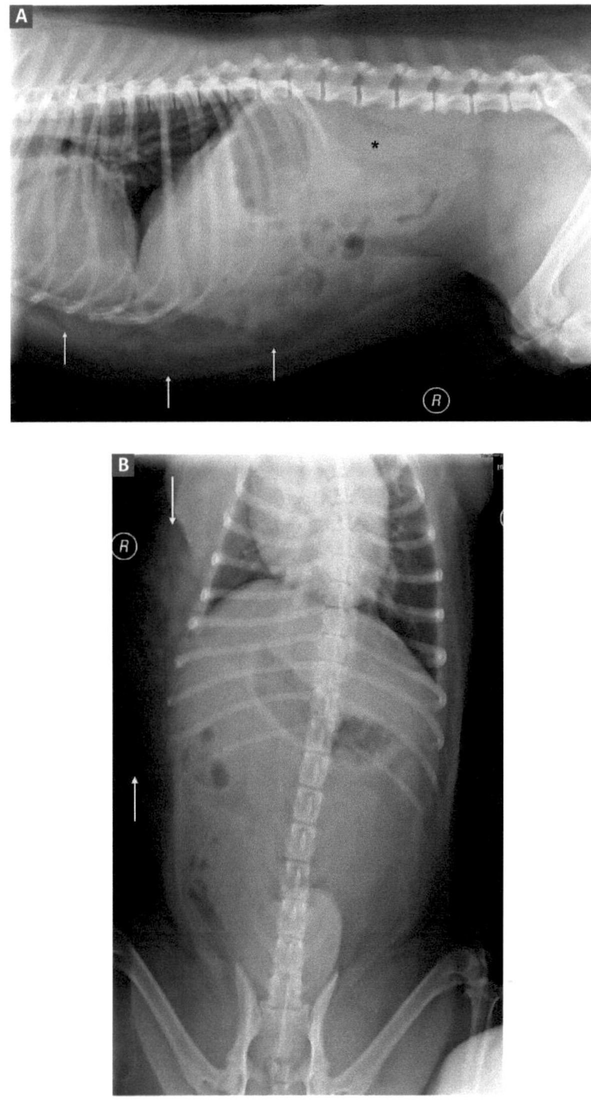

Figure 21. Lateral (**A**) and VD (**B**) radiographs of the abdomen of a dog with an abdominal wall rupture. Note the subcutaneous herniation of the loops of the small intestine (arrows) and the retroperitoneal effusion (asterisk).

The external oblique muscle can be identified by the presence of fat on both sides of it. The internal oblique and transverse muscles are visualised as a continuation of the rib cage. The most frequent pathologies of the abdominal wall are hernias and traumatic tears (Fig. 21). Displacement of abdominal organs through defects in the abdominal wall can be identified radiographically but is better assessed by ultrasonography or CT. The most easily displaced organs are the loops of the small intestine and the urinary bladder, along with the omentum. The presence of gas with a rounded or tubular morphology in these types of abdominal wall defects may indicate the presence of small intestinal loops. However, sometimes it is difficult to differentiate them from other causes of the presence of gas such as penetrating wounds or abscesses, although in these cases the appearance of the gas is usually irregular and heterogeneous.

Abdominal Lymph Nodes

The abdominal lymph nodes are divided into two groups.

1. **Parietal**: these are retroperitoneal and include the renal, aortic lumbar, medial iliac, internal iliac and sacral lymph nodes. They drain into the lumbar lymphatic trunk, which ends in the cisterna chyli. The medial iliac lymph nodes are the largest. They are located at the bifurcation of the abdominal aorta ventral to the L6 and L7 vertebrae. They drain the urogenital tract, pelvis and hindlimbs.
2. **Visceral**: these include the peritoneal and hepatic, splenic, gastric, pancreaticoduodenal, jejunal and colic lymph nodes.

Normal abdominal lymph nodes are not visible on radiographs. However, enlargement of the medial iliac lymph nodes is easy to identify radiographically as masses in the caudal retroperitoneum, ventral to L6–L7.

Liver

The liver is the largest organ in the abdominal cavity. It is located in the cranial abdomen, just caudal to the diaphragm, and cranial to the stomach, pancreas, transverse colon and right kidney.

The liver is located mostly within the costal arch. On a right lateral radiograph of the abdomen, its caudoventral margin, which corresponds to the left lateral lobe, extends slightly caudal to the costal arch (Fig. 22). However, its position may vary slightly depending on the respiratory phase, age, breed and thoracic conformation of the animal, and the amount of fat in the falciform ligament. In deep-chested animals, it is located entirely within the costal arch. In animals with a large amount of fat in the falciform ligament, the liver may be displaced dorsally. In puppies, the caudoventral margin of the liver generally extends more caudal to the costal arch physiologically because the size of the liver relative to body weight is greater than in adults. The caudoventral margin of the liver has regular edges and angular morphology. In cats, the ventral margin of the liver may sometimes appear rounded as a result of the overlap of the gallbladder. Liver lobes cannot be differentiated on radiographs, although sometimes they can be separated and visualised better if there is a large amount of fat between them.

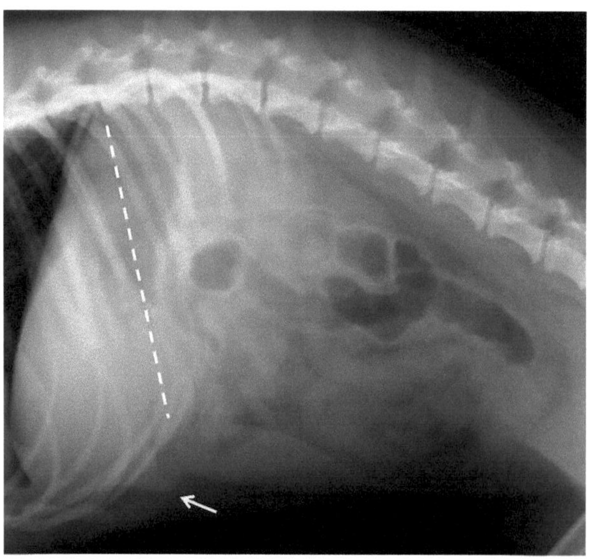

Figure 22. Lateral radiograph of the abdomen of a dog showing the normal size and position of the liver in this species. The dotted line marks the gastric axis. The arrow points to the caudoventral margin of the liver.

Changes in Liver Size

Increased Size (Hepatomegaly)

Liver size can be assessed by the position of the gastric axis. This axis is an imaginary line extending from the gastric fundus to the pyloric antrum. It is usually perpendicular to the thoracolumbar spine, where the gastric axis intersects with it (Fig. 22).

Hepatomegaly can be focal or generalised.

- **Generalised hepatomegaly**: a caudal displacement of the gastric axis occurs. It may be accompanied by dorsal displacement of the pyloric antrum and other adjacent organs. The caudoventral angle of the liver is usually rounded and protrudes more caudally from the costal arch. It is a very frequent and nonspecific radiographic sign. Causes of generalised hepatomegaly include venous congestion (right congestive heart failure), steroid liver disease (endocrinopathies such as Cushing's disease or diabetes, or iatrogenic), neoplasia (lymphoma, mastocytoma, histiocytic sarcoma, haemangiosarcoma, metastasis), acute hepatitis, severe nodular hyperplasia, lipidosis (in cats), feline infectious peritonitis, cholestasis and amyloidosis.
- **Focal hepatomegaly**: this is more difficult to assess radiographically. The position of the diaphragm, stomach and spleen helps evaluation of the left side of the liver. The right side of the liver is better assessed in the VD projection, as it causes a displacement of the pylorus towards the left side. Differential diagnoses of focal hepatomegaly include neoplasia (adenoma, carcinoma, haemangiosarcoma, lymphoma, histiocytic sarcoma, biliary cystadenoma, metastasis), granuloma, abscess, cyst, nodular hyperplasia, haematoma and torsion of a hepatic lobe.

Decrease in Size (Microhepatica)

In cases of microhepatica, the body and pylorus of the stomach appear cranially displaced, resulting in cranial displacement of the gastric axis. It should be kept in mind that, in some deep-chested breeds, the liver may normally be present in a relatively cranial and ventral position, and there may be a slight displacement of the gastric axis towards the skull. Decreased liver size usually occurs in cases of PSS, chronic hepatitis and cirrhosis.

Changes in Liver Radiopacity

- **Intrahepatic gas**: gas can enter the liver through the portal or systemic circulation or ascend through the biliary system. When gas appears in the portal vessels, simple radiographs show branching radiotransparent lines in the liver silhouette. The accumulation of gas in the portal system is usually the result of necrosis of the mucosa of the stomach or intestine. Emphysematous cholecystitis causes a build-up of gas in the right cranioventral part of the liver (Fig. 23). Liver abscesses sometimes also contain gas.
- **Liver mineralisation**: focal or multifocal mineralisation of the liver parenchyma may be associated with granulomas, abscesses, haematomas or neoplasms. Choleliths (gallstones) may also be visualised radiographically. The presence of stones in the intrahepatic bile ducts creates a pattern of branching lines of mineral opacity within the parenchyma (Fig. 24).

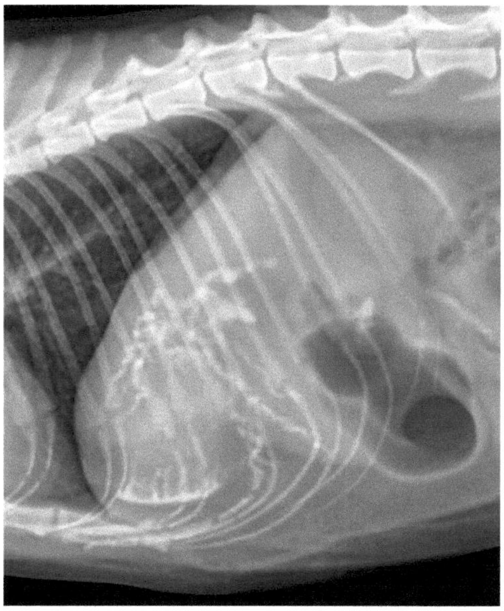

Figure 24. Calculi in the intrahepatic bile ducts. Note the linear, tortuous and branched appearance of mineral opacity structures in the liver area.

Hepatic Masses

CT is the technique of choice for characterising liver masses and determining their origin. The presence of a mass larger than 4.5 cm in diameter on cross-sectional images and with heterogeneous contrast enhancement in the late postcontrast or washout phase suggests the presence of malignancy (Leela-Arporn et al., 2019). Identification of the origin of liver masses is essential to determine whether it is possible to remove them surgically and to plan surgery appropriately. To do this, liver masses are classified into left division (left lateral and medial liver lobes), central (quadrate and right medial lobes) or right division (right caudate and lateral lobes) masses (Lamb et al., 2018).

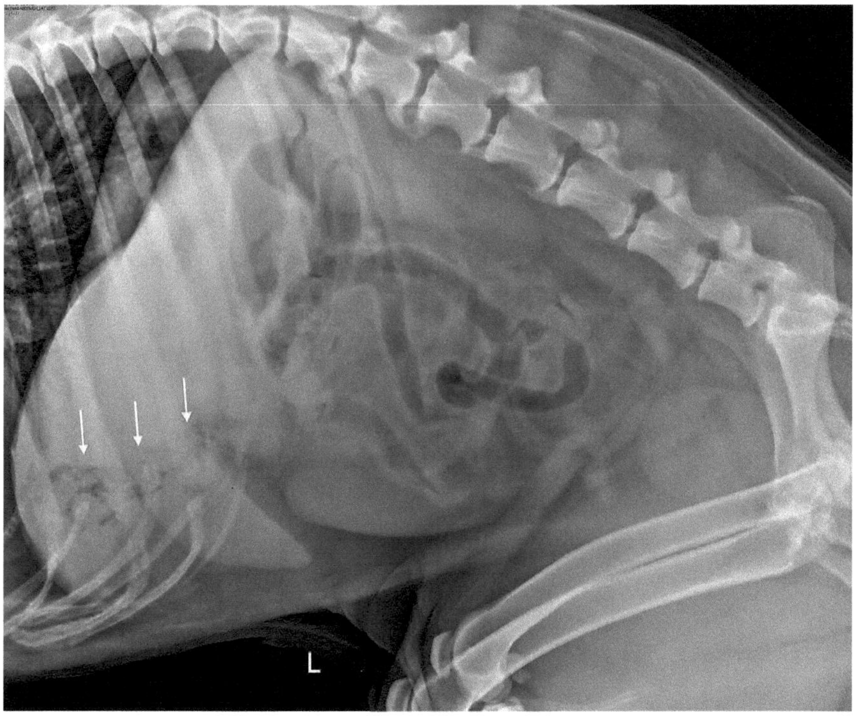

Figure 23. Lateral radiograph of the abdomen of a dog with emphysematous cholecystitis secondary to *Clostridium* infection. Multiple irregular gas bubbles are observed in the cranioventral aspect of the liver.

Criteria to be followed to determine the origin of a liver mass include:

- **any mass to the left of the midline is in the left division;**
- **any mass medial, lateral or dorsal to the portal vein is in the right division;**
- **dorsal displacement of the stomach is usually caused by a left division mass;**
- **displacement of the stomach to the left is usually caused by a right division mass; and**
- **hepatic lobar or portal veins can be used to distinguish right, central or left division masses (Fig. 25).**

Portosystemic Shunts

Radiographs are not specific for the diagnosis of PSS. Indirect signs of PSS that can be visualised on radiographs include a decrease in the size of the liver and the presence of bilateral renomegaly.

CT angiography (with arterial, portal and washout phases) is a rapid, noninvasive technique that allows the identification and characterisation of PSS.

Congenital Portosystemic Shunts

Congenital PSS consist of a single anomalous vessel that connects the portal circulation to the systemic circulation at the extra- or intrahepatic level. CT allows identification of the origin and insertion of the shunt, evaluation of its morphology and course, and assessment of the presence of other associated vascular malformations. General findings include:

- microhepatica
- renomegaly
- calculi in the urinary system
- enlarged and tortuous hepatic arteries
- periportal oedema (Fig. 26)
- reduction of the size of the cranial portal vein at the exit of the shunt or of the intrahepatic portal branches not associated with the shunt.

Depending on their location, congenital PSS can be:

- **extrahepatic**: these are classified according to their morphology, origin and insertion: splenocaval, splenophrenic, splenoazygous (Fig. 26), right gastric-caval, right gastric-caval with caudal shunt loop, and right gastric-azygous with caudal shunt loop (Nelson and Nelson, 2011). Multiple specific variations of PSS that do not fit this general classification have also been described; or
- **intrahepatic**: these are classified as follows (Plested et al., 2020):
  - left division: a tortuous vessel originating from the left portal branch and inserted into the left hepatic vein (HV) or the left phrenic vein

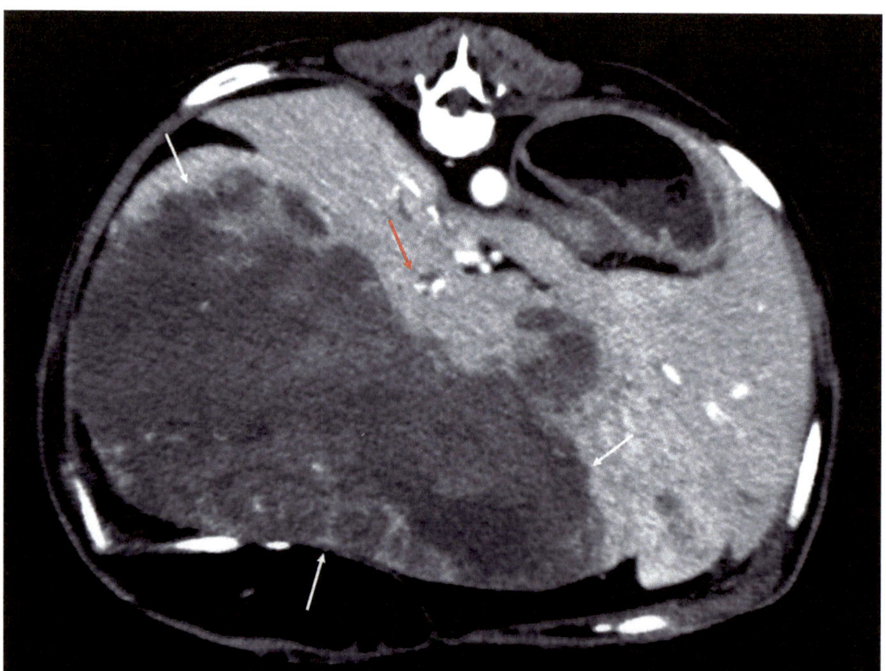

Figure 25. Postcontrast cross-sectional CT image of the abdomen of a dog in a soft tissue window (WW: 350 HU, WL: 40 HU) at the level of the liver. A large mass is visualised in the right medial and caudate lobes of the liver (delineated by the white arrows), which is hypoattenuated with respect to the rest of the liver parenchyma and shows mild, heterogeneous enhancement. The mass is vascularised by the right medial and caudate portal and hepatic veins (red arrow). The definitive diagnosis was hepatocellular carcinoma.

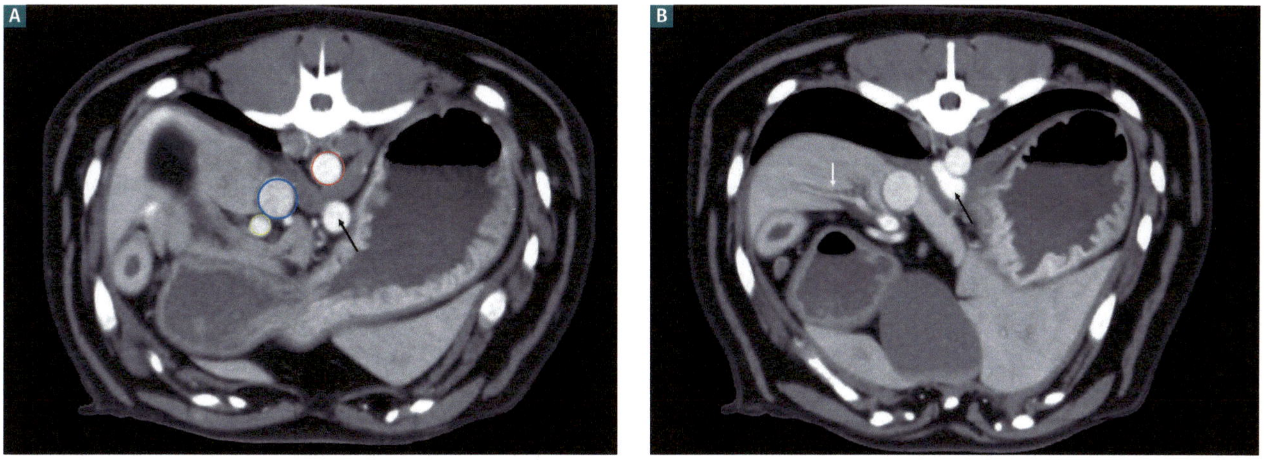

Figure 26. Splenoazygous extrahepatic shunt. **A**. An anomalous vessel (black arrow) of large size is visualised medial to the lesser curvature of the stomach. The yellow circle corresponds to the portal vein, the blue to the caudal vena cava and the red to the aorta. **B**. The shunt (black arrow) is directed dorsally and cranially with an insertion into the azygos vein, located to the right of the aorta in the caudodorsal aspect of the thorax. Note the hypoattenuated halo around the portal vein, compatible with periportal oedema (white arrow). Postcontrast portal phase cross-sectional CT images of the abdomen of a dog in a soft tissue window (WW: 350 HU, WL: 40 HU).

- central division (Fig. 27): connects the left portal branch with the quadrate HV, central HV, right medial dorsal HV or directly with the ventral aspect of the intrahepatic caudal vena cava. A short and very dilated abnormal vessel is visualised in the central portion of the liver
- right division: these are the most common type. These are tortuous vessels that originate from the right portal branch and insert at the level of the right lateral or right quadrate HV.

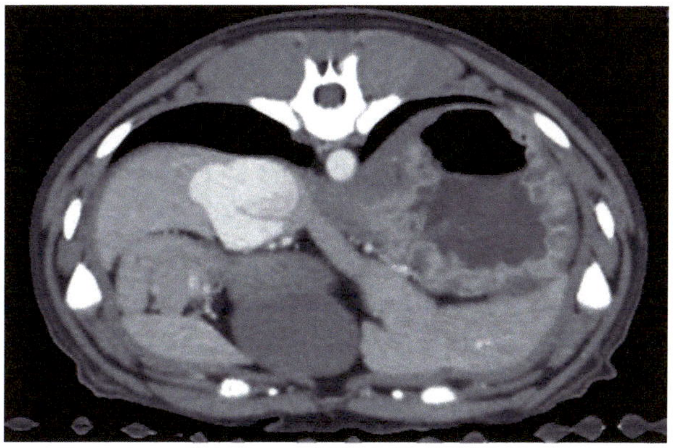

Figure 27. Central division intrahepatic shunt. Postcontrast portal phase cross-sectional CT image of the abdomen of a dog in a soft tissue window (WW: 350 HU, WL: 40 HU).

Acquired Portosystemic Shunts or Acquired Collateral Circulation

This refers to the opening of pre-existing collateral vessels that connect the portal and the systemic circulation (Fig. 28).

Acquired PSS are usually secondary to the presence of portal hypertension, such as in cases of chronic hepatitis or cirrhosis, portal vein hypoplasia or aplasia, portal thrombosis or portal vein compression, although they have also been described in cases of obstruction of the caudal vena cava or splenic vein (Specchi and Bertolini, 2020).

They are usually multiple and are often seen as a nest of very small, tortuous vessels medial and caudal to the left kidney, along the splenic hilum or the root of the mesentery, and at the level of the stomach wall or oesophagus (gastric and oesophageal varicose veins). Large acquired tortuous vessels, such as spleno-gonadal shunts, can also be visualised in animals with portal hypertension (Bertolini, 2010).

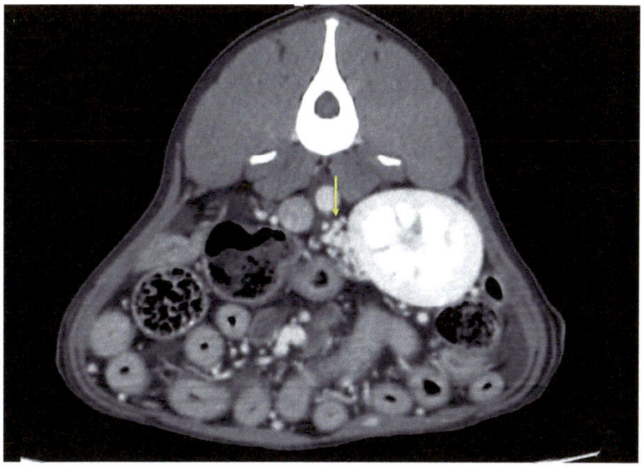

Figure 28. Multiple acquired shunts in the medial aspect of the left kidney. Multiple small, very tortuous vessels are visualised. Postcontrast portal phase cross-sectional CT image of the abdomen of a dog in a soft tissue window (WW: 350 HU, WL: 40 HU).

Spleen

The spleen is a very mobile organ of variable size depending on the species, size and breed of the animal. The head of the spleen is the most fixed part of the organ because it is attached to the stomach by the gastrosplenic ligament. The position of the body and tail of the spleen in the abdomen can vary depending on the degree of distension of the digestive tract or urinary bladder and the conformation of the animal. In the dog, the head of the spleen is visualised on VD radiographs in the left cranial abdomen, caudolateral to the gastric fundus and craniolateral to the left kidney, as a triangular structure with regular, well-defined margins and soft tissue opacity. The tail of the spleen in the dog is usually visualised on lateral radiographs in the cranioventral abdomen, caudal to the liver and pylorus, or in the middle or caudal abdomen, cranial to the bladder (Fig. 29). In the cat, the spleen can be seen on VD radiographs in the same position as in the dog and it sometimes extends along the left abdominal wall. On lateral radiographs, if there is a sufficient amount of intra-abdominal fat, it can be visualised in the craniodorsal abdomen, between the gastric fundus and the left kidney (Fig. 30).

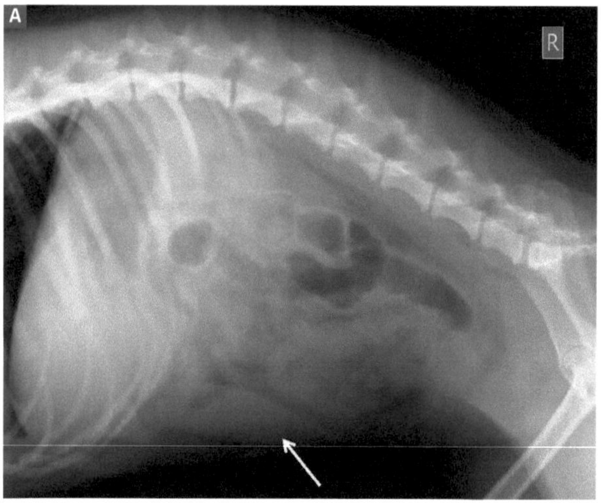

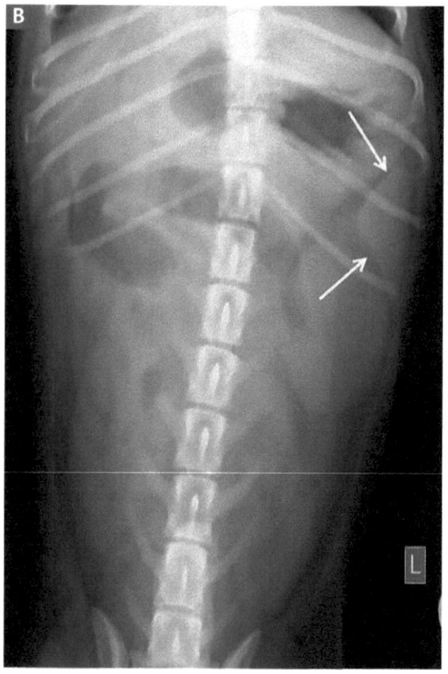

Figure 29. Lateral (**A**) and VD (**B**) radiographs of the abdomen of a dog, indicating the location of the spleen (white arrows).

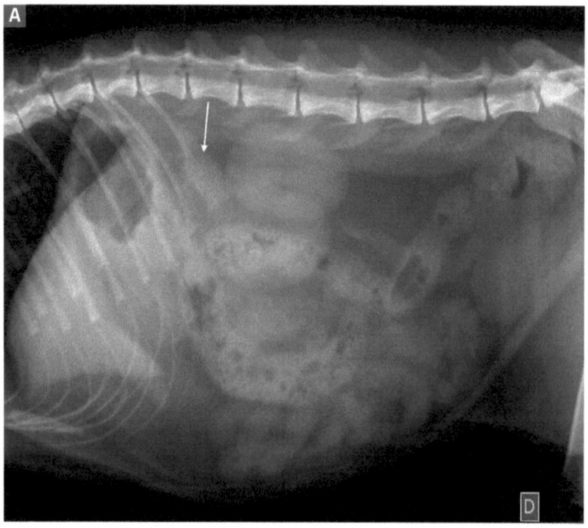

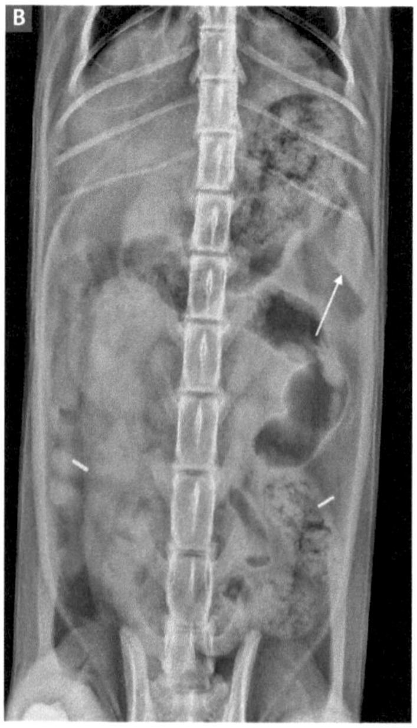

Figure 30. Lateral (**A**) and VD (**B**) radiographs of the abdomen of a cat, indicating the location of the spleen (white arrows).

Assessment of splenic size on radiographs is subjective, especially in the dog, and is generally based on the presence of rounded, mass effect margins on adjacent structures. In the cat, the spleen has less variability in size, and visualisation of the tail of the spleen in the ventral abdomen on a lateral radiograph is considered to be indicative of splenomegaly. The presence of generalised splenomegaly is a nonspecific radiographic finding.

Differential diagnoses include both benign lesions (nodular hyperplasia, extramedullary haematopoiesis, congestion, thrombosis, infarction, portal hypertension, torsion, infection) and malignant lesions (lymphoma, histiocytic sarcoma, mastocytoma, leukaemia, multiple myeloma).

If a **splenic torsion** is present, a significant and generalised increase in the size of the spleen, and an abnormal position of the organ, is observed radiographically. The head of the spleen is generally indistinguishable from its normal position on a VD projection, or a C-shaped soft tissue opacity is observed in the cranial abdomen on both VD and lateral projections. Sometimes it can appear as a mass in the middle of the abdomen. The presence of peritoneal effusion, which is often present in many cases of splenic torsion, may obscure these findings. If splenic necrosis (emphysematous necrosis) also occurs, the presence of gas in the parenchyma may be observed. Splenic torsion may occur primary or secondary to a gastric torsion/volvulus. CT can also be used for the diagnosis of splenic torsion (Fig. 31) (Hughes et al., 2020).

Typical findings include:
- spleen increased in size, with rounded and C-shaped margins
- absence of enhancement in the postcontrast phase
- whirl sign of the splenic hilum with the centre markedly hyperattenuated in the precontrast phase
- peritoneal effusion.

The presence of **focal or multifocal lesions** in the splenic parenchyma on both radiographs and CT is a nonspecific finding, and therefore differential diagnoses may include both benign (e.g. nodular hyperplasia, haematoma) and malignant (primary neoplasia or metastasis) lesions.

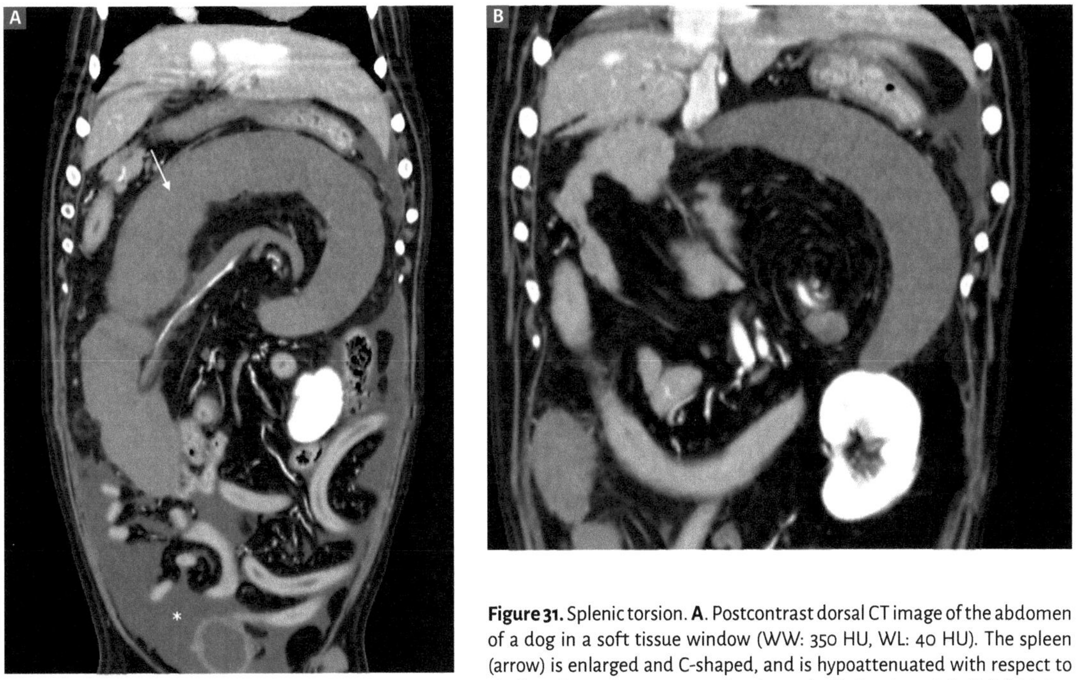

Figure 31. Splenic torsion. **A**. Postcontrast dorsal CT image of the abdomen of a dog in a soft tissue window (WW: 350 HU, WL: 40 HU). The spleen (arrow) is enlarged and C-shaped, and is hypoattenuated with respect to the liver. Note the presence of peritoneal effusion (asterisk). **B**. Whirl sign of the splenic vessels.

Bibliography

- Agut, A., Soler, M. (2014) Masas abdominales. In: Agut, A. (ed). *Diagnóstico por Imagen en Pequeños Animales*, pp. 277–282. Multimédica Ediciones Veterinarias.
- Bertolini, G. (2010) Acquired portal collateral circulation in the dog and cat. *Vet Radiol Ultrasound*, 51(1):25–33.
- Fields, E.L., Robertson, I.D., Osborne, J.A., et al. (2012) Comparison of abdominal computed tomography and abdominal ultrasound in sedated dogs. *Vet Radiol Ultrasound*, 53(5):513–517.
- Frank, P.M. (2018) The peritoneal space. In: Thrall, D.E. (ed). *Textbook of Veterinary Diagnostic Radiology*. 7th ed, pp. 764–791. Elsevier Saunders.
- Hughes, J.R., Johnson, V.S., Genain, M.A. (2020) CT characteristics of primary splenic torsion in eight dogs. *Vet Radiol Ultrasound*, 61(3):261–268.
- Lamb, C.R., Steel, R., Lipscomb, V.J. (2018) Determining the anatomical origin of canine hepatic masses by CT. *J Small Anim Pract*, 59(12):752–757.
- Leela-Arporn, R., Ohta, H., Shimbo, G. et al. (2019) Computed tomographic features for differentiating benign from malignant liver lesions in dogs. *J Vet Med Sci*, 81(12):1697–1704.
- Nelson, N.C., Nelson, L.L. (2011) Anatomy of extrahepatic portosystemic shunts in dogs as determined by computed tomography angiography. *Vet Radiol Ultrasound*, 52:498–506.
- Ng, J., Linn, K.A., Shmon, C.L., et al. (2020) The left lateral projection is comparable to horizontal beam radiography for identifying experimental small volume pneumoperitoneum in the canine abdomen. *Vet Radiol Ultrasound*, 61(2):130–136.
- Plested, M.J., Zwingenberger, A.L., Brockman, D.J., et al. (2020) Canine intrahepatic portosystemic shunt insertion into the systemic circulation is commonly through primary hepatic veins as assessed with CT angiography. *Vet Radiol Ultrasound*, 61(5):519–530.
- Schwarz, T., Saunders, J. (eds). (2011) *Veterinary Computed Tomography*. 1st ed. Wiley-Blackwell.
- Specchi, S., Auriemma, E., Morabito, S., et al. (2017) Evaluation of the computed tomographic "sentinel clot sign" to identify bleeding abdominal organs in dogs with hemoabdomen. *Vet Radiol Ultrasound*, 58(1):18–22.
- Specchi, S., Bertolini, G. (2020) CT angiography identifies collaterals in dogs with splenic vein obstruction and presumed regional splenic vein hypertension. *Vet Radiol Ultrasound*, 61(6):636–640.
- Thierry, F., Chau, J., Makara, M., et al. (2018) Vascular conspicuity differs among injection protocols and scanner types for canine multiphasic abdominal computed tomographic angiography. *Vet Radiol Ultrasound*, 59(6):677–686.
- Thrall, D.E. (2018) Principles of radiographic interpretation of the abdomen. In: Thrall, D.E. (ed). *Textbook of Veterinary Diagnostic Radiology*. 7th ed, pp. 754–763. Elsevier Saunders.
- Thrall, D.E., Robertson, I.D. (2011) *Atlas of Normal Radiographic Anatomy and Anatomic Variants in the Dog and Cat*. 2nd ed. Elsevier Saunders.

Notes

Radiography and Computed Tomography of the Abdomen: Digestive, Urinary and Reproductive Systems

Agustina Ansón Fernández

Digestive System

Radiographs are an excellent modality of choice when approaching the diagnosis of pathologies of the digestive system. A routine study should include right lateral, left lateral and ventrodorsal (VD) projections. Dorsoventral (DV) projections are used only in cases where a VD projection cannot be performed, and to assess gastric content in both plain and contrast studies.

Stomach

The stomach is a hollow organ that is divided into four regions: fundus, body, pyloric antrum, and pyloric canal. It has two curvatures (greater and lesser) that extend from the cardia to the pylorus. The greater curvature is longer and has a convex shape. The lesser curvature is concave and in a medial position. The angular notch is an area of more marked angulation in the lesser curvature between the body and the pyloric antrum. The stomach is located in the cranial abdomen caudal to the liver. In the dog, the gastric fundus is located in the left side of the abdomen, the body is located centrally and the pylorus (antrum and canal) is on the right side. In the cat, both the fundus and the body are located in the left side of the abdomen, while the pylorus occupies a more central position. The gastric axis is perpendicular to the thoracolumbar spine.

The empty stomach is U-shaped, although if it is distended this shape is not seen. It has folds in the mucosa that can be visualised if gas is present in the stomach and it is neither completely distended nor collapsed. Gastric folds are more prominent in the fundus and body and smaller in the area near the pylorus, and are visible in both dogs and cats. In a non-distended stomach the gastric folds are more tortuous, and they become more regular and parallel to the gastric curvature as the degree of distension increases (Terragni et al., 2014). In cats, the gastric wall may also occasionally display an area of fatty opacity with a striated appearance that corresponds to fat in the submucosal layer. The thickness of the stomach wall cannot be assessed radiographically because the opacity of the fluid in the stomach adds to the opacity of the gastric wall, making both indistinguishable (Frank, 2018).

The stomach normally contains gas, food, or fluid. However, it is possible for the stomach to be completely empty, and this makes it difficult to differentiate it from the liver. The gastric content and appearance of the stomach can vary depending on the projection (Table 1). In a **right lateral projection**, the gastric fundus will be in a dorsal position relative to the pylorus, so the gas present in the stomach will be located at the level of the gastric fundus and the fluid will be located in the most ventral portion, the pylorus. In this case, if the pylorus is completely filled with fluid, it will be visualised as a rounded structure in the cranioventral abdomen that should not be confused with an abdominal mass (Fig. 1 A). In a **left lateral projection**, the pylorus is located dorsally while the fundus will be in a more ventral position relative to the pylorus. Gas will therefore be located at the level of the pylorus in this lateral projection (Fig. 1 B). If the stomach does not contain any gas the pylorus will appear small; if it contains mostly ingested material, the pylorus will be heterogeneous in appearance. In a **VD projection**, gas is present at the level of the pylorus and sometimes also in the body of the stomach, while fluid accumulates at the level of the fundus. In a **DV projection**, the gas is located in the gastric fundus while the fluid accumulates in the pylorus and body.

Table 1. Distribution of gas and fluid in the stomach depending on radiographic projection.

Projection	Gas	Fluid
Right lateral	Fundus	Pylorus
Left lateral	Pylorus	Fundus
VD	Pylorus and body	Fundus
DV	Fundus	Pylorus and body

Small Intestine

The **duodenum** has a relatively fixed position in the abdomen, as it is located in the right cranial abdomen and extends

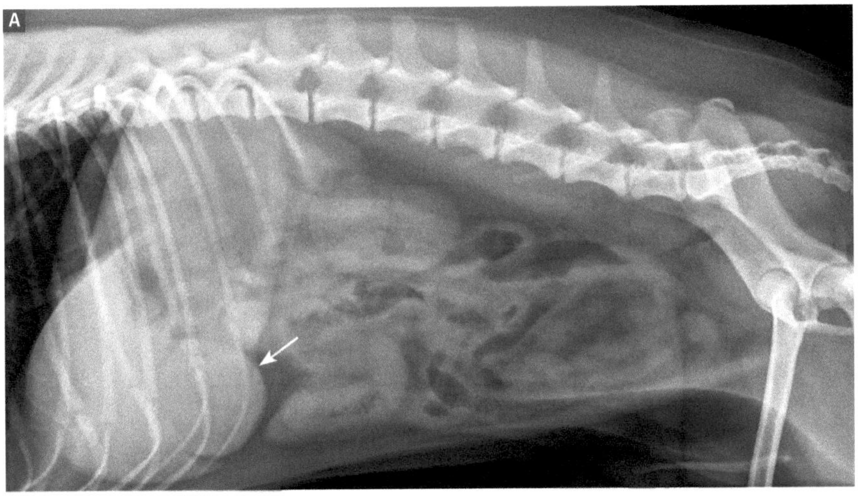

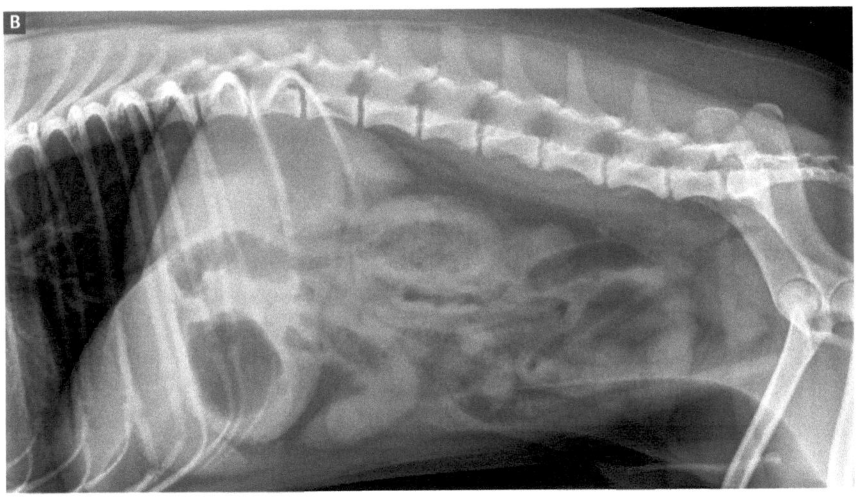

Figure 1. A. Right lateral projection of the abdomen of a dog. The pyloric antrum is visualised as a rounded mass of soft tissue opacity in the cranioventral abdomen (white arrow). **B**. Left lateral projection of the abdomen of the same animal. The pyloric antrum and the proximal duodenum contain gas.

along the right abdominal wall to the middle third of the abdomen. It can be visualised more clearly in the left lateral projection, because the gas present in the pylorus can extend into the duodenum and facilitate its visualization, and also in the VD projection. Peyer's patches are located at the antimesenteric border of the duodenum and, sometimes, if the duodenum contains gas, they can be seen as depressions of the mucosal surface known as pseudoulcers (Fig. 2). The **jejunum** is the most mobile portion of the small intestine. In general, in the dog, it occupies the middle and central abdomen. In the cat, especially in obese cats, the jejunum tends to cluster in the middle, ventral and right abdomen. The jejunum ends at the **ileum**, which is located in the right middle abdomen and is indistinguishable from the jejunum on plain radiographs. In cats, the small intestine can present a "string of pearls" appearance due to strong peristaltic contractions (Fig. 3). This phenomenon is known as hypersegmentation and is best observed in contrast studies. The normal content of the small intestine in both dogs and cats includes gas, digested food and fluid (Thrall and Robertson, 2011).

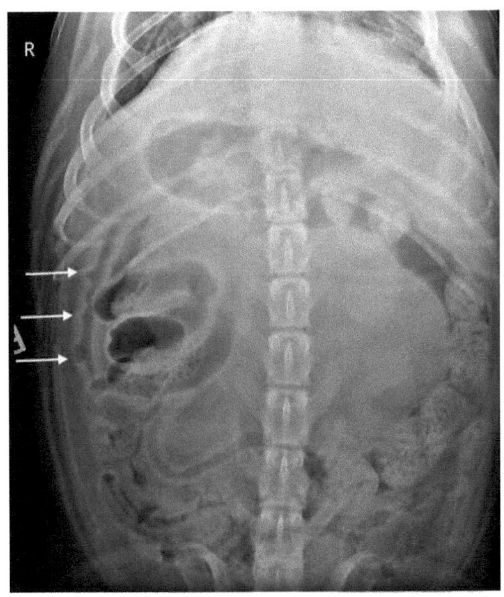

Figure 2. VD radiograph of the abdomen of a dog showing equidistant radiolucent indentations in the antimesenteric wall of the duodenum (white arrows) compatible with Peyer's patches.

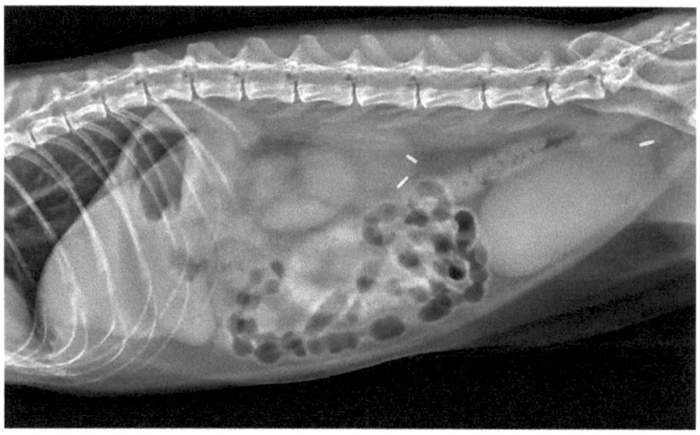

Figure 3. Lateral radiograph of the abdomen of a cat. The small intestine has a "string of pearls" appearance due to the strong intestinal peristaltic contractions in this species.

The size of the small intestine in the dog is assessed using the ratio of the maximum serosa-to-serosa intestinal diameter to the height of the central portion of the fifth lumbar vertebra (ID:L5 ratio), which should be less than 1.6 in normal dogs. In the cat, due to less variability among breeds, a maximum serosa-to-serosa diameter of 12 mm is considered normal. The wall thickness of the small intestine, as with the stomach, cannot be assessed radiographically.

Large Intestine

The junction of the small and large intestine occurs at the level of the ileocolic valve, which is located in the middle of the right abdomen. The caecocolic valve is also located in the same area in the dog. In the dog, the **caecum** has an inverted C shape and can be identified on radiographs if it contains gas. The cat has no caecocolic valve. The caecum in the cat is a comma-shaped caecum or diverticulum that continues directly into the colon and can rarely be identified on plain radiographs. The **ascending colon** is located in the right abdomen, medial to the duodenum and the right lobe of the pancreas, and extends cranially to the right colic flexure. The **transverse colon** extends from the right to the left abdomen, between the right and left colic flexures, and is located caudal to the stomach and the left lobe of the pancreas. The **descending colon** extends from the left colic flexure down the left abdomen to the pelvic cavity, where it continues as the **rectum**. Sometimes the descending colon is completely or partially located in the right abdomen. This may be due to distension of the stomach or the urinary bladder, or the presence of redundant colon, which is of no clinical significance. The normal diameter of the colon in the dog does not usually exceed the length of the seventh lumbar vertebra (L7). In the cat, its size is assessed by the ratio of the maximum diameter of the colon to the maximum length of the fifth lumbar vertebra (colon:L5 ratio), which should be less than 1.28 in normal cats. The large intestinal wall thickness cannot be assessed radiographically. Normal colon content in both species consists of gas and faeces.

Digestive System Contrast Techniques

Gastrointestinal Transit

Gastrointestinal transit is used to assess intestinal motility and gastric emptying time, and for the diagnosis of obstructions (Fig. 4). The patient should be fasted for 24 hours before the procedure and the colon should be empty, for which enemas

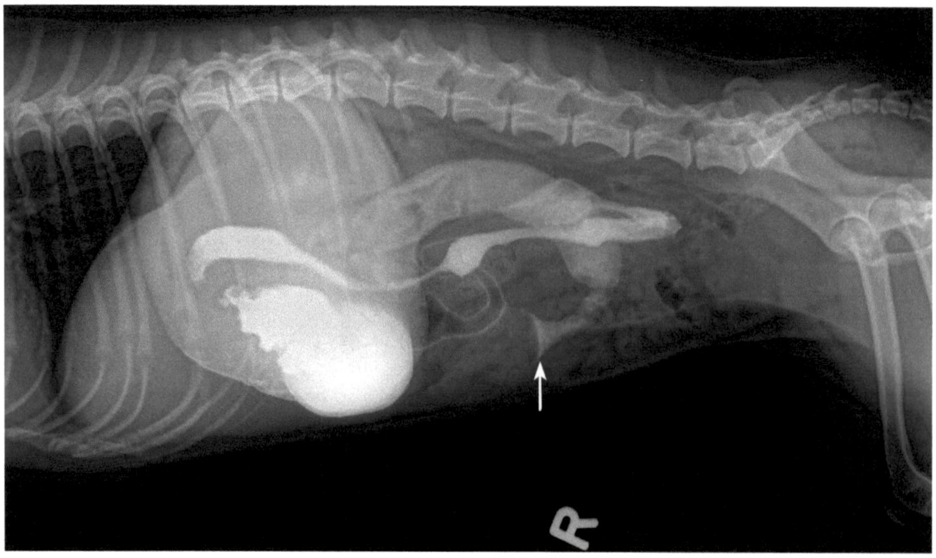

Figure 4. Lateral radiograph of the abdomen of a dog taken 30 minutes after oral administration of barium. Distension of the stomach, duodenum and proximal jejunum is visualised. The contrast stops at the level of an intraluminal structure in the jejunum, which it is unable to bypass. These findings are consistent with complete mechanical obstruction due to a foreign body.

can be used. This procedure is performed without sedation or anaesthesia so as not to affect gastrointestinal motility. If this is not possible, acepromazine can be used in dogs, and diazepam or ketamine in cats. Barium sulphate contrast medium is used at a dose of 8–12 ml/kg orally for small and medium dogs, 5–7 ml/kg for large dogs and 12–20 ml/kg for cats, and is preferably administered via a gastric tube (Terragni et al., 2014). Four projections (right lateral, left lateral, VD and DV) should be performed immediately after administration of the contrast, mainly to assess the gastric content. Subsequently, periodic radiographs (two orthogonal projections) should be performed until the contrast reaches the colon or a diagnosis is made. Orthogonal radiographs should also be taken after 24 hours to ensure that all the contrast has reached the colon. The main advantage of barium over other contrast media is that it is not absorbed by the mucosa of the gastrointestinal tract, so it does not lose opacity or definition as it moves along the intestine. The use of barium is contraindicated if intestinal perforation is suspected because it can cause granulomatous peritonitis. In this case, the use of an iodinated contrast medium is recommended; however, this type of contrast is absorbed through the mucosa, so obtaining a definitive diagnosis, especially in cases of distal obstructions (e.g. in the ileum), can be complicated.

Gastric emptying should begin within the first hour after barium administration and should be completed within a maximum of 8 hours in dogs and 5 hours in cats. **Intestinal transit time** is 2–4 hours in the dog and 1 hour in the cat. Gastrointestinal transit times are shorter when iodinated contrast is used.

Normally, in the small intestine of cats, especially in the duodenum, a characteristic "string of pearls" appearance can be observed due to strong peristaltic contractions (hypersegmentation) (Fig. 3). In the canine duodenum, pseudoulcers are visualised on the antimesenteric border that correspond to Peyer's patches (Fig. 2).

Pneumogastrography

Pneumogastrography is used to identify masses or foreign bodies in the stomach. For this technique, 20 ml/kg of air is introduced into the stomach and radiographs are then taken.

Barium Enema

A barium enema is used to identify intraluminal masses or areas of stenosis. This procedure is performed under general anaesthesia. Fasting the patient for 24 hours prior to the procedure is required and the colon should be empty, for which enemas can be used. A dose of 8 ml/kg of barium sulphate diluted 1:2 with warm or room-temperature water is introduced using a Foley catheter placed directly in the rectum. The anus is sealed using Allis clamps to prevent retrograde movement of the contrast medium. Orthogonal projections should be obtained. Subsequently, the contrast can be drained and the same volume of air then introduced (double contrast technique), to allow better visualisation of the wall of the colon.

Pneumocolon

The pneumocolon technique is used to locate the colon and differentiate it from the rest of the digestive tract (Fig. 5). Air is administered by using a syringe placed directly into the anus

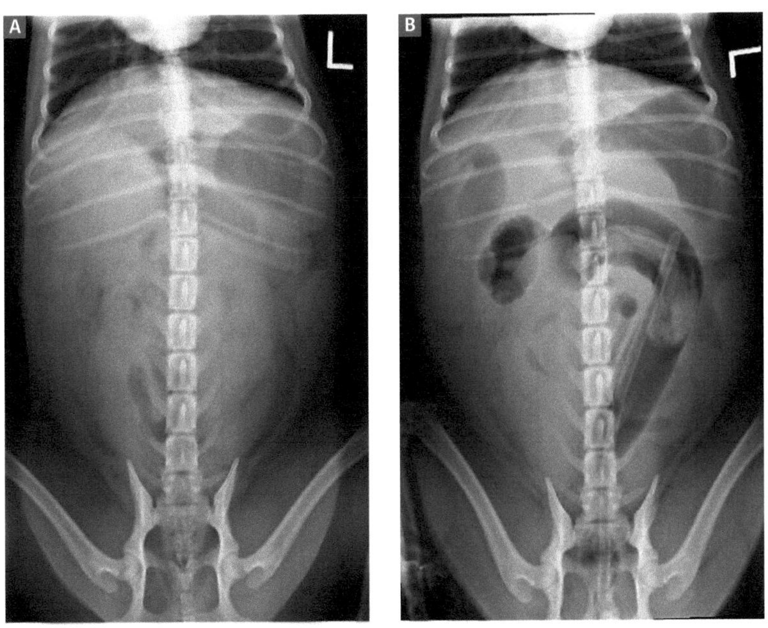

Figure 5. Ventrodorsal radiographs obtained before (**A**) and after (**B**) pneumocolonography. A tubular structure with soft tissue opacity is visualised within the transverse and descending colon, compatible with ileocolic intussusception. Note the meniscus sign in the caudal aspect.

or through a Foley catheter until the colon is distended. When performing this technique, it is usually not necessary to seal the anus with Allis clamps.

Computed Tomography of the Digestive System

Computed tomography (CT) can be useful for evaluation of the digestive system and for the diagnosis of gastrointestinal neoplasms, especially in large dogs or large breeds (weighing more than 25 kg), in which radiographic and ultrasonographic evaluation of the abdomen is challenging (Fields et al., 2012). A complete evaluation of the gastrointestinal tract requires a CT scan using dual phase contrast. A postcontrast phase is recommended at 30 seconds after contrast administration to achieve good enhancement of the mucosal surface of the small and large intestine, and another at 60 seconds to evaluate the gastric wall (Fitzgerald et al., 2017). The accuracy of CT in the diagnosis of pathology of the gastric wall improves when it is performed after oral administration of water (30 ml/kg) (hydro-CT) or air followed by intravenous administration of contrast (Fig. 6) (Terragni et al., 2012).

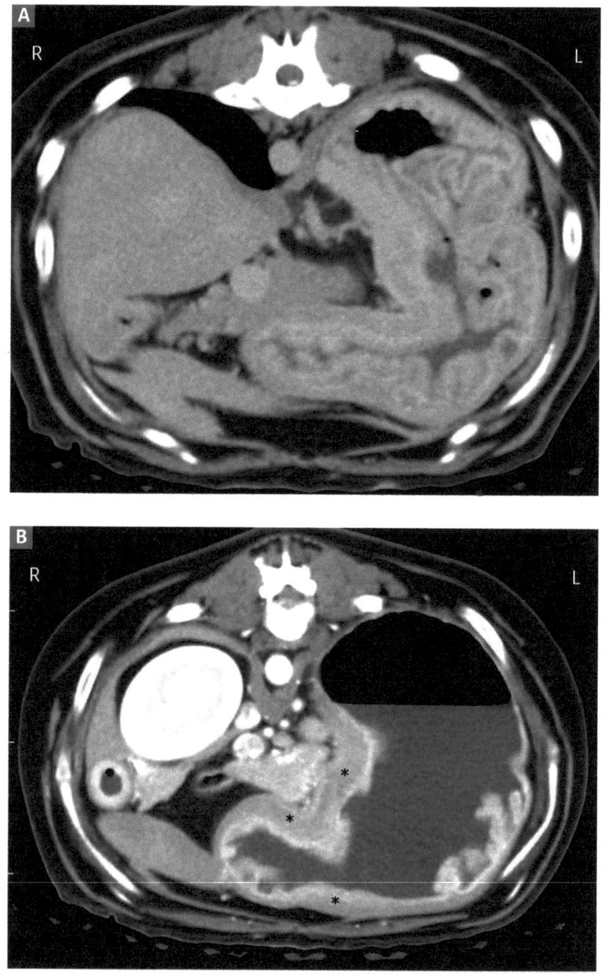

Figure 6. Cross-sectional CT images of the cranial abdomen of a dog before (**A**) and after (**B**) intragastric introduction of water (hydro-CT). The thickening of the wall (asterisks) is more easily recognisable after the hydro-CT has been performed. Images courtesy of Amalia Agut.

Digestive Tract Pathologies

Gastric Dilatation

In gastric dilatation, the stomach is observed to be dilated, usually with gas, secondary to aerophagia (e.g. due to dyspnoea) or functional ileus (e.g. due to pain, pancreatitis or postsurgical abdomen). The stomach is in its normal position (Fig. 7).

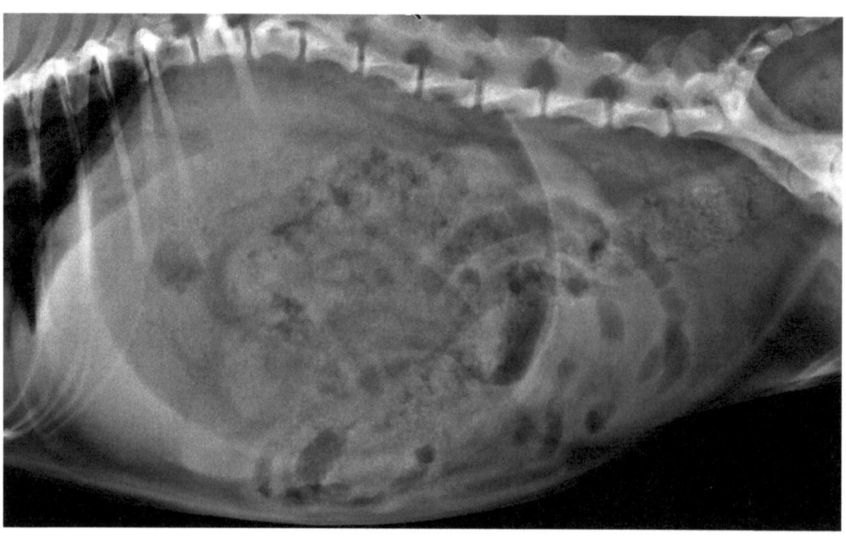

Figure 7. Right lateral radiograph of the abdomen of a dog showing gastric dilatation.

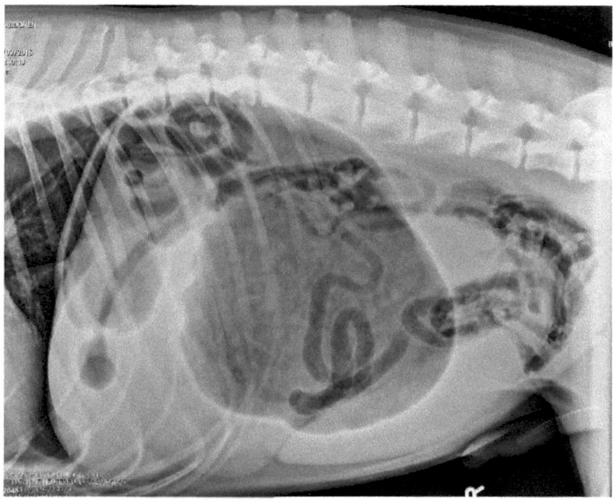

Figure 8. Right lateral radiograph of the abdomen of a dog showing gastric volvulus. Note the dorsal and cranial position of the pylorus and the compartmentalisation sign.

The most common radiographic findings of a volvulus or gastric torsion are (Fig. 8):

- **The stomach is distended with gas and liquid or with gas only.**
- **The pylorus is located in the cranial left dorsal abdomen, while the fundus is located in the caudal right ventral abdomen, except in cases where the torsion is 360°. The pylorus generally has a tubular morphology and can be easily distinguished from the rest of the stomach.**
- **Presence of the compartmentalisation sign. This refers to a band of soft tissue that projects into the lumen of the stomach as a result of the folding of the stomach and divides the stomach into two compartments.**
- **Distension of the caudal oesophagus and the loops of the small intestine.**
- **Splenic torsion can also be present.**
- **Loss of serosal detail, usually in the cranial abdomen, due to steatitis or regional effusion.**
- **Gastric pneumatosis: the presence of gas at the level of the stomach wall is very rare but has a high specificity for predicting gastric wall necrosis (Fischetti et al., 2004).**
- **Pneumoperitoneum: may be present in cases of gastric wall necrosis.**
- **Microcardia, hypovascular lungs and decreased caudal vena cava size may also be seen in these cases as a consequence of hypovolaemic shock.**
- **In cases in which the gastric torsion is 360°, the stomach will be in a normal position on radiographs. Diagnosis in these cases is reached by physical examination (e.g. inability to pass a gastric tube through the cardia) or by exploratory laparotomy. This type of gastric torsion is very uncommon. In a study of 220 dogs, only 2.5% had a 360° rotation (Fischetti et al., 2004).**

Gastric Dilatation-volvulus

Gastric dilatation-volvulus (GDV) is a common and life-threatening condition that primarily affects large-breed dogs. It has also been described in cats, although it is much less common. In cats and brachycephalic breeds of dog, the presence of a hiatal hernia appears to be a predisposing factor. GDV is characterised by acute dilatation of the stomach and rotation on its longitudinal axis. It requires immediate medical and surgical treatment, so a quick diagnosis is essential. In most cases, a right lateral radiograph of the abdomen is sufficient to reach a diagnosis. Owing to the instability and state of shock that patients with gastric torsion usually present with, performing additional radiographic projections is not recommended if the right lateral projection is diagnostic. The radiographic appearance of a volvulus or gastric torsion depends on the degree of rotation and distension of the stomach.

Chronic Gastric Instability

Chronic gastric instability is defined as the presence of a flaccid stomach resulting in an abnormal and intermittent gastric position. It has also been described in the literature as volvulus or partial gastric torsion, chronic gastric torsion or gastric torsion without dilatation. Clinical signs are usually less specific and less acute than in cases of gastric volvulus (e.g. weight loss, chronic vomiting, lethargy and abdominal pain). The radiographic findings described are variable and depend on the time at which the study is performed. The position of the stomach can vary from craniodorsal displacement of the pylorus in the lateral projection to displacement of the cardia to the right of the midline in the VD projection or displacement of the fundus to the left of the midline (Fig. 9). It is also possible for the stomach to appear normal in position and size, making it impossible to establish a diagnosis by plain radiography. A combination of radiography (plain and contrast), abdominal ultrasonography and endoscopy can aid definitive diagnosis of chronic gastric instability (Paris et al., 2011). The use of CT for diagnosis has also been described (White et al., 2020).

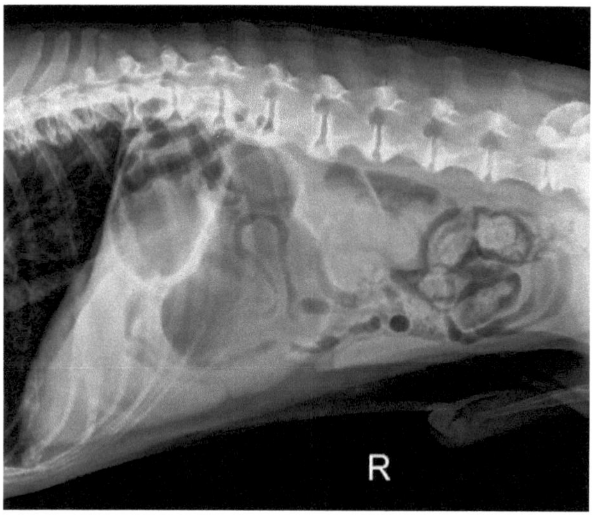

Figure 9. Right lateral radiograph of the abdomen of a dog diagnosed with chronic gastric instability. The study was conducted as part of an annual check-up. The animal showed no clinical signs when the radiographs were taken; however, the radiographic image is compatible with gastric torsion.

Gastric Foreign Bodies

Gastric foreign bodies with metal or bone opacity can be easily identified in the stomach (Fig. 10). Foreign bodies with soft tissue opacity may be more difficult to diagnose and differentiate from food, a fairly common finding in dogs and cats when performing abdominal radiographs.

If the stomach contains gas or the foreign body has a characteristic shape, it may be useful to identify them. A left lateral radiograph is essential in cases in which the presence of a foreign body in the stomach or proximal duodenum needs to be ruled out (Fig. 11). If the stomach contents are indistinguishable from food and the patient is clinically stable, follow-up radiographs obtained after 8–12 hours of fasting can help to differentiate them. Performing a pneumogastrogram or orally administering a small amount of barium may also aid diagnosis.

Gastric Masses

Gastric tumours are rare in dogs and cats, accounting for less than 1% of neoplasms in these species (Gualtieri et al., 1999). Gastric masses protruding into the lumen can be recognised on radiographs if the stomach contains air and does not contain a large amount of food (Fig. 12) (Burk and Ackerman, 1996). However, radiographs are not usually helpful for identifying intramural or diffuse lesions. In contrast studies, intraluminal masses appear as filling defects that are best visualised once most of the contrast has left the stomach. The most common malignant gastric neoplasms include adenocarcinoma (the most common type in dogs), leiomyosarcoma, stromal cell tumour and lymphoma (the most common type in cats). Benign gastric masses include leiomyoma, polyps, mucosal hyperplasia and adenoma. CT is a useful imaging technique in the diagnosis of these pathologies, especially in large-breed dogs in which the stomach is difficult to evaluate by ultrasonography (Fields et al., 2012). Hydro-CT improves the visualisation of gastric masses.

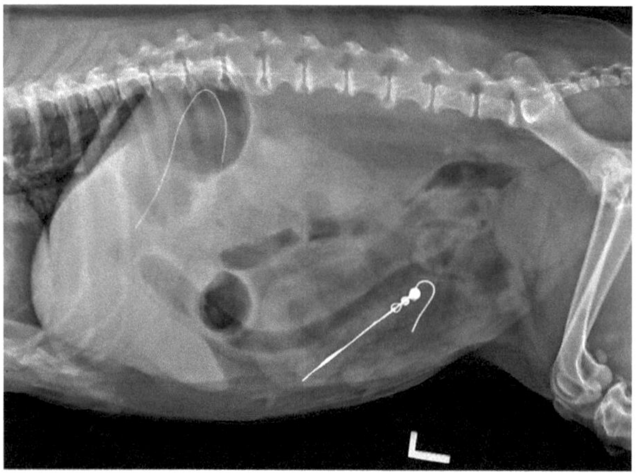

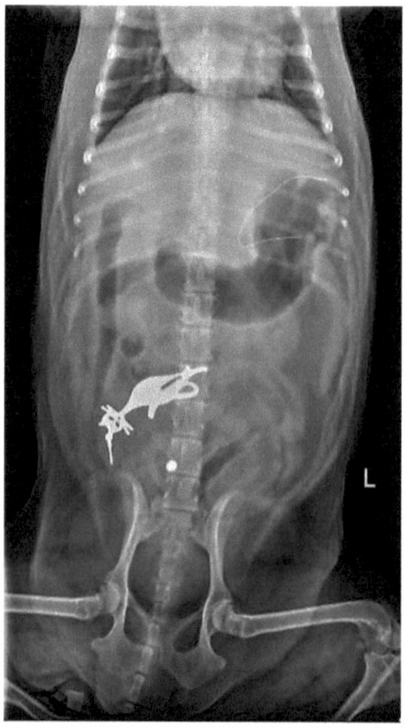

Figure 10. Metallic foreign bodies in the stomach and small intestine of a dog.

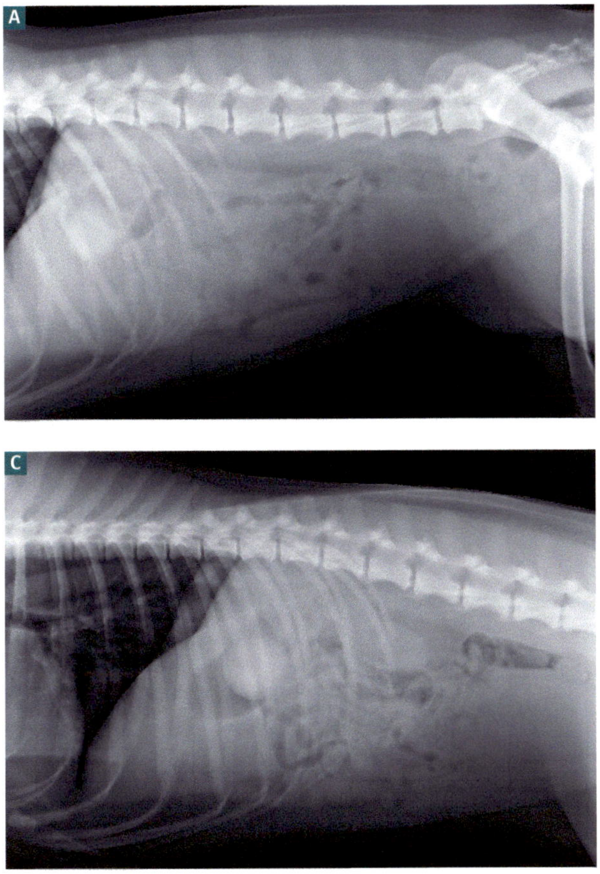

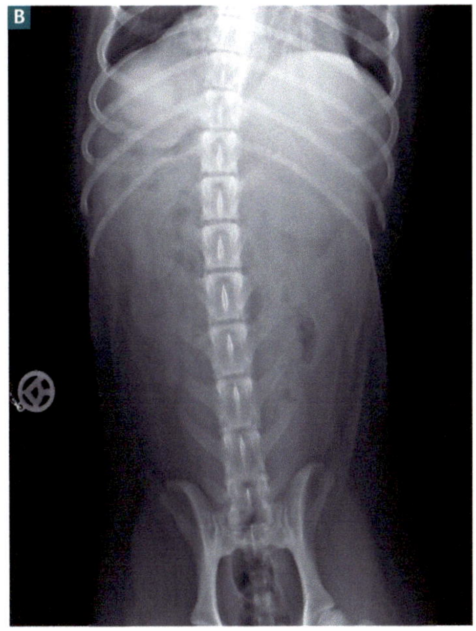

Figure 11. Right lateral (**A**), VD (**B**) and left lateral (**C**) projections of the abdomen of a dog with a foreign body (a ball) in its stomach. The foreign body can be clearly visualised in the left lateral projection.

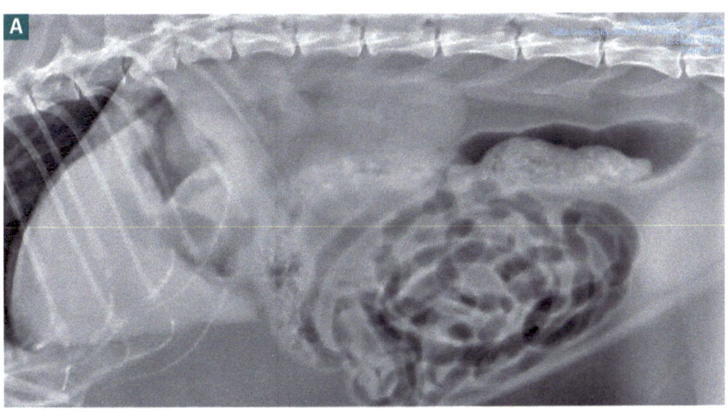

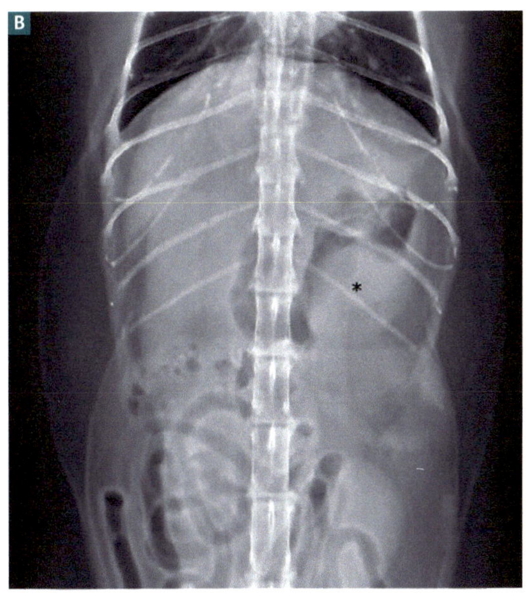

Figure 12. Right lateral (**A**) and VD (**B**) projections of the abdomen of a cat. A mass is present in the area of the greater curvature of the stomach (asterisk).

Hypertrophic Pyloric Stenosis

Hypertrophic pyloric stenosis has been described in breeds such as the Boxer, Boston Terrier and Bulldog, in which it is congenital. Other breeds, such as the Lhasa Apso, Shih Tzu, Pekingese and Poodle, are predisposed to the acquired form of this pathology (Walter and Matthiesen, 1993). Plain radiographs show signs of partial chronic obstruction such as gastric dilatation or delayed gastric emptying. In contrast studies, the **string sign**, which consists of a fine thread of barium extending between the pyloric antrum and the proximal duodenum and represents the thinning of the pyloric canal lumen, can be observed. The **beak sign**, which is the presence of a prominence (beak) just where the area of stenosis begins, where the barium attempts to enter the pyloric canal, may be seen. The **nipple sign** refers to a protrusion in the minor curvature of the pyloric antrum. It corresponds to the shape of a prominent peristaltic wave due to difficulty in gastric emptying (Frank, 2018).

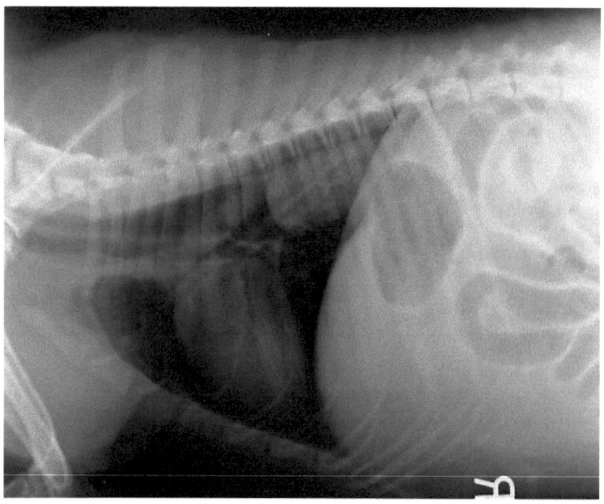

Figure 13. Gastro-oesophageal intussusception in a dog. Note the meniscus sign.

Gastro-oesophageal Intussusception

Gastro-oesophageal intussusception is an intussusception of the stomach into the caudal oesophagus, with or without other abdominal organs (e.g. spleen, duodenum, pancreas). It has been described mainly in young dogs (less than 3-months-old) with a pre-existing condition such as megaoesophagus, chronic vomiting or hiatal hernia. It is a medical emergency that requires immediate surgery because there is serious vascular compromise. On plain radiographs, an ovoid mass of large size and soft tissue opacity is visualised in the caudal oesophageal region, which usually presents a blunt cranial end outlined by gas present in the oesophagus (**meniscus sign**) (Fig. 13).

Mechanical Ileus

The lumen of the digestive tract can be obstructed by foreign bodies, intussusceptions, adhesions, masses originating in the wall or extrinsic lesions that compress the tract from outside. Mechanical obstruction may be complete or partial, and acute or chronic. In cases of complete obstruction, the main radiographic finding is dilatation of the loops proximal to the point of obstruction. As a consequence of the obstruction, two populations of intestinal loops are visible, one dilated and the other collapsed or empty (Fig. 14). The ID:L5 ratio helps assess the presence of dilated intestinal loops in the dog. A ratio of 1.95 represents a 77–80% chance of obstruction, while a ratio of 2.07 indicates a 86–90% chance of diagnosis of an intestinal

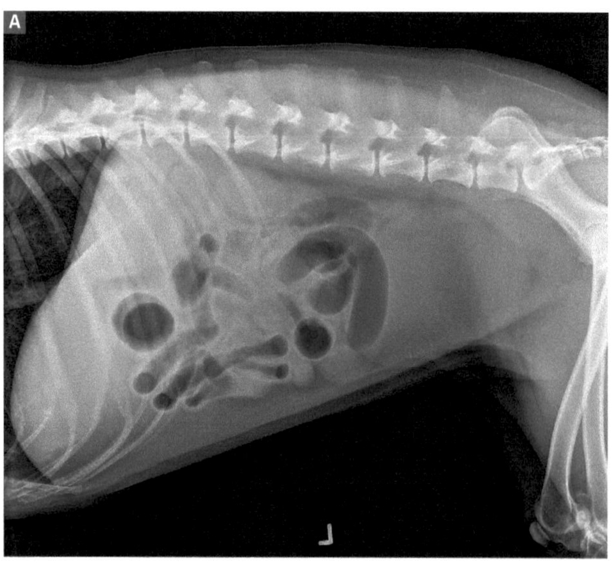

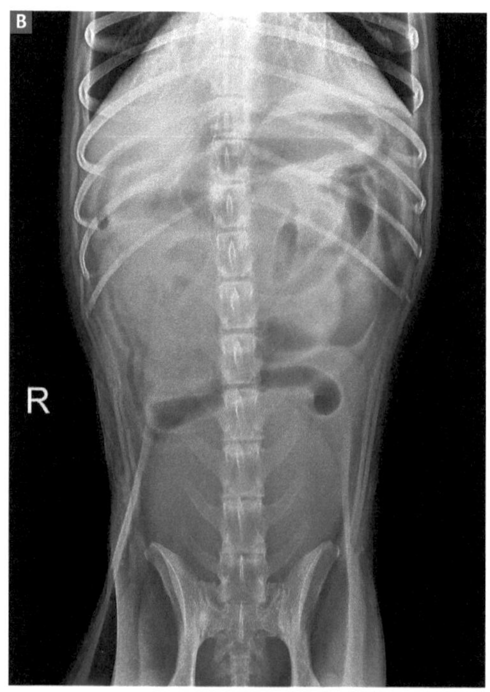

Figure 14. Lateral (**A**) and VD (**B**) radiographs of a dog with a mechanical intestinal obstruction. Two populations of small intestinal loops are observed.

obstruction (Finck et al., 2014). A mechanical obstruction at the level of the distal intestine, for example, in the ileum or ileocolic valve, can be difficult to diagnose and differentiate from a functional ileus because all or almost all of the intestinal loops may be dilated. In these cases, ultrasonography or a contrast study is more helpful.

Partial obstructions or those at the level of the duodenum generate less obvious changes on plain radiographs. In these cases, follow up radiographs (after 12–24 hours) are necessary, in addition to ultrasonography or a contrast study to reach a diagnosis. Left lateral radiographs are essential for the diagnosis of mechanical obstruction at the level of the proximal duodenum. If the partial obstruction is chronic, for example, in cases of intestinal neoplasms that grow slowly and obstruct the intestinal lumen progressively, they can generally be identified by the presence of the **gravel sign** (the accumulation of multiple small radiopaque structures in the lumen, proximal to the point of obstruction) (Fig. 15). The most common intestinal neoplasms include adenocarcinoma, lymphoma, mastocytoma, stromal cell tumour, leiomyoma and leiomyosarcoma.

Linear foreign bodies usually consist of a portion that is fixed in the pylorus (more frequent in dogs) or under the tongue (more frequent in cats) while most of the foreign body advances through the small intestine due to peristaltic contractions. Therefore, unlike other types of foreign body, they do not produce intense distension of intestinal loops. Instead, they result in plication and an abnormal pattern of gas distribution in the small intestine; the gas is trapped in the folds of the intestine and acquires a small rounded or geometric (e.g. teardrop, comma or crescent) gas bubble shape (Fig. 16).

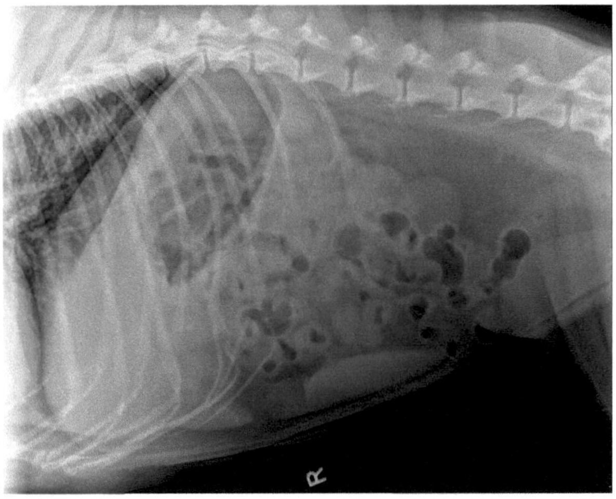

Figure 16. Lateral radiograph of a dog with a linear foreign body. Note the geometric morphology of the gas in the intestinal loops.

An **intussusception** is the invagination of a segment of intestine (intussusceptum) within the lumen of an adjacent segment (intussuscipiens). It is usually associated with concurrent pathologies such as parvovirus or parasitic infection, neoplasms or a foreign body. It most frequently occurs at the ileocolic level. Intussusception can cause chronic complete

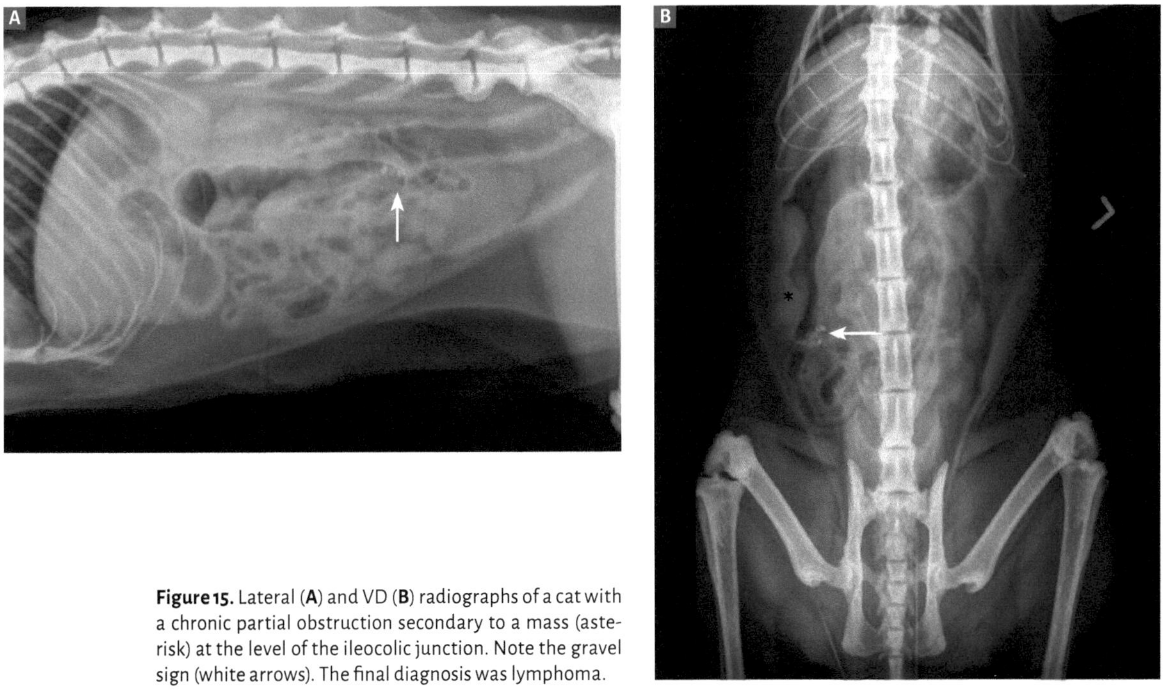

Figure 15. Lateral (**A**) and VD (**B**) radiographs of a cat with a chronic partial obstruction secondary to a mass (asterisk) at the level of the ileocolic junction. Note the gravel sign (white arrows). The final diagnosis was lymphoma.

or partial obstruction and can therefore present variable radiographic signs depending on the point and degree of obstruction: these signs include the presence of two populations of small intestinal loops, generalised distension of intestinal loops if it is at the ileocolic level or the presence of the **gravel sign** if it is a chronic partial obstruction. Sometimes the **meniscus sign** (described earlier for gastro-oesophageal intussusception) can be observed (Fig. 13).

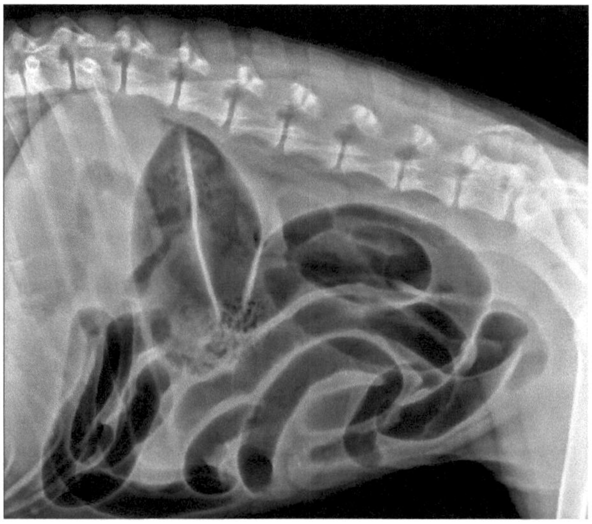

Figure 17. Lateral radiograph of a dog with functional ileus. Generalised distension of the small intestinal loops can be seen. The final diagnosis was mesenteric torsion and intestinal ischaemia.

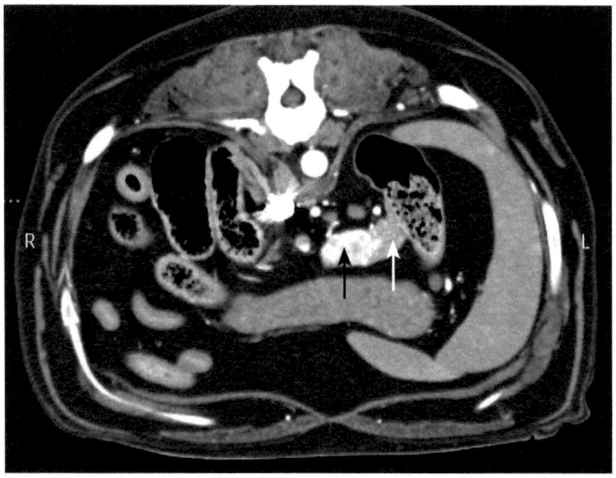

Figure 18. Postcontrast (arterial phase) cross-sectional CT image of the cranial abdomen of a dog at the level of the left pancreatic lobe (white arrow). A nodule that is hyperattenuated relative to the rest of the pancreatic parenchyma is observed (black arrow). The final diagnosis was insulinoma.

Functional Ileus

Functional ileus is characterised by a generalised and uniform dilatation of the digestive tract due to a lack of peristalsis. The main causes of the cessation of peristalsis are vascular or neuromuscular abnormalities. Diseases that cause functional ileus include viral enteritis (e.g. parvovirus), peritonitis, vascular compromise (e.g. intestinal or mesenteric volvulus, thrombosis), spinal trauma (neurological damage) and diseases of the autonomic nervous system (e.g. dysautonomia). Radiographically, a generalised distension of the intestinal loops with gas is usually visualised (Fig. 17).

Pancreas

The pancreas is not visible radiographically in the dog. In the cat, if there is sufficient intra-abdominal fat, the left lobe of the pancreas can be visualised caudal to the gastric fundus, medial to the spleen and lateral to the left kidney in a VD projection. In lateral projections it usually overlaps the spleen in the craniodorsal abdomen, between the stomach and the left kidney. CT angiography is useful for the diagnosis of pancreatic neoplasms. Adenocarcinomas usually present as masses that are hypoattenuated relative to the rest of the pancreatic parenchyma in all postcontrast phases. Insulinomas, on the other hand, are usually small masses that protrude slightly from the pancreatic surface and show marked enhancement during the arterial contrast phase. In a recent study, 20 out of 21 dogs with insulinoma exhibited hyperattenuation of insulinoma during the arterial phase, and the sensitivity of the arterial phase for detecting insulinoma was 94% (Coss et al., 2021) (Fig. 18).

Urinary System

Kidneys

The kidneys are located in the retroperitoneal space. The left kidney is located at the level of vertebrae L1–L3 and the right kidney is located slightly more cranially at the level of T12–L1. This variation in the position of the kidneys is more evident in the dog than in the cat. The kidneys are oval in shape and have a uniform soft tissue opacity and regular, rounded margins. In cats, a radiolucent central area can be seen that corresponds to an accumulation of fat in the renal pelvis (Fig. 19). Renal size can be assessed on VD radiographs, to avoid the magnification of one kidney relative to the other that occurs on lateral radiographs. Normal kidney length in the dog is between 2.5 and 3.5 times the length of the body of L2 (Lobacz et al., 2012).

Normal kidney length is 2.4–3.0 times the length of L2 in unneutered cats, and somewhat smaller in neutered cats (1.9–2.6 times the length of L2) (Shiroma et al., 1999).

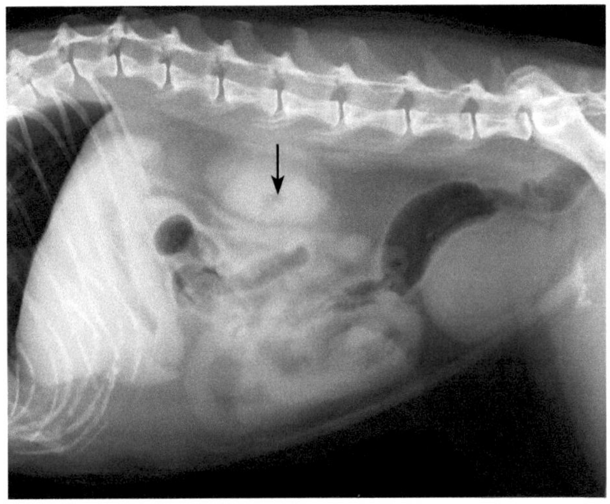

Figure 19. Lateral radiograph of the abdomen of a cat. The arrow indicates a radiolucent central area in the kidneys compatible with fat in the renal pelvis.

Ureters

The ureters are retroperitoneal structures that are not visible on plain radiographs in most cases; however, they can be visualised in obese cats with a large amount of retroperitoneal fat. Excretory or intravenous urography and CT allow visualisation and evaluation of the ureters.

Urinary Bladder and Urethra

The urinary bladder is located in the caudal abdomen and should have soft tissue opacity. The urinary bladder is usually positioned more cranially in the cat than in the dog, which causes the visible portion of the urethra in the caudal abdomen to be longer in the cats than in the dog. The size of the urinary bladder varies depending on the volume of urine it contains. To fully evaluate the lower urinary tract using radiography, the caudal abdomen, pelvis, perineum and (in male animals) penis should be included. To do this, a lateral projection should be obtained with the animal in a neutral position and, in the case of male dogs, an additional projection with the hindlimbs displaced cranially in such a way that they do not overlap with the path of the urethra should be taken.

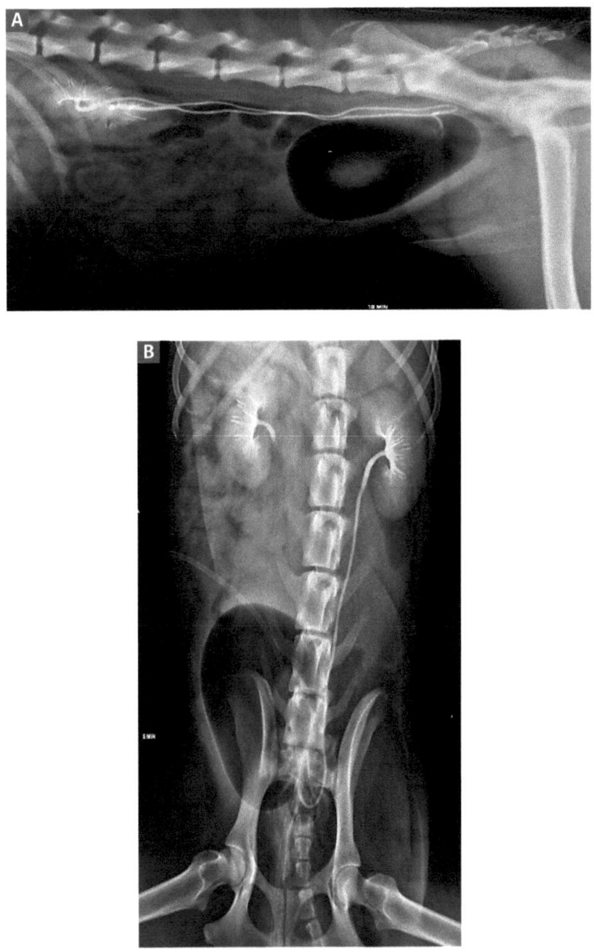

Figure 20. Lateral (**A**) and VD (**B**) radiographs of the abdomen of a cat following negative contrast cystography and excretory urography.

Urinary System Contrast Techniques

The patient should be fasted for 24 hours and the colon should be empty, for which an enema can be used. Contrast techniques are performed under general anaesthesia or deep sedation. Plain radiographs (two orthogonal projections) should be taken before contrast is administered.

Excretory or Intravenous Urography

Excretory urography is used to assess the shape, size and position of the kidneys, ureters and bladder, and to assess the glomerular filtration rate semiquantitatively. Pneumocystography (negative contrast cystography) prior to intravenous contrast administration is recommended to improve visualisation of the ureterovesical junction (Fig. 20). Intravenous iodinated contrast medium should be administered at a dose of 600–800 mg I/kg. VD radiographs should be performed at 30 seconds, 1–2 minutes and 5 minutes after contrast administration, and VD and lateral radiographs should be performed every 5 minutes starting at 10 minutes. Oblique projections can be obtained to evaluate the ureterovesical junction.

Positive Cystography

Positive cystography is mainly used to differentiate the urinary bladder from urine and in cases of suspected bladder rupture. The bladder is catheterised and completely emptied. Iodinated contrast medium is then introduced at a concentration of 150 mg I/ml until the bladder is distended.

Pneumocystography

Pneumocystography is used to complement other contrast techniques for imaging the urinary system and can also be used to differentiate the bladder from urine. The bladder is catheterised and completely emptied, after which air (6–12 ml air/kg) is introduced until the bladder is distended.

Retrograde Urethrography in Males and Retrograde Vaginourethrography in Females

These techniques are used in cases of haematuria, dysuria, suspected ectopic ureters, urinary tract obstruction, prostate disease, and to visualise the urethra and masses in the pelvic cavity and caudal abdomen. A previous pneumocystogram is recommended. In males, the catheter is placed at the distal end of the urethra and iodinated contrast medium is administered in boluses of 1 ml in cats and 10–20 ml in dogs. Lateral radiographs are performed with the hindlimbs directed cranially. Oblique lateral radiographs can also be performed. In females, a Foley-type catheter is placed in the vaginal vestibule and the vulva is then sealed with atraumatic forceps (Allis type). Administration of a 20–30 ml bolus of iodinated contrast medium is recommended until complete opacification of the vagina and urethra is achieved (Fig. 21).

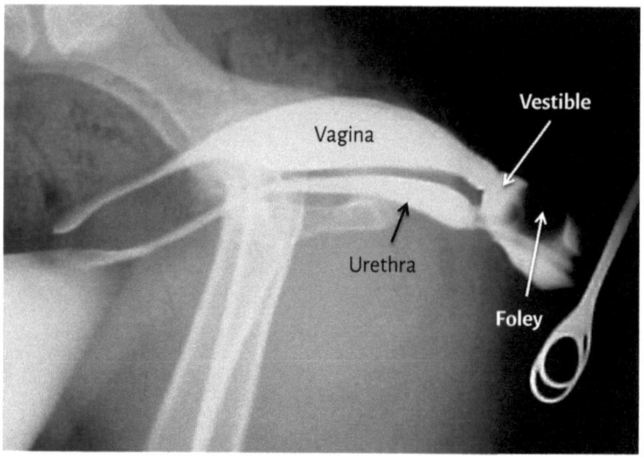

Figure 21. Retrograde vaginourethrography in a bitch.

Computed Tomography of the Urinary System

CT allows evaluation of the entire urinary system. It is also the imaging technique of choice for the diagnosis of ectopic ureters because it allows identification of their location of insertion and determines whether they are intra- or extramural. The CT protocol for evaluation of the urinary system includes:

- prior enema
- avoiding catheterisation before or during CT so that the presence of gas does not hinder diagnosis
- deep sedation/general anaesthesia
- administration of iodinated contrast into the cephalic vein at a dose of 800 mg I/kg
- positioning the animal in ventral recumbency with the pelvis elevated by means of a radiolucent wedge placed so as to avoid compressing the caudal abdomen.

The phases included in the study are as follows.

- **Precontrast**: with a soft tissue and bone algorithm, including the entire abdomen, pelvis, perineal area and penis. This is used to evaluate the morphology of the urinary system and the presence of mineralisation or calculi. The presence of lipiduria can also be detected.
- **Arterial**: used only if vascular malformations (e.g. idiopathic renal haematuria) are suspected. Occurs 2–3 seconds after the start of contrast injection. An automatic injector and a dynamic study are required.
- **Parenchymatous**: occurs 1 minute after the start of contrast injection. Used to evaluate the presence of masses, infarcts and cysts and the wall of the ureters, bladder and urethra.
- **Excretory**: used to evaluate the renal pelvis, ureters and ureterovesical junction. Occurs at 2–5 minutes after the start of contrast injection. However, in the case of ectopic ureters, this phase can last up to 20–30 minutes depending on the glomerular filtration rate and how distended the collecting system is. Therefore, performing the bolus tracking technique is recommended: this consists of placing a region of interest in the most caudal aspect of the ureter visible in the precontrast study and starting to acquire CT images once 150 Hounsfield units are reached in that region. This ensures that the excretory phase is occurring at the time of the study.

Four-dimensional CT has recently been described for use in the diagnosis of ectopic ureters; this technique had a sensitivity of 97% and a specificity of 94.6% (Schwarz et al., 2021).

Retrograde CT urethrography has also recently been described in dogs. The retrograde technique requires the use of an automatic injector (Kang et al., 2020). A case has also been described in a dog in which an antegrade technique was performed by using an acoustic gel drum positioned over the urinary bladder to cause urination and filling of the urethra during the CT study (Kang et al., 2019).

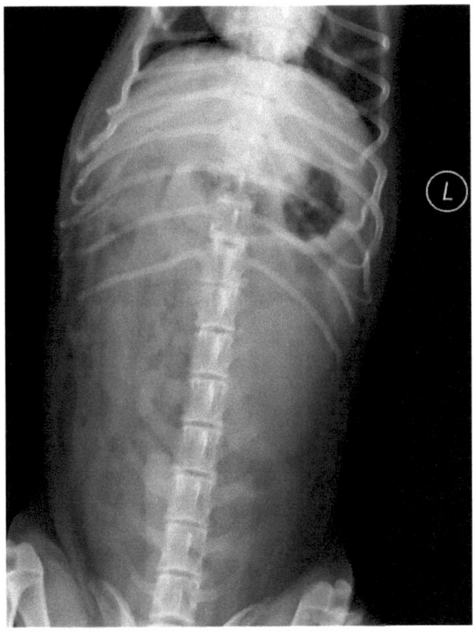

Figure 22. Left unilateral renomegaly in a dog. The final diagnosis was perirenal pseudocyst.

Pathologies of the Urinary System

Renomegaly

Renomegaly can be unilateral or bilateral, and the affected kidney can have regular or irregular margins. Differential diagnoses to consider include:

- **unilateral renomegaly** (Fig. 22)
  - hydronephrosis: regular margins
  - perirenal pseudocyst: regular margins
  - haematoma or subcapsular abscess: regular or irregular margins
  - neoplasm: more frequent in the dog and of epithelial type, usually has irregular margins
  - compensatory hypertrophy: usually secondary to chronic kidney disease in the contralateral kidney. Therefore, a small and irregular kidney and a slightly enlarged kidney with regular margins are usually observed.
- **bilateral renomegaly** (Fig. 23)
  - lymphoma (cats): regular or irregular margins
  - polycystic kidney disease: irregular margins
  - feline infectious peritonitis (cats): regular margins
  - leptospirosis (dogs): regular margins
  - bilateral perirenal pseudocysts: regular margins
  - hydronephrosis: regular margins
  - portosystemic shunt (mild): regular margins.

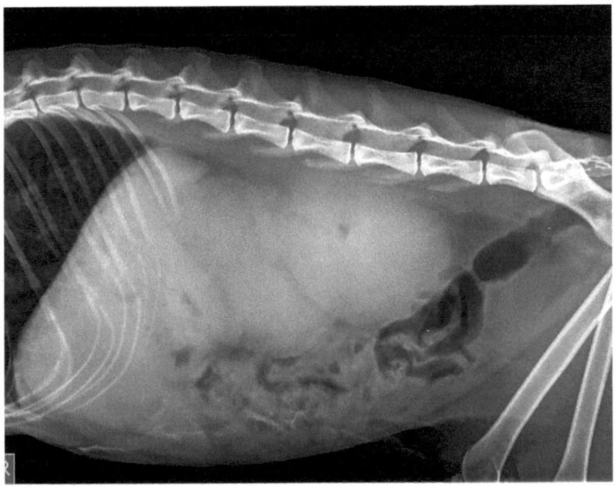

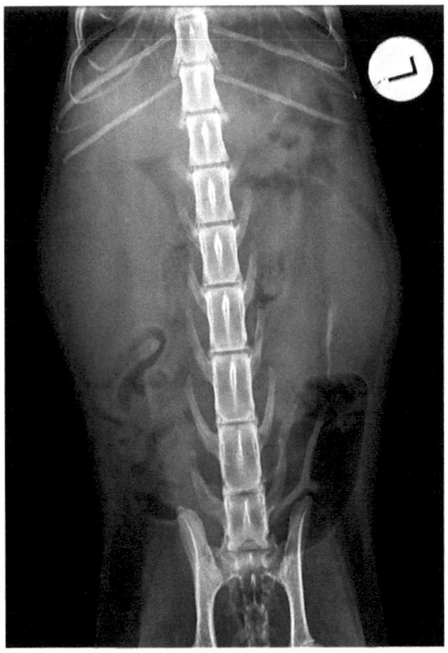

Figure 23. Bilateral renomegaly in a cat. The final diagnosis was feline infectious peritonitis.

Urinary Calculi

Urinary calculi (Fig. 24) with calcium content can be visualised on plain radiographs, although sometimes this can be difficult. Factors that make it difficult to identify urinary calculi include the presence of faeces in the descending colon or mineral structures in the gastrointestinal tract, and decreased serosal visualisation in lean animals or puppies (physiological). In addition, other areas of mineralisation may be apparent in the retroperitoneal space ,such as adrenal mineralisation or mineralised ovarian granulomas secondary to neutering, and these could be confused with ureteral calculi. Deep circumflex arteries are visualised as one or two small, rounded radiopaque structures in the caudal retroperitoneal space and should not be confused with ureteral calculi. If the intestinal loops or colon overlap the urinary bladder, it may be impossible to differentiate urinary calculi from gastrointestinal material such as small fragments of bone or stones. To differentiate these, a radiograph can be performed while applying compression to the caudal abdomen with a wooden spatula (or any other radiolucent material) to displace the gastrointestinal tract away from the bladder. The penile bone can sometimes be identified in male cats (in 38% of cats on radiographs and in 78% on CT) and should not be confused with a urethral calculus. Tumours of the prostate, bladder or urethra or paraprostatic cysts may mineralise and be mistaken for calculi.

Cystourethrography is the radiographic contrast technique of choice for the identification of radiotransparent calculi in the bladder or urethra. Urinary obstructions in cats may result in the presence of perivesical free fluid, which is seen as decreased visualisation of the serosa and increased regional attenuation. Most of the urinary calculi found in dogs and cats,

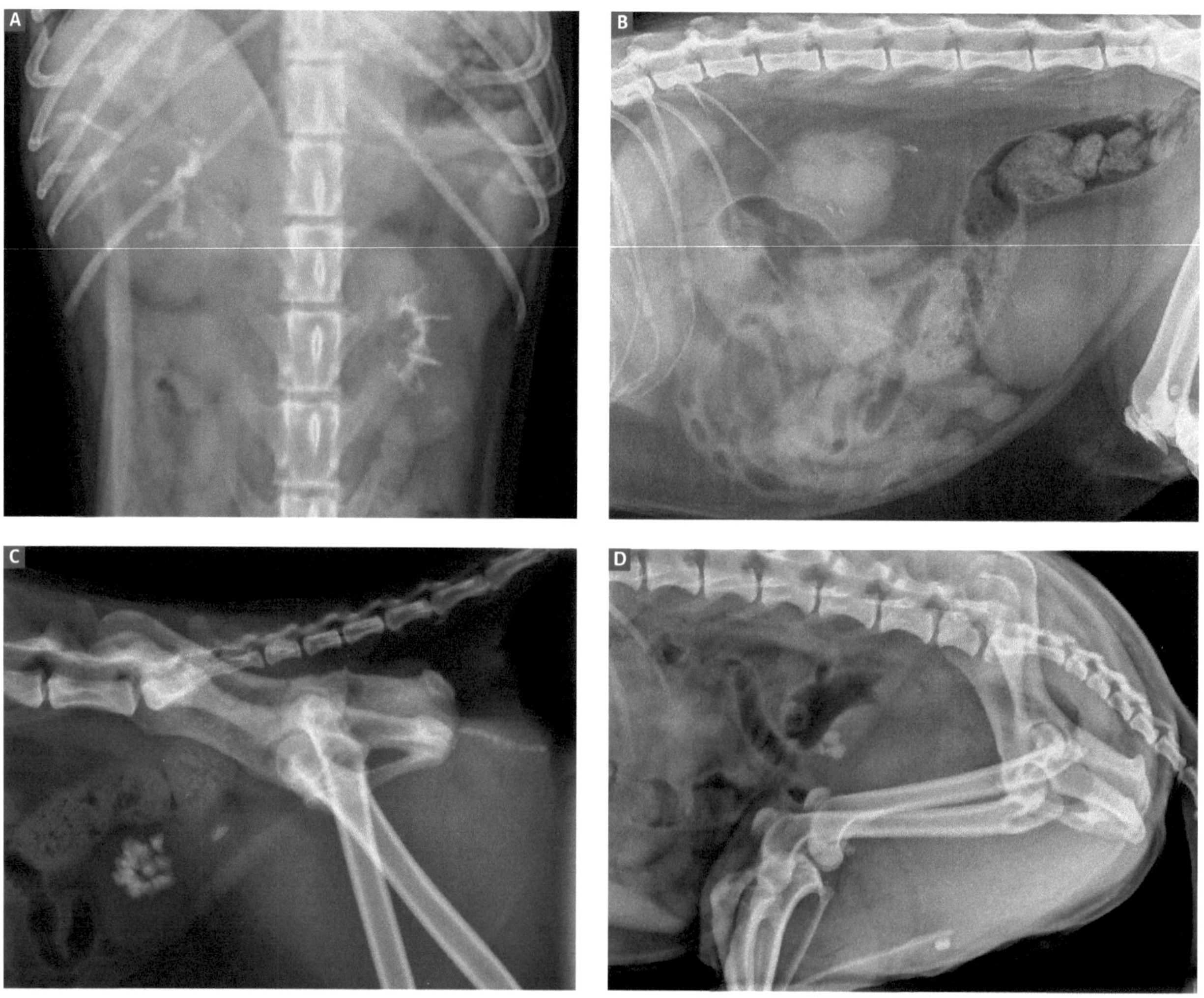

Figure 24. Urinary calculi. **A**. In the kidneys of a dog. **B**. In the ureters of a cat. **C**. In the bladder and urethra of a cat. **D**. In the bladder and urethra of a dog.

such as **calcium oxalate** and **struvite**, are radiopaque and are usually visualised on plain radiographs. **Cystine** and **urate** stones are radiotransparent. Very small calculi (<1 mm) are not usually visualised on plain radiographs regardless of their composition. Plain radiographs have a 13% chance of a false negative for detecting calculi. The composition of calculi cannot be determined by their morphology on radiographs.

Neoplasia

The most frequent neoplasms of the urinary system are **urothelial carcinomas**, which are usually located at the level of the trigone or bladder neck. They are not usually visualised on plain radiographs, although they can become mineralised. These neoplasms can metastasise to the medial iliac lymph nodes, which become enlarged in the caudal retroperitoneal space, and also to the last lumbar vertebrae, the sacrum or the pelvis, appearing as an irregular periosteal reaction or osteolysis in these bone structures. A filling defect can usually be observed in the caudodorsal aspect of the bladder during a positive cystogram.

Ectopic Ureter

Ectopic ureter is by far the most common congenital anomaly of the upper urinary tract. It is more common in dogs than in cats and in females than in males. It can be unilateral or bilateral, and can be associated with other congenital anomalies such as ureterocoele or renal dysplasia. The ureterovesical junction is located at the level of the bladder trigone in the dog and in the bladder neck or proximal urethra in the cat. In the dog, the ureterovesical junction has a hook shape with a caudomedial flexure. Differentiation between extramural and intramural ectopic ureters is crucial because intramural ureters can be resolved using minimally invasive laser treatment, whereas extramural ureters require surgical reimplantation. CT is the imaging technique of choice for the diagnosis of ectopic ureters (Fig. 25).

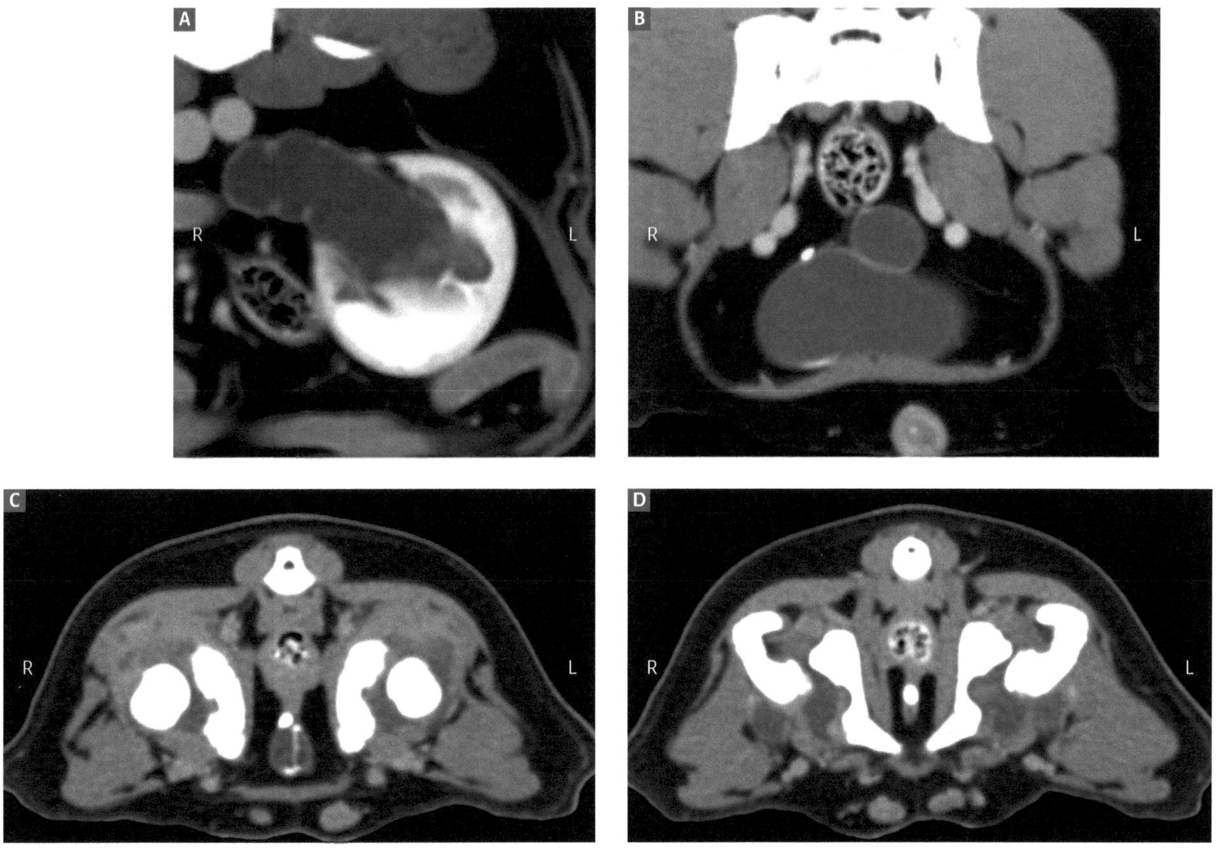

Figure 25. Cross-sectional CT images of different cases of ectopic ureter. **A**. Hydronephrosis and hydroureter. **B**. Severe left hydroureter; **C**. Note the normal insertion of the left ureter and the slight distension and caudal continuation of the right ureter. **D**. Compatible with a unilateral intramural ectopic ureter with insertion at the level of the urethra.

Ureterocoele

Ureterocoele is a congenital abnormality consisting of a focal dilatation of the distal portion of the ureter. It may be associated with an ectopic ureter (ectopic ureterocoele). It may be an incidental finding but has also been associated with obstruction and recurrent urinary tract infections. In contrast studies it is visualised as a filling defect in the bladder lumen.

Retrocaval Ureter

Retrocaval ureter is a congenital malformation characterised by one or both ureters following a spiral path around the caudal vena cava. Retrocaval ureter (or ureters) may be incidental but has been found to be associated with a higher rate of urinary tract infections and may predispose to ureteral obstruction. It is rare in dogs but occurs in 20–30% of cats. It can be diagnosed using CT.

Intrapelvic Bladder

An intrapelvic bladder is one in which the trigone is in an intrapelvic location and is usually accompanied by a short urethra. It may be associated with recurrent urinary tract infections and in some cases incontinence. The diagnosis can be established using contrast techniques. The degree of bladder distension affects the location of the trigone; therefore, the bladder must be adequately distended during cystography before an intrapelvic bladder can be diagnosed (Fig. 26).

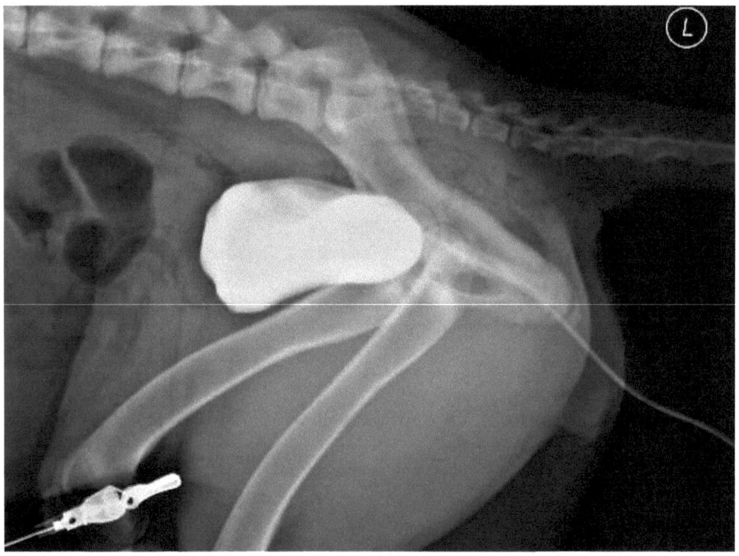

Figure 26. Positive contrast cystography in a dog with an intrapelvic bladder. Note the rounded shape of the bladder neck and its intrapelvic location.

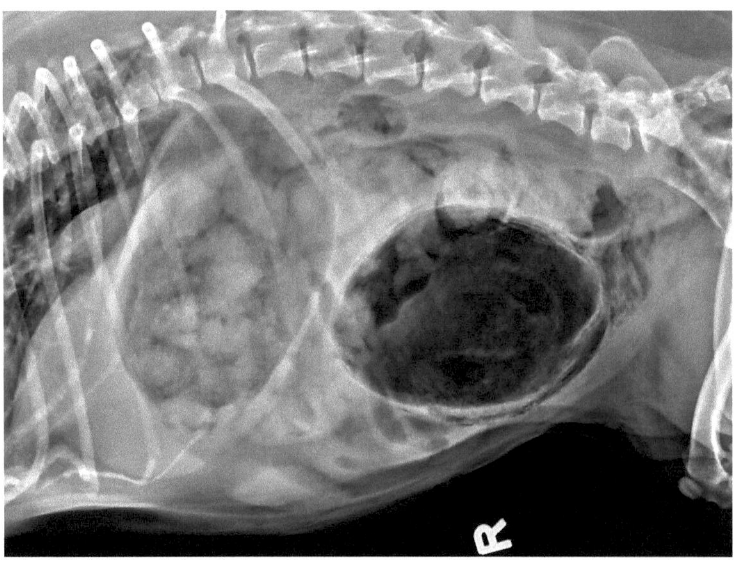

Figure 27. Emphysematous cystitis in a dog. Gas is observed in the bladder lumen and wall.

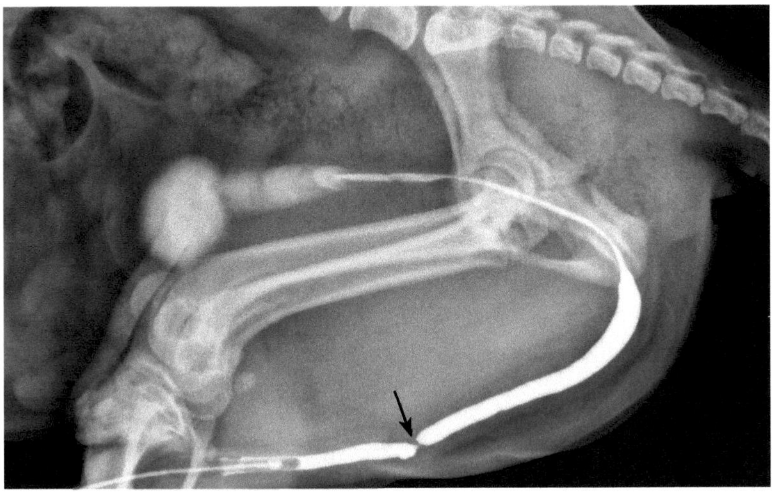

Figure 28. Retrograde urethrography in a puppy with congenital urethral stenosis (black arrow).

Emphysematous Cystitis

Emphysematous cystitis is characterised by gas in the bladder lumen and walls (Fig. 27) due to the presence of gas-producing microorganisms. It develops in diabetic patients with glycosuria because glucose in urine is an excellent source of energy for the growth of these microorganisms.

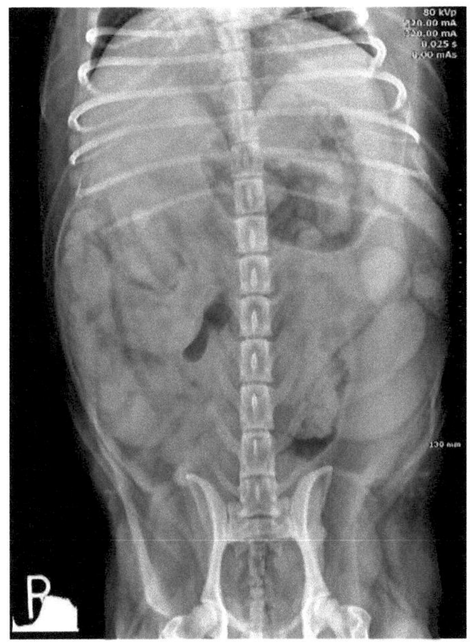

Urethral Stenosis

Urethral strictures (Fig. 28) can be congenital or secondary to trauma or calculi. They are diagnosed using retrograde urethrography. The normal urethra narrows slightly through the pelvis and then widens again in the prostate gland in males. True filling defects or stenosis should be visible on multiple images. Air bubbles can mimic filling defects but will move to different locations in the urethra as contrast medium is injected. It is important to take several radiographs while injecting contrast to differentiate between true lesions and artefacts.

Reproductive System

Uterus and Ovaries

The ovaries and uterus are not visible radiographically, except in some cases when there is a large amount of intra-abdominal fat, in which the body of the uterus can be seen between the descending colon and the bladder. When the uterus is distended, for example, in cases of pyometra, tubular structures with soft tissue opacity are visualised bilaterally in the caudal abdomen, which can be confused with distended small intestinal loops (Fig. 29). If the cervix is sufficiently distended, it can cause a mass effect between the bladder and the descending colon.

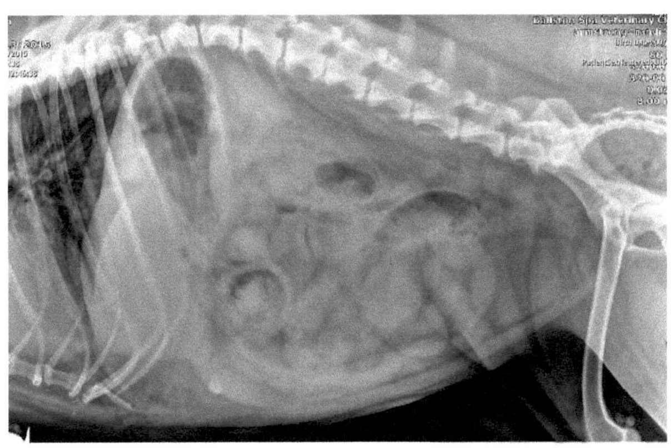

Figure 29. Pyometra in a bitch.

Prostate

Most lesions of the prostate are visualised radiographically as **prostatomegaly**, so changes are nonspecific. However, radiography allows the evaluation of associated abnormalities, such as compression of the colon or rectum, possible lymphadenopathy or metastatic bone lesions associated with prostatic neoplasia (Fig. 30). The presence of prostatomegaly with mineralisation in neutered dogs is indicative of neoplasia. **Paraprostatic cysts** are those of prostatic origin that are located outside the prostate. Radiographically, they are visualised as mass-like structures with soft tissue opacity in the caudal abdomen. They can cause dorsal displacement of the urinary bladder and may even spread cranially to the bladder. Their location can also be intrapelvic or perineal. The cyst capsule may become mineralised, resulting in an "eggshell" appearance (Fig. 31). If they are not mineralised it can be difficult to differentiate them from the prostate or bladder. If this is the case, ultrasonography and contrast studies are required to establish the diagnosis. Paraprostatic cysts are usually associated with prostatomegaly.

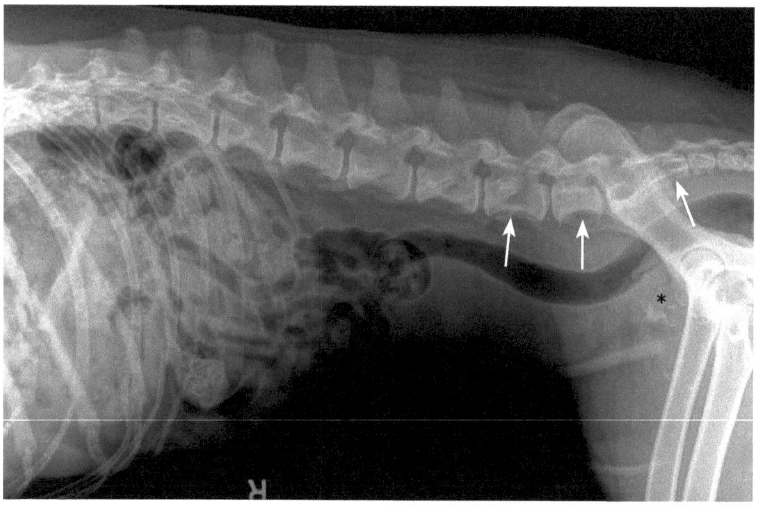

Figure 30. Prostatic carcinoma in a neutered dog with metastasis to the lumbar vertebrae. An amorphous mineralisation is visualised in the prostate (asterisk), as well as a periosteal reaction in L6, L7 and the sacrum, in addition to lysis of the ventral cortex of L7 (white arrows).

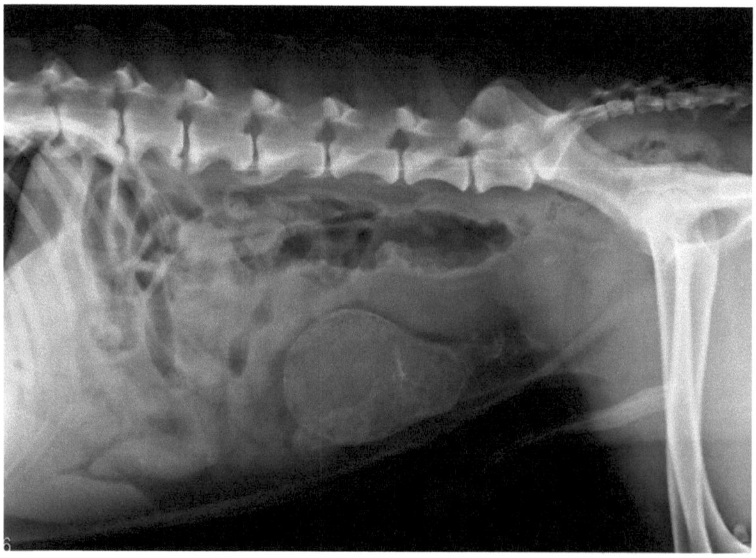

Figure 31. A mineralised paraprostatic cyst in a dog. The prostate is enlarged and the bladder is displaced dorsally.

Bibliography

- Agut, A., Soler, M. (2014) Sistema gastrointestinal. In: Agut, A., et al. (eds). *Diagnóstico por Imagen en Pequeños Animales*, pp. 403–420. Multimédica Ediciones Veterinarias.
- Burk, R.L., Ackerman, N. (1996) The abdomen. In: *Small Animal Radiology and Ultrasonography*, pp. 215–426. Saunders.
- Coss, P., Gilman, O., Warren-Smith, C., et al. (2021) The appearance of canine insulinoma on dual phase computed tomographic angiography. *J Small Anim Pract*, 62(7):540–546.
- Fields, E.L., Robertson, I.D., Osborne, J.A., et al. (2012) Comparison of abdominal computed tomography and abdominal ultrasound in sedated dogs. *Vet Radiol Ultrasound*, 53(5):513–517.
- Finck, C., d'Anjou, M.A., Alexander, K., et al. (2014) Radiographic diagnosis of mechanical obstruction in dogs based on relative small intestinal external diameters. *Vet Radiol Ultrasound*, 55(5):472–479.
- Fischetti, A.J., Saunders, H.M., Drobatz, K.J. (2004) Pneumatosis in canine gastric dilatation-volvulus syndrome. *Vet Radiol Ultrasound*, 45(3):205–209.
- Fitzgerald, E., Lam, R., Drees, R. (2017) Improving conspicuity of the canine gastrointestinal wall using dual phase contrast-enhanced computed tomography: a retrospective cross-sectional study. *Vet Radiol Ultrasound*, 58(2):151–162.
- Frank, P.M. (2018) The stomach. In: Thrall, D.E. (ed). *Textbook of Veterinary Diagnostic Radiology*. 7th ed, pp. 754–763. Elsevier Saunders.
- Gualtieri, M., Monzeglio, M.G., Scanziani, E. (1999) Gastric neoplasia. *Vet Clin North Am Small Anim Pract*, 29(2):415–440.
- Kang, K., Jang, M., Choi, K.U., et al. (2019) Antegrade and retrograde CT urethrography with virtual urethroscopy in a dog with urethral narrowing after bilateral triple pelvic osteotomy. *Vet Radiol Ultrasound*, 62(5):48–53.
- Kang, K., Kim, K., Oh, D., et al. (2020) Retrograde CT urethrography using a power injector quantitatively reveals effects of bladder distension on urethral size in healthy male Beagle dogs. *Vet Radiol Ultrasound*, 61(3):302–311.
- Lobacz, M.A., Sullivan, M., Mellor, D., et al. (2012) Effect of breed, age, weight and gender on radiographic renal size in the dog. *Vet Radiol Ultrasound*, 53(4):437–441.
- Paris, J.K., Yool, D.A., Reed, N., et al. (2011) Chronic gastric instability and presumed incomplete volvulus in dogs. *J Small Anim Pract*, 52(12):651–655.
- Schwarz, T., Bommer, N., Parys, M., et al. (2021) Four-dimensional CT excretory urography is an accurate technique for diagnosis of canine ureteral ectopia. *Vet Radiol Ultrasound*, 62(2):190–198.
- Shiroma, J.T., Gabriel, J.K., Carter, R.L., et al. (1999) Effect of reproductive status on feline renal size. *Vet Radiol Ultrasound*, 40(3):242–245.
- Terragni, R., Vignoli, M., Rossi, F., et al. (2012) Stomach wall evaluation using helical hydro-computed tomography. *Vet Radiol Ultrasound*, 53(4):402–405.
- Terragni, R., Vignoli, M., van Bree, H.J., et al. (2014) Diagnostic imaging and endoscopic finding in dogs and cats with gastric tumors: a review. *Schweiz Arch Tierheilkd*, 156(12):569–576.
- Thrall, D.E., Robertson, I.D. (2011) *Atlas of Normal Radiographic Anatomy and Anatomic Variants in the Dog and Cat*. 2nd ed. Elsevier Saunders.
- Walter, M.C., Matthiesen, D.T. (1993) Acquired antral pyloric hypertrophy in the dog. *Vet Clin North Am Small Anim Pract*, 23(3):547–554.
- White, C., Dirrig, H., Fitzgerald, E. (2020) CT findings in dogs with gastric malposition: 6 cases (2016-2019). *J Small Anim Pract*, 61(12):766–771.

Normal Ultrasonographic Appearance and Common Pathologies of the Liver, Biliary System, Spleen and Gastrointestinal Tract

Amalia Agut Giménez

Ultrasound Technique for the Abdominal Cavity

When planning an abdominal ultrasonographic study, fasting the patient before the examination is recommended so that the gastrointestinal tract is empty, as a full stomach will impair thorough examination of the liver. If the animal is very nervous or in pain, it should be sedated or given an analgesic to relax it, because panting or abdominal tension makes ultrasound examination difficult.

The entire ventral abdomen from the xiphoid process to the pelvic brim should be clipped as far dorsally as is necessary to facilitate examination of the retroperitoneal organs. Most abdominal ultrasound examinations are performed with the animal in dorsal recumbency, although they can also be performed with the animal in right or left lateral recumbency, or even with the animal standing. The presence of a large amount of gas in the gastrointestinal tract or a large amount of liquid in the peritoneal cavity, which causes intestinal loops containing gas to float, makes it difficult to examine the nondependent side adequately. Instead, it has to be examined from the dependent side, for which either a table with an access hole must be used or the animal must be examined while standing. A similar difficulty occurs when there are very heavy masses present (Novellas and Espada, 2014).

Liver

Technique

To perform ultrasound examination of the liver, the animal should be positioned in dorsal or lateral recumbency (Fig. 1). For most medium-sized and large dogs, a microconvex transducer of 5–8 MHz is generally used. Higher frequencies (8–12 MHz) are used for small-breed dogs and cats. Sometimes a frequency of 3 MHz is necessary for examining giant-breed dogs.

Sagittal and transverse sections of all parts of the right, left and midline liver should be routinely examined. The examination should begin by placing the transducer on the ventral midline caudal to the xiphoid process, directing the transducer craniodorsally and cranioventrally and moving the transducer to the right and left. Next, the transducer is oriented in a transverse plane to scan the liver from ventral to dorsal, and angling the beam to the right and left sides. This approach can usually be used to examine the entire liver, but sometimes it will be necessary to use an intercostal approach from the 10th to the 12th intercostal space on both the right and left sides. The intercostal approach is useful in cases of microhepatica, when the stomach is full of gas or in deep-chested breeds of dog. The right intercostal approach is very useful for visualising the caudal vena cava, portal vein, common bile duct and the lymph nodes of the porta hepatis region (d'Anjou and Penninck, 2015; Larson et al., 2020).

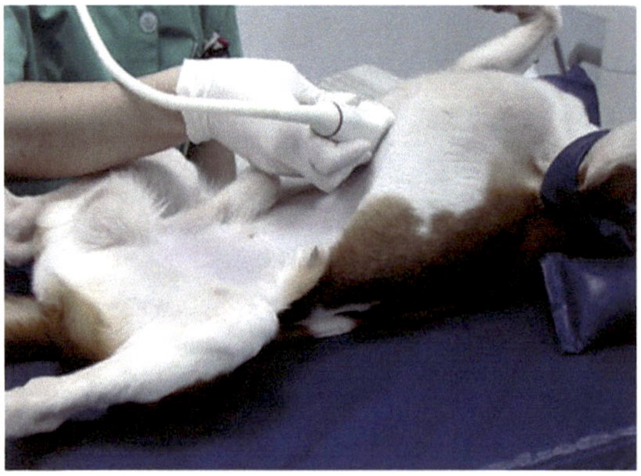

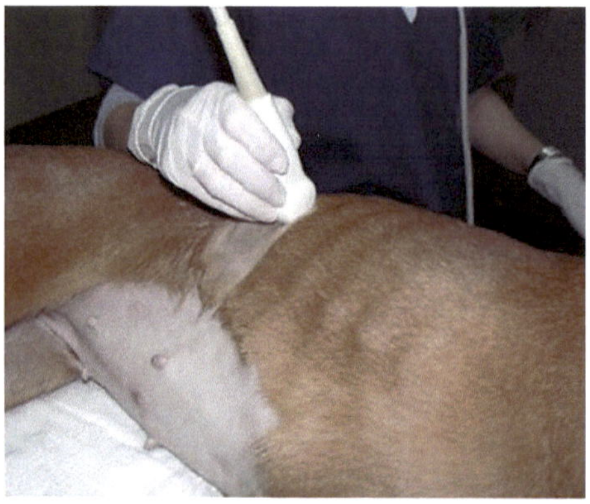

Figure 1. Positioning of the animal for ultrasonography exam of the liver.

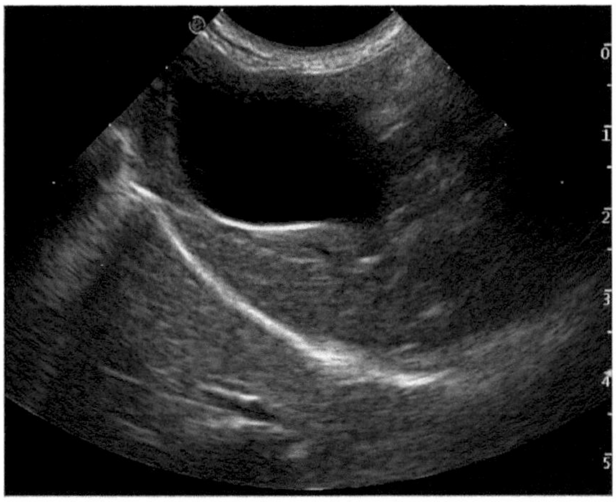

Figure 2. Sagittal section of the liver. A hyperechoic curvilinear line can be seen, which is the diaphragm. The gallbladder can be seen as an ovoid structure with anechoic content and a hyperechoic wall.

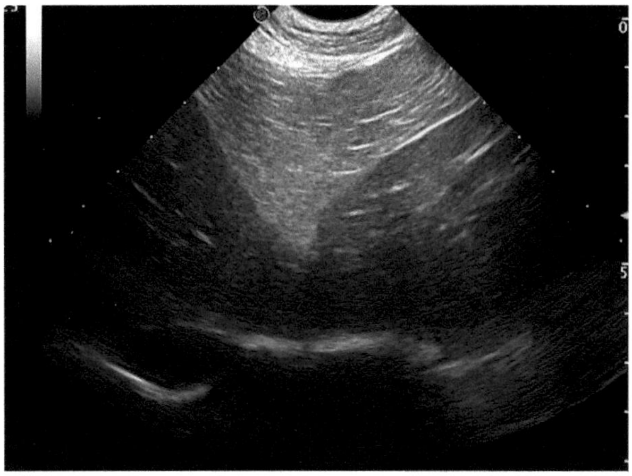

Figure 3. Transverse section of the liver. The fat within the falciform ligament can be seen, and is hyperechoic with respect to the hepatic parenchyma.

Normal Ultrasonographic Appearance

Localisation of the Liver

The liver is bordered cranially by the diaphragm, ventrally by the falciform ligament, and caudally by the right kidney on the right side, the stomach centrally, and the spleen on the left side.

During ultrasound examination, an echogenic curvilinear line is observed cranially to the liver, which is normally called the diaphragm (Fig. 2) but is actually the interface between the liver and the lung. The diaphragm itself is observed only when there is fluid in both the peritoneal and pleural cavities.

The fat of the falciform ligament is located ventral to the liver. In the dog, it can be of variable echogenicity, and can be isoechoic, hypoechoic or hyperechoic with respect to the liver (Fig. 3). In obese cats, the falciform fat is usually isoechoic or hypoechoic with respect to the liver parenchyma (Larson et al., 2020).

Parenchyma

In dogs and cats, the liver is composed of four lobes, four sublobes and two processes:

- right lobe, which includes lateral and medial sublobes
- quadrate lobe
- left lobe, which includes lateral and medial sublobes. This is the largest lobe and can constitute up to half of the total volume of the liver
- caudate lobe, which includes caudate and papillary processes.

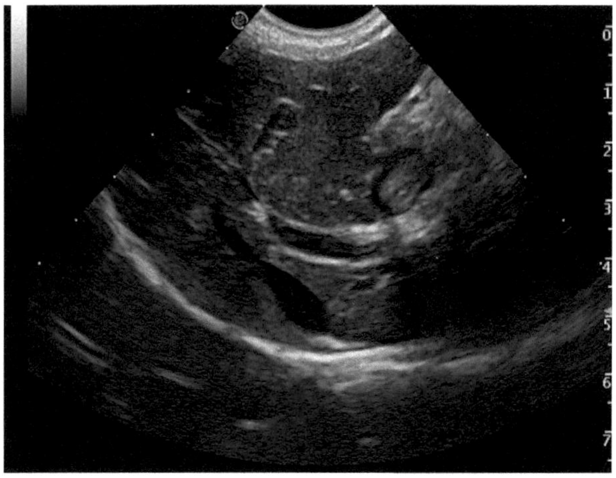

Figure 4. Transverse section of the liver. The portal vein can be identified by its hyperechoic walls, but the walls of the hepatic vein cannot be seen.

The gallbladder is surrounded by the right medial, quadrate and left medial lobes. The caudate lobe extends dorsally and caudally, ending with the renal fossa, which is occupied by the cranial pole of the right kidney. The liver lobes cannot be differentiated ultrasonographically, unless there is peritoneal effusion with a considerable amount of fluid, in which case the divisions between the different lobes may be visible.

The normal liver parenchyma has a medium, uniform echogenicity, interrupted by only the hepatic and portal veins (Fig. 4). The hepatic artery and bile duct lie adjacent to the portal vein but cannot be visualised. The echogenicity of the liver is equal to or slightly greater than that of the cortex of the right kidney, and it is hypoechoic with respect to the spleen. It has a coarser echotexture than the spleen (Larson et al., 2020).

Size

Measurement of the size of the liver by ultrasound is a subjective assessment. The same criteria as those used with radiographs can be applied, in which the liver should not extend past the costal arch. In dogs, the breed and body shape of the dog need to be taken into account; in cats there is less variability because cats are generally similar in size.

An increase in liver size is suspected when the distance between the diaphragm and the stomach is larger than expected, there is an increase in the extent of the liver in the area ventral to the stomach or ventral to the right kidney, and rounding of the margins of the liver is seen.

A decrease in liver size is suspected when a small amount of liver parenchyma is seen, when the distance between the diaphragm and the stomach is smaller than expected, or when the extent of the liver in the area ventral to the stomach or ventral to the right kidney is smaller than usual.

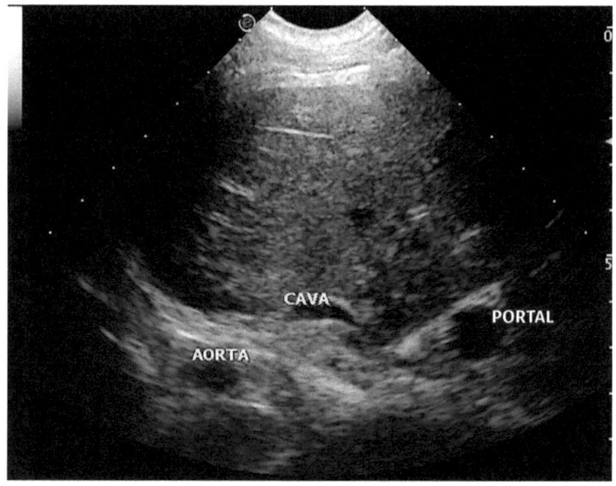

Figure 5. Ultrasound image of the liver obtained with a right intercostal approach. The location of the portal vein, caudal vena cava and aorta can be seen.

Hepatic Vascularisation

The afferent flow from the liver is formed by two systems: the **portal vein**, which represents 80% of the flow that reaches the liver, and the **hepatic arteries**. Efferent flow goes through the hepatic veins to the caudal vena cava.

The porta hepatis (or hilum of the liver) is located in the central part of the liver to the right of the midline, and is the area where the **portal vein**, **hepatic artery** and **bile duct** enter and exit the liver. Of these three structures, the portal vein is the easiest to identify. The intrahepatic portal veins are a continuation of the portal vein itself from where it enters the liver at the porta hepatis. When the main portal vein enters the liver, the first division to emerge from it is the right intrahepatic branch. The main portal vein continues cranially, with the central branch emerging next, and the portal vein then continues as the left intrahepatic branch. The hepatic artery is smaller and can be identified using colour Doppler. The common bile duct is located ventral to the porta hepatis and is more difficult to visualise in dogs than in cats.

The intrahepatic portal veins are the most easily visualised vessels in the hepatic parenchyma because their walls are hyperechoic due to the presence of connective tissue and fat around the wall. By contrast, the walls of the hepatic veins are not observed unless the ultrasound waves are completely perpendicular to the walls, in which case they can also appear as hyperechoic.

The **caudal vena cava** is more easily observed in images obtained using the right intercostal approach, where it is visualised dorsal to the portal vein (Fig. 5). The **hepatic veins** (both right and left branches) are normally seen entering the caudal vena cava just caudal to the diaphragm, and appear as anechoic tubular structures.

Extrahepatic Portal Vascular System

The extrahepatic part of the portal vein is located ventral and to the left of the caudal vena cava. The portal vein has a less rectilinear path than the caudal vena cava. The ratio of the diameters of the portal vein and the aorta (PV/Ao ratio) is 0.7–1.25 in both cats and dogs. Portal flow is almost constant, with an average velocity at the level of the porta hepatis of 15–20 cm/s in the dog and 10–18 cm/s in the cat.

The portal vein is formed by the confluence of the cranial and caudal mesenteric veins and the splenic vein. It also receives small tributary vessels such as the gastroduodenal vein, a few centimetres caudal to the entrance to the liver. All tributary veins increase in diameter as they approach the portal vein, and the flow from all of them is hepatopetal (towards the liver). The flow in the portal vein is normally parabolic and relatively constant (d'Anjou, 2007).

Gallbladder and Biliary System

The gallbladder is located to the right of the midline, near the diaphragm, and is visualised as a rounded or elongated (depending on the plane) anechoic structure bordered by a hyperechoic line that is the wall of the organ (Fig. 2). In cats, the gallbladder is occasionally bilobed. The size of the gallbladder is variable depending on how long the animal has been fasted. The gallbladder often contains mobile echogenic content (biliary sludge) in animals that are not showing clinical signs of gallbladder pathology; however, the idea that this biliary sludge indicates hypomotility or delayed emptying of the bile is gaining support.

The intrahepatic biliary tree is not visualised in normal patients. The common bile duct (CBD), which represents the continuity of the cystic duct and bile ducts, is more easily visualised in cats than in dogs. It is located ventral to the portal vein, surrounded by hyperechoic tissue. It can measure up to 4 mm in diameter in cats and 3 mm in dogs. The CBD runs parallel to the portal vein until it enters the duodenum through the major duodenal papilla. In dogs, the CBD and pancreatic duct enter separately, whereas in the cat they join before emptying into the duodenal papilla. The wall thickness of the gallbladder and CBD should not be more than 1 mm (Larson et al., 2020).

Ultrasonographic Abnormalities of the Liver Parenchyma

Liver abnormalities can be classified as:

- diffuse
- focal or multifocal.

Diffuse Liver Diseases

Normal liver echotexture is assessed subjectively; therefore, it is important to be aware of and know how to use the ultrasound equipment controls well to obtain normal liver echogenicity.

Diffuse liver diseases may cause an increase or decrease in echogenicity, or mixed echogenicity (Table 1). There are also pathologies that do not alter the echogenicity of the liver, such as lymphoma, disseminated mastocytoma, acute hepatitis and acute cholangiohepatitis. As well as the echogenicity of the liver, its size and shape must also be evaluated (Table 2).

Increased Echogenicity

When the liver is more echogenic than normal, the portal veins are less visible due to the general increase in echogenicity. The liver will be hyperechoic with respect to the renal cortex and spleen. The differential diagnoses of the pathologies that produce an increase in echogenicity are shown in Table 1.

In addition to its echogenicity, the size and the borders of the liver should be evaluated. Generally, in lipidosis (Fig. 6), steroid liver disease or lymphosarcoma, the liver will be enlarged and will have rounded edges. A biopsy or fine-needle aspiration is necessary to reach a definitive diagnosis.

Table 1. Differential diagnosis for diffuse hepatic abnormalities.

Hyperechoic	Hypoechoic	Mixed echogenicity
· Chronic hepatitis · Cirrhosis · Fibrosis · Lipidosis · Lymphoma · Mastocytoma · Steroidal hepatopathy	· Acute cholangiohepatitis · Acute hepatitis · Amyloidosis · Histiocytic neoplasia · Leukaemia · Lymphoma · Passive congestion	· Amyloidosis (cats) · Hepatocutaneous syndrome (superficial necrolytic dermatitis) · Chronic hepatitis · Hepatocellular carcinoma · Lymphoma · Metastasis · Necrosis · Cirrhosis · Steroidal hepatopathy · Nodular hyperplasia · Extramedullary haematopoiesis

Table 2. Differential diagnosis of pathologies that can cause changes in the size and shape of the liver.

Increase	Decrease	Asymmetrical increase
· Amyloidosis · Diffuse primary or metastatic neoplasia · Lipidosis · Round cell neoplasm · Vacuolar hepatopathy · Vascular congestion	· Cirrhosis · Congenital portosystemic shunt · Fibrosis · Microvascular dysplasia · Portal vein hypoplasia	· Abscess · Cyst · Granuloma · Hepatic lobe torsion · Primary neoplasia · Metastatic neoplasia

Decreased Echogenicity

Diffuse liver diseases can result in a hypoechoic liver, in which the liver is of lower echogenicity than the renal cortex and the walls of the portal vein appear more prominent (Fig. 7).

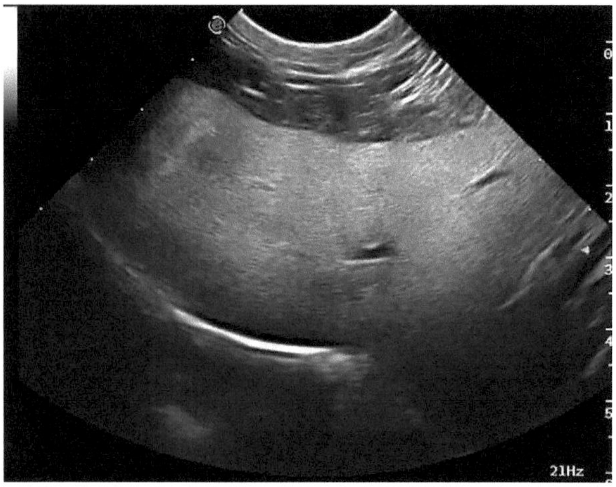

Figure 6. Transverse section of the liver of a cat with lipidosis. An increase in the echogenicity of the liver can be seen, and the portal veins cannot be visualised.

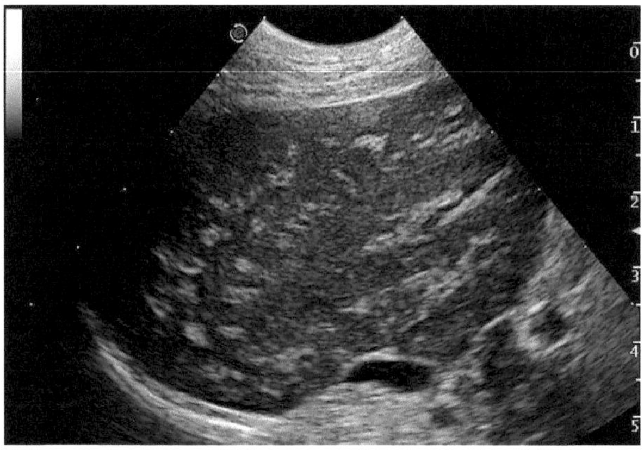

Figure 7. Liver with reduced echogenicity. The portal veins can be seen to be more prominent than normal.

The list of differential diagnoses for pathologies that cause decreased echogenicity is shown in Table 1. A biopsy or fine-needle aspiration are necessary to reach a definitive diagnosis.

Mixed Echogenicity

A liver with mixed echogenicity presents a diffusely speckled appearance that is generally characterised by a hyperechoic parenchyma with poorly defined hypoechoic areas, although there may also be hyperechoic nodules, making it difficult to differentiate one area from another.

The differential diagnoses of pathologies that cause mixed echogenicity of the liver are shown in Table 1. A biopsy or fine-needle aspiration is necessary to reach a definitive diagnosis (d'Anjou and Penninck, 2015).

Focal Parenchymal Diseases

Focal lesions in the liver commonly vary in size. They are called **nodules** when the lesion is less than 3 cm, and **masses** when they are larger. Focal lesions may be anechoic, hypoechoic, hyperechoic, isoechoic, mixed or have a "bullseye" pattern (Table 3). "Bullseye" lesions are nodules with a hyperechoic centre surrounded by a hypoechoic ring (Fig. 8). These lesions are usually neoplastic metastases when they occur in several abdominal organs (liver, spleen, kidney). They can occur as solitary or multiple lesions (Cuccovillo and Lamb, 2002).

The same pathology can present with more than one appearance; changes in the parenchyma can be seen, but because of the variability of appearance of the lesions sometimes it is difficult to establish a diagnosis. Therefore, biopsy or fine-needle aspiration is necessary to reach a diagnosis.

In addition to its echogenicity, the morphology and borders of the lesion should be evaluated, as well as its vascularisation.

Nodular Hyperplasia

Nodular hyperplasia is a common pathology that occurs in up to 70% of older dogs. These regenerative nodules can vary

Table 3. Differential diagnosis of multifocal lesions in the liver.

Anechoic	Hypoechoic	Hyperechoic	Mixed echogenicity
· Cyst · Necrosis · Abscess · Cystic tumour · Biloma	· Nodular hyperplasia · Haematoma · Lymphoma · Complex cyst · Metastasis · Primary neoplasia · Necrosis	· Nodular hyperplasia · Metastasis · Myelolipoma · Granuloma · Primary neoplasia · Mineralisation or cholelithiasis · Gas · Extramedullary haematopoiesis	· Nodular hyperplasia · Metastasis · Abscess · Haematoma · Primary neoplasia

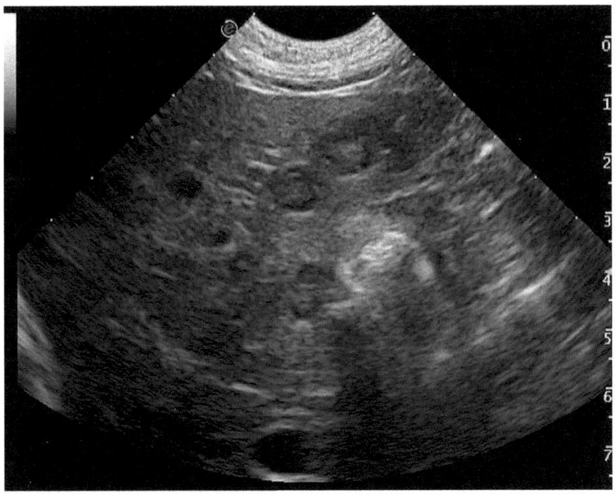

Figure 8. Several "bullseye" lesions can be seen, compatible with hepatic metastasis or nodular hyperplasia. The histopathological diagnosis was metastasis.

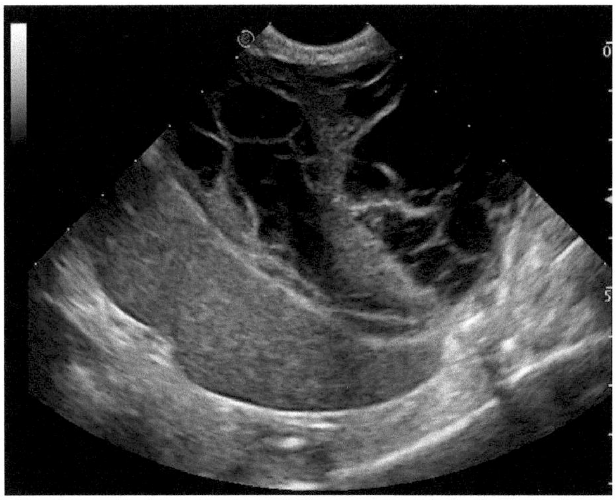

Figure 9. Ultrasound image of a septate cystic structure consistent with a haematoma, although a neoplasm cannot be completely ruled out.

in echogenicity and size (5–15 mm) and they can have well or poorly defined margins. They cannot be differentiated ultrasonographically from nodules caused by vacuolar hepatopathy or extramedullary haematopoiesis.

Cysts

Hepatic cysts are usually incidental findings, and usually cause clinical signs only when they are large and produce some mechanical compression of surrounding structures. Typically, hepatic cysts are rounded structures with a thin, well-defined, anechoic wall and posterior enhancement.

They can be solitary or multiple, congenital or acquired, and can affect both the parenchyma and the biliary tract (bilomas).

Sometimes, the cysts do not meet the criteria described above and the possible differential diagnoses are much broader, ranging from traumatic, toxic or inflammatory processes to neoplasms.

Complex cystic lesions may be haematomas, abscesses, cystic metastases, haemorrhages or necrotic tumours.

Haematomas

The ultrasonographic appearance of a haematoma changes over time. Acute haemorrhage of less than 24 hours is echogenic. During the first week, the haematoma becomes hypoechoic and better defined; in the following weeks the fluid disappears and is replaced by granulation tissue.

Sometimes, haematomas cannot be differentiated ultrasonographically from other lesions, such as abscesses, necrosis and neoplasms (Fig. 9).

Abscesses

Hepatic abscesses are uncommon in dogs and cats. They may be associated with infections of other organs or be due to penetrating foreign bodies, torsion of a liver lobe or hepatic neoplasia.

The ultrasonographic appearance of abscesses varies according to how long they have been present; they can appear as anechoic, hypoechoic, hyperechoic or with mixed echogenicity. Occasionally there may be gas present producing a reverberation artefact.

Granulomas

Hepatic granulomas or pyogranulomas can be detected in both dogs and cats, particularly in cases of fungal diseases, feline infectious peritonitis or feline eosinophilic fibroplasia. Granulomatous lesions tend to be hyperechoic and heterogeneous.

Mineralisation

Areas of mineralisation in the liver parenchyma are usually due to chronic granulomas, dystrophic mineralisation in the biliary tree, or secondary to ascending inflammation or cholecystitis. Ultrasonographically, hyperechoic areas with acoustic shadowing are observed.

Gas

Intraparenchymal gas is visualised as hyperechoic areas with reverberation artefact. Gas may be seen in the biliary tree and gallbladder after surgery, in the wall of the gallbladder in diabetic dogs with emphysematous cholecystitis, inside the biliary tree secondary to an ascending infection, inside a liver abscess or in a hepatic lobe torsion.

Hepatic Lobe Torsion

Torsion of a hepatic lobe is rare. It leads to congestion, haemorrhage and necrosis, and can present different ultrasonographic appearances (hypoechoic, mixed echogenicity, hyperechoic foci with reverberation when gas is present) that can resemble those of abscesses and neoplasms.

Neoplasms

Metastatic tumours in the liver from primary tumours of the pancreas, spleen and gastrointestinal system are more common in the dog, whereas primary liver tumours are more common in cats.

Primary liver tumours are usually solitary masses affecting one lobe, or they can be multifocal, involving several lobes. The most common **malignant primary tumour** of the liver in the dog is **hepatocellular carcinoma** (Fig. 10). Typically, the liver is also affected in cases of disseminated histiocytic sarcoma, lymphosarcoma and mastocytoma.

The most common **metastatic tumours** are **sarcomas** of the spleen or gastrointestinal tract, or **carcinomas** that originate in the stomach, pancreas, thyroid gland or mammary glands. The most common **benign tumour** is hepatocellular adenoma.

The ultrasonographic appearance of liver tumours is highly variable, making it difficult to differentiate benign from malignant masses on ultrasound examination. The patterns described are hepatomegaly, poorly defined hypoechoic areas, hypoechoic nodules, "bullseye" lesions and generalised changes in echogenicity, both hypoechoic and hyperechoic. In cases of malignant tumours, lymphadenopathy is usually present (Larson et al., 2020).

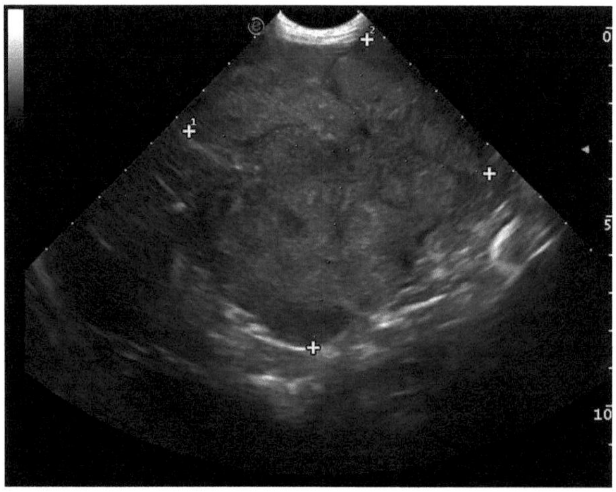

Figure 10. Ultrasound image of a hepatic mass with mixed echogenicity and a heterogeneous echotexture. The histopathological diagnosis was hepatocellular carcinoma.

Ultrasonographic Abnormalities of the Biliary System

Ultrasonography is widely used to assess abnormalities and diseases of the biliary system.

In addition to congenital anomalies, from an ultrasonographic point of view, gallbladder abnormalities can be divided into:

- luminal abnormalities
- wall abnormalities.

Congenital Abnormalities

Bilobed gallbladders are uncommon and are more often seen in cats than dogs, as incidental findings. A bilobed gallbladder is partially divided but has a single cystic duct.

Gallbladder agenesis is another rare abnormality in dogs. It occurs more frequently in small-breed dogs, which may show no clinical signs or have alterations in the activities of liver enzymes. Gallbladder agenesis must be differentiated from fibrosis of the gallbladder wall, in which the wall is unable to distend but the lumen is visible.

Luminal Abnormalities

Biliary Sludge and Calculi

Biliary sludge is made up of aggregations of calcium bilirubinate and cholesterol suspended in a mucin-rich bile. It is observed ultrasonographically as an echogenic material inside the gallbladder (Fig. 11). It is frequently visualised in dogs, in which it is not necessarily linked to hepatobiliary disease. However, when seen in cats, it is associated with biliary pathologies. Although biliary sludge is usually an incidental finding in dogs, it is currently thought to be due to alterations in gallbladder motility. It is therefore always important to assess whether the content of the gallbladder is mobile or not, in order to make treatment recommendations.

Cholelithiasis (gallbladder calculi; gallstones) or **choledocholithiasis** (bile duct calculi) may be an incidental finding with no clinical significance. However, biliary obstruction due to calculi can occur, especially in cats. Ultrasonographically, calculi will be observed as hyperechoic material or structures with acoustic shadowing, which will be more evident the larger the size of the calculus and the higher its calcium content. Calculi may develop as a result of factors including biliary stasis, cholecystitis and diet. In the cat, calculi are usually associated with cholangitis or cholangiohepatitis.

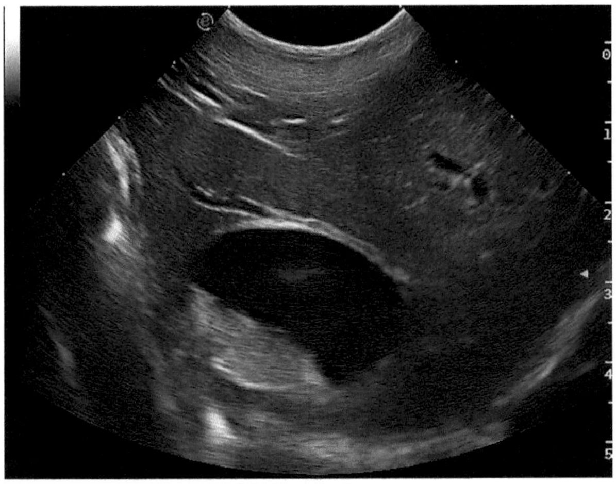

Figure 11. Ultrasound image of a sagittal section of the liver of a dog. Hyperechoic content with respect to the hepatic parenchyma can be seen on the dependent side. This content does not cause acoustic shadowing and was therefore diagnosed as biliary sludge.

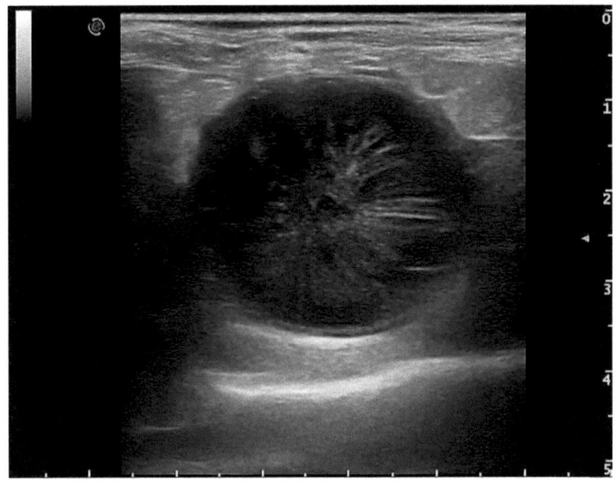

Figure 12. Ultrasound image of the gallbladder in a dog in which a mucocoele can be seen. The gallbladder contains hyperechoic striations that appear organised, with a stellate or "kiwi fruit" appearance.

In both dogs and cats, choleliths are made up of a mixture of calcium, cholesterol and bilirubin, and are visible on plain radiographs.

As a complication of cholelithiasis, in addition to biliary obstruction, gallbladder perforation may occur.

Biliary Mucocoele

Mucocoeles are a major cause of hepatobiliary disease. A mucocoele is an abnormal collection of bile salts and mucus inside the gallbladder that can cause biliary obstruction, necrosis of the gallbladder wall and gallbladder rupture. They are common in dogs but not in cats.

The pathogenesis of mucocoele is unknown, although multiple factors have been suggested that result in the abnormal retention of bile salts, decreased biliary motility (contractility of the gallbladder) and excessive secretion of mucus by the biliary epithelium. Factors associated with the development of mucocoele are endocrinopathies (hyperadrenocorticism, hypothyroidism), hyperlipidaemia and breed predispositions.

Ultrasonography is the most commonly used technique to diagnose mucocoele. Six types of ultrasonographic patterns have been described, which have no relationship to the clinical picture. The most typical patterns are the stellate or "kiwi fruit" appearance, in which there is a central area of immobile echogenic content and linear striations (Fig. 12), and the amorphous pattern, where the gallbladder is completely filled with immobile echogenic material. Striation marks represent the fracture lines between accumulations of mucus. The gallbladder wall is thickened and very distended.

Distension of the gallbladder can lead to necrosis of the wall and the leakage of bile into the peritoneal cavity, resulting in increased echogenicity of the peripheral mesentery, which is in contact with the gallbladder wall. Abnormal mucus accumulation can extend to the cystic and bile ducts, leading to extrahepatic biliary obstruction.

Animals with mucocoeles sometimes show no clinical signs; however, the condition can evolve to cause wall necrosis and perforation, and for these reasons monitoring the mucocoele or preventative surgical removal are recommended. Cases of mucocoele that resolve after medical treatment have also been described (Pike et al., 2004).

Wall Abnormalities

Cystic Mucinous Hyperplasia

Cystic mucinous hyperplasia is characterised by hyperplasia of the gallbladder epithelium where cysts containing mucus develop in the wall and protrude into the lumen. These cysts are usually incidental findings and have always been observed in animals with mucocoele.

Polyps and Neoplasms

Polyps are seen as pedunculated masses that protrude into the gallbladder lumen.

Neoplasms of the gallbladder are rare in both dogs and cats. They can present different ultrasonographic appearances and are sometimes difficult to differentiate from hepatic neoplasms. Biliary cystadenoma and cystadenocarcinoma of older cats have the typical appearance of cysts.

Cholecystitis

Cholecystitis can present various ultrasonographic appearances. The wall of the gallbladder may be normal or thickened symmetrically or asymmetrically, and it may be entirely hyperechoic or present a double layer (a hypoechoic line between two hyperechoic lines) (Fig. 13). In cases of cholecystitis, biliary sludge may also be present.

Cholangitis

Cholangitis is an inflammatory process that affects the periportal region, in which infiltration of the epithelium of the duct or ductal lumen occurs. It can affect both dogs and cats, and is more frequent in cats, due to inflammatory liver disease.

In the cat, in many cases of cholangitis no ultrasonographic abnormalities are visualised. When they are present, thickening of the gallbladder wall, biliary sludge, choleliths, and dilation, thickening and a tortuous path of the bile duct can be seen. These changes can occur in all types of cholangitis/cholangiohepatitis. The liver parenchyma may have normal, hypoechoic, heterogeneous or hyperechoic echogenicity. Pancreatitis and inflammatory bowel disease can also occur in these cases.

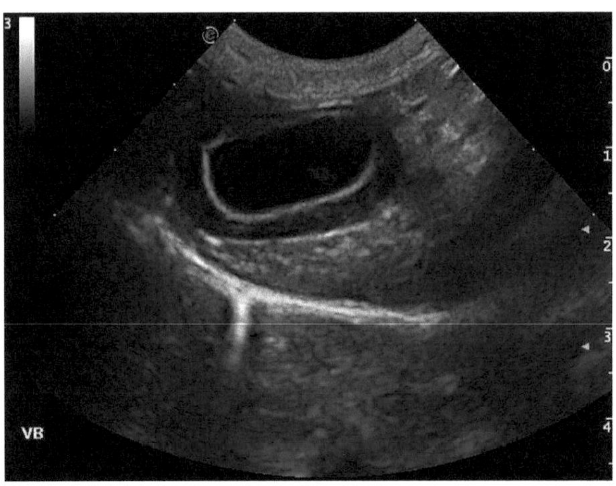

Figure 13. Ultrasound image of the gallbladder of a dog. A concentric thickening of the wall can be seen (double wall appearance), which can be seen in cases of oedema or inflammation.

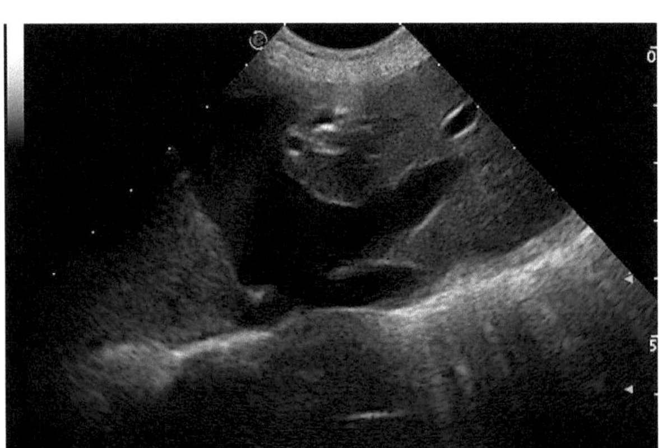

Figure 14. Ultrasound image of the liver of a dog with right-sided heart failure. The hepatic veins and caudal vena cava appear distended.

Cholangitis/cholangiohepatitis can also occur in dogs, in which ultrasonographic changes are seen at the biliary and hepatic level.

Extrahepatic Biliary Obstruction

Ultrasonography is a very useful technique to differentiate biliary obstruction from hepatocellular disease in animals presenting with jaundice. Causes of extrahepatic biliary obstruction are variable and include pancreatitis, gallstones, biliary mucocoele, neoplasia of the liver or adjacent organs, as well as foreign bodies in the duodenum. In cats, the most common causes are inflammatory disease (e.g. chronic pancreatitis, duodenitis), neoplasms of adjacent organs (duodenum, pancreas, bile duct) and cholelithiasis.

Ultrasonographic findings will depend on the duration and extent (percentage) of the obstruction. After 5–7 days of obstruction, anechoic tortuous tubular structures with hyperechoic walls are observed inside the liver parenchyma, producing the "too many tubes" ultrasonographic sign. Dilated intrahepatic bile ducts are ultrasonographically similar to portal veins but can be readily differentiated by using Doppler ultrasonography (Larson et al., 2020).

Vascular Disorders

Caudal Vena Cava and Hepatic Veins

Venous hepatic congestion is commonly caused by right-sided heart failure, producing an increase in pressure at the level of the caudal vena cava and hepatic veins. The caudal vena cava and hepatic veins appear dilated, and the liver is enlarged and diffusely hypoechoic (Fig. 14).

Portal Vein

Portosystemic Shunt

Congenital portosystemic shunts are one of the most common vascular abnormalities in dogs, and are also found in cats.

They can be divided into congenital and acquired.

- Congenital
    - **Intrahepatic** (usually in medium or large breeds of dog). They can be left, right or central. The most

frequent type is on the left side, due to persistence of the venous conduit. Ultrasonographically, dilated vascular structures are observed that connect the portal vein or one of its branches to a hepatic vein or the caudal vena cava (Fig. 15). The portal vein may appear to have a normal or increased diameter and a generally high flow velocity (≥50 cm/s) because there is very little resistance to flow due to the shunt being located cranial to the point of measurement.

- **Extrahepatic** (usually in small breeds). Extrahepatic shunts are more common than intrahepatic shunts and occur in small breeds of dog and in cats. Ultrasonographically, a dilated and tortuous vessel with hepatofugal (away from the liver) flow is observed, originating in the main portal vein or a tributary vein (often in the splenic or right gastric vein, but sometimes in the left gastric or gastroepiploic vein). Generally, these shunts empty into the caudal vena cava cranial to the right renal vein, or into the renal vein, azygos vein or phrenic vein. In animals with an extrahepatic congenital portosystemic communication (CPSC), the portal vein appears greatly reduced in size in the area cranial to the point of origin of the shunt. A PV/Ao ratio ≤0.65 is considered to be compatible with an extrahepatic CPSC (although the ratio is also reduced in primary portal hypoplasia), whereas a ratio ≥0.8 rules it out.

– Acquired: also associated with the presence of portal hypertension. These shunts are multiple and are located in the area caudal to the left kidney or in the splenic region. They are observed as long and tortuous vessels (d'Anjou, 2007).

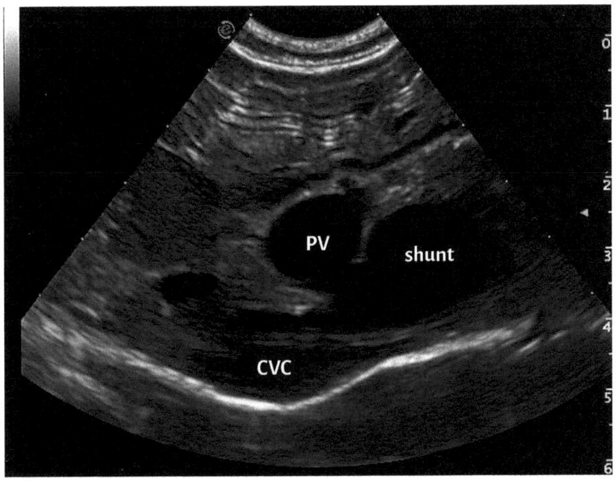

Figure 15. Ultrasound image of the liver of a 9-month-old Labrador. A large vessel (shunt) can be seen connecting the portal vein (PV) to the caudal vein cava (CVC). The diagnosis was a congenital intrahepatic shunt.

Portal Hypertension

Causes of portal hypertension can be:

- **prehepatic** (where something hinders the portal flow before it reaches the liver);
- **hepatic** (a problem at the level of the liver).

Ultrasonographically, the presence of free fluid can be observed, and in some cases oedema of the wall of the gallbladder and pancreas is also present. Portal hypertension leads to the formation of multiple portosystemic shunts (Mattoon and Duffy, 2020).

Portal Vein Thrombosis

Portal vein thrombosis has been described in cases of hyperadrenocorticism, hepatic neoplasms, protein-losing enteropathy and in autoimmune pathologies. The thrombus can appear anechoic, hypoechoic, isoechoic or hyperechoic, as well as homogeneous or heterogeneous, and fills the lumen and causes distension of the portal vein. It can also extend into the splenic vein, mesenteric vein, pancreaticoduodenal vein and caudal vena cava. In the event that the thrombus is anechoic, the use of colour or duplex Doppler is necessary for diagnosis.

Arteriovenous Fistula

Arteriovenous fistulas are uncommon, but have been described in both dogs and cats. They are a communication between the portal veins and the hepatic arteries and can produce an increase in pressure in the portal system, with the formation of acquired portosystemic collaterals. Ultrasonographically, dilated and tortuous vascular structures can be observed in or adjacent to the hepatic parenchyma (Larson et al., 2020).

Spleen

Technique

The spleen is examined by placing the transducer on the caudal part of the 13th left rib. The dorsal part of the spleen is usually located below the ribs if the stomach is empty, and in some cases an intercostal approach is necessary to visualise it (Fig. 16). The ventral part is mobile and can come into contact with the liver and, caudally, with the bladder. High-frequency transducers are needed to examine the spleen due to its flattened shape and superficial location (Mattoon and Duffy, 2020).

Normal Ultrasonographic Appearance

The spleen has an elongated, flattened shape, and is divided into three parts. The **head**, located dorsally, is hook shaped

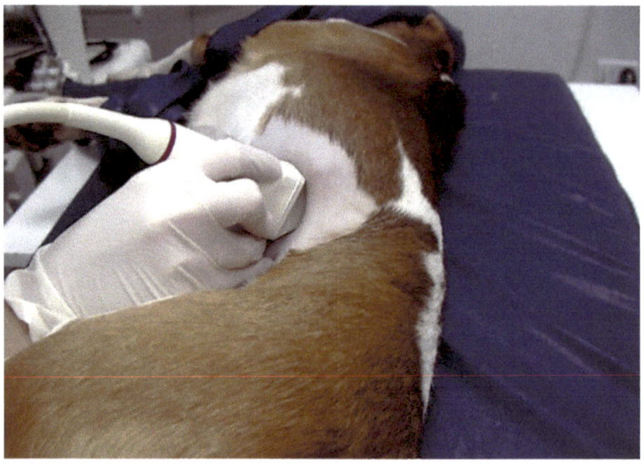

Figure 16. Positioning of the transducer for examination of the spleen.

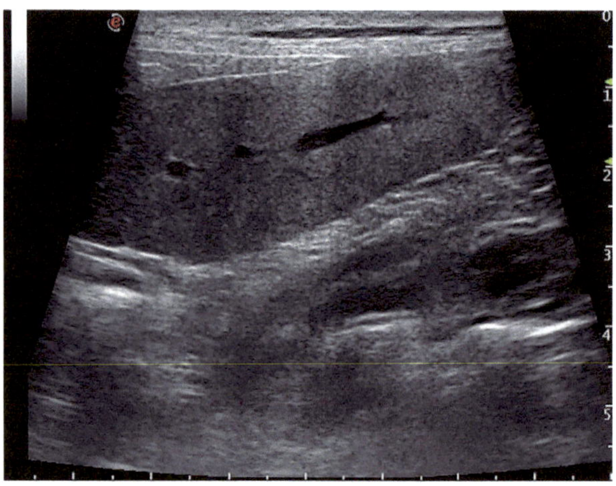

Figure 17. Ultrasound image of the body of the spleen in a dog. A fine, homogeneous echotexture can be appreciated.

and is located between the gastric fundus and the left kidney; the **body** is located in the mid-abdomen; and the **tail** is located towards the middle of the abdomen and slightly caudoventrally. Thus, the anatomical reference points used to locate the spleen are the stomach, the descending colon and the left kidney.

The splenic parenchyma has a very fine homogeneous echotexture (Fig. 17). It is hyperechoic with respect to the liver and renal cortex (Fig. 18). Occasionally, in cats it is isoechoic with respect to the renal cortex. The splenic veins can be visualised in the middle of the spleen as anechoic tubular structures. The splenic arteries are not visible in B mode (Hecht and Mai, 2015).

The size of the spleen is variable in dogs but more consistent in cats.

Abnormalities

Diffuse Parenchymal Disorders

Most of the time, the appearance of the spleen is the same in benign and malignant processes. For this reason, it is difficult to reach a diagnosis on the basis of ultrasound images only, and fine-needle aspiration is necessary (Hecht and Mai, 2015) (Table 4).

Splenic Torsion

Splenic torsion is a pathology that mainly affects large-breed dogs and does not usually occur in cats.

Splenic torsion can cause massive splenomegaly, with a diffuse anechoic pattern with hyperechoic lines. A diffuse hypoechoic

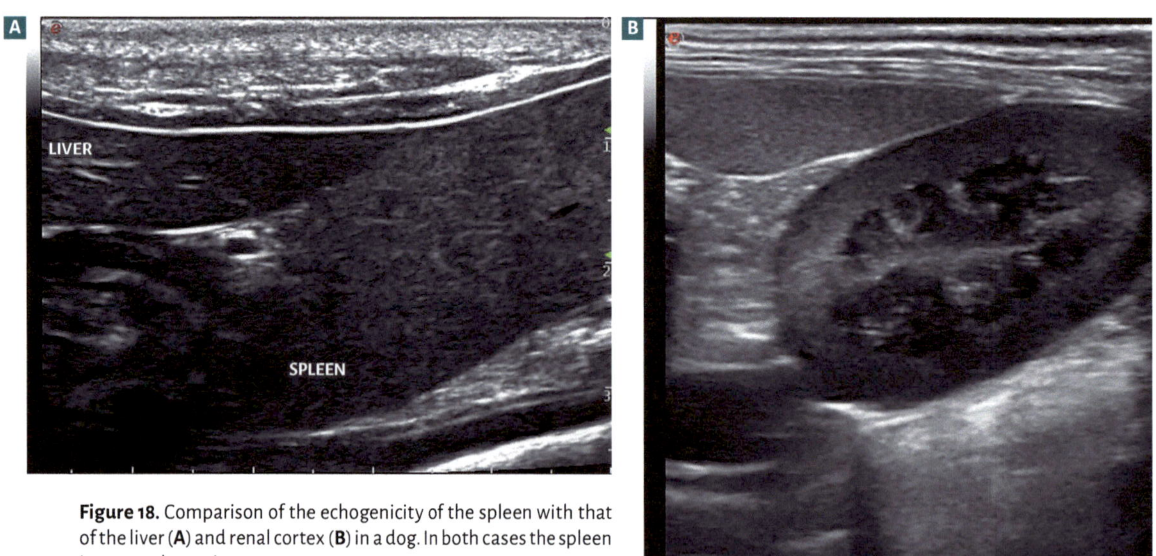

Figure 18. Comparison of the echogenicity of the spleen with that of the liver (**A**) and renal cortex (**B**) in a dog. In both cases the spleen is more echogenic.

Table 4. Differential diagnosis of diffuse splenic abnormalities.

Anechoic	Hypoechoic	Mixed echogenicity
· Sedation · Extramedullary haematopoiesis · Benign lymphoid hyperplasia · Acute splenic torsion · Haematopoietic neoplasia (mastocytoma, lymphoma, histiocytic sarcoma)	· Torsion · Massive infarct · Lymphoma (or other round cell tumour)	· Extramedullary haematopoiesis · Benign lymphoid hyperplasia · Splenitis · Neoplasia (round cell tumour)

Table 5. Differential diagnosis for focal/multifocal lesions of the spleen.

Anechoic	Hypoechoic	Hyperechoic	Mixed echogenicity
· Abscess · Cyst · Pseudocyst (trauma related)	· Lymphoma · Histiocytic sarcoma · Extramedullary haematopoiesis · Infarct · Benign nodular hyperplasia · Haematoma · Splenitis · Abscess · Neoplasia	· Myelolipoma · Calcified haematoma · Benign nodular hyperplasia · Extramedullary haematopoiesis · Granuloma · Haematoma · Splenitis · Abscesses · Neoplasia (primary, metastatic)	· Metastasis · Extramedullary haematopoiesis · Nodular hyperplasia · Haematoma · Splenitis · Abscess · Neoplasia

parenchyma can also be observed with small hyperechoic spots distributed throughout the parenchyma ("starry sky" pattern). The splenic veins in the hilum area can be seen to be enlarged and the omentum in the hilum area appears hyperechoic (Mai, 2006). Free fluid can sometimes also be visualised around the hilum area. In chronic torsions, hyperechoic areas can be seen with reverberation artefact representing the presence of gas, which can be due to infection with gas-producing bacteria or necrotic foci.

Extramedullary Haematopoiesis and Benign Lymphoid Hyperplasia

These two pathologies both produce generalised splenomegaly, and the splenic parenchyma can appear hypoechoic or heterogeneous.

Diffuse Neoplastic Diseases

Lymphoma and **mastocytoma** are included among these neoplasms. In these cases, the splenic parenchyma may have normal echogenicity or be hypoechoic. There may also be focal or multifocal lesions (Fig. 19).

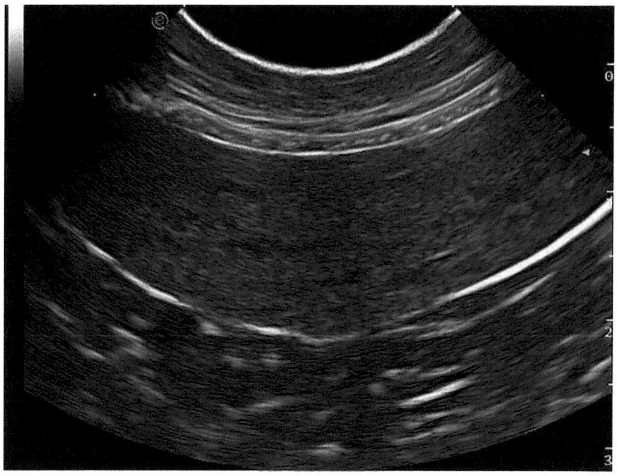

Figure 19. Ultrasound image of the spleen of a dog with lymphoma. The spleen has a mottled echotexture with hypoechoic foci distributed throughout the entire parenchyma. The diagnosis of lymphoma was made based on fine-needle aspiration.

Focal Parenchymal Abnormalities

Focal splenic lesions are easily detected by ultrasonography; however, it is difficult to reach a definitive diagnosis with this modality. The lesions can be small in size (nodules) or may become large masses. They can be hypoechoic, isoechoic, hyperechoic, of mixed echogenicity or have a "bullseye" appearance; they can be solitary or multiple; and they can represent neoplasms, metastases, haematomas, abscesses, infarcts or nodular hyperplasia (Table 5).

Extramedullary Haematopoiesis and Benign Lymphoid Hyperplasia

In both cases, the foci vary from hypoechoic to isoechoic, with well-defined borders (Fig. 20), and they do not protrude from the capsule. Ultrasonographically, the two cannot be differentiated, and cytology is necessary to distinguish between them.

Myelolipomas

Myelolipomas are observed as hyperechoic nodules of different sizes with a rounded shape and irregular borders. They can be located in the hilum area along the visceral border where the splenic vessels are located or, less frequently, inside the splenic parenchyma. They are benign lesions that are frequently seen in geriatric dogs and occasionally in geriatric cats.

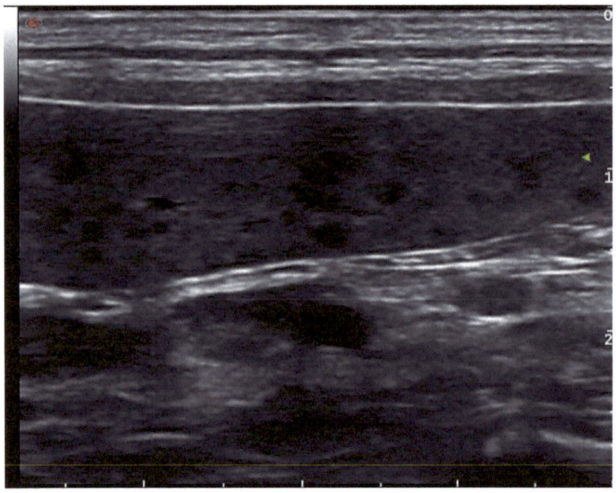

Figure 20. Ultrasound image of the spleen of a dog with lymphoid hyperplasia. A normal-sized spleen can be seen, with multiple hypoechoic nodules distributed throughout the whole parenchyma.

Focal Infarcts

Splenic infarcts occur secondary to thrombosis or embolism of the hepatic artery. In dogs, they have been described in association with pathologies including bacterial endocarditis, hyperadrenocorticism, kidney problems and neoplasms.

Ultrasonographically, initially they are observed as a hypoechoic focal lesion, which is not well defined, at the ends of the spleen, and generally with no flow seen on colour Doppler (Fig. 21). After 4–7 days, the lesion may be heterogeneous and may become hyperechoic. Differential diagnoses for this lesion include nodular hyperplasia, abscess, haematoma and neoplasia (Hecht and Mai, 2015).

Abscesses

Splenic abscesses are rare. They can be focal or multifocal, and their ultrasonographic appearance varies from hypoechoic to mixed lesions with poorly defined borders. Gas may also be observed inside these lesions as hyperechoic areas with reverberation artefact.

Haematomas

Haematomas can occur due to abdominal trauma, coagulation disorders or splenic neoplasms (haemangiosarcoma or lymphoma). They can be observed within the parenchyma, in the subcapsular region. The margins of the spleen may be altered from their normal appearance if the lesion is very large or close to the surface of the organ.

The ultrasonographic appearance of the lesion varies depending on how long it has been present: it can appear as anechoic, hypoechoic or of mixed echogenicity. Haematomas

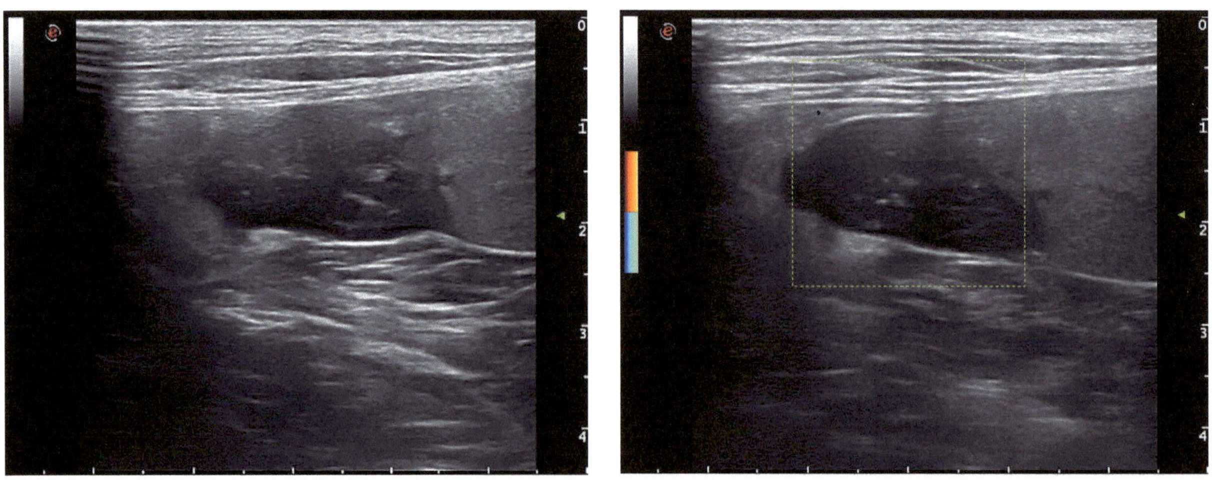

Figure 21. Ultrasound image of a splenic infarct. At the head of the spleen, an area that is hypoechoic relative to the rest of the parenchyma can be seen, and no flow is detected when power Doppler is applied.

have also been described to have internal septations and cavitations; in these cases it is difficult to differentiate them from haemangiosarcomas using ultrasonography alone.

Primary Neoplasms

Haemangiosarcoma is the most common neoplasm of the spleen in the dog. Other splenic neoplasms in the dog include histiocytic sarcoma, malignant histiocytosis, leiomyosarcoma and fibrosarcoma. In the cat, the most common splenic neoplasms are mastocytoma, lymphoma and, less frequently, haemangiosarcoma.

The ultrasonographic appearance of splenic neoplasms is variable. Splenomegaly or focal masses can also be observed, which are generally poorly defined; they can be anechoic, hypoechoic, have a "bullseye" pattern or be complex/mixed in appearance.

In the case of haemangiosarcoma, they usually have several anechoic or hypoechoic areas distributed throughout the parenchyma and are usually accompanied by haemoabdomen (Fig. 22). When the masses are very large, the hypoechoic central areas are compatible with areas of necrosis. The differential diagnosis would include haematoma and nodular hyperplasia, depending on the size and ultrasonographic appearance of the lesion.

Lymphoma usually has a diffuse appearance, but sometimes it can also present small hypoechoic nodules that give a "Swiss cheese" or "honeycomb" appearance, which can distort the appearance of the spleen. These patterns can also appear in cases of histiocytic sarcoma and extramedullary haematopoiesis. It can also be accompanied by haemoabdomen. In dogs, the regional lymph nodes are enlarged.

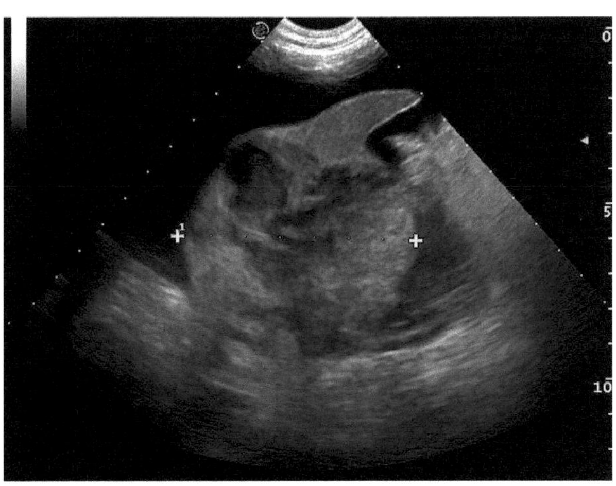

Figure 22. Ultrasound image of a splenic haemangiosarcoma with haemoabdomen. A mass with mixed echogenicity is seen in the body of the spleen, and there is disruption of the splenic capsule.

Malignant histiocytosis, **malignant fibrous histiocytoma** and **histiocytic sarcoma** present with multiple well-defined hypoechoic nodules that can distort the splenic capsule. Lymphadenopathy is also observed.

Mastocytoma causes splenomegaly, with hypoechoic nodules that can be solitary or multiple. Occasionally, the spleen may also appear normal in terms of its echogenicity. In cats, there may be only splenomegaly accompanied by a diffuse decrease in echogenicity, or multiple hypoechoic or hyperechoic nodules.

Metastatic carcinoma in cats appears as well-defined anechoic or hypoechoic nodules that may be solitary or multiple. In dogs, "bullseye" nodules can be observed (Cuccovillo and Lamb, 2002).

Multiple myeloma is a systemic disease. In the dog, multiple hyperechoic nodules can be seen in the spleen, whereas in the cat the spleen may have a normal appearance.

Gastrointestinal Tract

Ultrasonographic examination of the gastrointestinal tract can provide important information, despite the limitations to imaging imposed by gas inside the tract.

Technique

Gas and food in the gastrointestinal tract can interfere with the transmission of ultrasound waves, producing artefacts. Fasting the animal for at least 6–12 hours before ultrasonographic examination is therefore recommended to reduce the amount of gas and food in the tract.

The transducers used are high frequency: 7.5–10 MHz in dogs and 10–12 MHz in cats. Animals are typically examined in dorsal recumbency; however, placing the animal in right and left lateral recumbency can help displace gas and fluid in the stomach to enable better visualisation of deeper structures.

A **systematic examination** should be conducted.

- The **stomach** should be examined first, using transverse (longitudinal to the body plane) and longitudinal (transverse to the body plane) sections (Fig. 23). The stomach is located just caudal to the liver; therefore, the transducer is placed caudal to the xiphoid process and moved from the fundus area (left) to the pyloric area (right).
- The pylorus and pyloroduodenal junction are close to

the midline in most cats. In deep-chested dogs, a right dorsal intercostal approach may be necessary to better visualise the pyloroduodenal junction (Fig. 24).

– After observing the pyloroduodenal junction, the orad portion of the **descending duodenum** is visualised. The descending duodenum is followed caudally, keeping it in a longitudinal plane, along the right lateral wall (Fig. 25). Occasionally, in deep-chested dogs, an intercostal approach may be necessary to identify the cranial aspect of the duodenum. When using this approach, the right kidney can be used as an anatomical reference to identify the duodenum, as it is located ventral or ventrolateral to the kidney. In cats, the descending duodenum is located in the midline or just to the right of the midline.
– The **jejunum** is assessed in its entirety by shifting the transducer from cranial to caudal and from right to left across the entire abdomen.
– The **ileum**, in both the dog and the cat, is short and is located on the right side in the middle of the abdominal cavity, medial to the right kidney. The ileum can be located

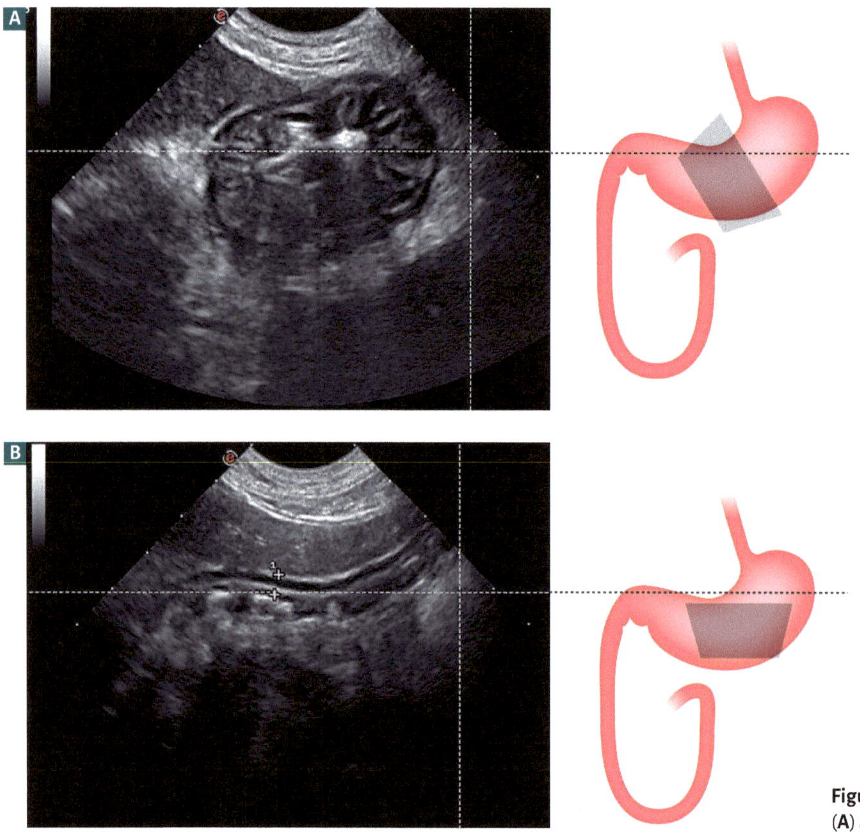

Figure 23. Positioning of the transducer in the transverse (**A**) and longitudinal (**B**) planes of the stomach.

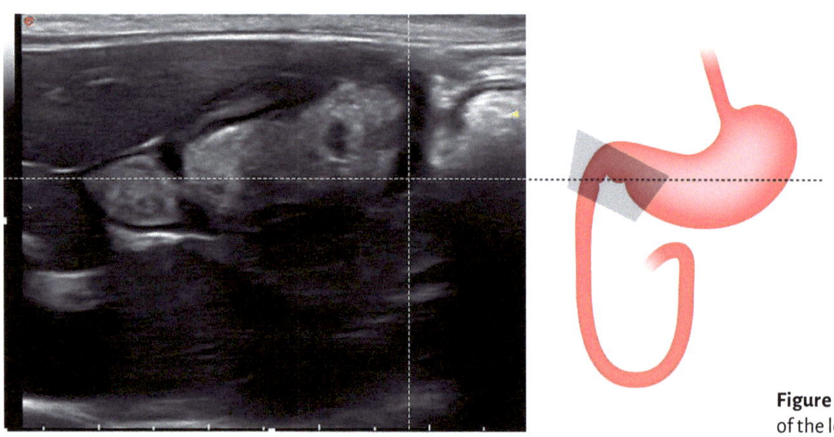

Figure 24. Positioning of the transducer to obtain an image of the longitudinal plane of the pyloroduodenal region.

using the transverse colon or the ileo(caeco)colic junction as a reference (Fig. 26).

– The **transverse colon** is immediately caudal to the body of the stomach; the **ascending colon** is located to the right of the midline, continuing in the cranial direction from the ileo(caeco)colic junction; the **descending colon** is located on the left side. Using the urinary bladder as a reference point, the colon is immediately dorsal to it. Finally, to locate the transverse colon, the transducer must be displaced cranially (Fig. 27) (Neelis et al., 2020).

Normal Ultrasonographic Appearance

When performing an ultrasonographic examination of the gastrointestinal tract, the layers of the organs that make up the tract, their echogenicity and thickness, content and motility must be evaluated.

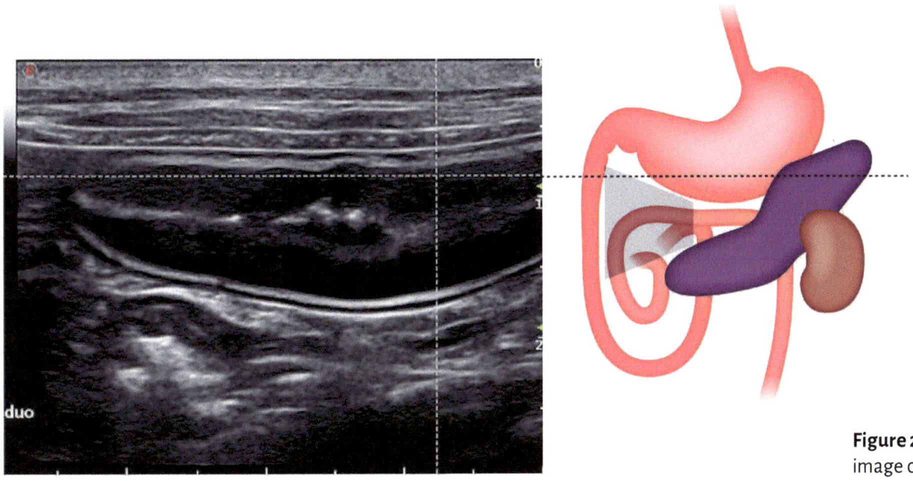

Figure 25. Positioning of the transducer to obtain an image of the longitudinal plane of the duodenum.

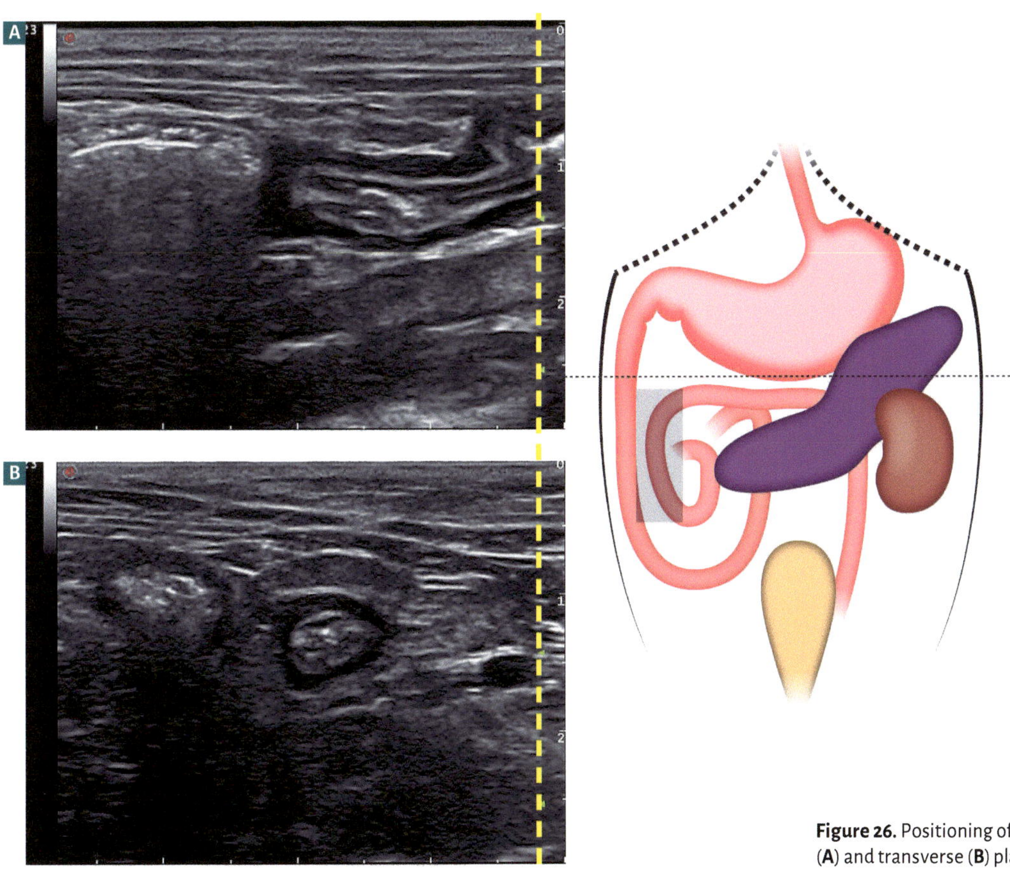

Figure 26. Positioning of the transducer in the longitudinal (**A**) and transverse (**B**) planes of the ileocolic region.

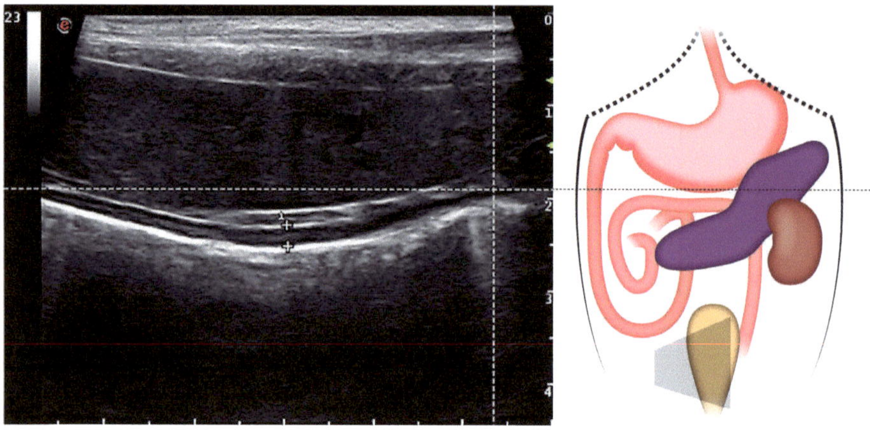

Figure 27. Positioning of the transducer to obtain an image of the longitudinal plane of the colon.

If a high-resolution transducer is used, the different **layers of the stomach** (Fig. 28) and **intestine** (Fig. 29) can be visualised. Normally, five layers are distinguished, which correspond to:

- the luminal–mucosal (hyperechoic) interface
- the mucosa (hypoechoic)
- the submucosa (hyperechoic)
- the muscular layer (hypoechoic)
- the serosa (hyperechoic).

The **gastric wall thickness** is variable depending on the degree of distension of the stomach, ranging between 2 mm and 5 mm. It is measured from the central hyperechoic line (luminal–mucosal interface) to the serous external hyperechoic line. **Gastric folds** can be seen when the stomach is empty. The folds are very prominent in cats and are hyperechoic due to the layer of fat present in the submucosa.

The **duodenum** can be up to 5 mm thick, with an average of 2–3 mm, and the thickness of the jejunum measures 3 mm. Peristalsis can be evaluated ultrasonographically; contractions in the stomach occur at a rate of six per minute, whereas in the small intestine three to six contractions occur per minute (Penninck and d'Anjou, 2015).

The ultrasonographic appearance of the **small intestine** depends on the type and amount of luminal content. When it is empty, a "mucosal pattern" is observed and the intestinal lumen appears as a hyperechoic line ("mucosal band") surrounded by the hypoechoic "halo" of the intestinal wall. The hyperechoic line represents mucus and small air bubbles that are trapped at the mucosal–luminal interface. When there is fluid in the intestinal lumen ("liquid pattern"), an anechoic area that appears tubular in sagittal images and circular in transverse images is observed between the walls of the intestine. Gas-filled intestinal loops cause a highly echogenic interface with distal acoustic shadowing or reverberation ("gas pattern") (Fig. 30).

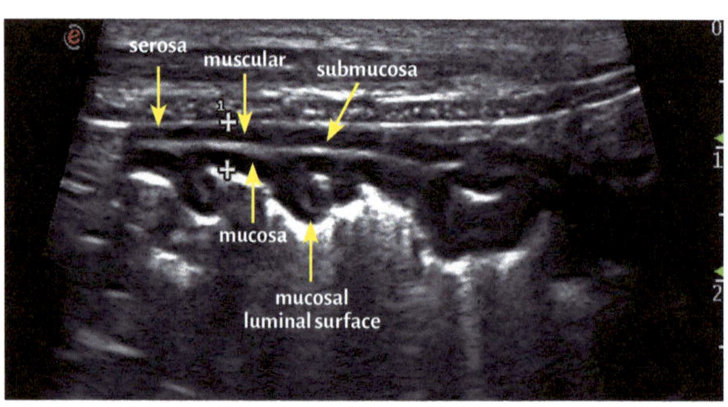

Figure 28. Ultrasound image in a longitudinal plane of the stomach wall, in which the different layers can be seen.

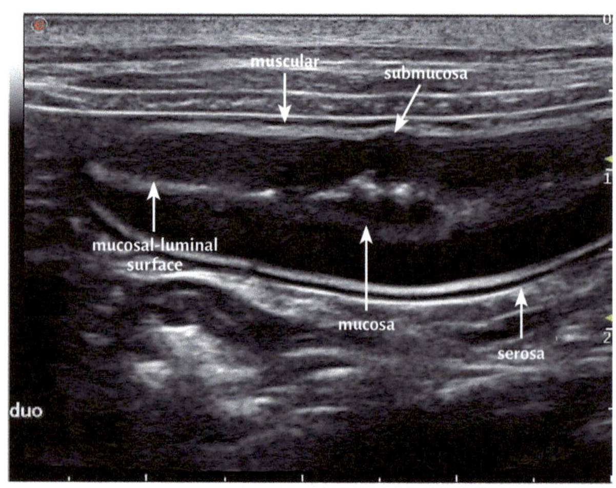

Figure 29. Ultrasound image in a longitudinal plane of the duodenal wall, in which the different layers can be seen.

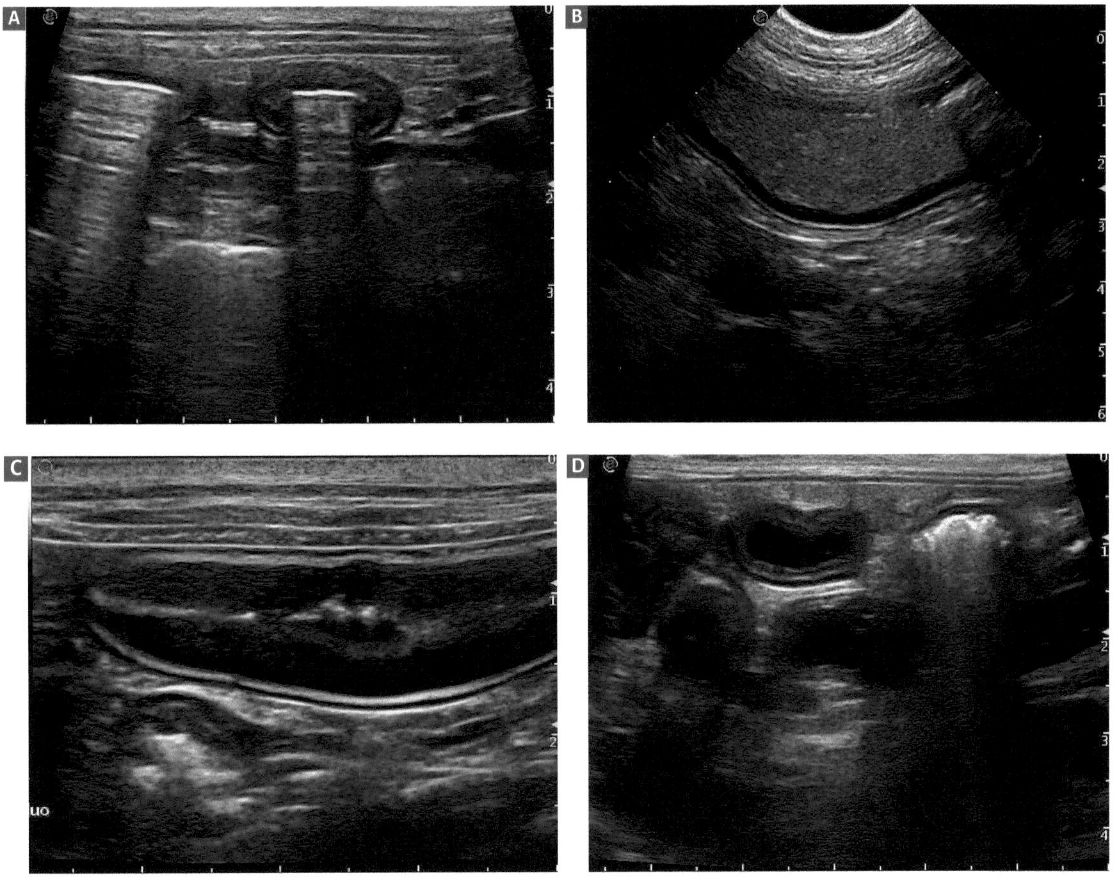

Figure 30. Ultrasound images of the small intestine. Different patterns can be observed depending on the content: **A**. air/gaseous; **B**. food; **C**. mucus; **D**. liquid.

Regarding the thickness of the small intestinal wall in the dog, correlation with the weight of the animal has been observed (Table 6), and the duodenum is the thickest part. In cats, the thickness depends on the part of the intestine; the ileum is the thickest part (Table 7) (Penninck and d'Anjou, 2015).

In the cranial area of the descending duodenum, the **major duodenal papilla** can be seen (Fig. 31). In the cat, the width of this papilla ranges from 2.9 mm to 5.5 mm, and it has a maximum thickness of 4 mm in the transverse plane (Penninck and d'Anjou, 2015).

Table 6. Normal thickness of the intestinal wall for different parts of the intestine in the dog.

Body weight (kg)	Duodenum (mm)	Body weight (kg)	Jejunum (mm)
<20	≤5.1	<20	≤4.1
20–29.9	≤5.3	20–39.9	≤4.4
≥30	≤6	≥40	≤4.7

Table 7. Normal thickness of the intestinal wall for different parts of the intestine in the cat.

Intestinal wall	Thickness (mm)
Duodenum	2.0–2.4
Jejunum	2.1–2.5
Ileum	2.5–3.2

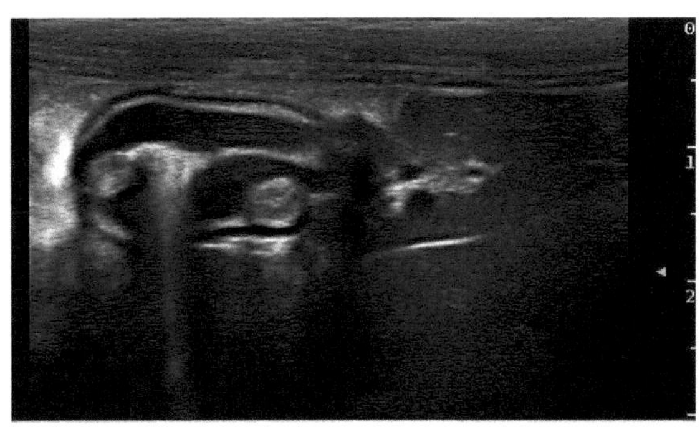

Figure 31. Ultrasound image of the normal duodenal papilla in a dog. The duodenal papilla can be seen as a hyperechoic area in the submucosa of the proximal area of the duodenum.

In cats, the **ileum** has a prominent submucosal and muscular layer, whereas in dogs only the submucosa is present.

The **colon** usually has the thinnest wall of all the intestinal segments, and stratification of the wall is normally impossible to visualise due to distension of the colon with air and faeces. Air and faeces result in a hyperechoic reverberation artefact with the colonic contents causing partial and irregular acoustic shadowing (Fig. 27). An empty colon can appear undulating, and the layers in the wall can be distinguished (Neelis et al., 2020).

Gastric Disorders

Gastric Dilation

When the stomach progressively distends or dilates, its wall becomes thinner, and it is difficult to see the stratification of the wall. The gastric content can range from hypoechoic to hyperechoic depending on its composition. If the stomach is dilated with gas, it will cause a reverberation artefact, making it impossible to visualise abnormalities of the dorsal area of the gastric wall or lumen.

Pyloric Obstruction

Causes of pyloric obstruction include pyloric stenosis, foreign bodies, inflammatory diseases and neoplasms.

Congenital hypertrophic pyloric stenosis causes a circumferential thickening of the pylorus. Ultrasonography shows an increase in thickness of both the gastric wall (to >6–7 mm) and the muscle layer, and is considered pathological when the muscle thickness measures more than 4 mm. It is more common in dogs than in cats.

Chronic hypertrophic gastropathy can cause muscle or mucosal hypertrophy. The thickness of the pyloric wall of affected dogs ranges from 9 mm to 15.3 mm, and the thickness of the muscle layer ranges from 3 mm to 5.4 mm (Fig. 32).

Gastric foreign bodies are usually diagnosed radiographically if they are radiopaque, although they can sometimes be diagnosed by ultrasound examination. Generally, foreign bodies are hyperechoic with an intense distal acoustic shadow, although some foreign bodies allow ultrasound waves to travel through them. If the foreign body is surrounded by liquid, it can be seen easily. Foreign bodies vary in shape and size (Biller et al., 1994). Most foreign bodies, such as balls or stones, are easily identified by ultrasonography as they produce a bright interface associated with strong acoustic shadows. However, the echogenicity of balls may vary depending on their physical characteristics. Linear foreign bodies are seen as a hyperechoic line extending into the duodenum. Gastric trichobezoars (hairballs) are common in cats; they are visualised as an irregular, hyperechoic gas interface with a strong acoustic shadow. In cases where there is gastric perforation, signs of peritonitis can be seen.

Wall Thickening

Wall thickening is seen in cases of **inflammation** and **neoplasms**. The distribution, symmetry, extent of thickening and appearance of the layers of the wall help to differentiate non-malignant processes from neoplasms.

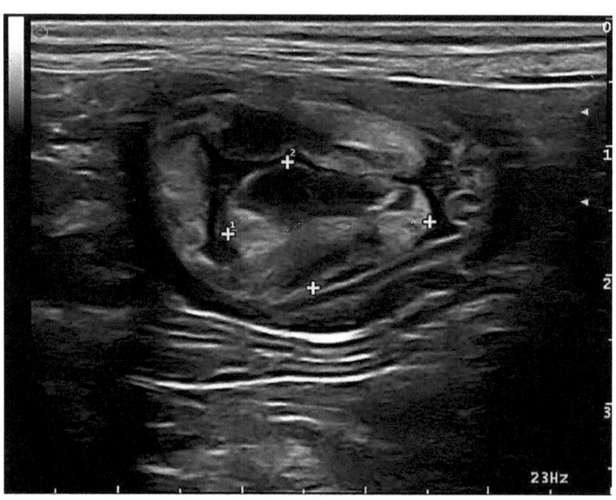

Figure 32. Hypertrophic pyloric gastropathy in a dog with chronic vomiting. In the ultrasound image, obtained in a transverse plane, thickening of the wall of the pylorus can be seen.

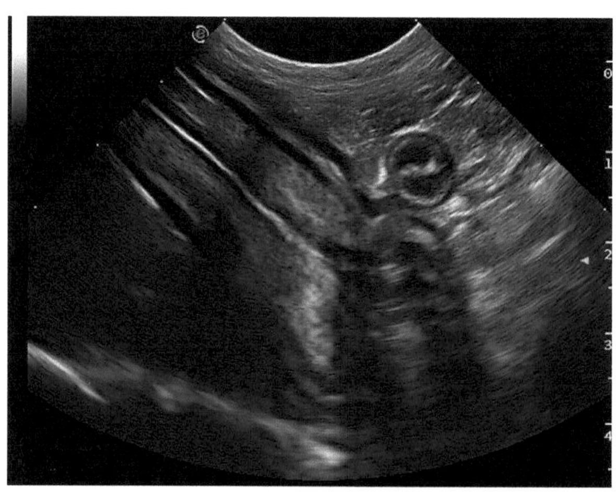

Figure 33. Oedema of the gastric wall in a dog with chronic vomiting. Thickening of the gastric wall can be seen with preservation of the layers.

Nonmalignant pathologies tend to be diffuse, and cause minimal or moderate thickening with preservation of the layers (Fig. 33), whereas neoplasms are characterised by focal thickening or mass-like lesions with loss of the layers (Willard, 2012). However, sometimes the ultrasonographic signs observed in inflammatory and neoplastic processes overlap. In these cases, either ultrasound-guided aspiration or biopsy is necessary to reach a diagnosis.

Inflammation

Acute gastritis is rarely diagnosed by ultrasonography unless it is associated with a foreign body. **Chronic gastritis** can affect the normal ultrasonographic appearance of the stomach; the most frequent finding is a diffuse thickening of the wall, with a hyperechoic or hypoechoic appearance. The loss of layers can occur in very serious cases, and the stomach can be observed to be full of fluid.

Uraemia-induced gastritis has an ultrasonographic appearance similar to that of other inflammation, but a hyperechoic line may be visible at the mucosal–submucosal interface, representing mineralisation that does not produce an acoustic shadow. The differential diagnosis for this finding includes gastric wall haemorrhage and oedema due to hypoalbuminaemia.

Neoplasms

The most common diffuse neoplasms in small animals are **lymphomas**, especially in cats. The ultrasonographic findings are loss of the wall layers with wall thickening, a hypoechoic wall and a focal mass effect with regional lymphadenopathy.

Another systemic infiltrative neoplasm is **mastocytoma**, which has a similar ultrasonographic appearance to lymphoma.

Focal benign and malignant **neoplasms** can cause obstruction in the area of the pyloric antrum.

Benign gastric polyps (adenomatous hyperplasia) can be incidental findings but, depending on their size and pedunculated shape, can cause obstruction. The ultrasonographic appearance of polyps is a lesion at the level of the antrum with its origin in the mucosa; they are usually hyperechoic or of mixed echogenicity, and there is no alteration of the layers or lymphadenopathy.

Malignant neoplasms can be focal or diffuse. Ultrasonographically, loss of layers and thickening of the wall (8–25 mm, mean 15 mm) and local lymphadenopathy (Fig. 34) are seen. Larger lesions are usually ulcerated. The most common neoplasms are adenocarcinomas, carcinomas and lymphomas, usually associated with lymphadenopathy. Lymphomas can be focal or diffuse, with loss of layers and hypoechoic wall thickening. Leiomyomas or leiomyosarcomas can be difficult to differentiate in the early stages because both originate in the muscle layer. Leiomyosarcomas tend to have mixed echogenicity whereas leiomyomas are hypoechoic; biopsy is needed to reach a definitive diagnosis (Fig. 35) (Gaschen, 2011; Willard, 2012).

Ulcers

The typical ultrasonographic appearance of ulcers includes focal wall thickening with or without layer loss, and with or without an ulcerated crater. Ulcerated craters sometimes accumulate gas, which is visualised as small hyperechoic foci causing a reverberation artefact.

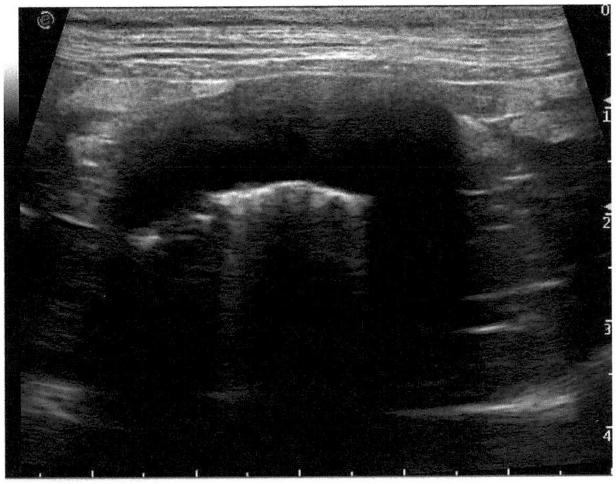

Figure 34. Gastric adenocarcinoma. Loss of layers and concentric thickening of the wall can be seen.

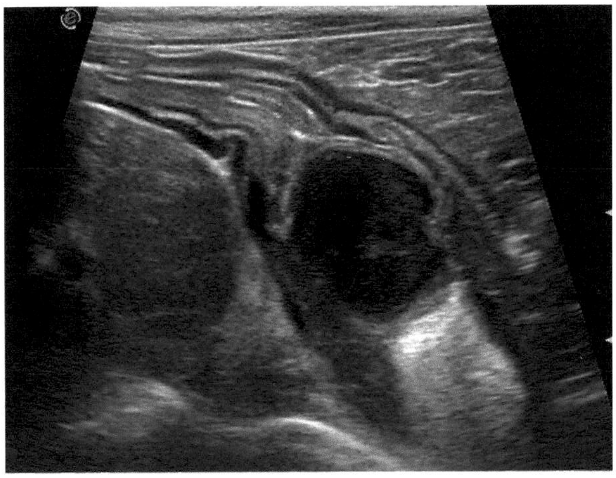

Figure 35. Gastric leiomyoma in a dog. A well-defined hypoechoic mass can be seen in the wall of the stomach.

Sometimes ulcers are associated with neoplasms; therefore, when ulcers are identified it is advisable to perform an ultrasound-guided puncture or biopsy of the area.

Small Intestinal Abnormalities

Intestinal Corrugation

Intestinal corrugation has been described in the duodenum and jejunum of dogs and cats. This pattern has been defined as an undulating or "wavy" wall, which is best identified by observing an undulating hyperechoic line at the mucosal–luminal interface or in the submucosa, or both (Fig. 36). This appearance is not a specific sign and can occur in several diseases, such as pancreatitis, inflammatory diseases, peritonitis, neoplasms and intestinal ischaemia.

Dilation

Dilation of the small intestine may be due to a functional disorder or a mechanical obstruction.

A **functional disorder** is one in which paralysis of the intestinal musculature (paralytic ileus) prevents the progression of the intestinal contents along the intestine. Functional disorders can result in localised or generalised dilation of the small intestine. **Mechanical obstruction** of the intestine can also result in localised or generalised dilation of the small intestine. The degree of dilation depends on the location and duration of the obstruction and whether it is total or partial.

In functional obstruction, the intestinal loops are dilated and are all of a uniform size, whereas in mechanical obstruction some loops are dilated and others are of normal size.

Mechanical Obstruction

Partial or complete obstruction of the small intestine may be caused by a foreign body, stenosis, granuloma, abscess, intussusception or tumour. Other less frequent causes are strangulation of the intestine in an abdominal hernia or mesenteric laceration and torsion of the mesenteric root.

Foreign Bodies

In small animals, foreign bodies are the main cause of **mechanical obstruction.** Distension of the small intestine with fluid, gas or a combination of both is indicative of mechanical ileus (obstruction). The degree of intestinal distension depends on whether the obstruction is partial or complete, and the duration and location of the obstruction. When the entire small intestine is dilated, it is important to differentiate diffuse intestinal disease (e.g. parvovirus infection) from distal obstruction of the small intestine. Visualisation of a small portion of normal, nondistended small intestine (distal to the obstruction) is a clue to the possible existence of a distal obstruction. Some foreign bodies, such as balls or stones, are easily identified by ultrasonography due to their characteristic shape and the presence of an acoustic shadow (Fig. 37). However, the echogenicity of balls may vary depending on their physical characteristics. Most foreign bodies produce a bright interface associated with strong shadows. Sometimes, the contour of the interface can help to identify the type of foreign body present in the intestine (Penninck and d'Anjou, 2015).

In cases where the **intestinal wall is pierced** by a foreign body, such as a stick, the ultrasonographic appearance is a local thickening and focal loss of wall layers. In addition, reactive mesenteric fat, peritoneal effusion, free gas in the abdomen, a fluid-filled intestine and decreased motility may be observed.

Linear foreign bodies are more commonly seen in cats but can also be seen in dogs. The types of foreign material ingested include string/yarn, cellophane, pieces of cloth and tights. This type of mechanical obstruction presents with an accordion-like folding of the small intestine visible on radiographs. Linear foreign bodies can also be diagnosed by ultrasonography by recognising the characteristic folded appearance of the small intestine (Hoffman, 2003). Ultrasonographic signs are an abnormal undulating trajectory of the intestine and the presence of a bright linear interface within the intestinal lumen (Fig. 38). The affected intestine may be dilated with fluid and gas or may simply appear thickened and stacked. Linear gastroduodenal foreign bodies can be observed in the stomach. Secondary problems associated with the linear foreign body, such as peritonitis, may be suspected if gas or free fluid is detected in the abdomen or if the mesentery is hyperechoic with little ultrasonographic detail and if there is lymphadenopathy. Aspiration of free peritoneal fluid may be helpful in assessing whether peritonitis is present.

The presence of **gastrointestinal parasites** can mimic the appearance of a linear foreign body. The ultrasonographic appearance of a gastrointestinal nematode is a hyperechoic linear structure without acoustic shadowing, with a hypoechoic centre.

Intussusception

Intussusception is the invagination of a portion of the intestine into the lumen of an adjacent intestinal segment. Intussusceptions normally occur within the jejunum, within the ileocolic junction or ileocaecal junction, or within the colon (colocolic), and rarely involve the stomach or duodenum. They

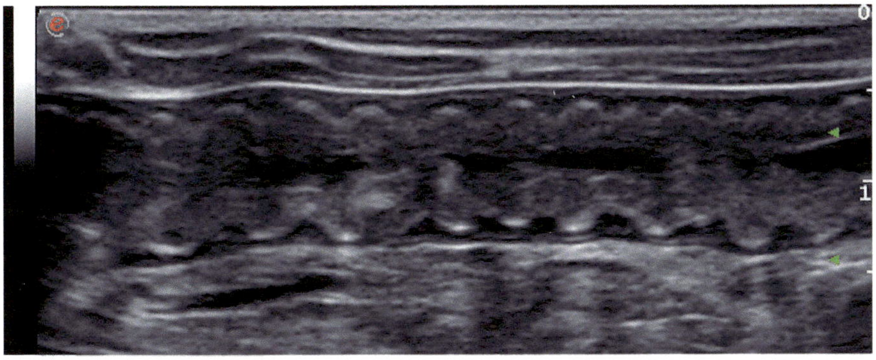

Figure 36. Ultrasound image of a corrugated intestinal loop secondary to peritonitis in a dog.

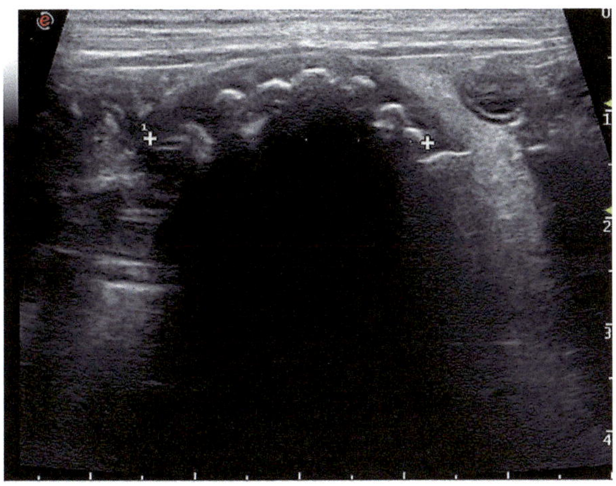

Figure 37. Ultrasound image of an intestinal foreign body. A hyperechoic structure with irregular edges, producing an acoustic shadow, can be seen.

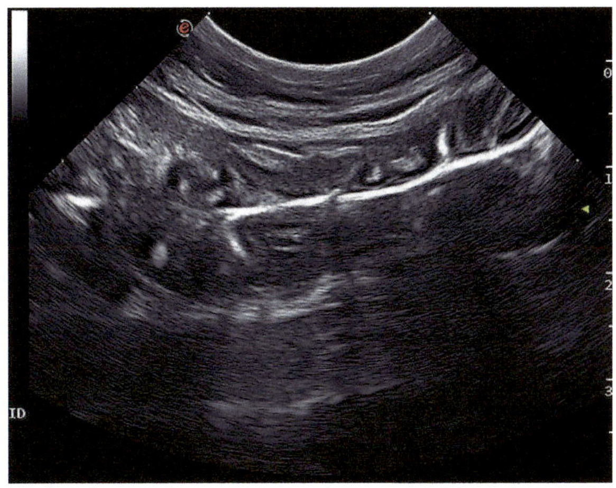

Figure 38. Ultrasound image of a linear foreign body in the intestine of a cat. There is intestinal plication, with a hyperechoic structure with acoustic shadow inside.

often occur in puppies or kittens secondary due to a primary intestinal disease such as parasitic enteritis or intestinal bacterial or viral infections. In older animals, intussusceptions may occur near pseudocysts, enlarged lymph nodes, foreign bodies or neoplastic masses.

Intussusceptions have a characteristic ultrasonographic appearance that in most cases allows a definitive diagnosis to be made with confidence. The most frequently observed ultrasonographic pattern in intestinal cross sections is that of a target-like mass with multiple concentric hyperechoic and hypoechoic rings around a hyperechoic centre representing the trapped mesentery (Fig. 39). In longitudinal sections, multiple hyperechoic and hypoechoic parallel lines are normally visible (Patsikas et al., 2003). Ultrasonographic patterns may vary along the affected intestine and with the duration of the process and the orientation of the plane of examination relative to the axis of the invagination. Thus, in some cases, the concentric or layered appearance is distorted and not as easily recognised due to inflammation and oedema. The presence of a thin, hypoechoic, outer, target-like ring is usually associated

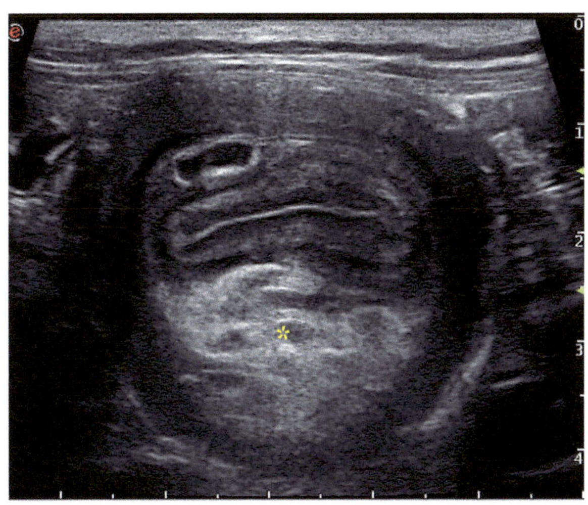

Figure 39. Ultrasound image showing an intussusception. Alternating intestinal hypoechoic and hyperechoic intestinal layers can be seen, with a hyperechoic centre (*), which corresponds to the mesentery.

with reducible intussusceptions. The appearance of fluid within the intussusception, the absence of peristaltic activity of the intestine and the presence of enlarged lymph nodes in the invaginated intestine are signs compatible with irreducible invaginations. However, visualisation of blood flow in the invaginated intestine using colour Doppler appears to be the most valuable factor in predicting whether the intussusception is reducible.

Wall Thickening

Wall thickening is frequently observed in cases of inflammatory diseases and neoplasia. The distribution, symmetry and appearance of the layers of the wall can help differentiate inflammatory diseases from neoplasms.

Inflammatory diseases tend to induce mild to moderate thickening of the wall with preservation of the layers, whereas **neoplasms** usually cause focal thickening or mass lesions with alteration or loss of the wall layers. The exception is lymphoma, which can diffusely infiltrate the intestine or cause mass lesions.

Lymphadenopathy is usually more pronounced with neoplasia, and this can also help differentiate between nonmalignant disease and neoplasia. However, ultrasound-guided aspiration or biopsy of the intestine and lymph nodes can help reach a final diagnosis.

Inflammatory Bowel Disease

The term inflammatory bowel disease (IBD) is used to describe a group of chronic gastrointestinal disorders in which there is an infiltration of inflammatory cells into the intestinal mucosa without a known cause.

IBD is classified according to the type of cell that predominates in the infiltrate in **lymphocytic plasmocytic enteritis** (most common) or **eosinophilic enteritis**. Another type of chronic enteritis with an allergic factor that should be included on the list of differential diagnoses is **food-responsive enteropathy.** These diseases do not always produce changes that are detectable by ultrasonography, and in most cases intestinal biopsy is needed to confirm the diagnosis and evaluate the severity of the lesions.

The intestinal wall thickness has been a criterion for determining activity (i.e. clinical manifestation of disease) in humans with IBD. However, intestinal wall thickness has not been shown to be a specific or sensitive feature for diagnosing IBD in dogs. Accordingly, the use of wall thickness measurements in isolation might produce false negative results for dogs with inflammation of the intestinal wall. In addition to the thickness, alteration of the distribution of the layers of the wall seems to be an important factor that allows inflammatory infiltration to be distinguished from neoplastic and granulomatous infiltration. However, loss of layer distribution has also been described in cases of severe enteritis and in haemorrhagic, necrotising or granulomatous infiltration.

At present, it seems that the most important ultrasonographic parameters that allow the identification of **dogs** with inflammatory bowel disease are the **echogenicity of the mucosa of the small intestine** and the **presence of secondary abnormalities of the intestine and adjacent organs**. Two patterns of increased mucosal echogenicity have been described:

- with hyperechoic speckels
- with hyperechoic striations.

Hyperechoic striations are associated with histopathological findings of dilated mucosal lymphatic ducts and are very specific to protein-losing enteropathy (Fig. 40). **Hyperechoic speckels** is a sensitive parameter for determining the presence of inflammatory disease but is not specific for differentiating the disease category and activity. Mottling within the mucosa may represent chronic changes that require a longer period to resolve. Normal hypoechoic intestinal mucosa in dogs with chronic diarrhoea is a sensitive and specific finding for the diagnosis of food-responsive disease. The presence of secondary abnormalities of the intestine, such as free abdominal fluid, pancreatic oedema or thickening of the gallbladder wall, as well as distension of the intestinal loops, is seen in dogs with protein-losing enteropathy, although it is not commonly seen in dogs with IBD (Gaschen, 2011).

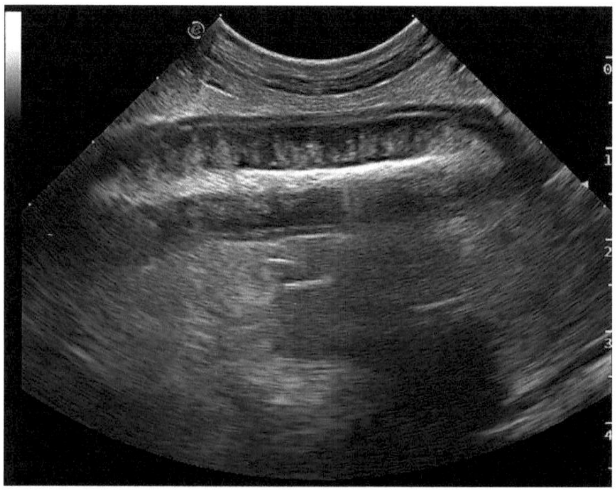

Figure 40. Ultrasound image of an intestinal loop in a Yorkshire Terrier with protein-losing enteropathy. Hyperechoic striations are seen in the mucosa, which correspond to lymphangiectasia.

In **cats**, a thickening of the muscle layer of the intestinal wall has been observed, which is associated with diffuse infiltrative intestinal diseases such as lymphoma and IBD (Fig. 41). A hyperechoic line in the mucosa parallel to the submucosa has also been described, and it is suggested that this band represents fibrosis. Occasionally, ultrasonographic abnormalities are observed in the ileocaecocolic region in cats, including lymphadenopathy, thickening of the muscle layer and the presence of hyperechoic fat. These abnormalities may be related to inflammatory or neoplastic processes, and therefore performing a biopsy of this area is recommended (Gaschen, 2011).

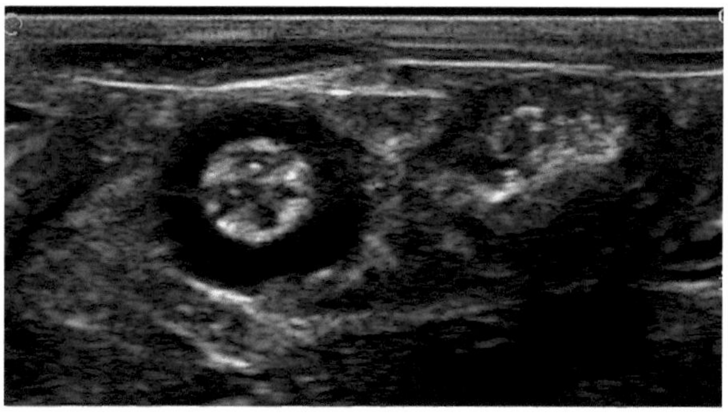

Figure 41. Inflammatory intestinal disease in a cat. Ultrasound image in a transverse plane of the ileum. A thickening of the muscular layer can be seen.

Small intestinal corrugation in the form of regular undulations of intestinal segments is a sensitive but nonspecific pattern observed in intestinal or abdominal disorders. It can be seen in association with enteritis (parvovirus, lymphocytic plasmacytic enteritis and haemorrhagic duodenitis), pancreatitis, peritonitis and ischaemia of the intestinal wall.

Neoplasms

Lymphomas, adenocarcinomas and mastocytomas are the most common intestinal tumours in the **cat**. **Adenocarcinomas and leiomyomas** are most common in the **dog.**

The most common ultrasonographic findings in intestinal neoplasms are thickening of the intestinal wall and a loss of the normal appearance of the wall layers. The changes associated with neoplasms are often focal, as in the case of the presence of masses, but they can also be diffuse, generally in the case of intestinal lymphoma. Metastases can occur either to regional lymph nodes or to the liver (Gaschen, 2011).

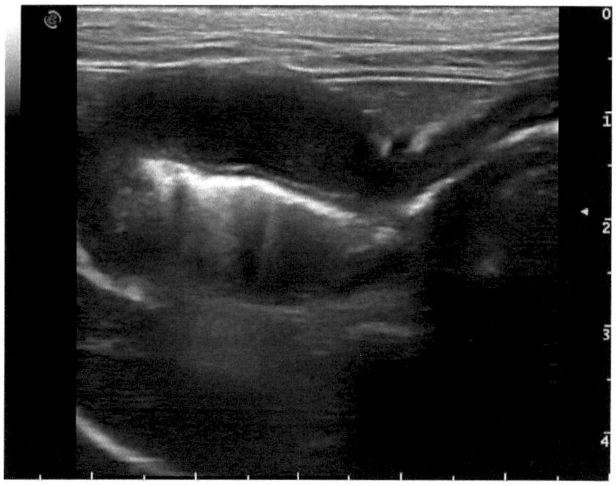

Figure 42. Nodular lymphoma in a cat. An intestinal loop with thickening of the wall can be seen in addition to loss of the wall layers. The perilesional tissue appears hyperechoic.

Lymphoma

Intestinal lymphoma can occur in two forms, diffuse and nodular.

- The **diffuse** type is characterised by infiltration of the lamina propria and submucosa with neoplastic lymphocytes. Ultrasonography shows a diffuse thickening of the intestinal wall (0.4–0.5 cm) without loss of the layers. Regional lymphadenopathy is also seen. The area affected most is the jejunum and ileum. It is difficult to differentiate between diffuse lymphoma and IBD.
- The **nodular** type presents ultrasonographically with transmural thickening together with a loss of the layers, decreased echogenicity of the intestinal wall, a localised decrease in motility and an increase in the size of regional lymph nodes (Fig. 42). In cats, the most common site for this neoplasm is in the ileocolic region.

Adenocarcinoma

Adenocarcinoma is considered to be the most common intestinal tumour in the dog. The most frequent ultrasonographic findings are transmural thickening with total loss of the layers. It is often associated with lymphadenopathy. In the dog, adenocarcinoma can be located anywhere in the small intestine but is found more frequently in the duodenum, whereas in the cat it is more often located in the jejunum and ileum.

Intestinal adenocarcinoma has an ultrasonographic appearance similar to that of nodular lymphoma; however, the lesion is usually smaller in adenocarcinoma than in lymphoma (Fig. 43). Biopsy of these lesions should be performed to reach a definitive diagnosis.

The spread of neoplasms through the mesentery and abdominal organs is known as **carcinomatosis**. Intestinal adenocarcinoma has been associated with carcinomatosis in dogs. The ultrasonographic signs that can be observed are hypoechoic nodular foci and irregularities on the surface of organs such as the liver and spleen.

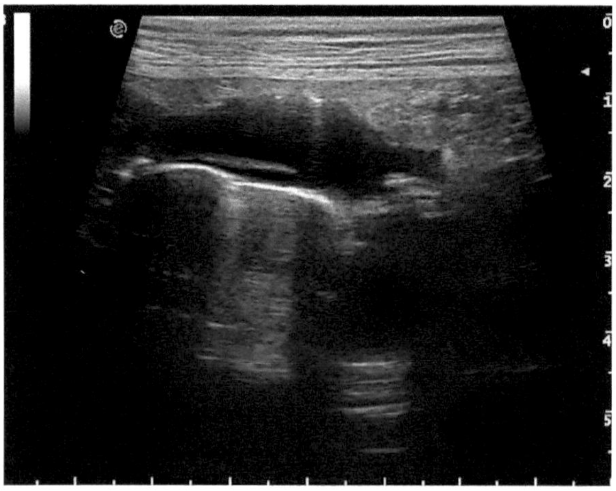

Figure 43. Intestinal adenocarcinoma in a dog. An intestinal loop with thickening of the wall can be seen, as well as loss of layers. The perilesional tissue appears hyperechoic. Small hyperechoic areas with reverberation artefact are apparent in contact with the intestine, compatible with areas of gas as a consequence of intestinal lacerations.

Mastocytoma

Intestinal mastocytoma is less differentiated than cutaneous mastocytoma. Lesions can be solitary or multiple, and range in length from 1 cm to 7 cm. Ultrasonographically, thickening of a part of the intestine is observed, which can sometimes appear to be like a mass.

Leiomyosarcoma

These types of tumours are locally very invasive and form large masses that produce a mass effect, with varying echogenicities. However, it is rare for them to metastasise.

Focal Nonneoplastic Masses

Fungal infections, abscesses, haematomas and foreign body granulomas can produce focal intestinal masses that can partially or completely obstruct the intestinal lumen. In the case of cats, gastrointestinal eosinophilic sclerosing fibroplasia, which is an inflammatory disease of unknown aetiology, should be considered. The main manifestation of the disease is a firm and irregular intramural mass, located in the gastrointestinal tract region.

In these cases, ultrasound-guided aspiration or biopsy of the intestine and lymph nodes can help in reaching a definitive diagnosis.

Large Intestinal Abnormalities

Many of the pathologies of the caecum and colon appear similar to those of the small intestine. The presence of air and faeces in the large intestine makes it more difficult to evaluate ultrasonographically.

Intussusception

Intussusceptions affecting the caecum or colon have a similar ultrasonographic appearance to that described above for the small intestine. Multiple concentric rings are seen in cross section, and a multilayered structure is seen in the longitudinal plane.

Diffuse Wall Thickening

Inflammation usually produces a medium, diffuse thickening similar to that seen in the small intestine. Neoplasms can also produce a diffuse, symmetrical thickening of the wall in the caecum or colon; lymphoma is the neoplasm most likely to cause this appearance.

Focal Wall Thickening

Eccentric thickening of the wall or thickening associated with focal masses usually indicates a neoplasm. The layers of the wall are often lost and the ultrasonographic appearance is similar to that of a neoplasm in the small intestine. Carcinoma and lymphoma are tumours of the caecum and colon.

Bibliography

- Biller, D.S., Partington, B.P., Miyabayashi, T., Léveillé, R. (1994) Ultrasonographic appearance of chronic hypertrophic pyloric gastropathy in the dog. *Vet Radiol Ultrasound*, 35(1):30–33.
- Cuccovillo, A., Lamb, C.R. (2002) Cellular features of sonographic target lesions of the liver and spleen in 21 dogs and a cat. *Vet Radiol Ultrasound*, 43(3):275–278.
- d'Anjou, M.A. (2007) The sonographic search for portosystemic shunts. *Clin Tech Small Anim Pract*, 22(3):104–114.
- d'Anjou, M.A., Penninck, D. (2015) Liver. In: Penninck, D., d'Anjou, M.A. (eds). *Atlas of Small Animal Ultrasonography*. 2nd ed, pp. 183–238. Wiley.
- Gaschen, L. (2011) Ultrasonography of small intestinal inflammatory and neoplastic diseases in dogs and cats. *Vet Clin North Am Small Anim Pract*, 41(2):329–344.
- Hecht, S., Mai, W.M. (2015) Spleen. In: Penninck, D., d'Anjou, M.A. (eds). *Atlas of Small Animal Ultrasonography*. 2nd ed, pp. 239–258. Wiley.
- Hoffman, K.L. (2003) Sonographic signs of gastroduodenal linear foreign body in 3 dogs. *Vet Radiol Ultrasound*, 44(4):466–469.
- Mai, W. (2006) The hilar perivenous hyperechoic triangle as a sign of acute splenic torsion in dogs. *Vet Radiol Ultrasound*, 47(5):487–491.
- Larson, M.M., Mattoon, J.S., Lawrence, Y., Sellon, R.K. (2020) Liver. In: Mattoon, J.S., Sellon, R. K., Berry, C.R. (eds). *Small Animal Diagnostic Ultrasound*. 4th ed, pp. 355–421. Elsevier.
- Mattoon, J.S., Duffy, M. (2020) Spleen. In: Mattoon, J.S., Sellon, R. K., Berry, C.R. (eds). *Small Animal Diagnostic Ultrasound*. 4th ed, pp. 422–460. Elsevier.
- Neelis, D.A., Mattoon, J.S., Slovak, J.E., Sellon, R.K. (2020) Gastrointestinal tract. In: Mattoon, J.S., Sellon, R. K., Berry, C.R. (eds). *Small Animal Diagnostic Ultrasound*. 4th ed, pp. 491–525. Elsevier.
- Patsikas, M.N., Papazoglou, L.G., Papaioannou, N.G., et al. (2003) Ultrasonographic findings of intestinal intussusception in seven cats. *J Feline Med Surg*, 5(6):335–343.
- Penninck, D., d'Anjou, M.A. (2015) Gastrointestinal tract. In: Penninck, D., d'Anjou, M.A. (eds). *Atlas of Small Animal Ultrasonography*. 2nd ed, pp. 259–308. Wiley.
- Pike, F.S., Berg, J., King, N.W., et al. (2004) Gallbladder mucocele in dogs: 30 cases (2000–2002). *J Am Vet Med Assoc*, 224(10):1615–1622.
- Willard, M.D. (2012) Alimentary neoplasia in geriatric dogs and cats. *Vet Clin North Am Small Anim Pract*. 42(4):693–706.

Normal Ultrasonographic Appearance and Main Pathologies of the Urinary and Reproductive Systems and Adrenal Glands

Amalia Agut Giménez

URINARY SYSTEM

Ultrasonography has become a routine technique for the evaluation of the urinary system as it is a rapid, noninvasive and relatively sensitive method for assessment of the kidneys and ureters. Changes in kidney size, architecture and echogenicity can be observed by ultrasonography. However, it does not provide any information on renal function.

Proximal Kidneys and Ureters

Technique

A 5 MHz probe is usually suitable for most dogs, and a 7.5 MHz probe for cats and miniature-breed dogs. The abdomen is usually prepared by clipping it and applying acoustic gel to the skin.

The **kidneys** are examined by placing the animal in dorsal recumbency and obtaining a sagittal section in this position; alternatively, the animal can be placed in either right or left lateral recumbency. In dogs, the left kidney is easier to visualise due to its more caudal position, and sometimes the spleen can be used as an acoustic window. The more cranial position of the right kidney and its position below the rib cage makes it harder to locate. The cat's kidneys are easier to examine due to their more caudal location.

Sagittal, dorsal and transverse sections of the kidneys should be obtained. The animal is placed in right or left lateral recumbency, depending on which kidney is to be evaluated, and the lateral part of the abdomen is prepared to obtain dorsal (frontal) and lateral transverse sections. To obtain good images of the right kidney, it must be examined at the 11th and 12th intercostal spaces. The presence of gas in the descending duodenum or faeces or other content in the ascending colon can affect the quality of the image.

The kidneys can also be examined with the animal in sternal recumbency or standing; this position is useful in animals that have ascites or large masses as it reduces the distance between the transducer and the organ (Widmer et al., 2020).

Normal Ultrasonographic Appearance

In a **dorsal plane** (Figs. 1 and 2), three areas of the kidney can be clearly distinguished. These regions consist of a bright echogenic central area corresponding to the renal sinus zone and peripelvic fat, around which a hypoechoic area representing

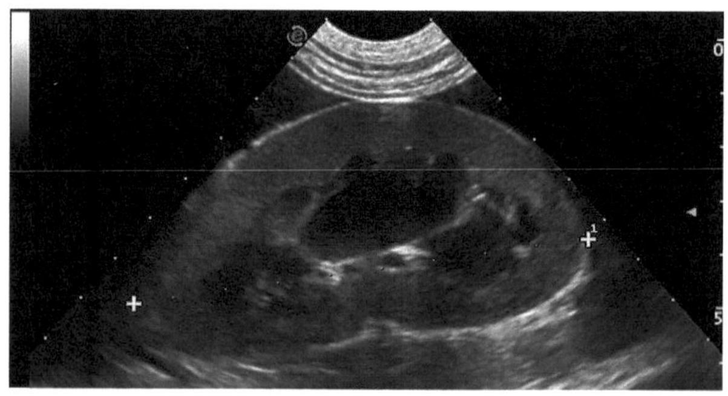

Figure 1. Appearance of a normal kidney in a dog, in a dorsal plane. There are three clearly differentiated areas: the renal sinus, medulla and cortex.

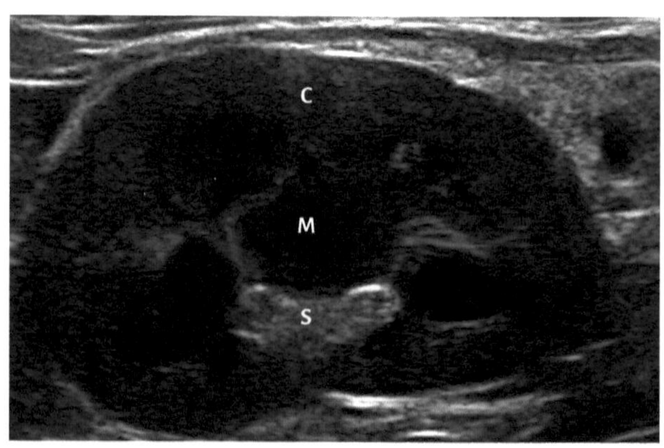

Figure 2. Appearance of a normal kidney in a cat, in a dorsal plane. S: renal sinus; M: medulla; C: cortex.

the renal medulla is seen, and an outermost zone of intermediate echogenicity, which is the renal cortex.

When the **sagittal plane** is examined from medial to lateral, the hyperechoic central zone of the renal sinus disappears and a hypoechoic central zone bordered by two hyperechoic lines appears. The central hyperechoic region represents the renal crest, and the dorsal and ventral echogenic lines are the pelvic diverticula (recesses) accompanied by the interlobular vessels (Fig. 3). Arcuate and intralobular arteries can sometimes be identified, with discrete echogenicity at the corticomedullary junction and in the cortex (d'Anjou and Penninck, 2015).

In the **transverse plane** (Fig. 4), echogenic lines representing the pelvic diverticula and interlobular vessels can be seen radial to the cortex from the central pelvic region. The medullary region appears separated into sections by the diverticula and vessels. This is the best plane to use for evaluation of the renal pelvis, which is not normally dilated, but occasionally a small amount of anechoic fluid can be seen (Fig. 4). In the transverse plane, the width of the renal pelvis can measure up to 2 mm in dogs and 1.6 mm in cats.

It is important to be able to recognise the **echogenicity of the kidney relative to that of the liver and spleen** in order to identify changes. The renal medulla is the least echogenic of these, followed by the cortex. The echogenicity of the renal cortex is similar to or slightly less than that of the hepatic parenchyma (Fig. 5), and slightly less than that of the splenic parenchyma (Fig. 6) when compared using a 5 MHz transducer and at approximately the same depth. The echogenicity of the renal cortex may be increased in neutered or pregnant cats. Fat around the kidney has an echogenicity similar to or greater than that of pelvic fat. The capsule has an echogenicity

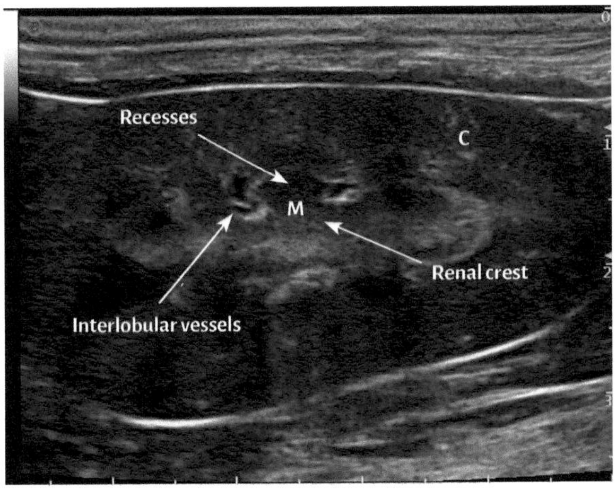

Figure 3. Appearance of a normal kidney in a dog, in a sagittal plane. A central hyperechoic region, the renal crest, is observed, and dorsal and ventral echogenic lines represent the pelvic diverticula (recesses) accompanied by the interlobular vessels. C: cortex; M: medulla.

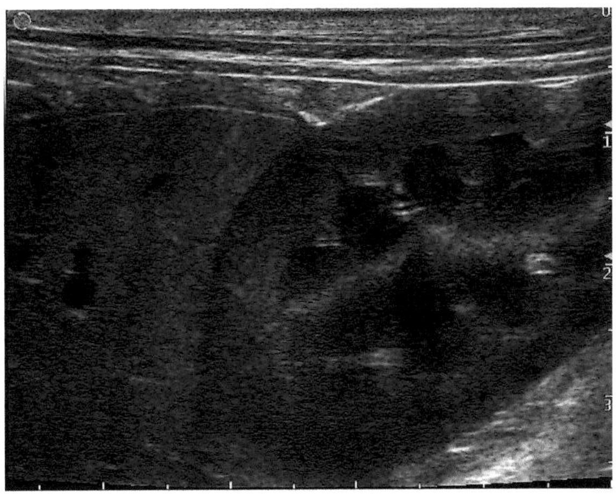

Figure 5. Ultrasound image of the renal cortex and the liver. The cortex of the right kidney is hypoechoic with respect to the liver.

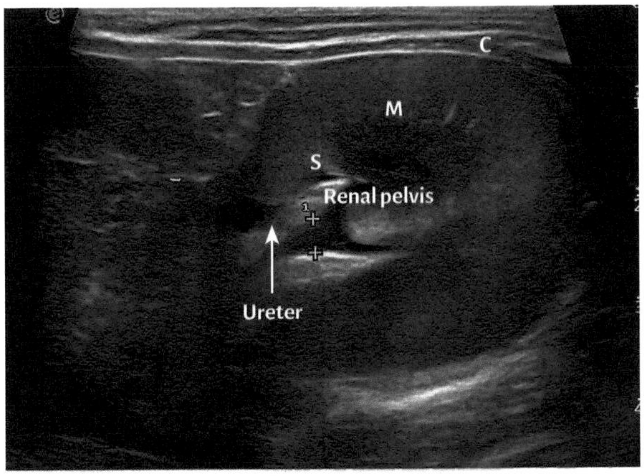

Figure 4. Appearance of a normal kidney in a dog, in a transverse plane. S: renal sinus; M: medulla; C: cortex.

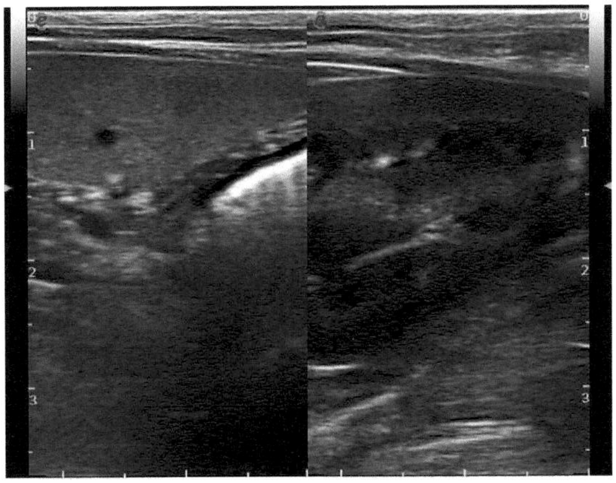

Figure 6. Ultrasound images of the renal cortex and the spleen. The cortex of the left kidney is hypoechoic with respect to the spleen.

similar to that of the perirenal fat and is not identifiable as a separate structure. The difference in the echogenicity of the medulla and the renal cortex is due to the structure of these regions: the renal medulla has a higher water content and less acoustic interface than the cortex. Sometimes a hyperechoic line can be observed in the corticomedullary junction, which is not a sign of any pathological change unless the animal presents clinical signs or abnormalities of renal parameters. In small breeds of dog, a broad hyperechoic band is seen in the corticomedullary junction that corresponds anatomically to the location of the arcuate arteries as branches from the interlobar arteries (Fig. 7) (Hart et al., 2013, Widmer et al., 2020).

The kidneys can be measured in any of the three planes. In cats, the length ranges between 3 cm and 4.3 cm. However, in dogs the measurements should be related to body weight and conformation, since there is a lot of variation among breeds. However, two articles have been published, one of which (Mareschal et al., 2007) investigated the ratio of the length of the kidney to the diameter of the aorta. This ratio is obtained by dividing the maximum length of the kidney by the maximum diameter of the aorta at the level of the kidney. Kidney size is considered to be decreased when this ratio is less than 5.5 and increased when it is greater than 9.1. Another published study compared the length of the kidney with the length of lumbar vertebra 5 (L5) or L6, with the normal ratio being between 1.3 and 2.7 (Barella et al., 2012).

The proximal and middle parts of the ureters extend along the retroperitoneal space, lateral to the aorta and caudal vena cava. When examining the urinary bladder, the distal ureters can be visualised and evaluated where they enter the ureteral papillae in the trigone region. Ureteral jets entering the bladder lumen can often be detected when examining the papilla area; the detection of jets can be improved with the use of colour Doppler (d'Anjou and Penninck, 2015).

Renal and Ureteral Disorders

Animals may present with clinical signs and alterations of renal function but not show any changes on ultrasonographic examination, or vice versa. Abnormalities that can be observed ultrasonographically are, in most cases, not specific to a given disease (d'Anjou and Penninck, 2015; Widmer et al., 2020). Thus, ultrasound-guided aspiration or biopsy of the kidneys is very useful in these cases.

Parenchymal Abnormalities

Diffuse Abnormalities

Congenital

Young cats and dogs may present with chronic renal failure due to both congenital and chronic diseases.

Familial nephropathies have been described in different dog breeds. These animals usually show kidney failure before 1 year of age. Ultrasonographically, the kidneys are small, with irregular margins, and diffusely hyperechoic, with loss of the corticomedullary junction. In addition, a small dilation of the renal pelvis may be observed (Fig. 8).

Another condition that can produce similar ultrasound images is **congenital renal dysplasia**. This abnormality may be

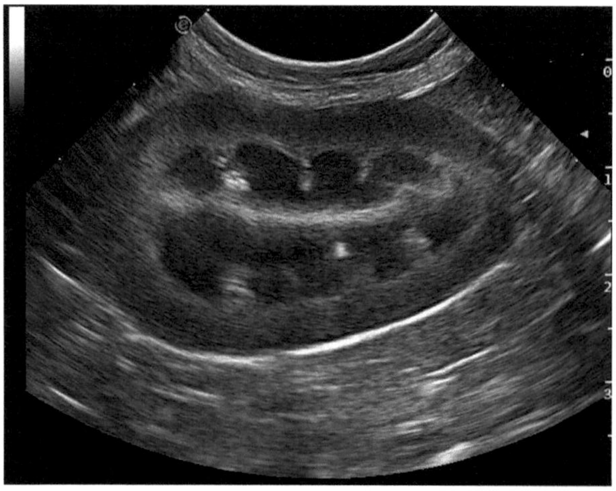

Figure 7. Sagittal section of the left kidney of a dog. A broad hyperchoic band is observed in the corticomedullary junction that corresponds anatomically to the area where the arcuate arteries branch from the interlobar arteries.

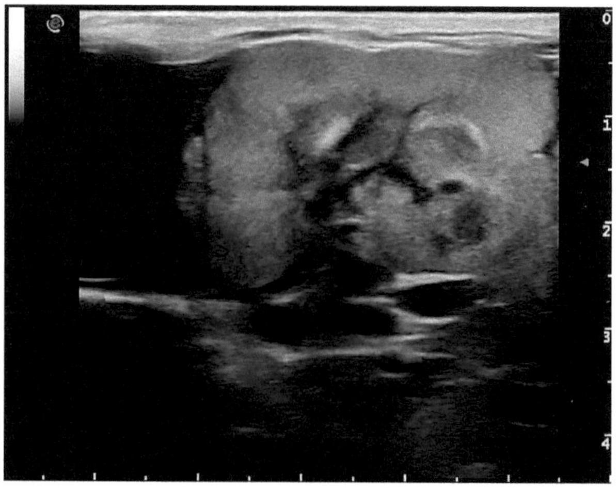

Figure 8. Sagittal image of the right kidney of a 2-month-old Pyrenean Mastiff with renal failure. The kidney is smaller than normal and has irregular borders, and loss of the corticomedullary junction and dilation of the renal pelvis can be seen. Both kidneys in this animal had the same appearance.

hereditary or can result from a neonatal infection, such as feline panleukopaenia virus or canine herpesvirus. Renal dysplasia is defined as the disorganised development of the renal parenchyma, resulting in deformed and fibrous kidneys. These kidneys can be normal in size or small, irregular in shape, and hyperechoic with loss of the corticomedullary junction (Cordella et al., 2020; Griffin, 2020).

Unilateral renal agenesis or hypoplasia is uncommon but has been described in dogs and cats. If there is only one kidney, compensatory hypertrophy of that kidney may occur. In this case, the kidney increases in size but retains the normal internal architecture.

Ectopic kidney is the abnormal location of one or both kidneys. The aetiology of this abnormality is unknown. Ectopic kidneys are classified based on their anatomical position: pelvic, iliac or abdominal. Ectopic kidneys are structurally and functionally normal, but may be smaller than normal. If the ureter is short it may be bent, predisposing to obstruction, secondary hydronephrosis or pyelonephritis (Widmer et al., 2020).

Acquired

Increased echogenicity is one of the most common findings in cats and dogs with chronic kidney disease (Fig. 9). Several diseases of the kidneys can be associated with increased cortical or medullary echogenicity (Table 1) (Sutherland-Smith and Penninck, 2015; Bragato et al., 2017). In some of these processes, the cortical echogenicity may be increased, producing an enhancement of the corticomedullary junction. This is very pronounced in cases of necrosis caused by ethylene glycol poisoning (Fig. 10).

In other cases, both the cortex and the medulla show increased echogenicity resulting in a loss of the corticomedullary junction; this is particularly evident in cases of chronic kidney disease (Table 1).

Table 1. Differential diagnoses of renal pathologies that cause increased echogenicity of the cortex and medulla.

	Dogs	Cats
Hyperechoic cortex	· Interstitial or glomerular nephritis · Pyelonephritis · Leptospirosis · Acute tubular necrosis · Ethylene glycol and grape poisoning · End-stage renal disease · Nephrocalcinosis	· Interstitial or glomerular nephritis · Ethylene glycol and lily poisoning · Diffuse renal lymphoma · Feline infectious peritonitis · Cryptococcosis · Amyloidosis
Cortex and medulla with increased echogenicity (loss of corticomedullary junction)	· Congenital renal dysplasia · Juvenile Boxer nephropathy · End-stage renal disease	· Congenital renal dysplasia · End-stage renal disease

In cases of severe renal disease, a hyperechoic band may be observed in the medulla, parallel to the corticomedullary junction, consistent with mineralisation, necrosis, congestion and haemorrhage. This so-called "medullary rim sign" has been observed in several processes (d'Anjou and Penninck, 2015; Cordella et al., 2020):

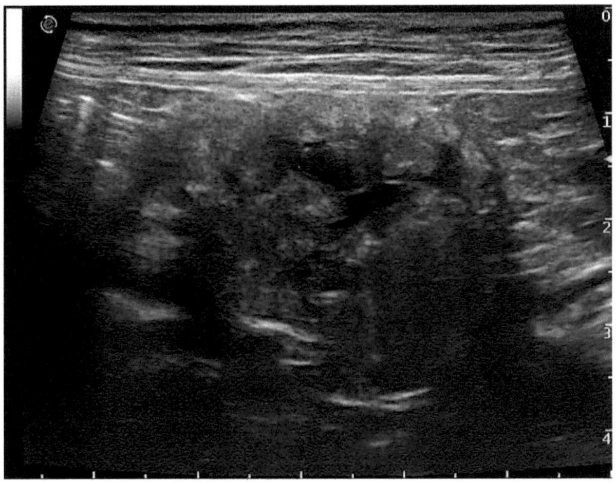

Figure 9. Appearance of a kidney in a dog with end-stage renal failure. Sagittal image of the left kidney showing an increase in echogenicity of the cortex, a decrease in size, irregular margins and loss of the corticomedullary junction.

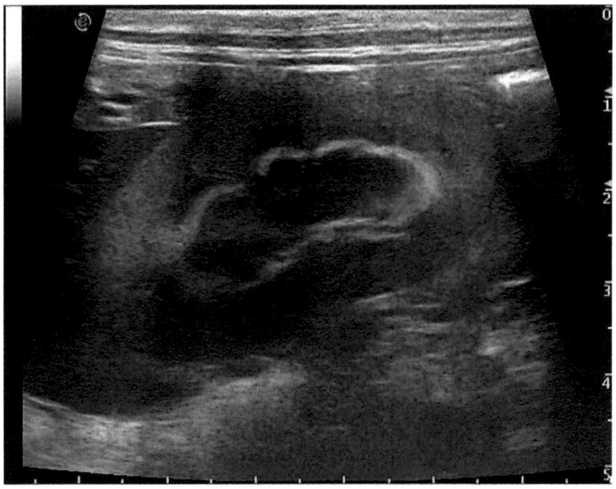

Figure 10. Acute renal failure due to ethylene glycol poisoning. There is an increase in the echogenicity of the cortex and a hyperechoic line is observed at the corticomedullary junction.

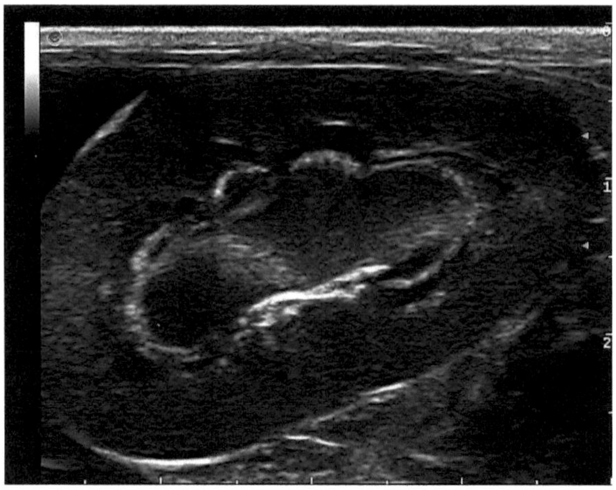

Figure 11. Appearance of the kidney of a cat with feline infectious peritonitis. The "medullary rim sign" is seen at the corticomedullary junction.

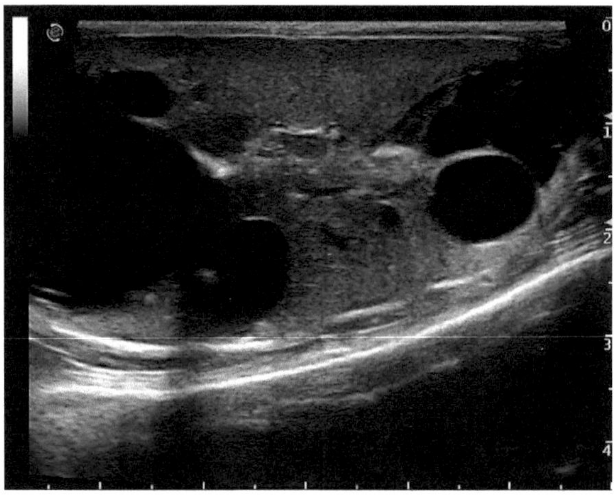

Figure 12. Polycystic kidney disease. Multiple cysts of different sizes are observed in the renal cortex.

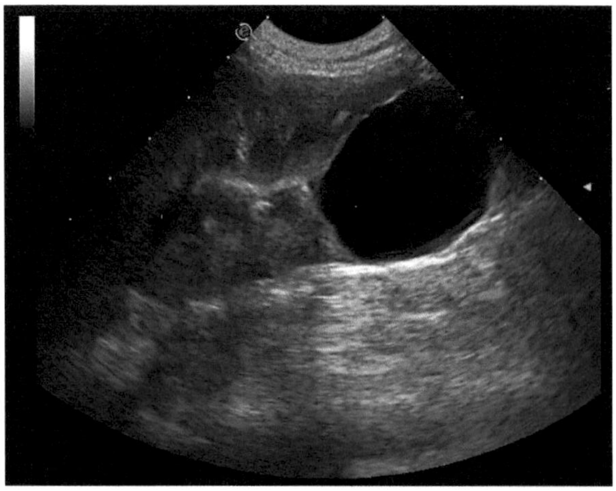

Figure 13. Solitary renal cyst at the caudal pole of the left kidney.

- acute tubular necrosis (ethylene glycol poisoning) (Fig. 10)
- nephrocalcinosis
- leptospirosis
- pyogranulomatous vasculitis (feline infectious peritonitis) (Fig. 11)
- lymphoma
- lymphoma in dogs (decreased echogenicity)
- normal dogs and cats (the renal profile is normal).

Focal Abnormalities

Focal abnormalities are easier to diagnose than diffuse disorders and are common in small animals. The most common are renal cysts, nephrolithiasis or dystrophic mineralisation, and cortical infarcts, followed by metastatic or primary neoplasia, granulomas and abscesses.

Renal Cysts

Renal cysts can be hereditary or acquired. Hereditary polycystic kidney disease occurs in Persian cats (Fig. 12) and in Cairn Terriers. Cysts can be solitary or multifocal, of different sizes, and unilateral or bilateral. Ultrasonographically, they are observed as oval or rounded structures, which are anechoic, with a thin hyperechoic wall and well-defined edges, and may present posterior enhancement (Fig. 13). Sometimes they are found incidentally during an ultrasonographic examination. Most cysts are located in the renal cortex or in the corticomedullary junction. They can also appear secondary to chronic kidney disease.

Solitary cysts can be very large and should be differentiated from cavitary or solid masses, abscesses or haematomas. Solid masses or nodules have internal echoes and are not associated with posterior enhancement. The cysts that are associated with cystadenocarcinomas are usually irregular and have heterogeneous echogenicity. Renal cystadenocarcinomas occur in female German Shepherd Dogs and are accompanied by nodular dermatofibrosis (d'Anjou and Penninck, 2015).

Renal Haematomas

Renal haematomas usually occur in young animals that have bleeding disorders or have recently undergone trauma. They may have anechoic, hypoechoic and hyperechoic components within the renal cortex or medulla. Differentiation between haematomas and neoplasms such as renal haemangiosarcoma by ultrasonography can be a challenge.

Renal Abscess

Renal abscesses can generally be differentiated from true cysts by the presence of echoes and sedimentation in the cavitary lesion and by their irregular contour. They may present posterior enhancement if the cellular content is low (Widmer et al., 2020).

Renal Infarcts

Renal infarcts are observed ultrasonographically as well-defined linear or triangular-shaped areas in the renal cortex perpendicular to the capsule (Fig. 14). The appearance of infarcts can vary; **chronic** infarcts are typically hyperechoic and a depression may appear in the capsule, and **acute** infarcts may initially be hyperechoic and then become hypoechoic.

Renal Mineralisation (Nephrocalcinosis)

Renal mineralisation may be observed in elderly dogs and cats. It appears ultrasonographically as hyperechoic foci with distal acoustic shadowing at the level of the renal diverticulum, pelvis and cortex.

Solid Mass-Type Lesions

Solid masses are generally malignant. They may be hypoechoic, hyperechoic, isoechoic or of mixed echogenicity. Although echogenicity patterns are not specific to tumour types, uniformly hypoechoic masses or nodules are often compatible with **lymphoma** and **malignant histiocytosis**. Hyperechoic masses are less common and are related to chondrosarcomas, haemangiosarcomas and metastatic adenocarcinomas.

The most common renal tumour in dogs is **carcinoma** (Fig. 15), and in the cat it is **lymphoma**. In this case the kidneys are enlarged, irregular and hyperechoic with a subcapsular hypoechoic halo (Fig. 16) (d'Anjou and Penninck, 2015; Griffin, 2020; Widmer et al., 2020).

Other pathological processes, such as abscesses and solid haematomas or granulomas, may appear to be neoplastic processes due to their solid appearance on ultrasonography; in most cases, fine-needle aspiration or biopsy is necessary to reach a diagnosis.

Size Alterations

An increase in kidney size is observed in neoplasms (usually lymphoma) and in the initial stages of pyelonephritis, portosystemic shunt, feline infectious peritonitis, urinary obstruction and polycystic kidney disease (Fig. 12).

A decrease in size appears in chronic conditions and is usually associated with changes in the shape of the kidneys (Fig. 9) (Bragato et al., 2017).

Accumulation of Renal Subcapsular Fluid

Large amounts of subcapsular fluid have been observed in the case of perirenal pseudocysts in cats (Fig. 17), which are also occasionally diagnosed in dogs. The kidney appears to float in the encapsulated fluid, and its shape, size and internal architecture may be normal or altered. Due to the presence of fluid, the kidney usually appears more echogenic than normal.

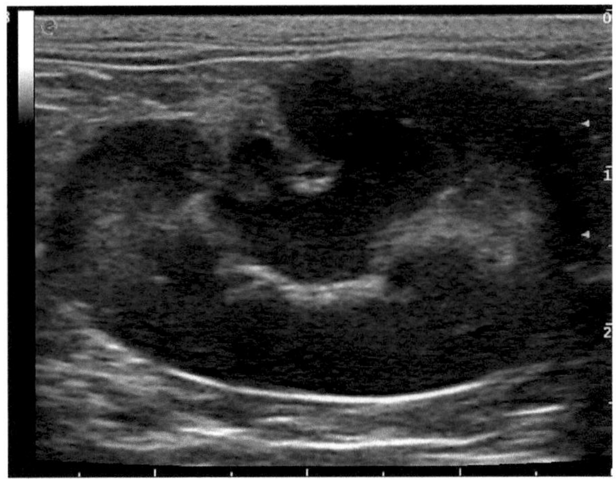

Figure 14. Ultrasound image of a renal infarct. A focal depression is seen in a hyperechoic triangular area, consistent with a renal infarct.

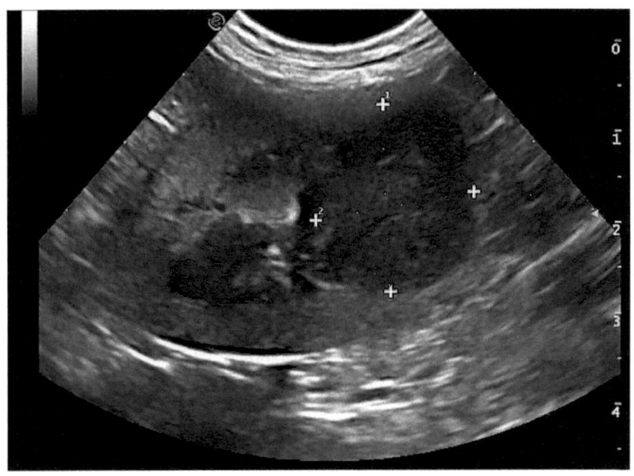

Figure 15. Ultrasonographic appearance of renal carcinoma. A hypoechoic mass is observed at the caudal border of the left kidney that alters the normal morphology of the kidney. cat. The kidney is enlarged, irregular and hyperechoic, with a subcapsular hypoechoic halo, and presents with pyelectasis.

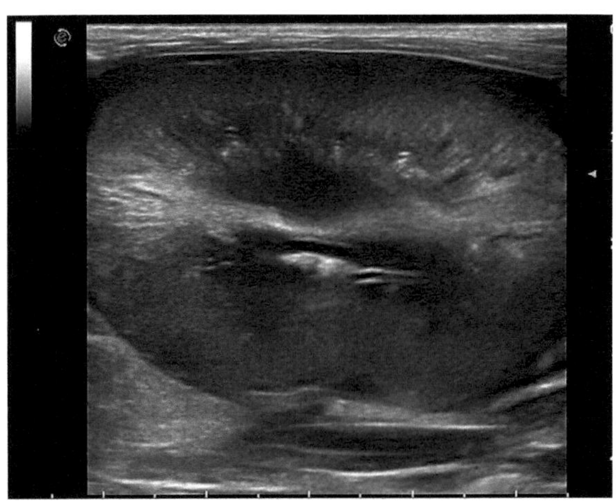

Figure 16. Ultrasonographic appearance of renal lymphoma in a cat. The kidney is enlarged, irregular and hyperechoic, with a subcapsular hypoechoic halo, and presents with pyelectasis.

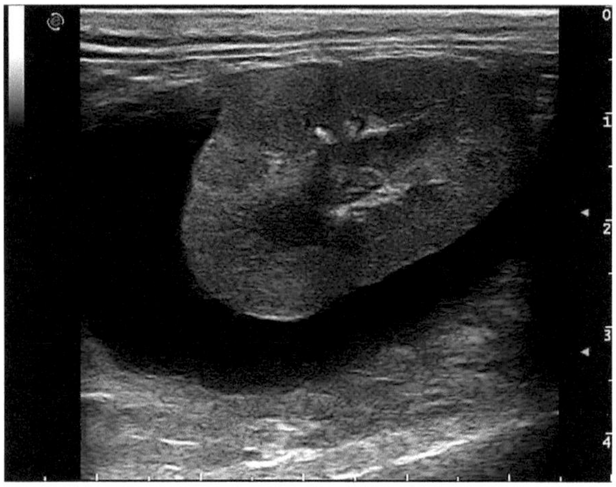

Figure 17. Ultrasonographic appearance of a perirenal pseudocyst. Longitudinal image of the left kidney showing a large amount of fluid around the kidney.

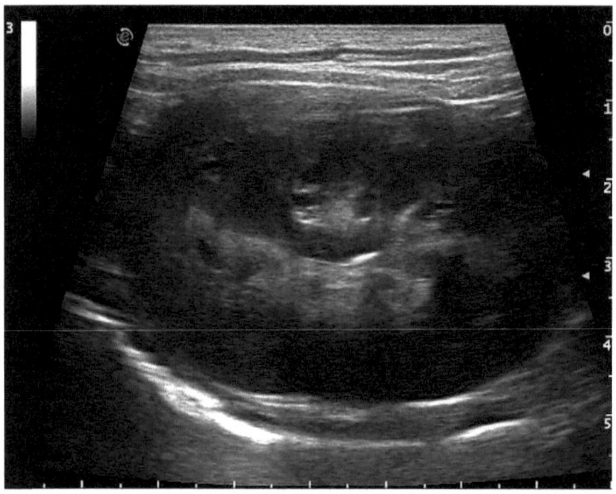

Figure 18. Ultrasound image of pyelonephritis. Increased echogenicity is observed in both the cortex and the medulla, with loss of the corticomedullary junction and pyelectasis.

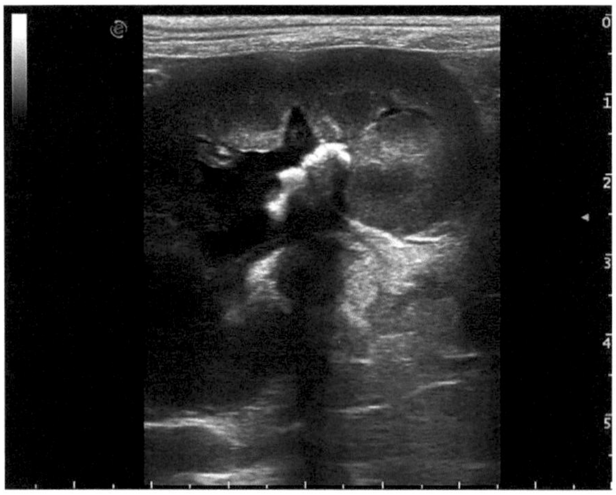

Figure 19. Ultrasonographic appearance of obstructive hydronephrosis. Longitudinal image of the left kidney showing a hyperechoic structure with an acoustic shadow in the centre of the dilated renal pelvis, consistent with a calculus.

Other causes of subcapsular fluid are the accumulation of urine, blood, exudate or transudate around the kidney. Renal coagulopathies or trauma can result in retroperitoneal bleeding. In feline infectious peritonitis and renal lymphosarcoma, small amounts of subcapsular fluid are often observed. Free peritoneal, retroperitoneal or subcapsular fluid can also be caused by ethylene glycol poisoning (Widmer et al., 2020).

Collecting System Abnormalities

Dilation of the collecting system is called **pyelectasis** or **hydronephrosis**. Hydronephrosis refers to when there is an obstruction of the collecting system.

When the height of the renal pelvis in the transverse plane is measured as greater than 13 mm on ultrasonographic examination, it is considered as a predictive reference measure to establish that there is obstruction (d'Anjou et al., 2011).

Pyelectasis

Pyelectasis is the dilation of the renal pelvis. It is observed ultrasonographically as an anechoic separation in the hyperechoic central zone of the renal sinus (Fig. 18). Pyelectasis can be observed in animals with increased diuresis (due to diuretic therapy or chronic kidney disease) and in animals with congenital malformations (ectopic ureter), pyelonephritis or lower urinary tract obstruction.

Pyelonephritis

Pyelonephritis can affect one or both kidneys and is usually the result of an ascending ureteral infection from the urinary bladder. Ultrasonographic changes observed in pyelonephritis are an increase in the size of the kidney, increased echogenicity of the cortex, and mild or moderate dilation of the renal pelvis and proximal ureter (Fig. 18). An echogenic line may also be visualised at the corticomedullary junction, as well as focal hyperechoic areas in the renal medulla, and focal hypoechoic or hyperechoic areas in the cortex.

In chronic cases, distortion of the renal pelvis and diverticula and a hyperechoic line at the corticomedullary junction can be observed (d'Anjou and Penninck, 2015; Widmer et al., 2020).

Hydronephrosis

Hydronephrosis occurs when the renal pelvis and the diverticula dilate, distorting and compressing the renal parenchyma. Renal diverticula are rounded and appear as finger-like anechoic projections extending from the anechoic renal pelvis (Fig. 19).

Hydronephrosis develops when there is an obstruction of urinary flow. In cases of severe hydronephrosis, a fluid-filled sac will be observed, with a very thin ring surrounding it that corresponds to the small amount of cortex that remains. Hydronephrosis may progress to pyonephrosis in cases where urinary stasis and consequent infection occur.

The differential diagnosis of causes of moderate or severe hydronephrosis includes congenital diseases, lower urinary tract obstruction, pelvic or ureteral obstruction by a calculus, an infiltrative mass in the bladder trigone or a retroperitoneal mass (Widmer et al., 2020).

Renal and Ureteral Calculi

Calculi in the kidney or ureter are observed as hyperechoic structures with an acoustic shadow (Fig. 19), whether they are radiopaque or radiolucent. Small calculi may not produce an acoustic shadow if they are smaller than the width of the ultrasound beam.

Ureteral Abnormalities

Hydroureter or dilation of the ureter usually occurs in combination with hydronephrosis in cases of urinary flow obstruction. Distended ureters are most easily seen in the area of the renal hilum; they are difficult to visualise in the bladder trigone unless they are very dilated. In cases of chronic obstructions, the ureter can become large and tortuous. Occasionally, colour Doppler or power Doppler can help to differentiate an abdominal vessel from a dilated ureter.

Dilation of the ureter is seen in cases of **ureteritis** and in cases of **obstruction**, either due to a calculus, where the calculus will appear as a hyperechoic structure with an acoustic shadow (Fig. 20), or in cases of neoplastic conditions of the urinary bladder that infiltrate the bladder trigone or the ureter. It is also seen in cases of ectopic ureter.

Congenital ectopic ureters can be unilateral or bilateral. They are more common in female dogs than in males, and may end in the urethra, vagina or colon. These ureters are often distended because there is a partial obstruction in the area where they empty or because there is intramural tunnelling or an ascending infection (Fig. 21). Hydronephrosis can also sometimes be observed in cases where ureteral distension is very marked (d'Anjou and Penninck, 2015; Widmer et al., 2020).

A **ureterocoele** is a focal cystic dilation in the distal submucosal portion of the ureter that protrudes into the bladder lumen. It can be classified as **orthotopic** when it is located in the normal area of the opening of the ureter or **ectopic** when it is located in the neck of the bladder or urethra. Ultrasonographic examination shows an anechoic, rounded structure with a thin wall protruding into the bladder lumen (d'Anjou and Penninck, 2015; Widmer et al., 2020).

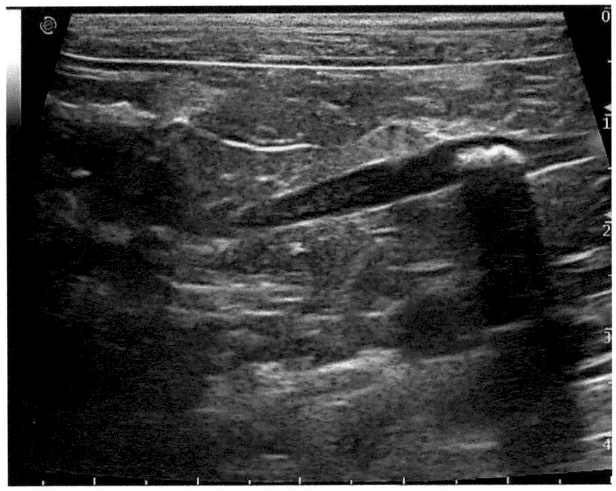

Figure 20. Ultrasound image of a dilated ureter due to a calculus. A hyperechoic structure with acoustic shadowing is observed.

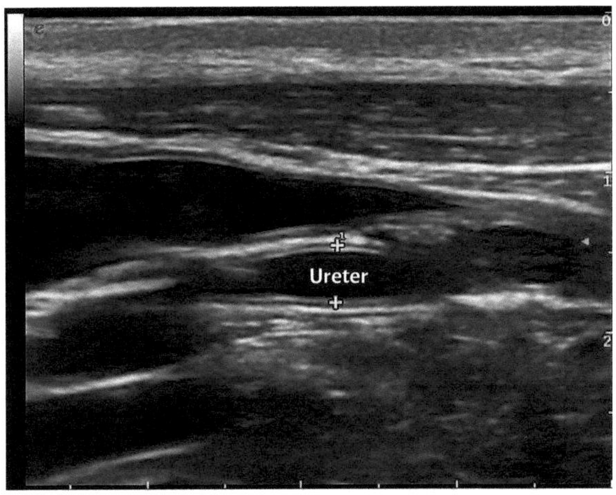

Figure 21. Ectopic ureter. Longitudinal ultrasound image of the area of the bladder trigone where, in the area dorsal to the trigone, a tubular structure with anechoic content that extends beyond the ureterovesical junction is observed. Colour Doppler showed that there was no flow in this structure, consistent with an ectopic ureter.

Retroperitoneal Abnormalities

Different types of fluid can accumulate in the retroperitoneal space on the periphery of one or both kidneys. Leptospirosis, acute renal failure due to nephrotoxicity or interstitial nephritis predispose to bilateral perirenal effusion; when the effusion is unilateral, it is more indicative of an obstruction or rupture of the renal pelvis or ureter.

Retroperitoneal transudate appears as anechoic to hypoechoic linear, triangular or oval foci adjacent to the kidneys. These changes can be seen with the accumulation of urine or blood, following trauma to the kidneys or ureters.

Urinoma is the accumulation of encapsulated urine as a result of traumatic extravasation.

Retroperitoneal exudate and **acute haemorrhage** are usually more echogenic due to their higher cell numbers. Inflammatory processes, such as acute pyelonephritis and ureteritis, can cause the retroperitoneal fat to appear hyperechoic.

Retroperitoneal abscesses can be caused by the migration of grass seeds. The ultrasonographic appearance is of thickened, irregular walls, often presenting as anechoic or hypoechoic masses, with or without septa with an ultrasound signal on the inside (Fig. 22).

Retroperitoneal masses can be secondary to **granulomas**, **neoplasms** or enlarged **sublumbar lymph nodes**. They can vary in size, shape and echogenicity. **Haemangiosarcoma** is a common neoplasm of the retroperitoneal space in the dog (Widmer et al., 2020).

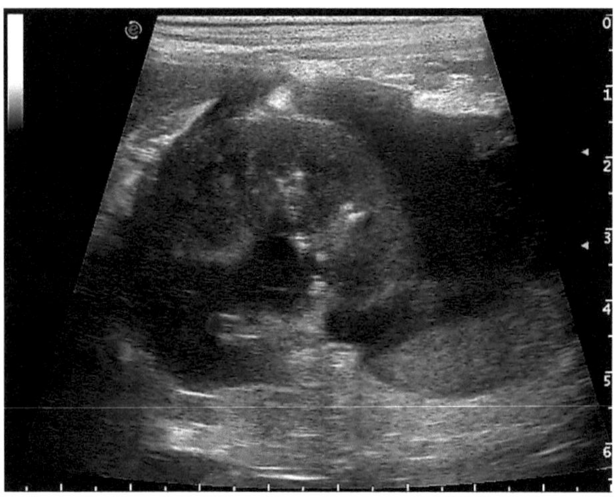

Figure 22. Ultrasound image of a retroperitoneal abscess. The kidney is observed to have a dilated pelvis and an ultrasound signal inside. At the subcapsular and retroperitoneal level, hypoechoic fluid is visualised and the perirenal fat is hyperechoic.

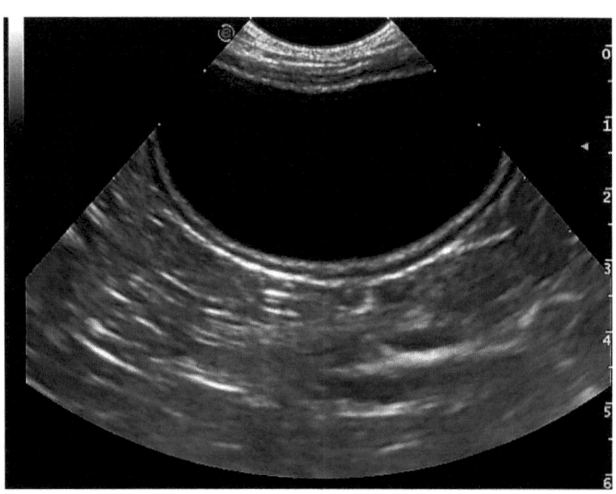

Figure 23. Ultrasound image of a normal distended urinary bladder in a transverse plane. Three layers can be identified: a hypoechoic central layer that is the muscle layer, an external hyperechoic layer representing the serosa, and an internal hyperechoic layer that is the mucosa–submucosa.

Urinary Bladder and Urethra

Technique and Normal Appearance of the Bladder

The bladder is easily examined when it is distended with urine and can serve as an acoustic window for the visualisation of adjacent structures such as the colon and uterus.

A linear or semiconvex transducer can be used with a frequency ranging from 5 MHz to 10 MHz. The bladder should be examined in both transverse and sagittal planes from the ventral wall of the abdomen. Sometimes the transducer must be positioned on the lateral part of the abdomen; this can cause reverberation artefacts to occur and simulate intramural abnormalities. These artefacts are resolved by changing the position of the transducer and obtaining images in other planes (Sutherland-Smith and Penninck, 2015).

The **wall** thickness of the bladder depends on the extent of bladder distension. If it is minimally distended (0.5 ml/kg), the thickness of the bladder wall should be 2.3 ± 0.43 mm. If slightly distended (2 ml/kg), the thickness of the wall should be 1.6 ± 0.29 mm. If the bladder is moderately distended (4 ml/kg), the thickness of the wall should be 1.4 ± 0.28 mm.

When the bladder is distended, it is well defined, its profile is regular and its wall is very thin (1–2 mm in dogs and 1.3–1.7 mm in cats). Three layers can be differentiated: a hypoechoic central layer, which is the muscle layer; an external hyperechoic layer, which is the serosa; and an internal hyperechoic layer, which is the mucosa–submucosa (Fig. 23). If the bladder is not very distended, its wall is thickened, and incorrect diagnoses may occur. Urine is generally anechoic with posterior reinforcement; occasionally, small echoes in suspension, corresponding to fat droplets, can be observed in cats (Sutherland-Smith and Penninck, 2015; Widmer et al., 2020; Griffin, 2020).

The bladder **trigone** should be examined carefully because it is an area where neoplasms commonly occur. Occasionally, two small protuberances can be seen in the dorsal part of the trigone; these represent the intramural portion of the ureters when they enter the bladder, termed the ureterovesical junction. Occasionally, bright echoes can be seen with turbulence from the ureters to the bladder, called "ureteral jets"; these are very useful when evaluating animals in which ectopic ureters are suspected (Sutherland-Smith and Penninck, 2015). This sign may be accentuated when the animal is undergoing diuretic therapy or fluid therapy.

There are several **artefacts** that are commonly visualised when the urinary bladder is examined. It is important to recognise these artefacts, as most of them look like pathological processes. Among them, the following are of particular note: lateral edge shadow, reverberation and partial volume.

- The **lateral edge shadow** artefact is caused by a refraction of the ultrasound beam due to the curvilinear shape of the cranial part of the bladder. This can produce an anechoic focal zone in the wall that may appear to be a loss of wall integrity or a diverticulum (Fig. 24). If the transducer is redirected, the artefact will disappear (Sutherland-Smith and Penninck, 2015).
- The **reverberation** and **partial volume** artefacts are manifested by the appearance of echoes in the bladder lumen. In the case of the partial volume artefact, these bright echoes may look like sediment. Reverberation is manifested by parallel horizontal linear echoes in the area near the transducer (Widmer et al., 2020). To avoid or reduce these artefacts, the gain should be adjusted, or harmonic ultrasound used.

Technique and Normal Appearance of the Urethra

The proximal urethra should also be examined routinely, when possible. It is seen as a thin-walled tubular structure that extends into the pelvis. The proximal part can be evaluated in most dogs and cats. In male animals, the prostatic urethra can also be seen inside the prostate gland (Fig. 25). The distal urethra is more difficult to assess. In male dogs, portions of the penile and perineal urethra can be examined using high-frequency transducers (Sutherland-Smith and Penninck, 2015).

Urinary Bladder Abnormalities

Mural Abnormalities

Cystitis

Cystitis produces an irregular, hypoechoic thickening of the wall, usually in the cranioventral area of the bladder (Fig. 26). The thickening can vary according to the severity of the pathology and the extent of distension of the bladder.

Polypoid Cystitis

On ultrasound examination of polypoid cystitis, a diffuse thickening of the bladder wall with multiple hyperechoic pedunculated masses that protrude towards the bladder lumen can be observed. These masses are located more frequently in the cranioventral part of the bladder (Fig. 27), and sometimes they have a similar appearance to neoplasms. Biopsy is recommended to reach a diagnosis (Sutherland-Smith and Penninck, 2015).

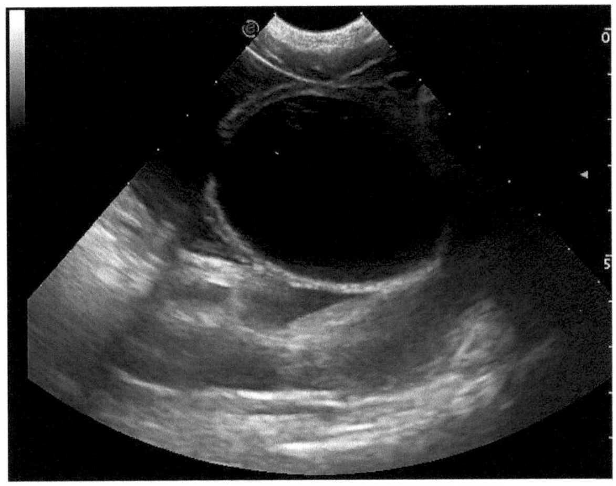

Figure 24. Ultrasound image of the bladder showing the lateral edge shadow artefact. Some of the wall is visualised and there appears to be a loss of wall integrity.

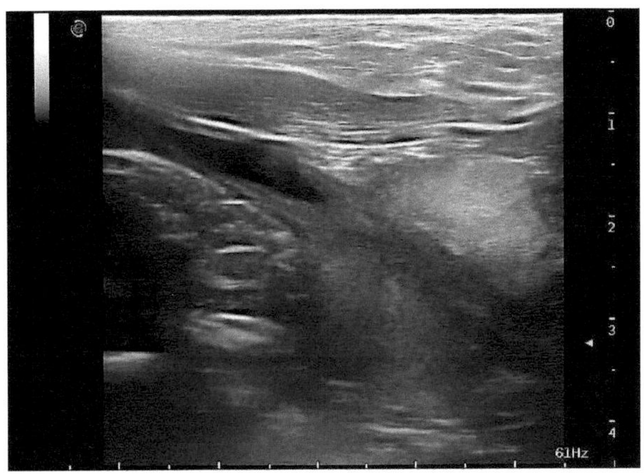

Figure 25. Ultrasound image of the urethra of a male dog in a longitudinal section.

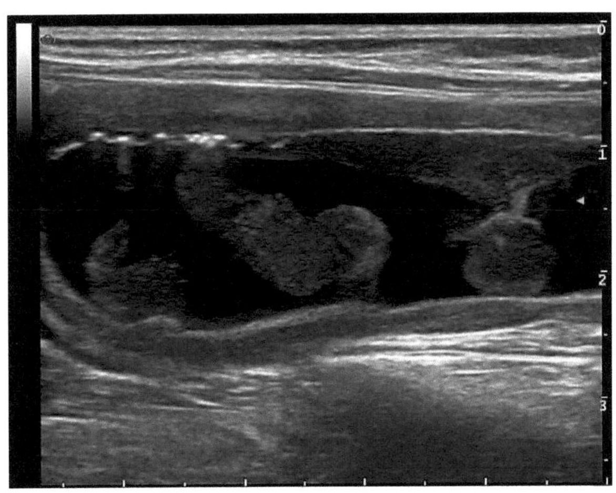

Figure 26. Emphysematous cystitis. Ultrasound image in the longitudinal plane of the urinary bladder. Thickening of the bladder wall is visualised, with persistence of the layers. There is echogenic content in the bladder in the form of masses consistent with clots. In the ventral area, hyperechoic lines are observed, with some reverberation compatible with gas.

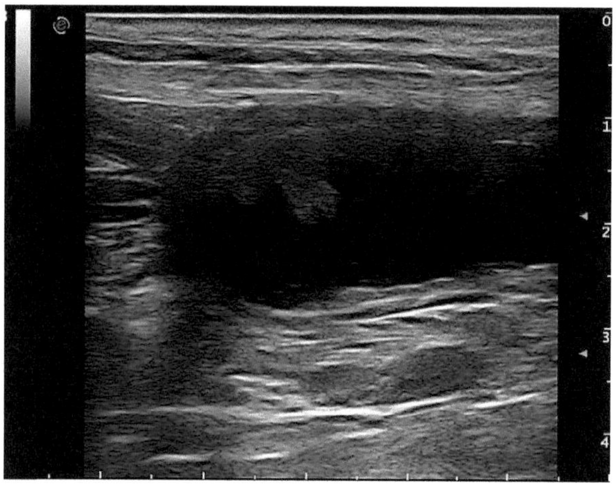

Figure 27. Polypoid cystitis. Ultrasound image in the longitudinal plane of the urinary bladder. Thickening of the bladder wall is observed, with several hyperechoic pedunculated masses that protrude towards the bladder lumen, located in the cranioventral part.

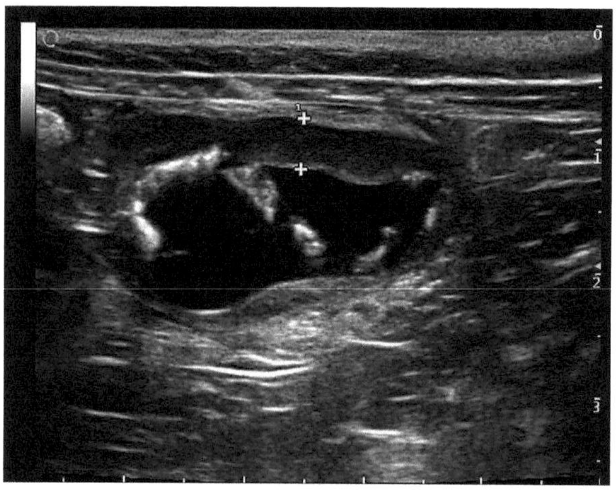

Figure 28. Pseudomembranous cystitis. Ultrasound image in a transverse plane of the urinary bladder. A nonhomogeneous thickening of the wall can be seen. Hyperechoic bands representing mucosal detachments with fibrin are observed extending from the ventral wall.

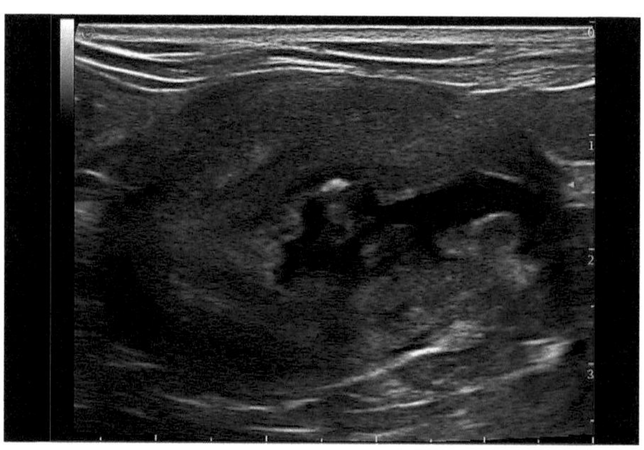

Figure 29. Transitional cell carcinoma. Ultrasound image of the urinary bladder in a longitudinal plane. Thickening of the wall is observed in the dorsal and ventral areas.

Emphysematous Cystitis

Emphysematous cystitis is most commonly seen in diabetic animals that have glycosuria. It is characterised by the presence of gas-forming bacteria such as *Escherichia coli, Aerobacter aerogenes, Proteus mirabilis* or *Clostridium* spp. in the bladder wall. The ultrasonographic appearance is of irregular, hyperechoic interfaces with a distal reverberation artefact. Intraluminal gas (sometimes seen in catheterised patients) is located in the nondependent part of the bladder (in the ventral area when the ultrasound examination is performed with the animal in dorsal recumbency) (Fig. 26) and altering the position of the patient will cause the position of this gas to vary, whereas if the gas is located in the bladder wall it will always be in the same place (Widmer et al., 2020).

Pseudomembranous Cystitis

Pseudomembranous cystitis is associated with diffuse ulcerations, necrosis and bladder wall haemorrhage, as well as with necrotic tissue and fibrin inside the bladder. Ultrasonographic findings are wall thickening and multiple intraluminal hyperechoic septa (Fig. 28) (Sutherland-Smith and Penninck, 2015).

Neoplasia

Transitional cell carcinoma is the most common neoplasm of the urinary bladder. It is characterised by an irregular mass with a wide base in the wall of the bladder that protrudes towards the lumen. The echogenicity of the mass is generally mixed, and can be hyperechoic, isoechoic or hypoechoic with respect to the bladder wall (Fig. 29). The mass is usually located in the bladder trigone area and in the dorsal bladder. Due to the location of the ureteral papillae in this area, it can sometimes be affected, causing unilateral or bilateral hydroureter. It is also common for the mass to extend into the proximal urethra and prostate. These tumours are typically highly vascular and present areas of dystrophic mineralisation.

Squamous cell carcinoma is a neoplasm of the urinary bladder of epithelial origin. Neoplasms of mesenchymal origin include botryoid rhabdomyosarcoma, chemodectoma, leiomyosarcoma, fibroid, fibrosarcoma, haemangioma, haemangiosarcoma, lymphoma and mastocytoma (Sutherland-Smith and Penninck 2015, Widmer et al 2020).

It is not possible to differentiate neoplasms of the urinary bladder by ultrasonography; a biopsy is necessary to reach a diagnosis.

The most **common urethral neoplasms** in dogs include **squamous cell carcinoma** and **adenocarcinomas**. Neoplasms of the proximal urethra often spread locally to the bladder and prostate.

The superficial medial, hypogastric, sacral and inguinal iliac lymph nodes should be checked when a neoplasm of the bladder or urethra is suspected.

Content Abnormalities

Calculi

Both radiopaque and radiotransparent calculi are observed ultrasonographically as hyperechoic foci with acoustic shadowing in the dependent area of the bladder (Fig. 30). The size and shape of calculi are variable, and there may be one or more present.

In cats, urinary calculi are usually more flattened and, sometimes, sediment can be observed on the dependent side of the bladder that also causes acoustic shadowing. The characteristics of the acoustic shadow produced by calculi depend on the size of the calculi and the frequency of the transducer; studies have found that they do not depend on the composition of the calculi (Widmer et al., 2020).

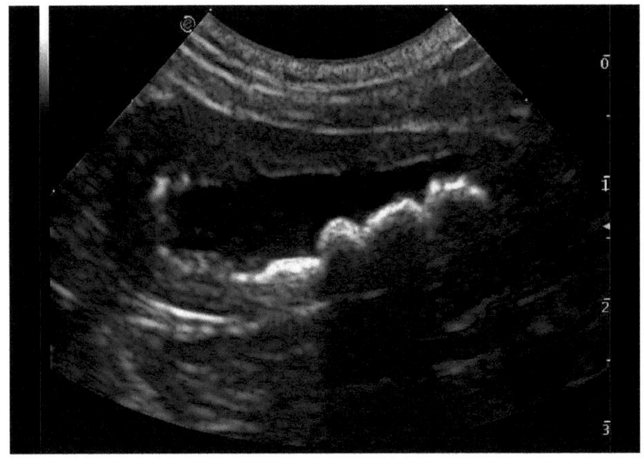

Figure 30. Bladder calculi. Ultrasound image of the urinary bladder in a longitudinal plane. Several hyperechoic foci with acoustic shadowing are visualised in the dependent area of the bladder.

The descending colon can overlap the interior of the bladder on ultrasound images, causing a distortion of its contour or the appearance of a mural mass, or mineralised fragments in the colon can produce acoustic shadowing and cause them to be mistaken for bladder calculi. There are several ways to distinguish calculi from an artefact associated with the colon; the easiest is to shake the transducer to move the structures inside the bladder and then stay still and assess whether the position of the calculus has changed. Another technique is to examine the animal in a standing position; in this case the colon remains dorsal whereas calculi in the bladder move ventrally due to gravity.

Blood Clots

Clots can occur due to trauma, coagulation disorders, neoplasms or cystitis. Immature clots are observed with heterogeneous shape and echogenicity; as they mature and become organised they appear more homogeneous and hyperechoic, without acoustic shadowing. They may adhere to the bladder wall, and in these cases it can be difficult to differentiate between a clot, a polyp or a mural mass (Fig. 26). On these occasions, the absence of colour Doppler flow signal can help to differentiate a clot from a neoplastic mass (Widmer et al., 2020).

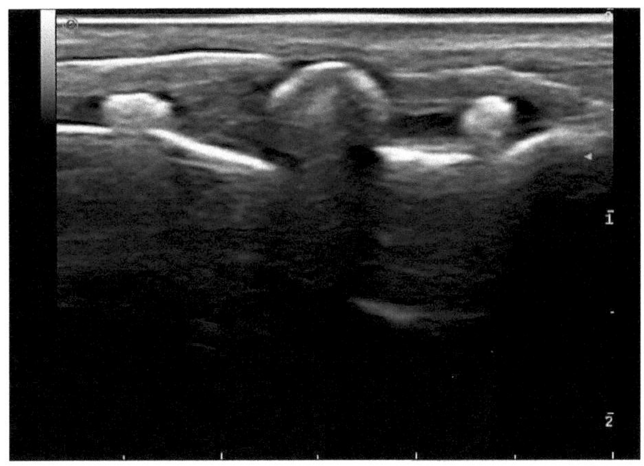

Figure 31. Calculi in the penile urethra. Ultrasound image of the penile urethra in a longitudinal plane of a dog with urinary obstruction. Three hyperechoic calculi with acoustic shadowing are observed.

Bladder Rupture

Positive retrograde cystourethrography is the technique of choice for diagnosing bladder rupture. However, ultrasonography is useful because free fluid in the abdomen can be observed with a varied echogenicity that is dependent on the cellularity of the urine. The area of the bladder wall that is ruptured will be thickened and hypoechoic, and the bladder will be partially distended.

Bladder rupture should be differentiated from refraction artefact associated with the cranial part of the bladder when there is free fluid present. In this case, the apparent defect is in the cranial area of the bladder, there is no thickening of the wall and the bladder is distended (Widmer et al., 2020).

Congenital Abnormalities

Congenital abnormalities of the urinary bladder are uncommon. They include urachal diverticulum, persistent urachus and urachal cysts (Sutherland-Smith and Penninck, 2015). Vesiculourachal diverticulum is visualised as a sac-like structure containing anechoic content in the cranioventral area of the bladder, to which it is attached.

Urethral Abnormalities

Dilated Urethra

The urethra may be dilated due to obstruction by a calculus or mass.

Calculi

Both radiopaque and radiotransparent calculi are observed ultrasonographically as hyperechoic foci with acoustic shadowing (Fig. 31). They are frequently located in the penile urethra (Sutherland-Smith and Penninck, 2015).

Female Reproductive System

In the dog, the use of ultrasonography to image the female reproductive system was initially limited to pregnancy diagnosis. However, it is now widely used to monitor foetal development, for pregnancy synchronisation, to predict the date of parturition, and in the diagnosis and monitoring of diseases of the reproductive tract.

For evaluation of the ovaries and uterus in dogs, a 7.5 MHz probe is recommended, whereas a 10 MHz transducer should be used for cats. However, a 5 MHz transducer may be used for the diagnosis of gestational age, pyometra and ovarian tumours.

Ovaries

Technique and Normal Appearance

The ovaries should be examined with the animal in dorsal or lateral recumbency, similar to the position used to evaluate the kidneys, obtaining two sections, one longitudinal and one transverse.

The caudal pole of the kidney and the adjacent area are examined in sagittal and transverse planes to locate the ovary (Fig. 32). The ovary may be in contact with the caudal pole of the kidney or up to 2 cm caudal, caudolateral, caudomedial or ventral to the caudal pole. The ovaries are hypoechoic, very small and difficult to locate because they are often surrounded by adipose tissue and there is gas interference.

The appearance of the ovary varies throughout the oestrous cycle. During anoestrus, the ovaries are not easy to find. They are small and of heterogeneous echogenicity. In pro-oestrus, the shape of the ovaries makes them easier to visualise and they are often located more caudoventral to the kidneys. They contain several small, anechoic follicles approximately 1 mm in size. At the end of pro-oestrus, during the preovulatory period, the size of the ovaries increases due to the large amount of fluid in the follicles, which makes them easier to visualise. Several or all of the anechoic follicles in the ovary are usually replaced by hypoechoic or echogenic structures at the time of ovulation, which tend to disappear (Fig. 33) (Pollard and Hecht, 2015; Mattoon et al., 2020).

Abnormalities

Ovarian Cysts

Cysts of the ovarian pouch are more common than those of the ovary itself; at the endocrine level these cysts are inactive and are of no clinical importance. A true ovarian cyst originates in the ovarian stroma or follicles. The ultrasonographic appearance is characterised by anechoic content with thin walls and posterior reinforcement (Fig. 34). They vary in size from small to large.

Ultrasonography cannot be used to differentiate between the different types of cysts, although follicular cysts may be associated with persistent or prolonged oestrus, whereas luteal cysts are more commonly found in older dogs and may be associated with persistent bleeding. They are generally associated with pathologies such as pyometra, cystic endometrial hyperplasia and hydrometra (Mattoon et al., 2020).

Ovarian Granuloma

Ovarian granulomas are seen as complex masses in the ovarian region and are associated with previous ovariohysterectomy. They can vary in size, shape, echotexture and echogenicity.

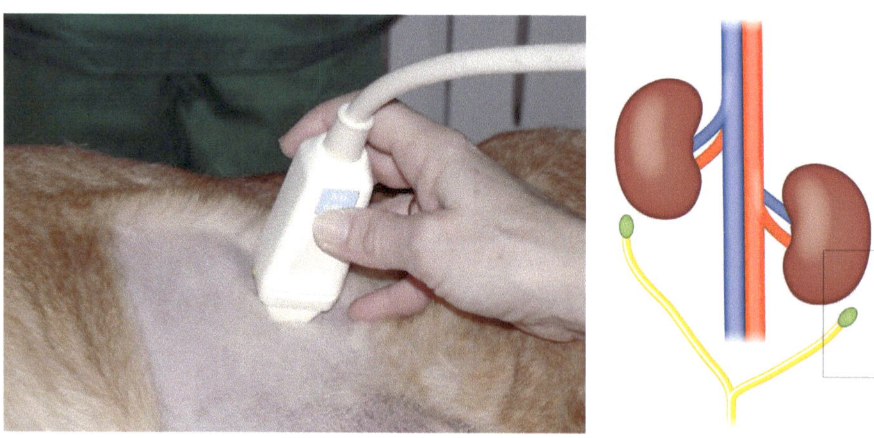

Figure 32. Diagram of the location of the ovaries relative to the kidneys, and positioning of the transducer for examination.

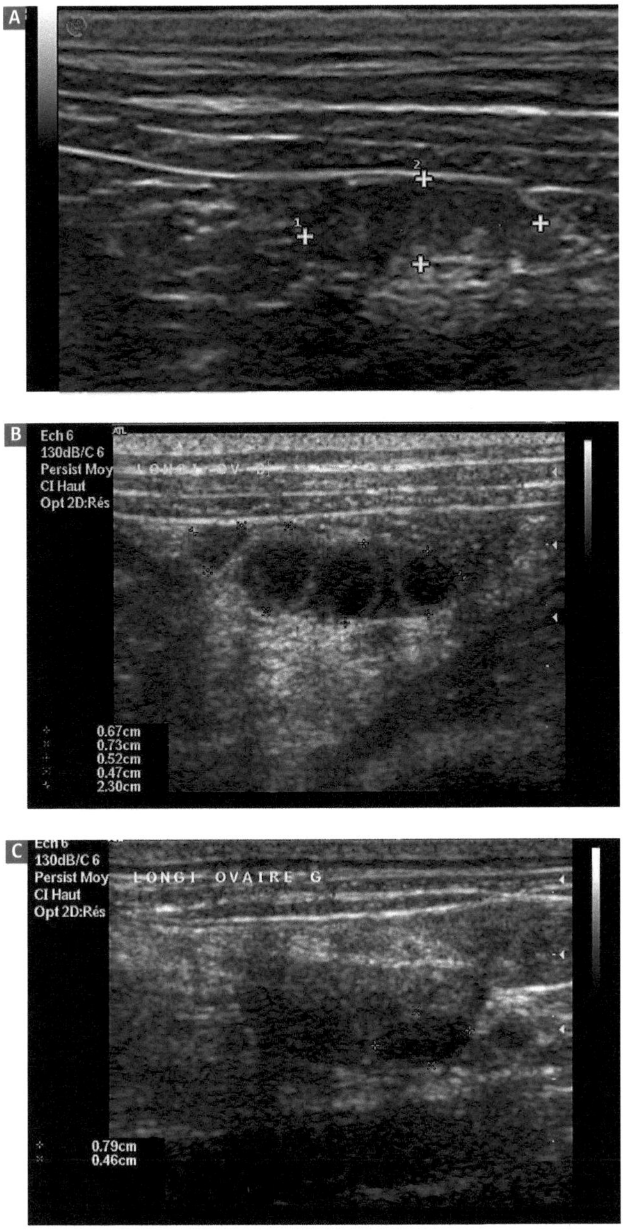

Figure 33. Appearance of the ovaries at different times of the oestrous cycle. **A**. Anoestrus. **B**. Pro-oestrus. **C**. Ovulation. Images B and C provided by Prof. Alain Fontbone.

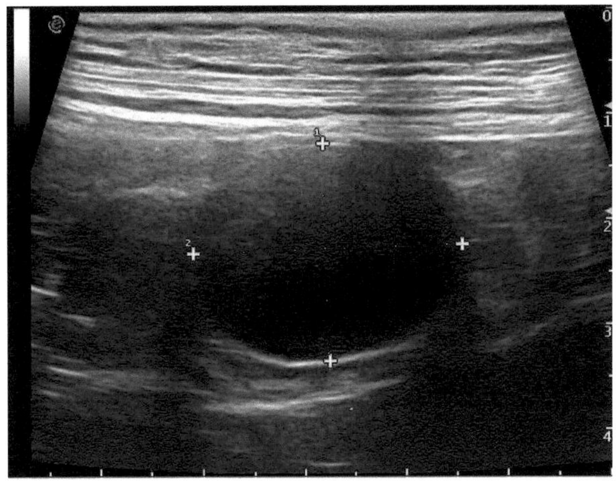

Figure 34. Ultrasonographic appearance of an ovarian cyst. Anechoic content is visualised, with thin walls and posterior enhancement.

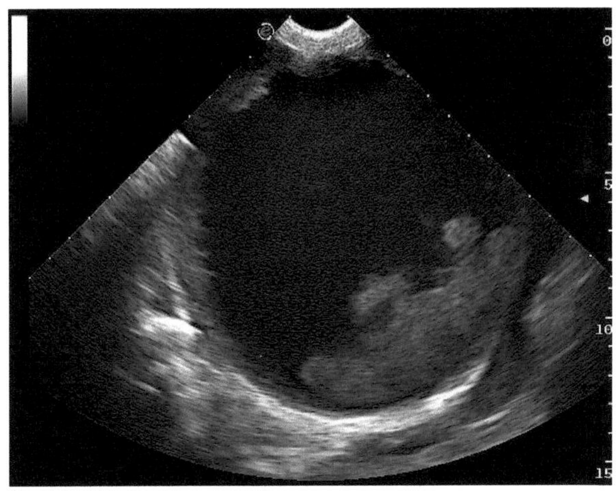

Figure 35. Ovarian carcinoma. A cystic structure with hypoechoic and echogenic content is observed.

Ovarian Neoplasia

Ovarian neoplasms are uncommon in the dog (Fig. 35). The most common are **granulosa cell tumours**, which can be large and cystic, and can sometimes be difficult to distinguish from ovarian cysts. However, sometimes there may be ascitic fluid present with neoplasms.

Ovarian tumours are usually large and characterised by hyperechoic fibrous tissue, heterogeneous neoplastic tissue and anechoic cystic regions. Unilateral tumours are more common, although bilateral adenocarcinomas have also been described (Pollard and Hecht, 2015).

Uterus

Technique and Normal Appearance

The animal can be placed in any position, either dorsal or lateral recumbency or standing. The urinary bladder must be full to serve as an acoustic window for evaluation of the uterine body (Fig. 36).

The neck of the uterus and the uterine body are located on the dorsal aspect of the caudal part of the bladder. They can be observed as a rectangular, solid, homogeneous and relatively hypoechoic structure in the longitudinal plane, and as a rounded structure in the transverse plane (Fig. 37). Moving cranially to the uterine body, it is possible to observe the bifurcation of the uterine horns. These have the same appearance as the uterine body but are smaller.

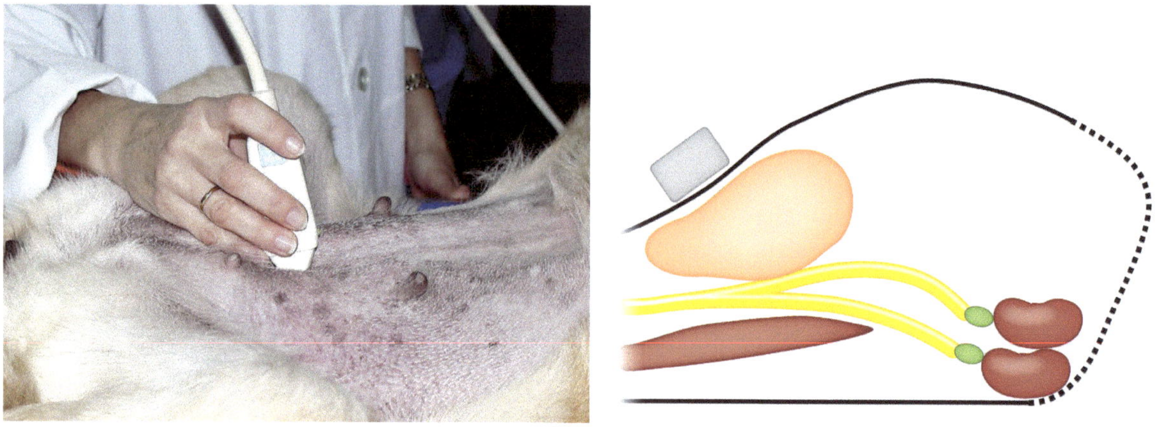

Figure 36. Diagram of the location of the uterus and positioning of the transducer for examination.

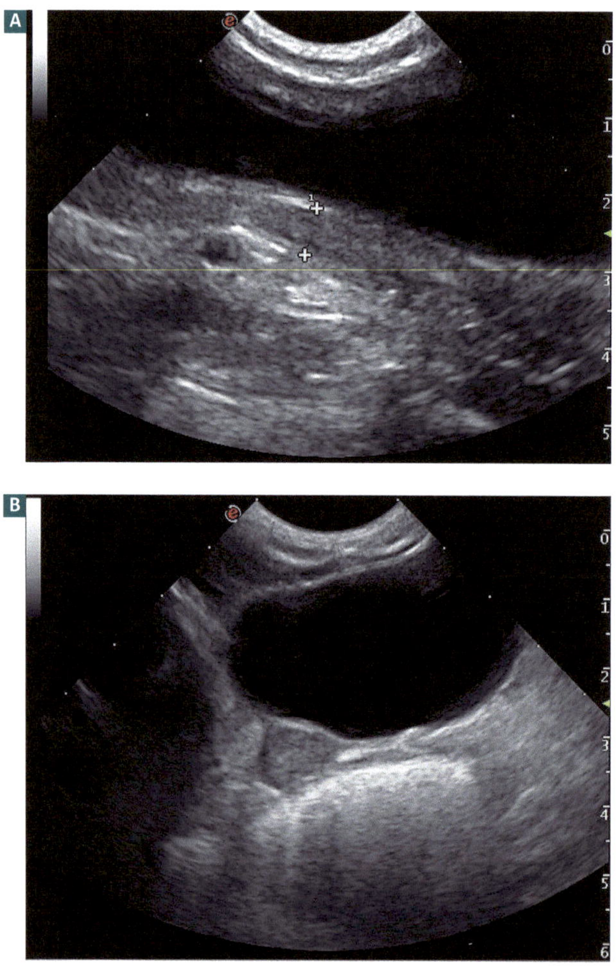

Figure 37. Ultrasonographic appearance of the uterus. **A.** Longitudinal plane: the uterus is visualised as a rectangular, solid, homogeneous and relatively hypoechoic structure. **B.** Transverse plane: the uterus is observed as a hypoechoic rounded structure.

In normal situations it is difficult to differentiate the layers of the uterine wall and the lumen. In dogs, during anoestrus, the uterine body is usually between 5 mm and 8 mm in diameter, but may be smaller in prepubertal animals and young adults. The uterus increases in size during oestrus compared with the other phases of the cycle (Pollard and Hecht, 2015).

Abnormalities

Cystic Endometrial Hyperplasia

Cystic endometrial hyperplasia is a common condition in middle-aged breeding bitches and can cause mucometra and pyometra.

Ultrasonographically, the uterine wall is thickened and small cysts of 1–4 mm can be identified inside the endometrium. In some cases there is also a small amount of fluid in the uterine lumen (Fig. 38).

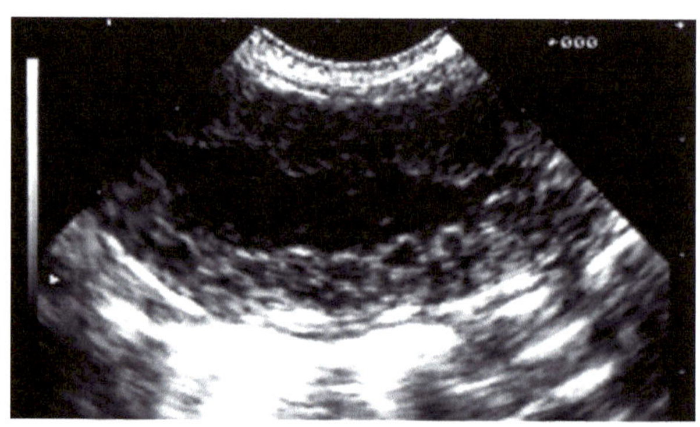

Figure 38. Cystic endometrial hyperplasia in a dog. The uterine wall is thickened and small cysts are seen inside the endometrium, as well as a small amount of fluid in the uterine lumen.

Mucometra, Hydrometra, Haemometra and Pyometra

All these terms refer to an accumulation of fluid with different characteristics inside the uterus (Fig. 39).

The term mucometra refers to when the uterus is distended with a considerable amount of fluid of a mucoid nature, whereas pyometra refers to the presence of pus in the uterus as a result of inflammation and bacterial infection. In most cases, these pathologies are suspected based on the clinical signs and the systemic repercussions that are present. In the case of pyometra, it is usually observed in elderly animals and is usually preceded by cystic endometrial hyperplasia.

The ultrasonographic appearance of these pathologies is an increase in the size of the uterus characterised by an accumulation of fluid. In the case of mucometra and hydrometra, the fluid content is anechoic, whereas in haemometra and pyometra it is more echogenic. The uterine walls may be smooth and thin, or thickened and irregular. Endometrial polyps are commonly observed. The walls are thinner when distension of the uterus is greater. In most cases, both horns are affected (Ortega-Pacheco et al., 2012).

Ultrasonographically, it can sometimes be difficult to differentiate between these changes, and this should be done based on the clinical signs.

Pyometra and Granuloma of the Uterine Stump

Stump pyometra may occur following the surgical removal of a uterus affected by pyometra. The appearance is similar to that of pyometra but located at the entrance to the pelvis.

In the case of uterine stump granuloma, the echogenicity is mixed, with hypoechoic areas due to pus accumulation and hyperechoic areas representing fibrous tissue (Pollard and Hecht, 2015).

Uterine Neoplasia

Neoplasms of the uterus (leiomyomas, leiomyosarcomas or adenocarcinomas) are uncommon. On ultrasonography, they present as mass-like lesions of different shapes and sizes attached to the wall of the uterus, projecting into the lumen; they can be echogenic or of mixed echogenicity if there is necrotic tissue or fibrosis present. They can produce an accumulation of fluid in the uterine lumen (Ortega-Pacheco et al., 2012).

Vaginal masses, when large, can extend through the pelvic canal into the abdomen.

Pregnancy Diagnosis

Ultrasonography is widely accepted as a routine method for the assessment of gestation in many species, as it allows the confirmation of pregnancy, assessment of embryonic viability and detection of abnormalities.

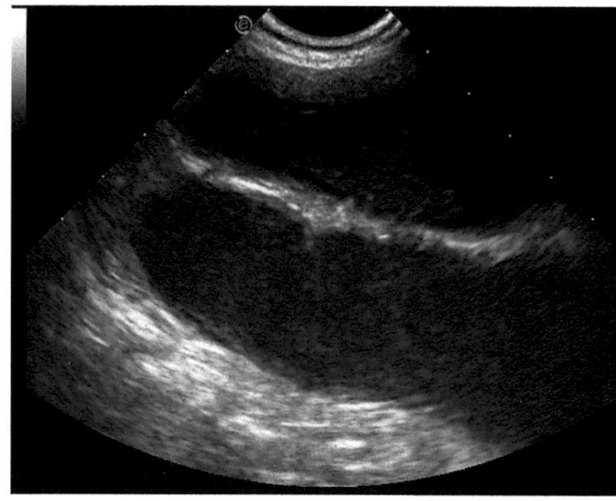

Figure 39. Pyometra. Ultrasound image of the uterine horns, which appear distended with hypoechoic content and have thin walls.

When considering the characteristics that can be detected by ultrasound for pregnancy diagnosis, it is important to remember that gestation does not necessarily begin on the day of mating in the bitch, and that events should be related to the day of the preovulatory surge in luteinising hormone (LH) or to the time of ovulation, which occurs 2 days after the LH surge. This is especially true in the case of the bitch, where a pregnancy can occur from the moment mounting occurs, and up to 5 days before ovulation (canine sperm has the ability to remain fertile in the bitch's tract for up to 6 or 7 days before fertilisation occurs). The day of the LH surge is considered day 0 of the cycle or of gestation. If ultrasound examinations are scheduled in relation to the time of mating rather than the time of ovulation, erroneous results may be obtained. Parturition usually occurs between 64 and 66 days after the LH surge.

In some bitches, pregnancy can be diagnosed at 17–18 days after ovulation and 18–19 days after the LH peak, meaning that it is accurate (in terms of obtaining a reliable diagnosis) to perform an ultrasound examination around day 20. First, an increase in the size of the uterus (on day 7 in the dog, day 4 in the cat) is detected, which is not specific to gestation but to hormonal changes. The first ultrasonographic sign for pregnancy confirmation is the detection of the embryonic sacs. On day 20 in the dog and day 11 in the cat, the embryonic sacs are observed as anechoic, rounded structures containing small, echogenic, comma-shaped embryos (Fig. 40). Although it is advisable to wait until day 30 for pregnancy diagnosis to have a high level of confidence in the diagnosis, between days 22 and 29 some embryonic cardiac activity is evident.

Ultrasonography is an accurate method for the diagnosis of pregnancy. There have been several recent studies in which ultrasonography was used to evaluate foetal development in relation to gestational age (Table 2). Based on these studies, the diameter of the embryonic sac is the most effective parameter to demonstrate gestational age of between 20 days and 37 days in the dog. Foetal head diameter followed by body diameter were the most effective parameters between days 38 and 60 (Fig. 41). The formulas to predict gestational age and the time to parturition in general are shown in Table 2, although there are specific formulas for certain breeds (Pollard and Hecht, 2015):

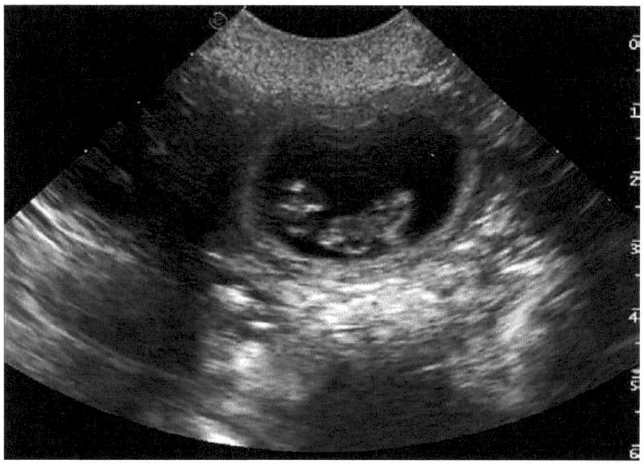

Figure 40. Ultrasonographic appearance of an embryonic sac. These are visualised as anechoic, rounded structures containing small echogenic embryos.

Table 2. Formulas for the estimation of gestational age (GA). (Table modified from Matton JS, Davidson A, Sellon RK, 2020).

GA	Less than 40 days	More than 40 days	Days before parturition
Dog	GA = (6 × ES) + 20	GA = (15 × HD) + 20 GA = (7 × BD) + 29	65 – GA
Cat		GA = (25 × HD) + 3 GA = (11 × BD) + 21	61 – GA

ES: embryonic sac diameter; HD: head diameter; BD: body diameter.

Estimation of the Number of Foetuses

Ultrasonography is not a reliable method for determining the number of foetuses. The most reliable estimate can be made before 30 days. Between 30 days and 50 days, estimates can be made with 18% certainty, and after 50 days with 8% certainty. Foetal resorption may be one of the causes of the disparity between the number of embryonic sacs observed and the number born in the litter.

Foetal Monitoring

Ultrasonography can be used to detect gestational abnormalities such as foetal resorption, abortion, foetal abnormalities, foetal stress and foetal death.

Comparison of one foetus with another may allow the identification of foetal abnormalities such as hydrocephalus or anasarca, among others.

Embryo Resorption and Abortion

If death of the foetus occurs before 25 days, a complete resorption of the embryo will happen, and if it occurs after 35 days, abortion will occur.

The ultrasonographic appearance of embryonic resorption is generally a decrease in the volume of the embryonic sac, an increase in the echogenicity of the fluid and an absence

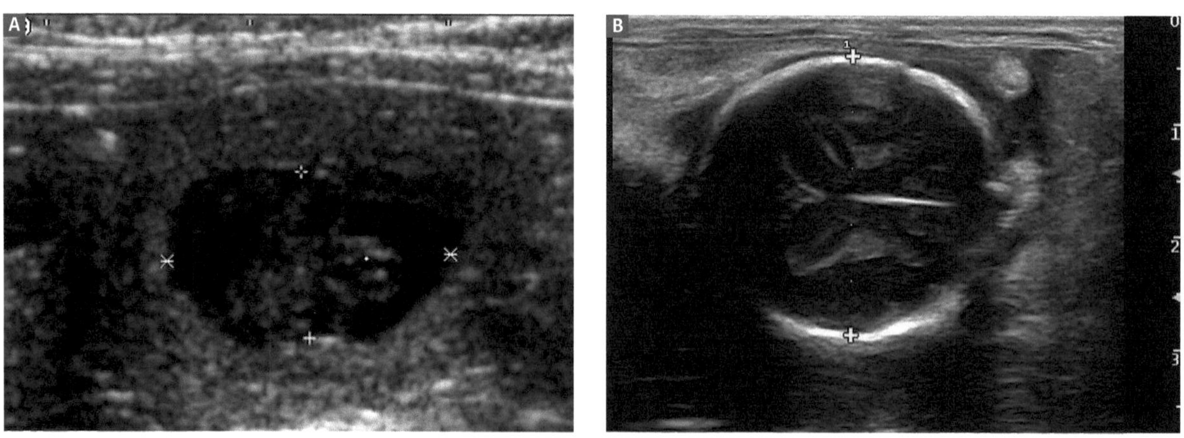

Figure 41. Method for taking measurements of embryonic sac diameter (**A**) and biparietal (foetal head) diameter (**B**).

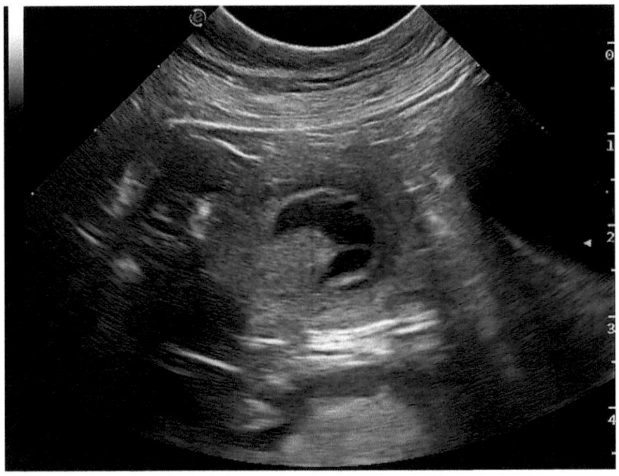

Figure 42. Embryonic resorption. A decrease in the volume of the embryonic sac, an increase in the echogenicity of the embryonic fluid and an absence of cardiac activity are seen.

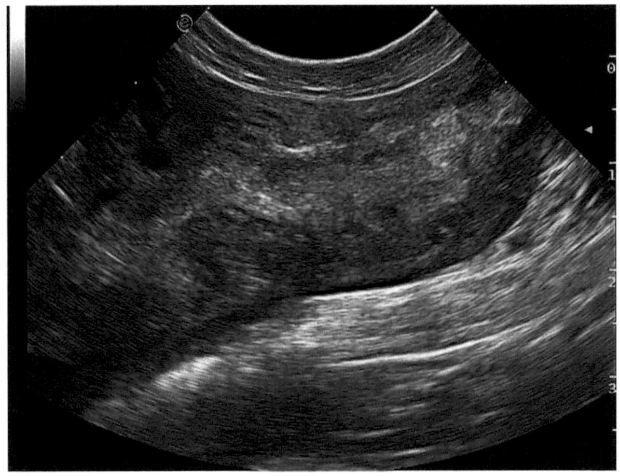

Figure 43. Postpartum uterus. The uterus is seen to be enlarged and has echogenic content.

of embryonic cardiac activity (Fig. 42). In addition, within 24 hours of embryonic death there is disintegration of the embryonic structures and collapse of the sac. The uterus is slightly enlarged in the area affected and the uterine wall is slightly more echogenic (Pollard and Hecht, 2015).

Foetal Stress

Foetal stress is recognised a by decreased heart rate (which indicates hypoxia); the foetal heart rate should be twice the mother's heart rate. Normal foetal heart rate should be >220 bpm (beats per minute). Foetal stress is considered to be present when the heart rate is below 180 bpm on days 58–62 of gestation. In most cases, bowel movements are also observed in all foetuses with a heart rate below 180 bpm (Mattoon et al., 2020).

Foetal Death

Signs of foetal death that can be detected by ultrasound are the absence of the foetal heartbeat, lack of foetal movement, reduced volume and increased echogenicity of foetal fluid, and the accumulation of gas within the foetal stomach, other foetal cavities or the uterus.

Postpartum Uterus

Involution of the uterus postpartum can be examined ultrasonographically. From days 1 to 4, the uterus is enlarged (2–3 cm in diameter at the sites of placentation and 1–1.5 cm between them), and its contents are of mixed echogenicity (Fig. 43). Unresorbed material and fluid can still be seen several weeks after birth.

In the first week postpartum, the uterine horns are visualised as multiple layers of different echogenicity and present enlarged areas at placental sites. Large variations in uterine diameter are observed between placental sites and interplacental areas. The uterus may return to a normal size when in anoestrus at 4–6 weeks postpartum; however, uterine involution is not complete ultrasonographically until 15 weeks postpartum (Mattoon et al., 2020).

Postpartum Disorders

The presence of retained foetuses may be suspected clinically due to the behaviour of the mother and a persistent vaginal discharge. Retained foetuses can be easily diagnosed with ultrasonography by visualising the presence of echogenic foetal skeletons. Foetal viability can be assessed as discussed above.

Retention of the placenta is rare and is diagnosed based on a persistent green discharge and signs of discomfort. The diagnosis of placental retention can be made ultrasonographically, but diagnosis can be complicated as soft tissue debris or blood clots may often persist within the uterus after parturition and may be indistinguishable from placental tissue debris.

Male Reproductive System

Ultrasonography is the technique of choice for evaluation of the prostate, as it allows the size of the gland to be measured and assessments to be made of the characteristics of the parenchyma.

Prostate

Technique and Normal Appearance

Transducers with a frequency of 7.5 MHz and 10 MHz are most suitable for the examination of the prostate. The animal is placed in dorsal recumbency to perform a transabdominal examination, and the transducer is placed on one side of the prepuce and just cranial to the pelvic edge, to obtain longitudinal and transverse sections (Fig. 44). It is recommended that the urinary bladder be full to displace the intestines and prostate cranially; if it is empty, it can be filled with warm physiological saline. A transrectal examination can also be performed, but this requires a special probe and only longitudinal sections can be obtained (Hecht and Pollard, 2015). The prostate is an ovoid, bilobed gland located at the neck of the bladder, surrounding the proximal urethra (Fig. 44). The prostate is located within or immediately cranial to the pelvic canal and is limited dorsally by the rectum. In entire dogs, the prostate presents a moderate, homogeneous echogenicity, with a fine to medium-coarse echotexture. In the longitudinal plane it has an oval shape, and a central hypoechoic line is observed that corresponds to the prostatic urethra. In the transverse plane, it has a more rounded shape; the two lobes can be identified and a there is a hyperechoic central band present due to the periurethral fibrous tissue, and a hypoechoic central duct that corresponds to the prostatic urethra (Fig. 44) (Hecht and Pollard, 2015; Mattoon and Davidson, 2020).

The size of the prostate varies with the size and age of the animal. It is assessed by measuring the maximum total diameter of the prostate on images in the transverse plane or by calculating the **prostate volume** using the ellipse volume formula:

$$\textbf{Volume} = \textbf{length} \times \textbf{width} \times \textbf{height} \times \textbf{0.523}$$

The length measurement is obtained in the longitudinal plane (Fig. 45) (Mattoon and Davidson, 2020).

In normal castrated dogs, the prostate appears smaller than in the entire dog. After castration, the prostatic parenchyma becomes more hypoechoic. The combination of reduced size and decreased echogenicity often makes it difficult to distinguish the margins of the gland from periprostatic fat (Fig. 46) (Hecht and Pollard, 2015).

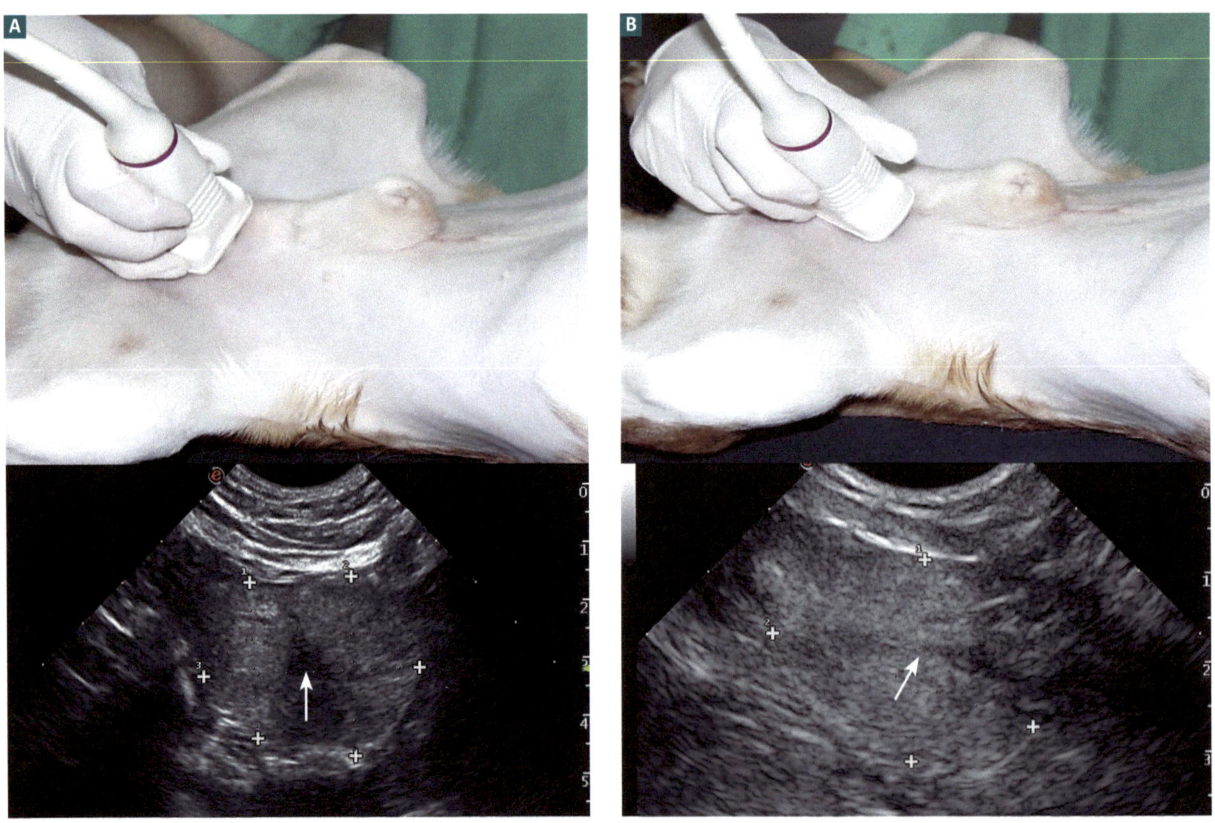

Figure 44. Positioning of the transducer for examination of the prostate in the transverse (**A**) and longitudinal (**B**) planes. The lower images show the corresponding ultrasonographic appearance of the prostate. A central hypoechoic line corresponding to the prostatic urethra (arrow) is observed.

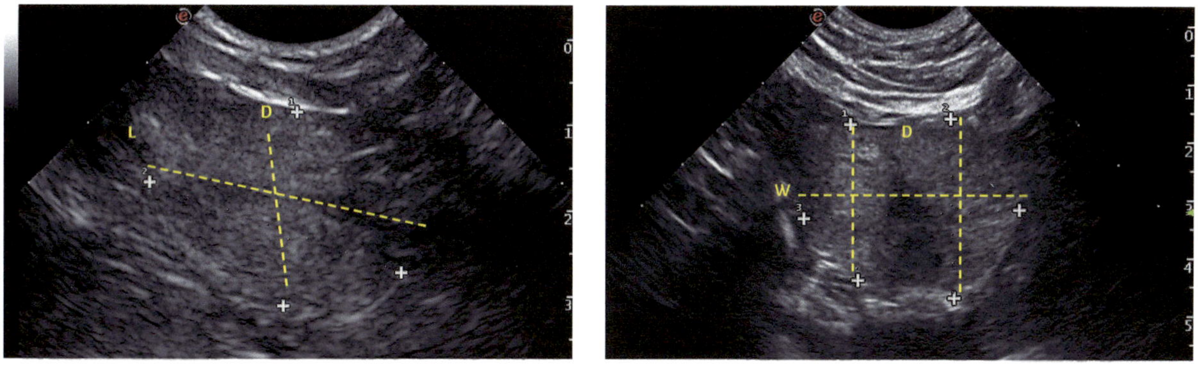

Figure 45. Method for obtaining measurements of prostate size.
L: length; W: width; D: depth.

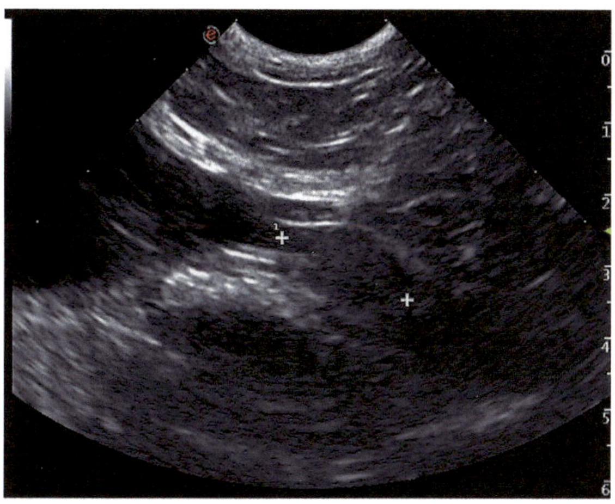

Figure 46. Prostate of a castrated dog. The prostatic parenchyma is more hypoechoic and the prostate is smaller in size than in an entire dog.

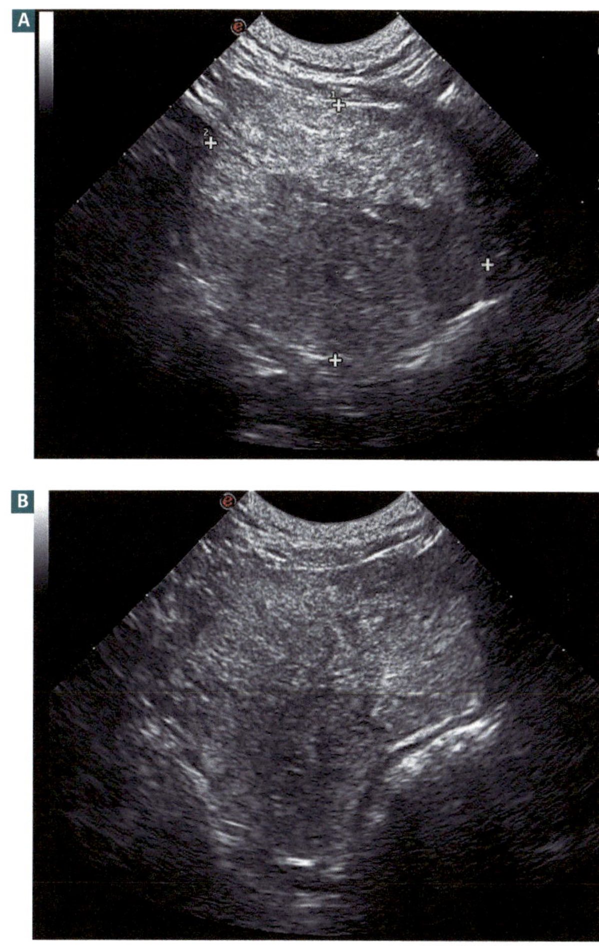

Figure 47. Benign prostatic hyperplasia. Longitudinal (**A**) and transverse (**B**) sections of the prostate. It is observed increased in size and the parenchyma is slightly hyperechoic and heterogeneous.

Abnormalities

Benign Prostatic Hyperplasia

At the onset of benign prostatic hyperplasia (BPH), there is usually a symmetrical enlargement of the prostate and a diffuse increase in its echogenicity, sometimes producing a heterogeneous echotexture. In many cases there are small cysts 1–2 mm in diameter. Usually, the normal contour of the prostate is maintained. However, if enlargement is significant, the prostate may lose its typical bilobed appearance (Fig. 47). There is generally no capsule disruption or enlargement of the medial iliac lymph nodes (Mattoon and Davidson, 2020).

Prostatitis

Prostatitis can be caused by ascending urinary tract infections or by septicaemia.

In cases of acute prostatitis, the prostate may be enlarged and may have either a symmetrical or an asymmetrical contour. The parenchyma is usually heterogeneous and has a hypoechoic appearance; in the most chronic cases, echogenicity increases in a patchy pattern (Fig. 48).

In chronic cases that do not resolve, patchy hypoechoic areas may appear, forming microabscesses with hypoechoic content and more irregular margins than the cysts observed in BPH.

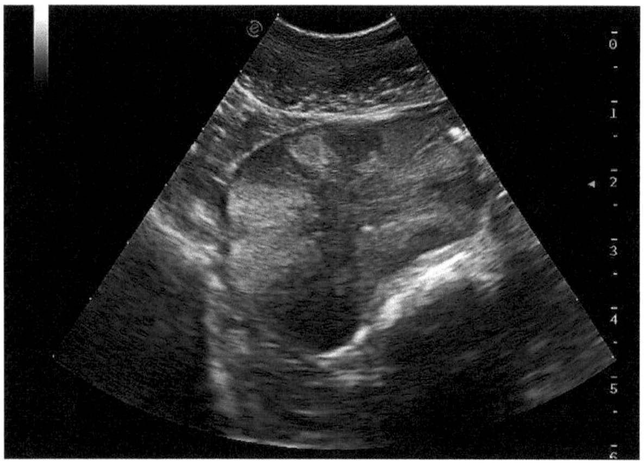

Figure 48. Chronic prostatitis. Ultrasound image of the prostate in the transverse plane. A heterogeneous echotexture with mixed echogenicity is observed.

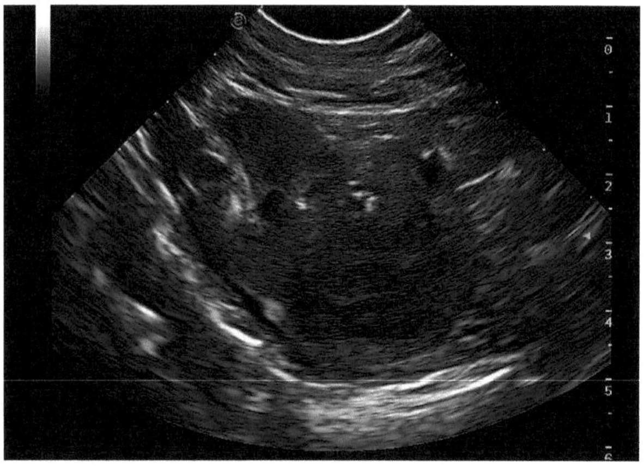

Figure 49. Prostatic neoplasm. Ultrasound image of the prostate in the longitudinal plane. The prostate has irregular margins, and a heterogeneous echotexture is visualised with hypoechoic irregular areas and zones of mineralisation. Ultrasound-guided fine needle aspiration resulted in a diagnosis of carcinoma.

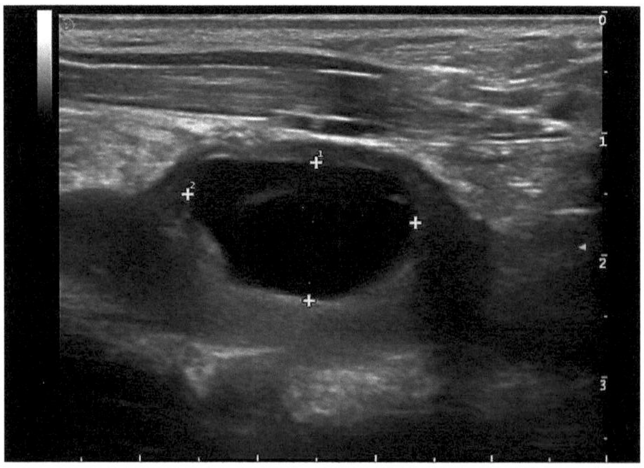

Figure 50. Intraprostatic cyst. Ultrasound image of the prostate in the longitudinal plane. A cystic structure is observed in the ventral area of the prostate, well defined by anechoic content that produces posterior enhancement.

The abscess cavities may increase in size and become calcified. There may also be perilesional peritoneal effusion and an increase in size of the medial iliac lymph nodes.

Ultrasonographically, sometimes prostatitis cannot be differentiated from a neoplasm and the two pathologies can even occur together; therefore, a biopsy or fine-needle aspiration of several areas of the prostate is necessary to reach a diagnosis (Hecht and Pollard, 2015).

Neoplasia

It is currently believed that prostatic neoplasms occur more often in castrated dogs than in entire dogs, although they can occur in both.

Prostatic neoplasia has a variable ultrasonographic appearance in both entire and castrated dogs. Adenocarcinomas and undifferentiated carcinomas are the most common neoplasms. At first, prostatic neoplasms usually appear as focal hypoechoic lesions and can be difficult to differentiate from other pathologies, including the patchy appearance seen in cases of BPH. In later phases, parenchymal changes are usually diffuse, the prostate is not symmetrical, and its margins become irregular. A markedly hyperechoic, heterogeneous parenchyma is generally visualised, with irregular anechoic areas and zones of calcification producing acoustic shadowing (Fig. 49). The neoplasm is locally aggressive and may extend into the urethra, bladder neck and medial iliac lymph nodes.

Metastases most commonly develop in the liver and spleen, as well as the lung, bones and lumbar spine (Mattoon and Davidson, 2020).

Intraprostatic Cysts

Cysts may be seen associated with BPH, prostatitis and neoplasia. Sometimes they are incidental findings without any associated clinical signs.

True cysts are characterised by anechoic content surrounded by a thin hyperechoic wall with posterior enhancement (Fig. 50). Prostatic cysts vary in size and number. Those that are less than 1 cm in diameter are considered to be normal accumulations of prostatic secretions; those that are larger and have irregular margins are considered abnormal and may correspond to intraprostatic cysts, haematomas, abscesses or neoplasms. Fine-needle aspiration is necessary to reach a definitive diagnosis (Hecht and Pollard, 2015).

Paraprostatic Cysts

Paraprostatic cysts are uncommon. They originate from the remains of the Müllerian ducts or as extensions of a prostatic lobe. They may be attached to the prostate by a thin base, or there may be broad fibrous adhesions. They can also communicate directly with the prostate gland and urethra. They can become very large and occupy virtually the entire abdomen.

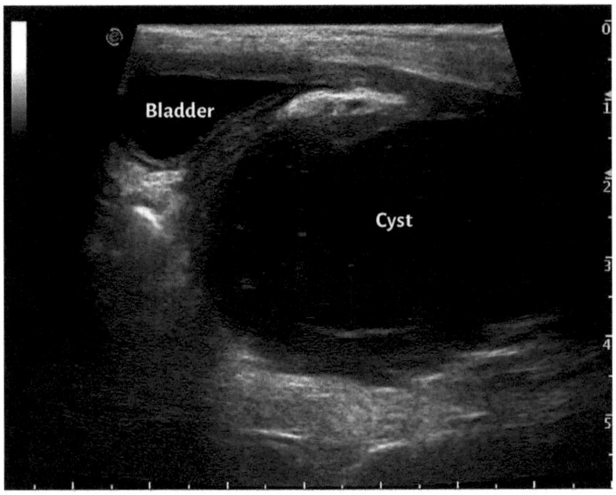

Figure 51. Paraprostatic cyst. Ultrasound image in the longitudinal plane. The urinary bladder and a dorsal cystic structure can be seen, with anechoic content and echoes inside that communicate with the prostate.

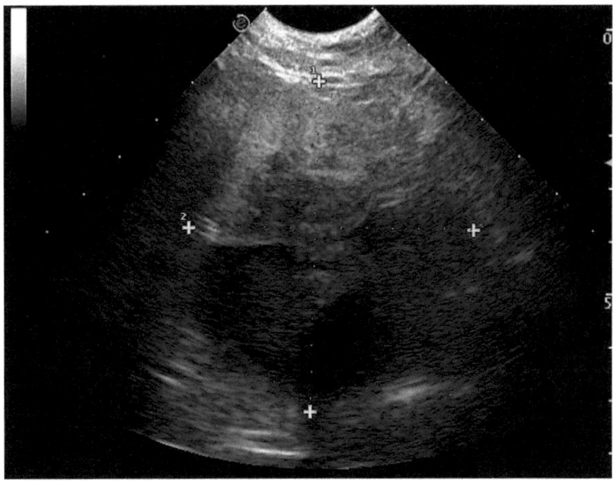

Figure 52. Prostatic abscess. Ultrasound image of the prostate in the transverse plane. A hypoechoic area with irregular edges is visualised in the dorsal and central region of the prostate.

Ultrasonographically, they are observed as anechoic cystic structures with walls that are thin and regular or thick and irregular. The anechoic content may have echogenic material inside, and sometimes internal septa are visualised (Fig. 51) (Hecht and Pollard, 2015).

Prostatic Abscesses

Abscesses present as large cystic areas with irregular margins and echoes inside (Fig. 52). It is difficult to differentiate an abscess from an intraprostatic cyst by ultrasonography, so fine-needle aspiration is necessary to reach a definitive diagnosis (Mattoon and Davidson, 2020).

Testes

Technique and Normal Appearance

Ultrasonographic examination of the testes is easy due to the anatomy of the dog's scrotum and the absence of hair in the area. High-resolution (7.5–10 MHz) or 5 MHz transducers with a standoff or pad can be used. In addition, in cases when both testes are intrascrotal, one testis can serve as an acoustic window to examine the one below it. The examination can be performed in the transverse, longitudinal and dorsal planes (Hecht and Pollard, 2015).

The two testes are the same size and oval in shape, and have a coarse, homogeneous echogenicity. There is a hyperechoic central band representing the mediastinum testis (a fibrous extension of the tunica albuginea). Each testis is bound by a hyperechoic capsule (the parietal and visceral tunics). The epididymis is composed of the head, body and tail. The head is found cranially, and the body is located dorsolateral to the testis, and is hypoechoic with respect to it (Fig. 53) (Hecht and Pollard, 2015; Mattoon and Davidson, 2020).

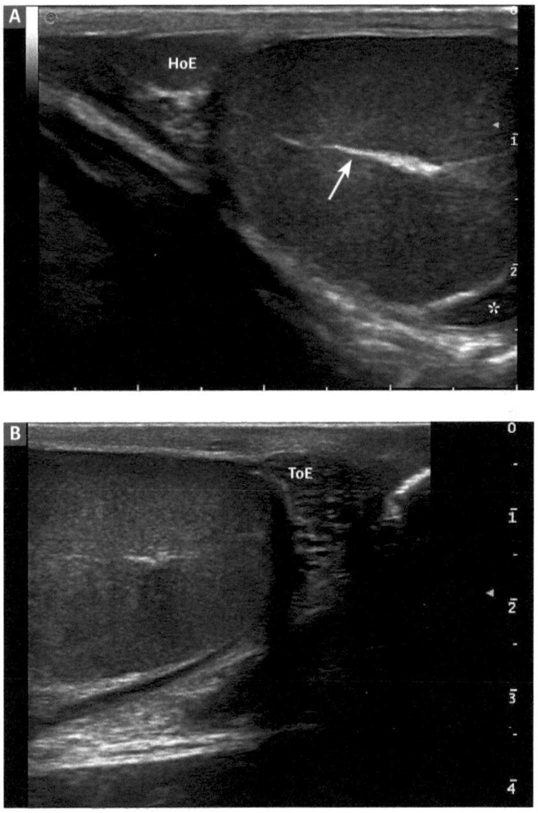

Figure 53. Ultrasonographic appearance of a normal testis in a longitudinal plane. Cranial (A) and caudal (B) areas. **A.** A hyperechoic central band (arrow) is observed representing the mediastinum testis; the head of the epididymis (HoE) in the cranial area and the body of the epididymis (*) are also observed. **B.** The tail of the epididymis (ToE) is observed in the caudal area.

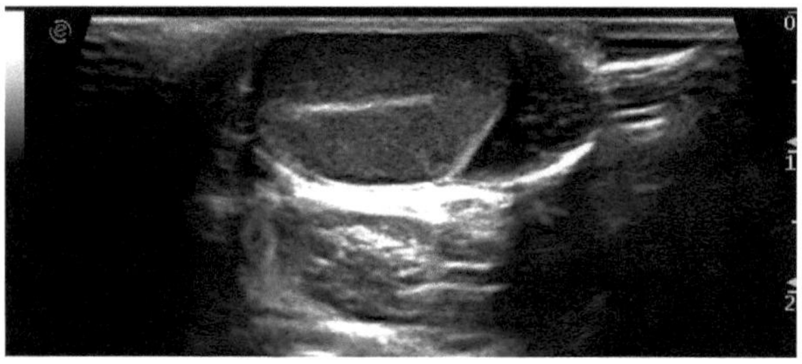

Figure 54. Intra-abdominal testis. Longitudinal plane of an undescended testis, which presents the same appearance as a normal descended testis but is smaller and hypoechoic.

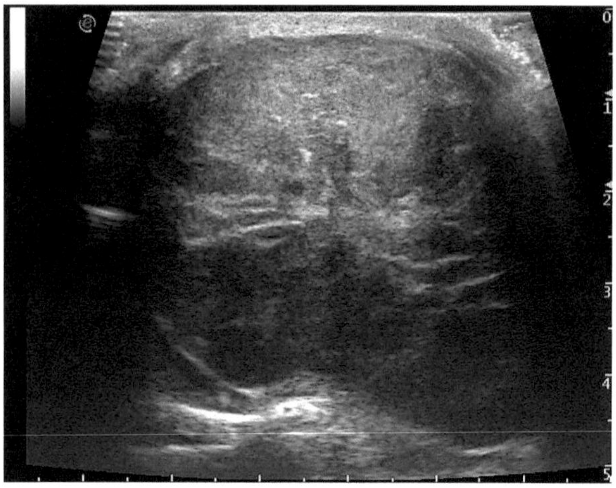

Figure 55. Testicular neoplasm: seminoma. Longitudinal image of the left testis of a 9-year-old German Shepherd Dog. The testis is enlarged and is observed to have heterogeneous parenchyma with a mixed echogenicity.

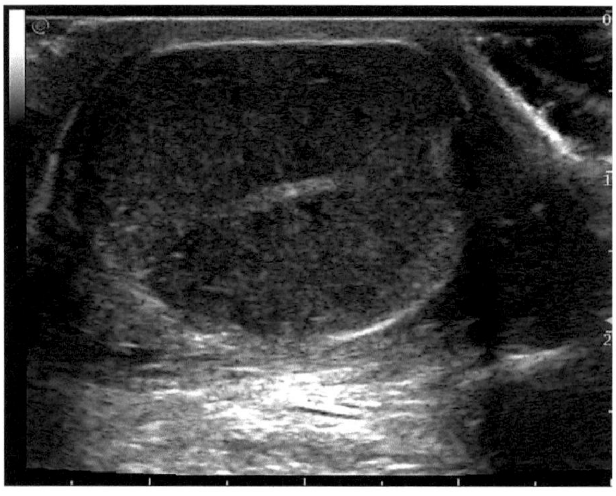

Figure 56. Orchitis. Longitudinal image of the right testis. It is larger than normal in size and hypoechoic but maintains the normal testicular structure.

Testicular volume can be accurately calculated by using the formula:

$$\textbf{Volume} = \textbf{length} \times \textbf{width} \times \textbf{height} \times \textbf{0.5236}$$

A positive association between testicular volume and body weight has been demonstrated in dogs. An increase in testicular dimensions has also been observed with age, peaking at 6 years old and decreasing thereafter.

The testes should be evaluated whenever a prostatic problem is identified.

Abnormalities

Undescended Testes

Undescended testes look similar to descended testes but are smaller and hypoechoic (Fig. 54). They should be located by evaluating the area from the bladder to the area caudal to the kidney. They are usually very superficial and can be recognised by the mediastinum testis, unless they have already become neoplastic (Felumlee et al., 2012).

Testicular Neoplasms

Testicular tumours may be benign or malignant, and may or may not be endocrinologically active. The ultrasonographic appearance of testicular tumours varies and is not specific to the type of tumour. However, they are easy to differentiate from normal testicular parenchyma.

They can be focal or diffuse. Thus, they can range from small, circumscribed nodules to large, complex masses with a heterogeneous ultrasonographic pattern and changes to the normal anatomy.

Sertoli cell tumours and **seminomas** are usually large and have mixed echogenicity; they can cause generalised testicular enlargement (Fig. 55). **Interstitial cell tumours** may appear as well-defined hypoechoic focal lesions. However, areas of haemorrhage and necrosis may occur in all types of tumours, which, ultrasonographically, will be visualised as poorly defined hypoechoic regions, as well as areas of mineralisation, which appear as hyperechoic foci with acoustic shadowing.

Orchitis

Orchitis is often associated with epididymitis. Ultrasonographically, orchitis can present different characteristics, from poorly defined anechoic areas to a diffuse hypoechoic pattern (Fig. 56). Generally, there is an increase in the size of the testes and epididymis, and fluid may accumulate between the visceral and parietal layers of the tunica vaginalis within the scrotum.

Testicular Degeneration

Testicular degeneration or atrophy is usually bilateral and caused by changes associated with ageing, although sometimes, when there is a neoplasm in one of the testes, the contralateral testis atrophies. The testicular parenchyma is hypoechoic or isoechoic with a decrease in size. A diffuse increase in echogenicity has also been described.

Testicular Torsion

In cases of torsion, ultrasonography shows a diffuse decrease in the echogenicity of the testicular parenchyma, and a simultaneous enlargement of the epididymis and spermatic cord, scrotal thickening and loss of the Doppler signal (Boza et al., 2011).

Colour Doppler ultrasonography is a sensitive technique for the evaluation of testicular vascularisation and can be used to differentiate testicular torsion from other pathologies, such as orchitis.

Adrenal Glands

Technique and Normal Appearance

The adrenal glands are small in size and are located in the craniodorsal area of the abdomen, in the retroperitoneal space. Due to their size, high-frequency transducers (usually 7.5 MHz) must be used to examine them.

In dogs, the **left adrenal gland** is located lateral or ventrolateral to the aorta and medial to the cranial pole of the left kidney. The **right adrenal gland** is located dorsal or dorsolateral to the caudal vena cava and medial to the cranial pole of the right kidney (Fig. 57). Both glands are flattened dorsoventrally; the left adrenal gland is shaped like a dumbbell and the right one is like an arrowhead or V shape.

The adrenal glands can be approached from the ventral or lateral area of the abdomen. The ipsilateral kidney is used as a reference point, and the transducer is then moved medially to locate the aorta and the left renal artery. The left adrenal gland is located cranial to the renal artery. The right adrenal gland is more difficult to visualise than the left because of its deeper, more cranial location under the ribs. The right kidney is visualised and the transducer is then moved to locate the caudal vena cava and, by fanning the transducer from the kidney to the caudal vena cava, the right adrenal gland is located (d'Anjou and Penninck, 2015).

Normal adrenal glands are hypoechoic and, on occasion, the medulla can be differentiated from the cortex. The medulla

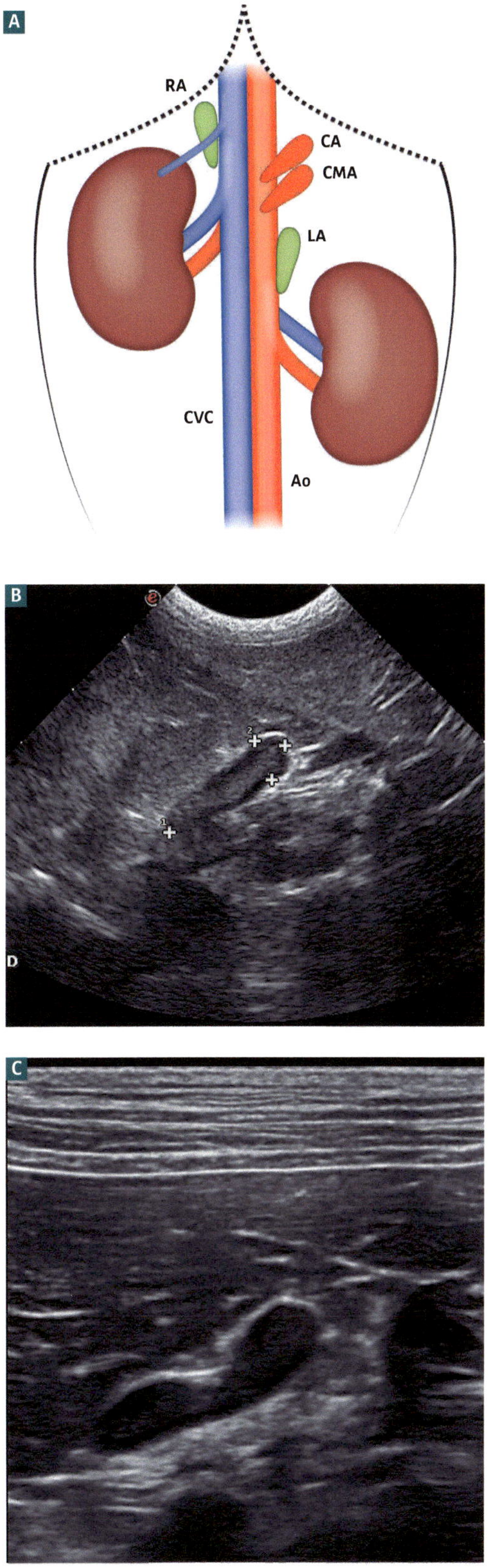

Figure 57. Location and appearance of normal adrenal glands. **A**. Diagram of the anatomical location of the adrenal glands. Ao: aorta; CVC: caudal vena cava; CMA: cranial mesenteric artery; CA: coeliac artery; RA: right adrenal gland; LA: left adrenal gland. **B**. Right adrenal gland. **C**. Left adrenal gland.

of the normal adrenal gland is slightly more hyperechoic than the cortex (d'Anjou and Penninck, 2015). The maximum length of a normal canine adrenal gland is 15–25 mm but the length varies according to the weight of the animal. The maximum diameter of the adrenal gland is the most sensitive measurement for detecting changes in size. The following diameters have been described in the dog (Soulsby et al., 2015):

- for dogs <10 kg: <0.54 cm
- for dogs between 10 kg and 30 kg: <0.68 cm
- for dogs >30 kg: <0.8 cm.

The ratio of the diameter of the adrenal gland to that of the aorta can also be calculated; mean values are 1.5 for dogs weighing 10 kg, 1.07 for dogs of 10–20 kg and 0.86 for dogs weighing over 20 kg (Agut et al., 2020).

In cats, the average adrenal gland diameter is 3.9 mm for cats <4 kg and 4.8 mm for those weighing between 4 kg and 8 kg (Perez-Lopez et al., 2020).

normal, a neoplasm should be suspected. They are normally hypoechoic and homogeneous, but may also appear irregular, with focal areas of increased echogenicity or a nodular appearance.

In animals with PDH treated with trilostane, the echogenicity of the adrenal glands changes, such that the difference in echogenicity between the cortex and the medulla is more pronounced. Both adrenal glands have also been reported to appear enlarged. Therefore, examination of the adrenal glands is recommended before starting trilostane treatment (Neelis et al.,.2020).

In dogs with hyperadrenocorticism caused by the administration of exogenous corticosteroids, the adrenal glands may appear smaller than normal or even not be visible (Fig. 59). These changes are reversible within approximately 1 month after the completion of treatment (Neelis et al., 2020).

Unlike in the dog, adrenal diseases are uncommon in the cat.

Adrenal Gland Abnormalities

Increase in Size

Ultrasonography of the adrenal glands is most useful in animals with hyperadrenocorticism, to differentiate between pituitary-dependent hyperadrenocorticism (PDH) and hyperadrenocorticism due to an adrenocortical tumour. In the typical case of a dog with PDH, both adrenal glands have a rounded appearance and their diameter is increased (Fig. 58); however, they can also be of a normal size (seen in approximately 30% of cases). Likewise, if the size of one of the adrenal glands is greater than 2 cm, even if its morphology is

Nodules and Masses

The ultrasonographic appearance of the nodules and masses found in the adrenal glands is not specific to a given condition. The most likely differential diagnoses are, depending on their size, hyperplasia, primary neoplasia or metastasis (Neelis et al., 2020).

Adrenal tumours are the most common of the endocrine tumours and can present various ultrasonographic appearances. As a general rule, ultrasonography cannot be used to differentiate between a benign and a malignant lesion, nor can it identify the tumour type. Mineralisation can occur in both

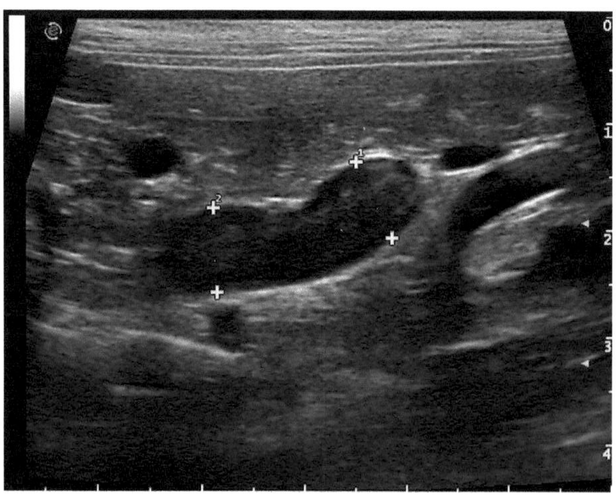

Figure 58. Pituitary-dependent adrenal hyperplasia. Left adrenal gland symmetrically increased in size.

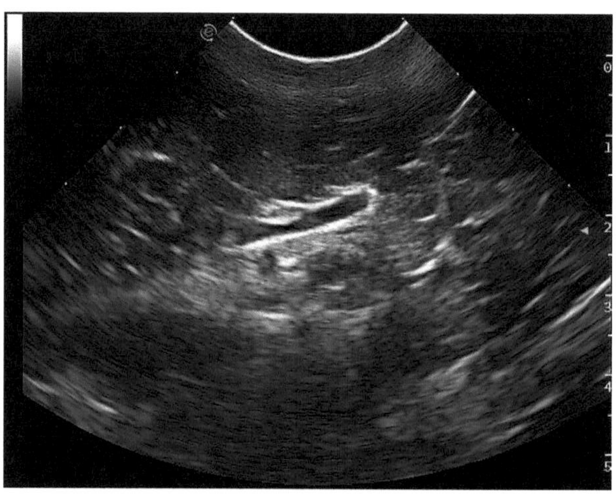

Figure 59. Ultrasonographic appearance of the left adrenal gland in a dog with hyperadrenocorticism caused by the administration of exogenous corticosteroids. The adrenal gland is observed to be small in size.

benign and malignant tumours, but has also been observed in hyperplastic adrenal glands; therefore, it is not a sign of adrenal neoplasia. Anechoic lesions are usually seen in large tumours, forming part of a mixed-echogenicity model, and may represent necrotic foci or bleeding associated with fast-growing tumours.

There is a high incidence of silent lesions of the adrenal glands in elderly dogs; they are often nodular hyperplasia, but they can also be neoplasms termed "incidentalomas".

When a nodule in the adrenal gland is observed in a dog that is showing signs of hyperadrenocorticism, the differential diagnosis is cortical adenoma, cortical adenocarcinoma and nodular hyperplasia (Fig. 60). Nodules or masses greater than 2 cm in size and/or with mineralisation are more likely to be neoplasms than hyperplasic nodules; in these cases, the findings are suggestive of adrenal-dependent hyperadrenocorticism. If the mass is larger than 4 cm, it is more likely to be malignant (Neelis et al., 2020).

When a nodule or a mass is found in an adrenal gland, there are various differential diagnoses:

- myelolipoma
- phaeochromocytoma
- metastatic tumour
- haematoma
- granuloma
- cyst.

Phaeochromocytoma is the second most common tumour of the adrenal glands (Pagani et al., 2016). Dogs with this type of tumour may present several clinical signs, some of which are similar to those of hyperadrenocorticism. These tumours can be of variable size and may have different ultrasonographic appearances similar to those described above, so it is impossible to differentiate them from adrenal tumours ultrasonographically.

Malignant tumours such as phaeochromocytoma can invade blood vessels near the adrenal glands (Fig. 61), the ipsilateral kidney or the musculature, and can also extend to the vertebrae, causing neurological signs. Invasive local lesions can be recognised ultrasonographically; however, it can sometimes be difficult to identify their origin. Other nonadrenal retroperitoneal masses, such as haemangiosarcoma and renal carcinomas, can sometimes be confused with adrenal tumours. In these cases, computed tomography or magnetic resonance imaging should be recommended to better define the extent of the mass.

To date, information regarding the appearance of the adrenal glands in cats with PDH and adrenal tumours is scarce, but it seems that everything described in dogs is applicable to cats as well.

Atrophy

In dogs with hypoadrenocorticism or Addison's disease, the adrenal glands are less than 3.2 mm in diameter (Wenger et al., 2010), making them difficult to identify. However, because it is sometimes difficult to find the adrenal glands, hypoadrenocorticism cannot be diagnosed with ultrasonography alone.

Treatment with mitotane results in a bilateral decrease in the size of the adrenal glands compared with their size before treatment. Adrenal glands that are smaller than normal can also be found in animals receiving long-duration corticosteroid treatments (Fig. 59).

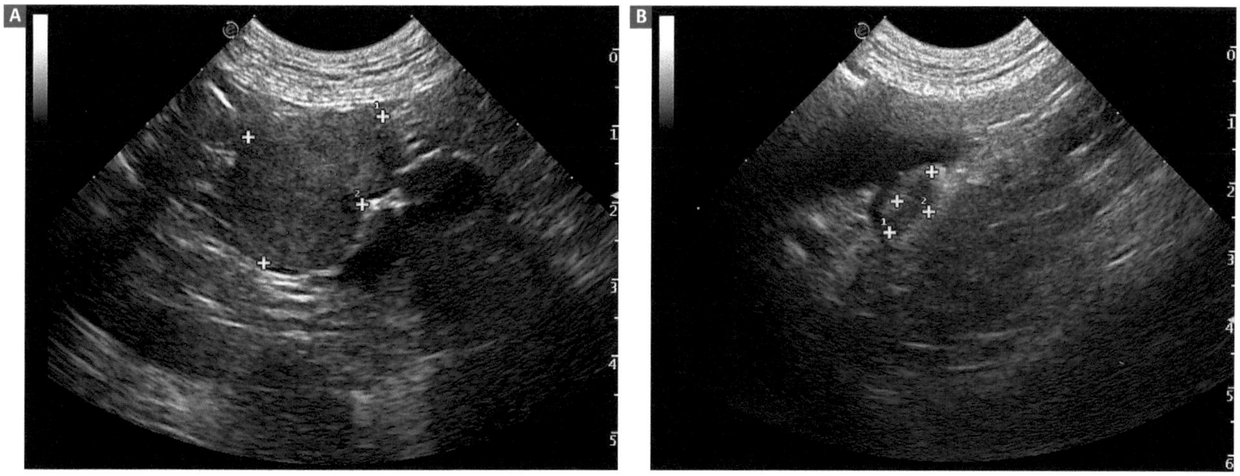

Figure 60. Adrenal-dependent hyperadrenocorticism. The left adrenal gland (**A**) appears abnormal and is observed as an echogenic mass (adenoma) of approximately 2 cm in diameter. The right adrenal gland (**B**) is seen to be reduced in size.

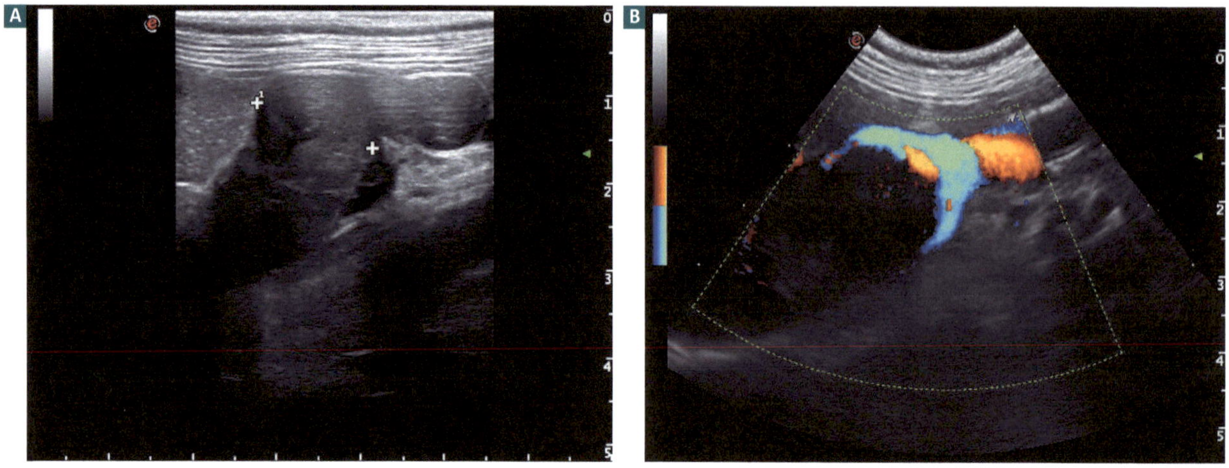

Figure 61. Adrenal phaeochromocytoma. **A**. Ultrasound image of a mass in the longitudinal plane at the level of the right adrenal gland. The mass is hypoechoic with respect to the liver and measures 1.5 cm in diameter. **B**. Ultrasound image of the caudal vena cava. A hypoechoic mass is observed in the lumen of the caudal vena cava, compatible with an invasion by the neoplasm.

Bibliography

- Agut, A., Martinez, M., Ansón, A., Soler, M. (2020) Ultrasonographic measurement of adrenal gland-to-aorta ratio as a method of estimating adrenal size in dogs. *Vet Record*, 186(19):e27.
- Barella, G., Lodi, M., Sabbadin, L.A., Faverzani, S. (2012) A new method for ultrasonographic measurement of kidney size in healthy dogs. *J Ultrasound*, 15(3):186–191.
- Boza, S., de Membiela, F., Navarro, A., et al. (2011) What is your diagnosis? Testicular torsion. *J Am Vet Med Assoc*, 238(1):37–38.
- Bragato, N., Borges, N.C., Fioravanti, M.C.S. (2017) B-mode and Doppler ultrasound of chronic kidney disease in dogs and cats. *Vet Res Commun*, 41(4):307–315.
- Cordella, A., Pey, P., Dondi, F., et al. (2020) The ultrasonographic medullary "rim sign" versus medullary "band sign" in cats and their association with renal disease. *J Vet Intern Med*, 34(5):1932–1939.
- d'Anjou, M.A., Bédard, A., Dunn, M.E. (2011) Clinical significance of renal pelvic dilatation on ultrasound in dogs and cats. *Vet Radiol Ultrasound*, 52(1):88–94.
- d'Anjou, M.A., Penninck, D. (2015) Kidneys and ureters. In: Penninck, D., d'Anjou, M.A. (eds). *Atlas of Small Animal Ultrasonography*. 2nd ed, pp. 331–362. Wiley.
- d'Anjou, M.A., Penninck, D. (2015) Adrenal glands. In: Penninck, D., d'Anjou, M.A. (eds). *Atlas of Small Animal Ultrasonography*. 2nd ed, pp. 387–402. Wiley.
- Felumlee, A.E., Reichle, J.K., Hecht, S., et al. (2012) Use of ultrasound to locate retained testes in dogs and cats. *Vet Radiol Ultrasound*, 53(5): 581–585.
- Griffin, S. (2020) Abdominal feline ultrasonography: What's normal? What´s abnormal? Renal pelvis, ureters and urinary bladder. *J Feline Med Surg*, 22(9):847–865.
- Hart, D.V., Winter, M.D., Conway, J., Berry, C.R. (2013) Ultrasound appearance of the outer medulla in dogs without renal dysfunction. *Vet Radiol Ultrasound*, 54(6), 652–658.
- Hecht, S., Pollard, R. (2015) Male reproductive tract. In: Penninck, D., d'Anjou, M.A. (eds). *Atlas of Small Animal Ultrasonography*. 2nd ed, pp. 423–454. Wiley.
- Mareschal, A., d'Anjou, M.A., Moreau, M., Alexander, K., Beauregard, G. (2007) Ultrasonographic measurement of kidney-to-aorta ratio as a method of estimating renal size in dogs. *Vet Radiol Ultrasound*, 48(5): 434–438.
- Mattoon, J.S., Davidson, A. (2020) Prostate and testes. In: Mattoon, J.S., Sellon, R. K., Berry, C.R. (eds). *Small Animal Diagnostic Ultrasound*. 4th ed. pp. 635–664. Elsevier.
- Mattoon, J.S., Davidson, A., Sellon, R.K. (2020) Ovaries and uterus. In: Mattoon, J.S., Sellon, R. K., Berry, C.R. (eds). *Small Animal Diagnostic Ultrasound*. 4th ed. pp. 665–688. Elsevier.
- Neelis, D.A., Mattoon, J.S., Sellon, R.K. (2020) Adrenal glands. In: Mattoon, J.S., Sellon, R. K., Berry, C.R. (eds). *Small Animal Diagnostic Ultrasound*. 4th ed. pp. 566–582. Elsevier.
- Ortega-Pacheco, A., Gutiérrez-Blanco, E., Jiménez-Coello, M. (2012) Common lesions in the female reproductive tract of dogs and cats. *Vet Clin N Am Small Anim Pract*, 42(3):547–559.
- Pagani, E., Tursi, M., Lorenzi, C., et al. (2016) Ultrasonographic features of adrenal gland lesions in dogs can aid in diagnosis. *BMC Vet Res*, 12:267.
- Pérez-López, L., Wägner, A.M., Saavedra, P., et al. (2020) Ultrasonographic evaluation of adrenal gland size in two body weight categories of healthy adult cats. *J Feline Med Surg*, 23(8) 804–808.
- Pollard, R., Hecht, S. (2015) Female reproductive tract. In: Penninck, D., d'Anjou, M.A. (eds). *Atlas of Small Animal Ultrasonography*. 2nd ed, pp. 403–422. Wiley.
- Soulsby, S.N., Holland, M., Hudson, J.A., Behrend, E.N. (2015) Ultrasonographic evaluation of adrenal gland size compared to body weight in normal dogs. *Vet Radiol Ultrasound*, 56(3):317–326.
- Sutherland-Smith, J., Penninck, D. (2015) Bladder and urethra. In: Penninck, D., d'Anjou, M.A. (eds). *Atlas of Small Animal Ultrasonography*. 2nd ed, pp. 363–386. Wiley.
- Wenger, M., Mueller, C., Kook, P.H., Reusch, C.E. (2010) Ultrasonographic evaluation of adrenal glands in dogs with primary hypoadrenocorticism or mimicking diseases. *Vet Record*, 167(6):207–210.
- Widmer, W.R., Mattoon, J.S., Vaden, S.L. (2020) Urinary tract. In: Mattoon, J.S., Sellon, R. K., Berry, C.R. (eds). *Small Animal Diagnostic Ultrasound*. 4th ed. pp. 583–634. Elsevier.

Ultrasonography of the Pancreas

Panagiotis (Pete) Mantis

Introduction

The pancreas is an elongated organ located caudal to the liver in the dorsal part of the cranial and right lateral abdominal regions, along the greater curvature of the stomach and the mesenteric border of the descending duodenum. It has a **right lobe** and a **left lobe**, connected by the **body**.

Indications for ultrasonographic examination of the pancreas include presenting signs such as vomiting and abdominal pain, diarrhoea, abnormal appetite, lethargy, weakness, icterus and fever. Indications also include changes in the complete blood count and serum biochemistry profile such as an inflammatory leucogram, thrombocytopaenia, elevated liver enzyme activities, hypoalbuminaemia, azotaemia, hyponatraemia, hyperlipidaemia, hypoglycaemia or hyperglycaemia, which may raise suspicion of pancreatic disease. The measurement of pancreatic lipase is considered the most sensitive test available for diagnosing acute pancreatitis in dogs and cats (Xenoulis, 2015).

Ultrasonography allows direct visualisation of the pancreas. However, it is limited by the difficulty in seeing the normal pancreas as a distinct structure in ultrasonographic studies and sometimes also by interference caused by the presence of gas in the gastrointestinal tract. Fasting the animal for 12 hours before the study may reduce gas interference.

Examination Technique

See also Mantis (2022).

The animal can be positioned in right lateral recumbency (for large dogs, left lateral recumbency is used) or dorsal recumbency (Fig. 1). For the technique described in this chapter, unless otherwise stated, right lateral recumbency, with the animal's head towards the ultrasound machine and the legs towards the examiner, should be considered standard (Fig. 1 A).

Usually, ultrasonographic examination of the pancreas is done as part of an examination of the whole abdomen. For examination of the whole abdomen, clipping the hair from the xiphoid to the pelvic inlet and halfway up the side of the abdomen is required. If only the pancreas is to be examined, the hair is clipped from the xiphoid to the umbilicus and halfway up the side. Use of an 8–12 MHz linear, microconvex or curvilinear transducer is recommended for small dogs and cats, whereas in large dogs a 5–8 MHz microconvex or curvilinear transducer is recommended because of the need for greater image depth.

Anatomical landmarks are used to identify the pancreas (Fig. 2). For the right pancreatic lobe, the landmarks are the right kidney, the descending duodenum and the pancreaticoduodenal vein that runs within the pancreas parallel to the descending duodenum. For the pancreatic body, the landmarks are the pyloric antrum of the stomach and the portal vein. For the left pancreatic lobe, the landmarks are the stomach, the transverse colon, the spleen and the left kidney, although the area between the splenic vein and the portal vein has been used as a landmark for identification of the left lobe.

Right Pancreatic Lobe in Small and Medium Size Dogs and in Cats

Position. The animal is positioned in right lateral recumbency with the head towards the ultrasound machine and the legs towards the examiner (Fig. 1 A).

Examination window. From the xiphoid to the umbilicus and two-thirds up the right abdominal wall in that area.

Orientation. The on-screen marker is on the left.

Transducer. A microconvex transducer of more than 8 MHz is recommended. A linear 8–12 MHz transducer, ideally with a small footprint, can also be used.

Technique. The transducer is positioned with the marker pointing towards the head of the animal (Fig. 1 A). It is placed parallel and close (up to 1 cm distance) to the table top, pointing towards the last rib, and is slid under the animal until it is two-thirds up the right lateral abdominal wall. The right kidney is identified. While maintaining the orientation of the transducer, the pressure is released, and the duodenum comes into view. Moving the probe slightly from right to left in a fanning motion will allow the pancreas to be visualised (Fig. 3). If the duodenum is not seen when the pressure

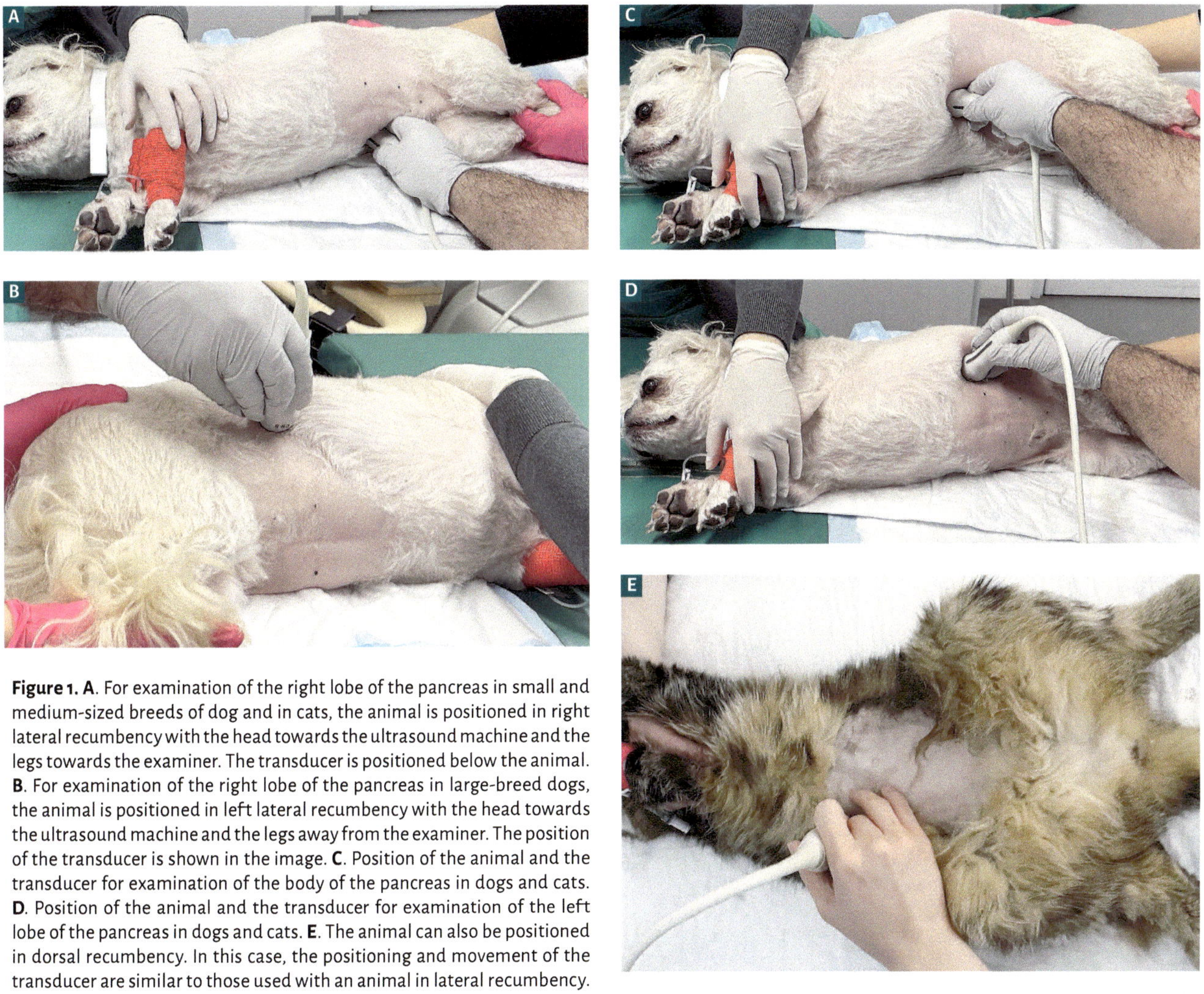

Figure 1. A. For examination of the right lobe of the pancreas in small and medium-sized breeds of dog and in cats, the animal is positioned in right lateral recumbency with the head towards the ultrasound machine and the legs towards the examiner. The transducer is positioned below the animal. **B**. For examination of the right lobe of the pancreas in large-breed dogs, the animal is positioned in left lateral recumbency with the head towards the ultrasound machine and the legs away from the examiner. The position of the transducer is shown in the image. **C**. Position of the animal and the transducer for examination of the body of the pancreas in dogs and cats. **D**. Position of the animal and the transducer for examination of the left lobe of the pancreas in dogs and cats. **E**. The animal can also be positioned in dorsal recumbency. In this case, the positioning and movement of the transducer are similar to those used with an animal in lateral recumbency. This position might be more practical for left-handed examiners.

is released, the transducer is fanned all the way to the right (towards the table) and then is fanned slowly towards the left (away from the table). The first loop of small intestine that is seen is usually the descending duodenum. Sliding and fanning the probe will allow the right lobe of the pancreas to be visualised and examined.

Right Pancreatic Lobe in Large Dogs

Position. The animal is positioned in left lateral recumbency with the head towards the ultrasound machine and the legs away from the examiner (Fig. 1 B).

Examination window. Right dorsal, from the ninth rib to caudal to the last rib.

Orientation. The on-screen marker is on the left.

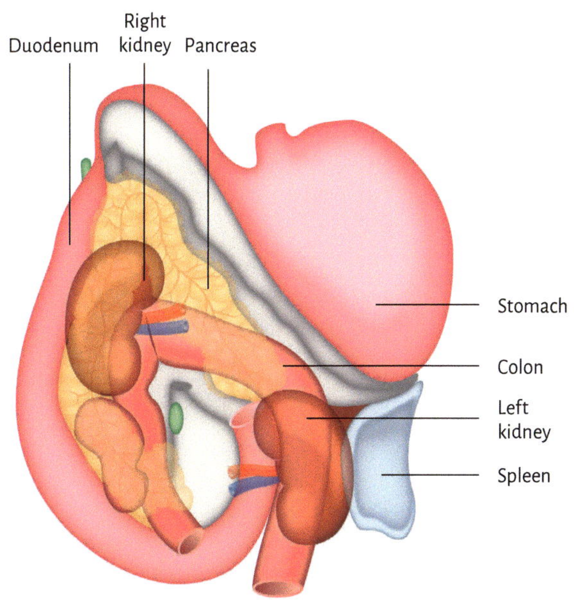

Figure 2. Anatomical landmarks for the identification of the pancreas.

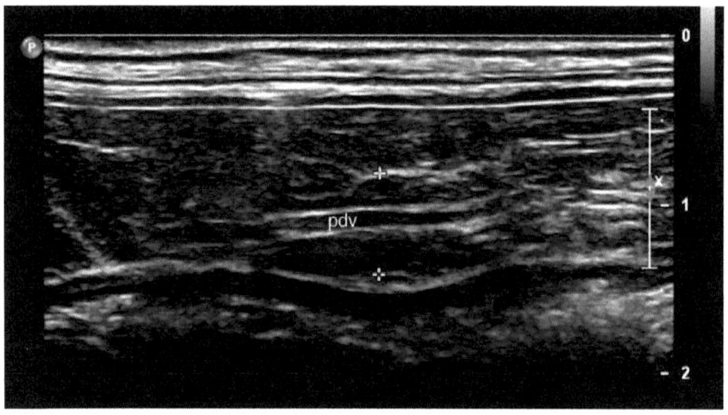

Figure 3. Normal right lobe of the pancreas in a dog (between the calliper marks). The pancreaticoduodenal vein (pdv) is visible within the pancreatic lobe.

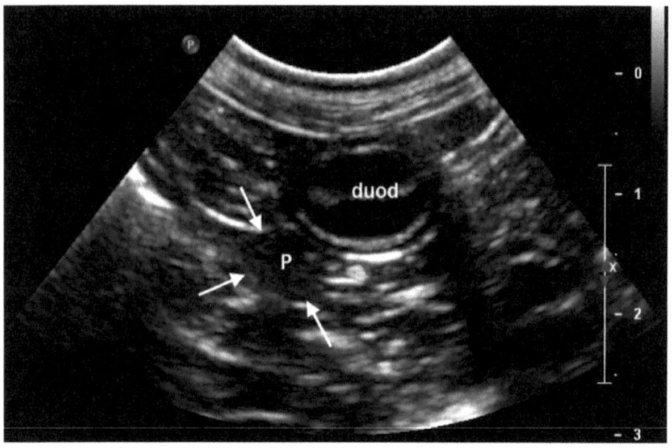

Figure 4. From the right dorsal approach in large-breed dogs, rotating the transducer anticlockwise, so the marker points towards the spine, allows identification of the right lobe of the pancreas (P, between the arrows) in transverse orientation below and to the left of the descending duodenum (duod), at approximately the 7 o'clock position on the screen. Sliding the transducer cranially and caudally allows examination of the pancreas. This orientation can be used if there are artefacts resulting from gas or matter in the lumen of the duodenum.

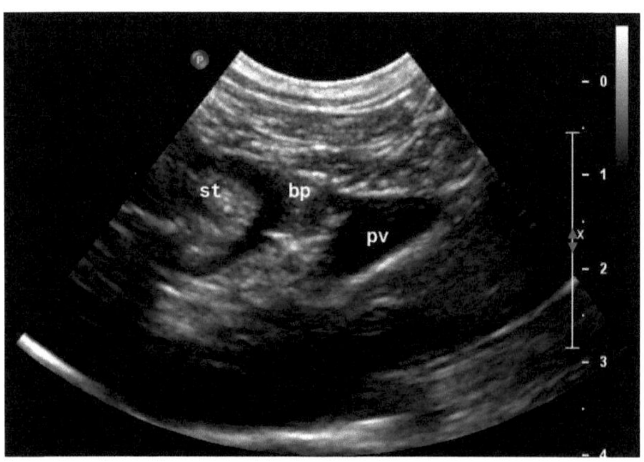

Figure 5. Image of the normal body of the pancreas (bp) in a dog. It can be seen between the stomach (st) and the portal vein (pv).

Transducer. A 5–8 MHz microconvex or curvilinear transducer is preferred.

Technique. The transducer is positioned with the marker pointing towards the animal's head. It is placed close and parallel to the spine, perpendicular to the skin. The right kidney is identified. While maintaining the orientation of the transducer, it is slided ventrally until the first loop of small intestine is visualised at the top of the screen. This is usually the descending duodenum. Slight fanning of the probe from dorsal to ventral will allow the pancreas to be located. If excess gas in the descending duodenum interferes with the examination, the transducer should be rotated anticlockwise (so that the marker on the transducer points to the spine); the pancreas is then visualised next to the descending duodenum, at the 7 o'clock position (Fig. 4). Sliding the transducer cranially and caudally allows examination of the right pancreatic lobe.

Body of the Pancreas in all Dogs and Cats

Position. The animal is positioned in right lateral recumbency with the head towards the ultrasound machine and the legs towards the examiner (Fig. 1 C).

Examination window. From the xiphoid to the umbilicus and one-third up the left and right abdominal wall in that area.

Orientation. The on-screen marker is on the left.

Transducer. A 5–10 MHz microconvex or curvilinear transducer is preferred.

Technique. The transducer is positioned with the marker pointing cranially (Fig. 1 C). It is placed in the midline, parallel to the table at the level of the pylorus of the stomach. Pressure is applied with the transducer, which is fanned all the way to the right side (towards the table). The transducer is then slowly fanned towards the left side until the portal vein is visualised. At this point, the body of the pancreas is visualised at approximately the 4 o'clock position (3–6 o'clock) in relation to the pylorus (Fig. 5).

Left Pancreatic Lobe in all Dogs and Cats

Position. The animal is positioned in right lateral recumbency with the head towards the ultrasound machine and the legs towards the examiner (Fig. 1 D).

Examination window. From the xiphoid to the umbilicus and two-thirds up the left abdominal wall in that area. More extensive clipping of the left abdominal wall may be required.

Orientation. The on-screen marker is on the left.

Transducer. 8–12 MHz for small dogs and cats, and 5–8 MHz for large dogs. Microconvex and linear (for small dogs and cats) transducers are preferred.

Technique. The transducer is positioned caudal to the last rib, perpendicular to the skin, with the marker pointing cranially (Fig. 1 D). The spleen is identified caudal to the last rib, and the splenic vein is visualised end on and is placed in the centre of the screen. The transducer is slowly moved dorsally towards the spine, maintaining its orientation, until the portal vein is visualised in the deep area of the image. The left lobe of the pancreas is located between the splenic and portal vein. The transducer is then rotated to examine the left pancreatic lobe longitudinally (Fig. 6).

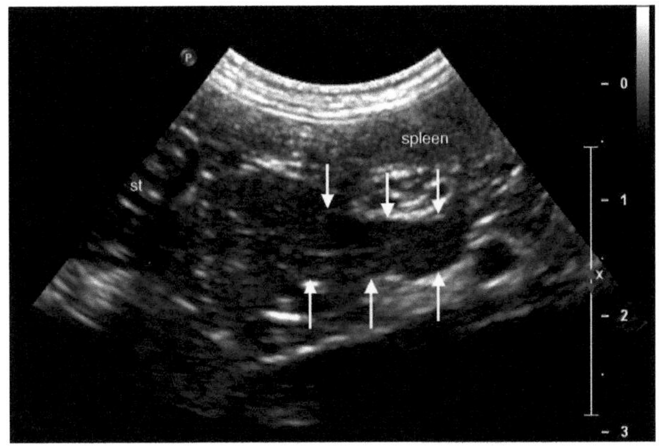

Figure 6. The normal left lobe of the pancreas (between the arrows) in a dog. Initially, the splenic vein (end on) and the portal vein are identified, and the space between them is examined to locate the left lobe of the pancreas. st: stomach.

Normal Appearance

The normal pancreas is difficult to identify ultrasonographically. The use of anatomical landmarks (Fig. 2) helps the examiner to identify and focus on specific lobes of the pancreas. For the right lobe, the important anatomical landmarks are the identification of the descending duodenum at the level of the right kidney and the pancreaticoduodenal vein within the lobe. The right lobe lies ventral to the right kidney and dorsomedial or medial to the descending duodenum. The pancreaticoduodenal vein runs through the right lobe parallel to the duodenum (Figs. 3 and 7) (Saunders, 1991; Saunders et al., 1992).

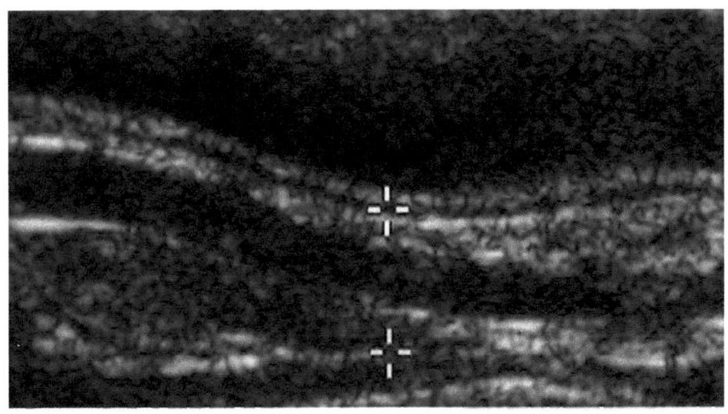

Figure 7. Close-up view of the normal right pancreatic lobe in a dog. Note the anechoic tubular pancreaticoduodenal vein passing through the lobe.

The pyloric antrum and portal vein are the anatomical landmarks for identifying the body of the pancreas, which lies ventral to the portal vein. The splenic vein, visualised end on below the spleen, and the portal vein, located deeper, are the anatomical landmarks for the left lobe of the pancreas. The left pancreatic lobe lies caudal to the greater curvature of the stomach. The splenic vein passes caudodorsal to the left lobe, which may extend to the cranial pole of the left kidney. It is usually easier to identify the body and left lobe of the pancreas in cats than in dogs.

The pancreas is usually isoechoic to slightly hyperechoic relative to the caudate lobe of the liver. Rarely, a normal-sized pancreas may appear homogeneously hyperechoic. Based on the author's experience, the normal pancreas is uniform in appearance and does not stand out as an organ with very well-defined margins. It is usually slightly hypoechoic in relation to the surrounding tissues (Fig. 3).

The pancreatic duct is a vessel-like structure and can be seen in the left lobe of the pancreas. The pancreatic duct might also be seen in the right lobe of the pancreas and can be distinguished from the pancreaticoduodenal vein by using Doppler ultrasonography (Lamb and Simpson, 1995). In cats, the mean diameter of the pancreatic duct increases with age (Larson et al., 2005; Hecht et al., 2006).

The thickness of the pancreas is usually less than 10 mm in dogs. In some large dogs it can measure up to 12 mm thick. In cats, the body and the left lobe of the pancreas can be up to 9 mm thick, while the right lobe is up to 6 mm thick (Hecht and Henry, 2007).

Pancreatic Disorders

Pancreatitis

The appearance of an inflamed pancreas varies considerably. Even if the pancreas appears normal on ultrasonography, acute pancreatitis cannot be excluded.

The most likely appearance in animals with **acute pancreatitis** is a pancreas that is thicker than normal and diffusely hypoechoic relative to the surrounding tissues (Figs. 8 and 9 A). The surrounding mesentery and omentum are usually hyperechoic (Figs. 8 and 9 A). Multifocal hypoechoic or hyperechoic regions may give the pancreas the appearance of mixed echogenicity. Additionally, cyst-like lesions may be identified in acute pancreatitis. In dogs, the right pancreatic lobe is more commonly affected (Penninck, 2008).

Localised ascites and thickening of the duodenal and/or gastric wall (more than 5 mm thick) may be present in the acute and subacute phases. Dilation of the common bile duct and enlargement of the gallbladder may also be present with pancreatitis (Fig. 9 B).

In cats, the findings are usually less obvious than in dogs, with the pancreatic body and left lobe showing the most severe changes (Penninck, 2008). Feline pancreatitis has been associated with hepatic lipidosis, inflammatory bowel disease and cholangiohepatitis (Akol et al., 1993; Weiss et al., 1996). Regional ascites and thickening of the duodenal and/or gastric wall may also be detected in these cases (Saunders et al., 2002).

In cases of **chronic pancreatitis**, the appearance of the pancreas is variable. The typical appearance consists of a mildly thickened pancreas with increased echogenicity, and less obvious or no changes in the surrounding mesentery.

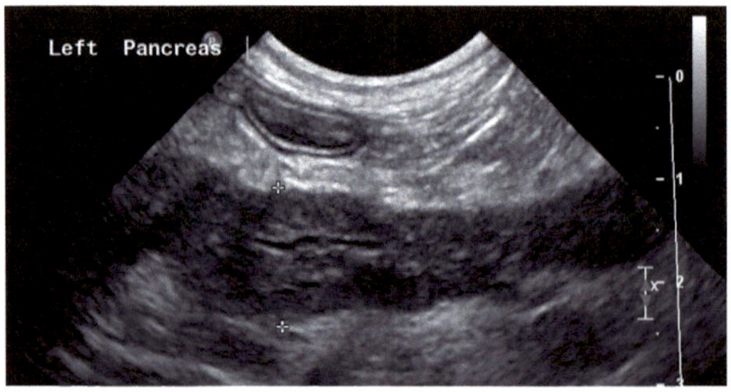

Figure 8. Thick hypoechoic left lobe of the pancreas in a dog (between the calliper marks). The pancreas is clearly visible and measures up to 14 mm in thickness.

In **haemorrhagic, necrotising pancreatitis**, the margins of the pancreas are poorly defined and irregular hypoechoic to anechoic areas may be seen. The adjacent mesentery is hyperechoic and hyperattenuating (Penninck, 2008).

It can be challenging to differentiate acute from chronic pancreatitis in dogs and cats, as it is difficult to evaluate the clinical relevance of unexpected pancreatic lesions seen on ultrasound examination.

Nodular Hyperplasia

Nodular pancreatic hyperplasia is commonly found in older dogs (Newman et al., 2005) and older cats (Hecht et al., 2007). It cannot be distinguished from neoplasia based solely on ultrasonographic findings (Fig. 10). Relatively well-defined hypoechoic or isoechoic nodules of variable size are visible. Nodular hyperplasia with the appearance of hypoechoic nodules up to 1 cm has been described in cats (Fig. 10 B) (Hecht et al., 2007). To distinguish pancreatic nodular hyperplasia from neoplasia, aspiration and/or biopsy for cytology and/or histopathology is required.

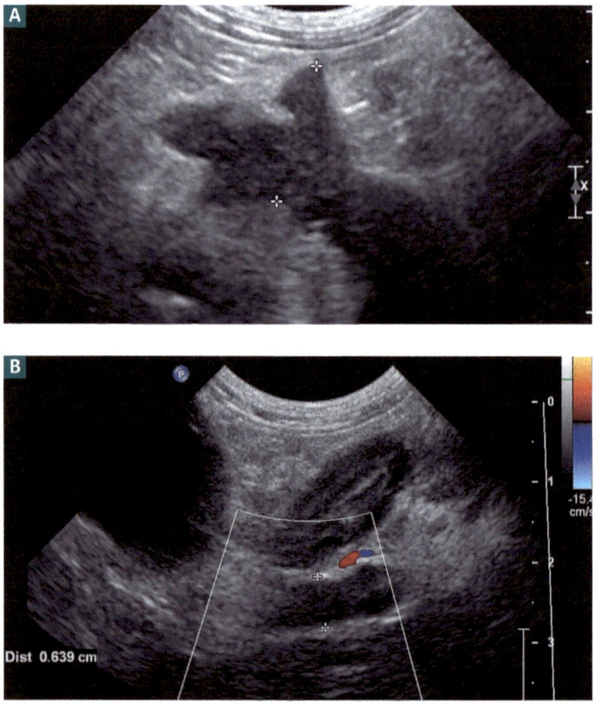

Figure 9. A. Hypoechoic body and right lobe of a dog with pancreatitis. Note the hyperechoic mesentery around the pancreas. **B.** Dilated common bile duct (between the calliper marks) in the same dog.

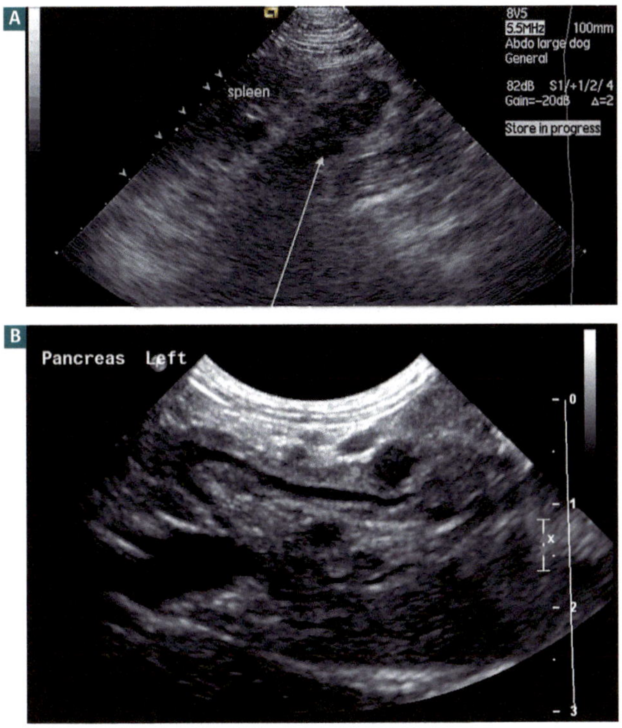

Figure 10. A. Nodular pancreatic hyperplasia in a 3-year-old Dobermann. **B**. Hypoechoic nodules in the pancreas of a 9-year-old Siamese cat with nodular hyperplasia.

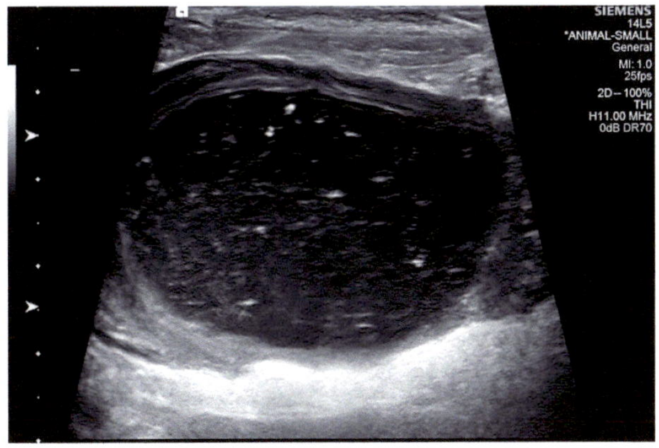

Figure 11. Pancreatic abscess in a dog. The wall is thickened and the fluid content is echogenic.

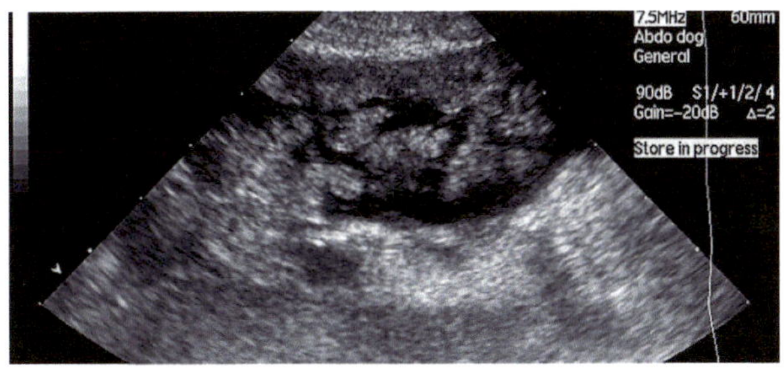

Figure 12. Pancreatic oedema in a Springer Spaniel. Note the hypoechoic to anechoic lines that highlight the pancreatic lobulation throughout the pancreas.

Cystic Lesions

Cystic lesions of the pancreas cannot be differentiated by ultrasonographic evaluation alone.

Information on **true pancreatic cysts** (**retention cysts**) in small animals is minimal. A true pancreatic cyst in a cat was described as being pedunculated and septate, with a thick wall (Coleman et al., 2005). Multiple recurrent cysts associated with pancreatitis, atrophy and endocrine dysfunction have also been reported in a cat (Branter and Viviano, 2010).

Pseudocysts are fluid-filled lesions associated with pancreatitis. They are anechoic or poorly echogenic cystic structures that often show acoustic enhancement, and can be found in both dogs and cats (Hines et al., 1996; Smith and Biller, 1998; Van Enkevort et al., 1999; Mattoon et al., 2021). The wall of pseudocysts is typically thicker and more irregular compared with that of true cysts. Pseudocysts can disappear spontaneously or persist and require surgical drainage. Large pseudocysts can cause extrahepatic biliary obstruction (Marchevsky et al., 2000).

Pancreatic abscesses (Fig. 11) are more common in dogs than in cats. They are usually a complication of pancreatitis. They contain pus and appear as cystic lesions with echogenic to almost anechoic fluid. They may even have the appearance of masses if the fluid they contain is very echogenic.

Oedema

Pancreatic oedema appears as hypoechoic or anechoic stripes that highlight the pancreatic lobulation and extend throughout the enlarged pancreas (Fig. 12). It can be associated with pancreatitis, but can also be caused by portal hypertension or hypoalbuminaemia (Lamb, 1999).

Neoplasia

Exocrine pancreatic tumours, such as **adenocarcinomas** (Fig. 13), are rare, but they are the most common type of pancreatic neoplasia in small animals. They usually affect older dogs and cats (Hawks et al., 1992; Bennett et al., 2001; Seaman, 2004; Hecht et al., 2007). The Airedale Terrier is considered to be predisposed to pancreatic adenocarcinoma (Priester, 1974).

Adenocarcinomas usually metastasise before clinical signs are apparent. They can compress the common bile duct, invade the adjacent gastric or duodenal wall, and metastasise to the liver (Lamb et al., 1995). Other tumours that can be seen in the pancreas of dogs and cats include cystadenomas, adenomas, lymphomas and metastatic carcinomas.

Endocrine tumours are uncommon. They include glucagonomas, insulinomas and gastrinomas. Insulinomas are the most common type in dogs. Insulinomas can appear as single or multiple nodules that are poorly echogenic and poorly defined, and are generally less than 2.5 cm in size (Fig. 14) (Lamb et al., 1995). They have variable visibility on ultrasonography. If insulinomas are not identified on ultrasound examination, they cannot be excluded. Most endocrine tumours are malignant and spread to the liver and regional lymph nodes. Insulinomas are extremely rare in cats (Mattoon et al., 2021).

Other Disorders

Pancreatic bladder refers to the cystic dilation of the pancreatic duct. It has been reported in cats (Garvey and Zawie, 1984). A cat with pancreatitis and pancreatolithiasis along with a **pseudobladder** (the term used instead of pancreatic bladder) has also been described (Bailiff et al., 2004). **Pancreatolithiasis** is the presence of calculi in the pancreatic ducts. They appear as hyperechoic structures associated with acoustic shadowing.

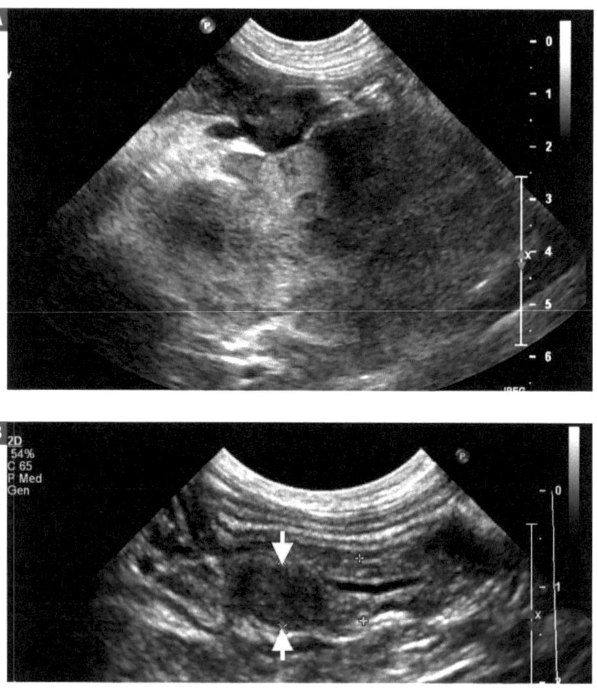

Figure 13. A. Pancreatic adenocarcinoma in a dog. A large, lobulated mass with mixed echogenicity is visualised. **B**. Pancreatic adenocarcinoma in a cat. A hypoechoic mass (between the arrows) is visible in the right lobe of the pancreas.

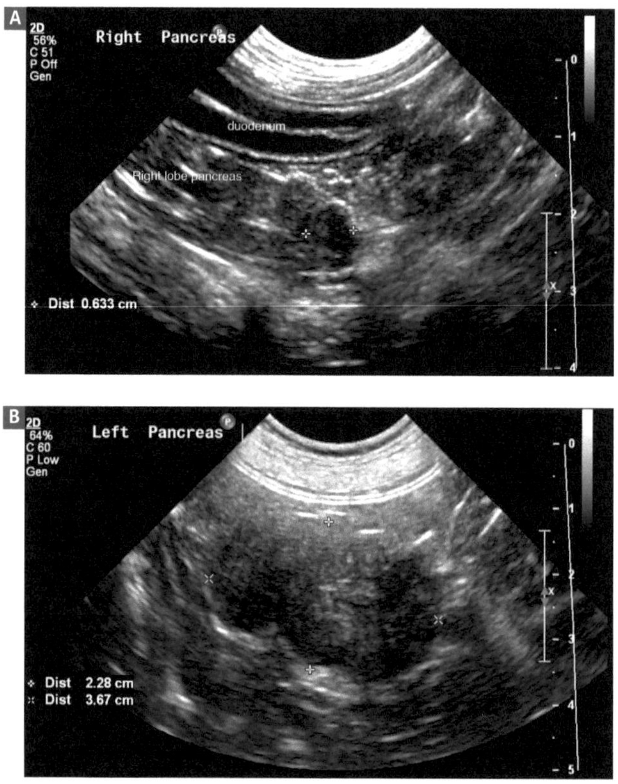

Figure 14. A. Hypoechoic nodular area (between the calliper marks) in the tip of the right lobe of the pancreas of a dog with insulinoma. **B**. Larger hypoechoic mass with mildly mixed echogenicity (between the calliper marks) in a dog. The mass was confirmed to be a large insulinoma.

Bibliography

- Akol, K.G., Washabau, R.J., Saunders, H.M., Hendrick, M.J. (1993) Acute pancreatitis in cats with hepatic lipidosis. *J Vet Intern Med*, 7(4):205–209.
- Bailiff, N.L., Norris, C.R., Seguin, B., Griffey, S.M., Ling, G.V. (2004) Pancreatolithiasis and pancreatic pseudobladder associated with pancreatitis in a cat. *J Am Anim Hosp Assoc*, 40(1):69–74.
- Bennett, P.F., Hahn, K.A., Toal, R.L., Legendre, A.M. (2001) Ultrasonographic and cytopathological diagnosis of exocrine pancreatic carcinoma in the dog and cat. *J Am Anim Hosp Assoc*, 37(5):466–473.
- Branter, E.M., Viviano, K.R. (2010) Multiple recurrent pancreatic cysts with associated pancreatic inflammation and atrophy in a cat. *J Feline Med Surg*, 12(10):822–827.
- Coleman, M.G., Robson, M.C., Harvey, C. (2005) Pancreatic cyst in a cat. *Vet J*, 53(2):157–159.
- Garvey, M.S., Zawie, D.A. (1984) Feline pancreatic disease. *Vet Clin North Am Small Anim Pract*, 14(6):1231–1246.
- Hawks, D., Peterson, M.E., Hawkins, K.L., Rosebury, W.S. (1992) Insulin-secreting pancreatic (islet cell) carcinoma in a cat. *J Vet Intern Med*, 6(3):193–196.
- Hecht, S., Penninck, D.G., Mahony, O.M., King, R., Rand, W.M. (2006) Relationship of pancreatic duct dilation to age and clinical findings in cats. *Vet Radiol Ultrasound*, 47(3):287–294.
- Hecht, S., Henry, G. (2007) Sonographic evaluation of the normal and abnormal pancreas. *Clin Tech Small Anim Pract*, 22(3):115–121.
- Hecht, S., Penninck, D.G., Keating, J.H. (2007) Imaging findings in pancreatic neoplasia and nodular hyperplasia in 19 cats. *Vet Radiol Ultrasound*, 48(1):45–50.
- Hines, B.L., Salisbury, S.K., Jakovljevic, S., DeNicola, D.B. (1996) Pancreatic pseudocyst associated with chronic-active necrotizing pancreatitis in a cat. *J Am Anim Hosp Assoc*, 32(2): 147–152.
- Lamb, C.R., Simpson, K.W. (1995) Ultrasonographic findings in cholecystokinin-induced pancreatitis in dogs. *Vet Radiol Ultrasound*, 36(2):139–145.
- Lamb, C.R., Simpson, K.W., Boswood, A., Matthewman, L.A. (1995) Ultrasonography of pancreatic neoplasia in the dog: a retrospective review of 16 cases. *Vet Rec*, 137(3):65–68.
- Lamb, C.R. (1999) Pancreatic edema in dogs with hypoalbuminemia and portal hypertension. *J Vet Intern Med*, 13(5):498–500.
- Larson, M.M., Panciera, D.L., Ward, D.L., Steiner, J.M., Williams, D.A. (2005) Age-related changes in the ultrasound appearance of the normal feline pancreas. *Vet Radiol Ultrasound*, 46(3):238–242.
- Mantis P. (2022) Practical small animal ultrasonography: abdomen. pp 67-79. Grupo Asis Biomedia, SL.
- Marchevsky, A., Yovich, J.C., Wyatt, K.M. (2000) Pancreatic pseudocyst causing extrahepatic biliary obstruction in a dog. *Aust Vet J*, 78(2):99–101.
- Mattoon, J.S., Slovak, J.E., Sellon, R.K. (2021) Pancreas. In: Mattoon, J.S., Sellon, R.K., Berry, C.R. (eds). *Small Animal Diagnostic Ultrasound*. 4th ed, pp. 461–490. Elsevier.
- Newman, S.J., Steiner, J.M., Woosley, K., Barton, L., Williams, D.A. (2005) Correlation of age and incidence of pancreatic exocrine nodular hyperplasia in the dog. *Vet Pathol*, 42(4):510–513.
- Penninck, D. (2008) Pancreas. In: Penninck, D., D'Anjou, M.A. (eds). *Atlas of Small Animal Ultrasonography*. 2nd ed, pp. 317–337. Wiley-Blackwell .
- Priester, W.A. (1974) Data from eleven United States and Canadian colleges of veterinary medicine on pancreatic carcinoma in domestic animals. *Cancer Res*, 34(6):1372–1375.
- Saunders, H.M. (1991) Ultrasonography of the pancreas. *Probl Vet Med*, 3(4):583–603.
- Saunders, H.M., Pugh, C.R., Rhodes, W.H. (1992) Expanding applications of abdominal ultrasonography. *J Am Anim Hosp Assoc*, 28(4):369–374.
- Saunders, H.M., VanWinkle, T.J., Drobatz, K., Kimmel, S.E., Washabau, R.J. (2002) Ultrasonographic findings in cats with clinical, gross pathologic, and histologic evidence of acute pancreatic necrosis: 20 cases (1994–2001). *J Am Vet Med Assoc*, 221(12):1724–1730.
- Seaman, R.L. (2004) Exocrine pancreatic neoplasia in the cat: a case series. *J Am Anim Hosp Assoc*, 40(3):238–245.
- Smith, S.A., Biller, D.S. (1998) Resolution of a pancreatic pseudocyst in a dog following percutaneous ultrasonographic-guided drainage. *J Am Anim Hosp Assoc*, 34(6):515–522.
- VanEnkevort, B.A., O'Brien, R.T., Young, K.M. (1999) Pancreatic pseudocysts in 4 dogs and 2 cats: ultrasonographic and clinicopathologic findings. *J Vet Intern Med*, 13 (4):309–313.
- Weiss, D.J., Gagne, J.M., Armstrong, P.J. (1996) Relationship between inflammatory hepatic disease and inflammatory bowel disease, pancreatitis, and nephritis in cats. *J Am Vet Med Assoc*, 209(6):1114–1116.
- Xenoulis, P.G. (2015) Diagnosis of pancreatitis in dogs and cats. *J Small Anim Pract*, 56(1):13–26.

Ultrasonography of the Abdominal Lymph Nodes

Raquel Salgüero Fernández

INTRODUCTION

The lymph nodes are an important part of the lymphatic system, which contributes to the immune system and water homeostasis. They are small in size and therefore not visible radiographically in normal circumstances. If they are pathologically greatly enlarged, they can be visualised as soft tissue structures producing a slight/moderate mass effect depending on their location. Therefore, ultrasonography is a necessary and essential tool for the evaluation of lymph nodes, as well as to guide the collection of samples, if necessary, depending on the individual case. As a general rule, ultrasonography is a noninvasive technique that provides real-time information about the soft tissue structures in the abdomen.

ANATOMY

The lymph nodes are the structural and functional unit of the lymphatic system. They are encapsulated organs that are linked by afferent and efferent lymphatic vessels. They have two fundamental functions, namely filtering lymph and being the germinal centre for lymphocytes.

Each lymph node is composed of an external **capsule** of connective tissue; a **cortex** attached to the capsule, which is divided into the outer cortex and inner cortex (also called the paracortex) and is composed of lymphoid follicles; and the **medulla**, the central part, which is composed of lymphoid tissue.

The abdominal lymph nodes are classified into parietal and visceral. The parietal lymph nodes include the aortic and iliosacral centres, and the visceral lymph nodes are divided according to the organs they drain (Bezuidebout et al., 2012).

Parietal Lymph Nodes

Aortic Lymph Centre

This centre (Fig. 1) is composed of the following lymph nodes.

- **Aortic lymph nodes**: these small lymph nodes are located in the retroperitoneal and sublumbar space along the aorta and caudal vena cava. Owing to their small size, most are not visible ultrasonographically unless they are abnormal or pathological.
- **Renal lymph nodes**: these are small and sometimes absent. They are located adjacent to the renal vessels bilaterally.

Iliosacral Lymph Centre

The iliosacral lymph centre is located at the caudal intrapelvic sublumbar level and is composed of the medial iliac, internal iliac and sacral lymph nodes (Fig. 2).

- **Medial iliac lymph nodes**: also called external iliac. These lymph nodes are located between the external iliac arteries and the circumflex arteries. Usually, one is seen on each side of the arteries; in some cases only one is present. They drain the skin of the entire abdominal wall, and the inguinal area, colon, rectum, anus, vagina, testes, prostate, bladder, urethra, aorta and meninges.
- **Internal iliac lymph nodes**: also called hypogastric. These are usually found in pairs, but there can be up to three or four. They are located caudal to the medial iliac lymph nodes, between the internal iliac arteries. Owing to their location, which is sometimes intrapelvic, they might not be visualised on routine ultrasound examinations. They drain the sublumbar muscles, the muscles of the hindlimbs, the lumbar and sacral vertebrae, and the testes, prostate, vagina, vulva, bladder and urethra.
- **Sacral lymph nodes**: these are the most caudally located lymph nodes. When present they are always located intrapelvically, but they may not be present in 50% of cases. They are located along the middle sacral artery in the pelvic canal, so they are also not visualised during routine ultrasound examinations.

Visceral Lymph Nodes

Iliac Lymph Centre

This centre (Fig. 3) is composed of the following lymph nodes.

- **Hepatic lymph nodes**: these are located to the right and left of the portal vein, approximately 1 cm from the hepatic hilum. They drain the stomach, duodenum, pancreas and liver. They vary in number, size and shape depending on the patient.

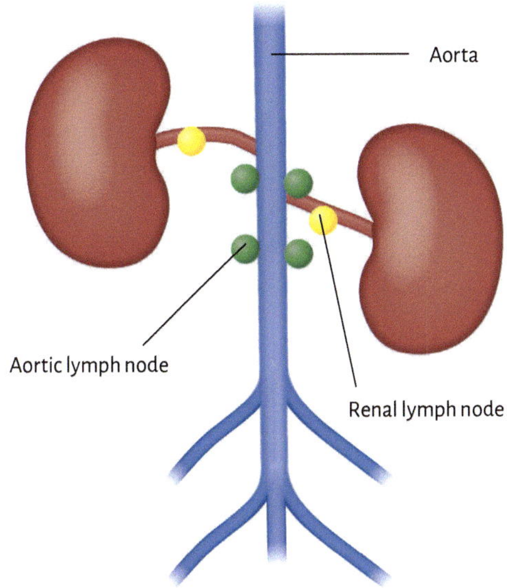

Figure 1. Diagram showing the aortic lymph centre, consisting of the renal lymph nodes (yellow circles) and the aortic lymph nodes (green).

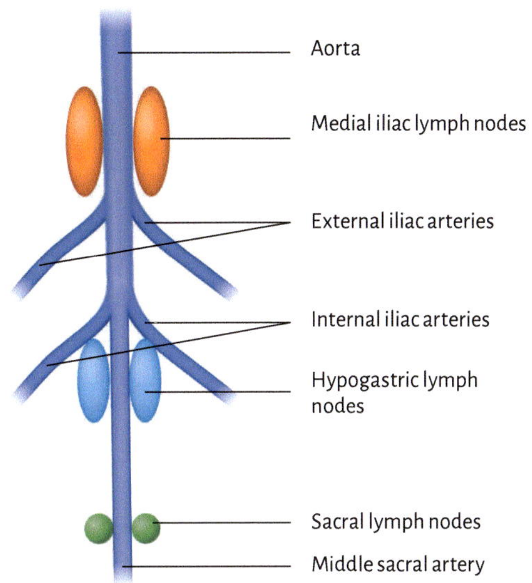

Figure 2. Diagram showing the iliosacral lymph centre, consisting of the medial iliac lymph nodes (orange ovals), the internal iliac or hypogastric lymph nodes (blue ovals) and the sacral lymph nodes (green circles).

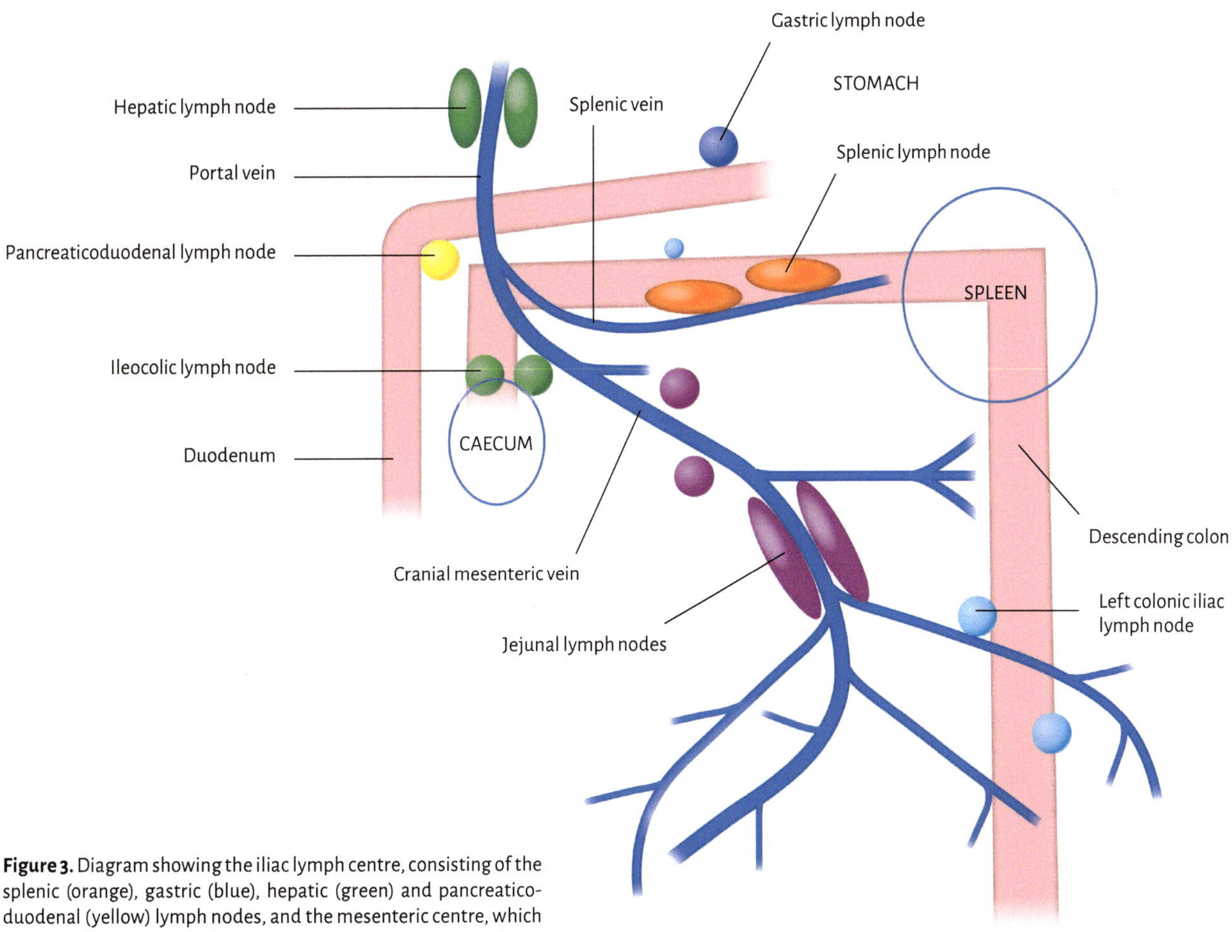

Figure 3. Diagram showing the iliac lymph centre, consisting of the splenic (orange), gastric (blue), hepatic (green) and pancreaticoduodenal (yellow) lymph nodes, and the mesenteric centre, which is composed of the jejunal (purple), ileocolic (dark green) and left colonic (light blue) lymph nodes.

- **Splenic lymph nodes**: this is a group of one or more lymph nodes along the splenic artery and vein. They drain the oesophagus, stomach, pancreas, liver, spleen, omentum and diaphragm.
- **Gastric lymph nodes**: these are located in the lesser curvature of the stomach, near the pylorus. They drain the oesophagus, stomach, diaphragm and omentum.
- **Pancreaticoduodenal lymph nodes**: these are located in the proximal area of the duodenum. They drain the duodenum, pancreas and omentum.

Mesenteric Lymph Centre

This centre (Fig. 3) is composed of the following lymph nodes.

- **Jejunal or cranial mesenteric lymph nodes**: there are multiple lymph nodes (two or three) located in the mid-abdomen along the mesenteric trunk, between the mesenteric veins and arteries. They generally have an irregular, elongated shape and are variable in size. They drain the jejunum, ileum and pancreas.
- **Colic lymph nodes**: these are located in the mesocolon and are divided into the middle, left and right colic lymph nodes. The right colic lymph node is in the dorsomedial aspect of the ascending colon at the ileocolic junction; the middle one is at the level of the transverse colon; and there are usually multiple left ones, which are located along the descending colon at the entrance to the pelvic canal. They all drain the ileum, caecum and colon.

Ultrasound Examination

Ultrasound examination of the lymph nodes should be included in all abdominal examinations. Ultrasound can even be used to evaluate the superficial and thoracic lymph nodes (which is beyond the scope of this chapter).

It is important to carry out an appropriate, comprehensive ultrasound examination, always guided by the anatomy of the different organs. The abdominal lymph nodes are deeper or more superficial depending on their location and size and the body condition of the patient, so it is important to use the most appropriate transducer in each case. Generally, a **microconvex/convex transducer** with frequencies between 8 mHz and 12 mHz should be used, or, for small dogs and cats, a higher-frequency linear transducer (10–15 mHz) (Fig. 4). In most cases, the conventional B mode is used.

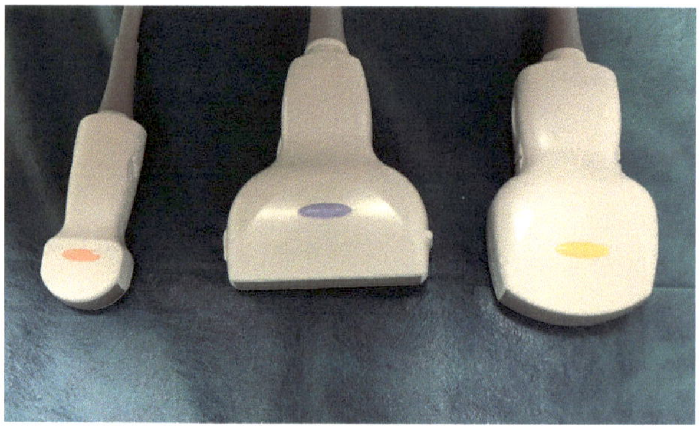

Figure 4. Examples of different ultrasound transducers (left to right: microconvex, linear and convex).

It is important to take into account that lymph nodes are sometimes not easily visualised ultrasonographically due to their echogenicity, which is similar to that of peritoneal fat, and their location adjacent to the gastrointestinal tract, which prevents their identification due to the presence of gas in the gastrointestinal tract, which produces a reverberation artefact limiting visualisation.

The lymph nodes that are visualised in most dogs and cats are the jejunal or cranial mesenteric lymph nodes, due to their larger size and their location around the mesenteric vessels, as well as the medial iliac lymph nodes. There are other lymph nodes that are not visualised on routine ultrasound examination of cats and dogs; for example, the splenic, renal and aortic lymph nodes are not usually visible, and the hepatic, gastric, renal and pancreaticoduodenal lymph nodes are seen in only some animals (Schreurs et al., 2008; Kinns, 2011).

Normal Ultrasonographic Appearance

There are multiple publications describing the normal appearance of the abdominal lymph nodes in dogs and cats, as well as differentiation between normal and pathological lymph nodes.

In this chapter, the different abdominal lymph nodes will be assessed, taking into account that most, as a rule, are homogeneous and range from isoechoic to hypoechoic compared with the adjacent abdominal fat, which makes it difficult to identify them, as mentioned above.

Factors to consider during ultrasound examination of the lymph nodes include their size, echogenicity and vascularisation.

Size

In the **dog**, there is quite a lot of variability in the normal size of the abdominal lymph nodes, although, as a rule, they should not be more than 1 cm in diameter.

- The **cranial jejunal/mesenteric** lymph nodes are usually present in pairs, although they can be multiple. They are the largest lymph nodes in the abdominal cavity and are oval in shape; they appear as elongated structures at the level of the mesenteric trunk. They are generally homogeneous in echogenicity, although some may present slight heterogeneity and be slightly hypoechoic relative to adjacent tissue or fat (d'Anjou, 2008) (Fig. 5).
  - The average normal size of these lymph nodes is 3.9 mm (range: 1.6–8.2 mm) length × 7.5 mm (range: 2.6–17 mm) diameter; they are larger in heavier and older animals (Agthe et al., 2009).
  - In most cases, vascular flow cannot be detected with colour Doppler.
- The **medial iliac** lymph nodes are usually present as pairs, with one located on each side of the iliac vessels, but single or multiple lymph nodes have also been described. They are usually spindle shaped and are identified in all dogs and most cats in normal circumstances (Mayer et al., 2010). In the author's opinion, these lymph nodes are best assessed using an acoustic window from a lateral position, to avoid abdominal fat. They have average measurements of approximately 2–4 cm long, 5 mm high and 6 mm diameter, although reported measurements vary among publications and lengths of up to 6 cm have been described in some cases (Llabrés-Díaz, 2004; Mayer et al., 2010) (Fig. 6). Citi et al. (2020) compared the length of the medial iliac lymph nodes with the diameter of the aorta to differentiate between normal and inflammatory lymph nodes, obtaining a cut-off value of 0.57 with a sensitivity of 78% and a specificity of 71%. In addition, they obtained a cut-off value of 0.69 to differentiate between normal and neoplastic lymph nodes, with a sensitivity of 89% and a specificity of 84%. However, this is not generally used in day-to-day practice.

In the **cat**, the size of the abdominal lymph nodes was described by Schreurs et al. (2008), providing a guide to their normal size: aortic 9.9 × 3.2 mm, renal 6.1 × 3.5 mm, hepatic 7.6 × 2.9 mm, splenic 8.4 × 3.2 mm, gastric 5.1 × 1.9 mm, pancreaticoduodenal 8.4 × 4.6 mm, jejunal 20.1 × 5 mm, ileocaecal 11.8 × 4.1 mm, colic 9 × 3.1 mm, medial iliac 13 × 4.5 mm, sacral 9.6 × 2.2 mm.

Colic lymph nodes can be visualised in healthy cats as circular structures; they are slightly more hypoechoic than the rest of the lymph nodes and may be surrounded by slightly reactive hyperechoic fat (Fig. 7).

In general, owing to the variation in the size of both lymph nodes and patients, the ratio of the short axis and the long axis of a lymph node (S/L ratio) can be used as a more objective measure of size; the normal ratio is 0.4 (Nyman, 2007). A ratio of <0.7 indicates that the lymph node is most likely normal or reactive. If the ratio is greater than 0.7, there may be a primary or metastatic neoplastic pathological process.

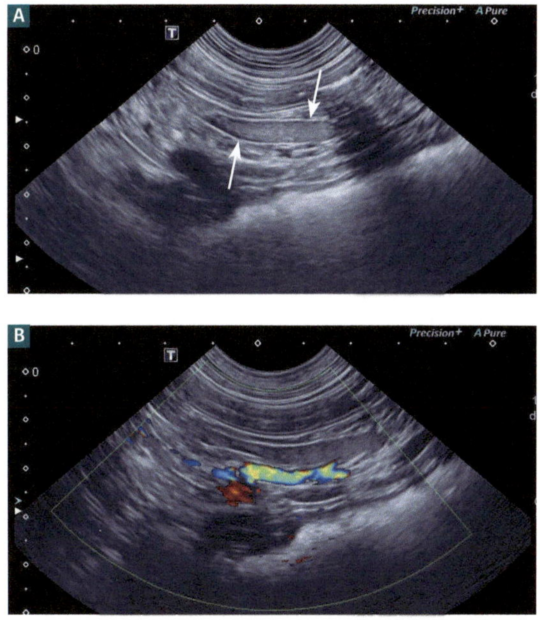

Figure 5. Ultrasound images showing a normal jejunal lymph node (arrows). **A.** B mode. **B.** Colour Doppler.

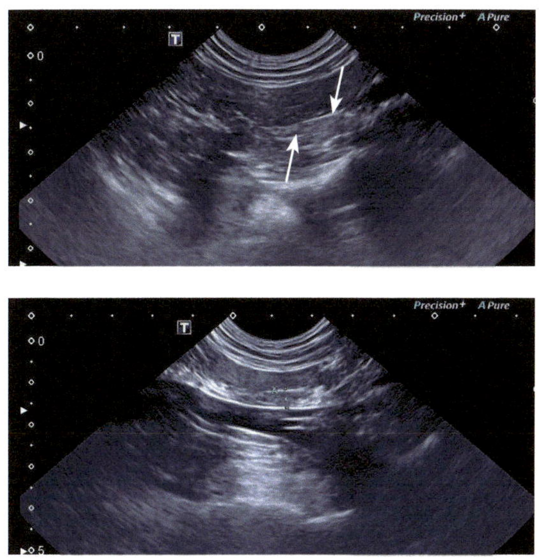

Figure 6. Ultrasound images showing the normal appearance of a medial iliac lymph node at the level of the bifurcation of the iliac arteries (arrows).

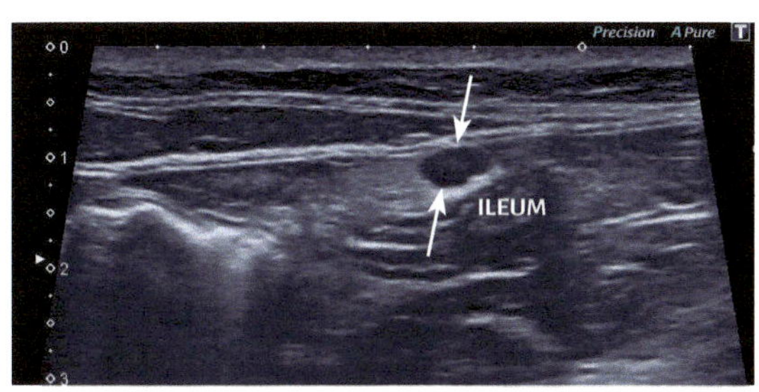

Figure 7. Ultrasound image showing an ileocaecal lymph node (arrows). Note the slight perinodal reaction.

In the author's experience, however, the S/L ratio is rarely used in day-to-day veterinary practice, and average measurements of the diameter of the lymph nodes are considered to be more useful, because their length is more variable.

Echogenicity

The echogenicity of lymph nodes is subjective and varies greatly depending on the patient and the ultrasound machine and transducer used. Normally, the lymph nodes are isoechoic or slightly hypoechoic relative to the adjacent mesenteric fat. They show a homogeneous pattern and echogenicity and, on some occasions, a thin hyperechoic capsule is observed surrounding them (Pugh, 1994).

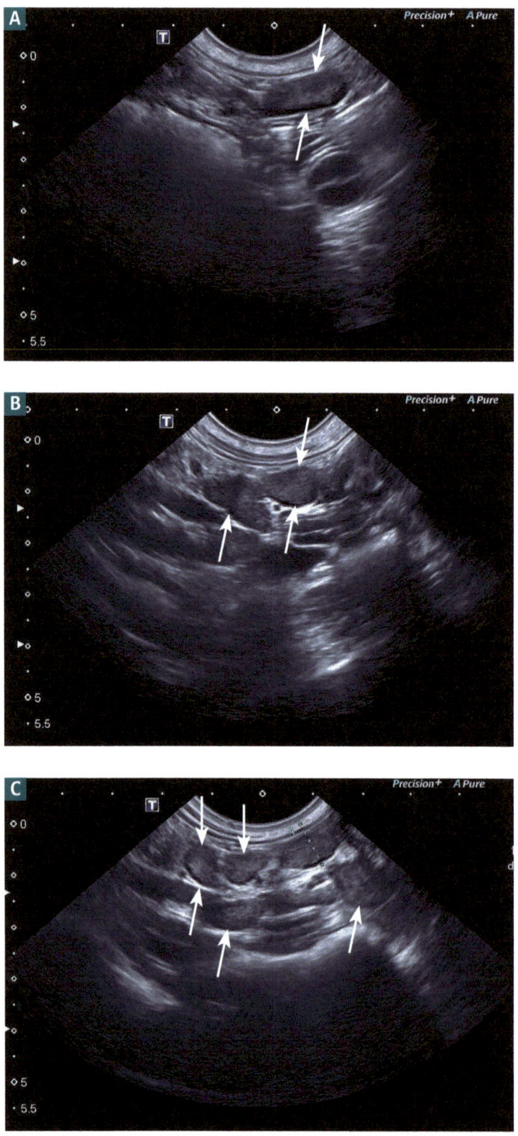

Figure 8. Images showing different ultrasonographic appearance patterns of the mesenteric lymph nodes in puppies (**A**, **B**, **C**).

In puppies, the cranial mesenteric lymph nodes have been identified as being larger than those described in adults, possibly due to their greater immunological activity, with an average length of 16.4 mm (range: 6.4–34.9 mm) and diameter of 6 mm (range: 2.3–5.7 mm). In addition, they can be of different shapes, although most are oval, and show different appearances on ultrasonography, namely homogeneously hypoechoic (66%) or centrally hyperechoic with a hypoechoic halo at the periphery (34%) (Fig. 8). However, in the case of the medial iliac lymph nodes, their size, shape and echogenicity are similar in puppies and adult dogs (length 13.6 mm, range: 7.2 × 28 mm; width 4.4 mm, range: 1.8 × 8.2 mm) (Agthe et al., 2009; Krol and O'Brien, 2012).

Vascularisation

Generally, conventional ultrasonography in B mode has higher spatial resolution, but Doppler ultrasonography allows the presence, number and distribution of vessels within the lymph node to be examined. Normal lymph nodes do not usually show vascularisation, but when they do, they have a discrete central vascularisation in the hilum area (Nyman and O'Brien, 2007).

The possibility of using spectral Doppler to determine the rates of flow in the lymphatic vessels has been investigated, with the aim of helping to differentiate between an anatomically normal, reactive or neoplastic lymph node, always taking into account other ultrasonographic characteristics such as size and echogenicity.

The Doppler indices that are determined are as follows.

- **Resistive index (RI)** = $(V_{systole} - V_{diastole}) / V_{systole}$
- **Pulsatility index (PI)** = $(V_{systole} - V_{diastole}) / V_{mean}$

Where $V_{systole}$ is the peak systolic velocity, $V_{diastole}$ is the end-diastolic velocity and V_{mean} is the mean velocity.

Prieto et al. (2009) observed a significant difference in the RI and PI values of neoplastic and nonneoplastic lymph nodes. The mean normal RI and PI for mesenteric lymph nodes were 0.58 and 0.81, respectively. For the medial iliac ones, the normal mean of RI and PI were 0.58 and 0.69, respectively.

It is important to mention that these measurements are very rarely performed in veterinary practice because some ultrasound scanners do not have Doppler and in addition, as mentioned above, the lymph nodes rarely present a vascularisation that can be measured. However, there are other characteristics that can help differentiate benign from neoplastic lymph nodes, and in most cases cytology or histology is necessary to obtain a definitive diagnosis.

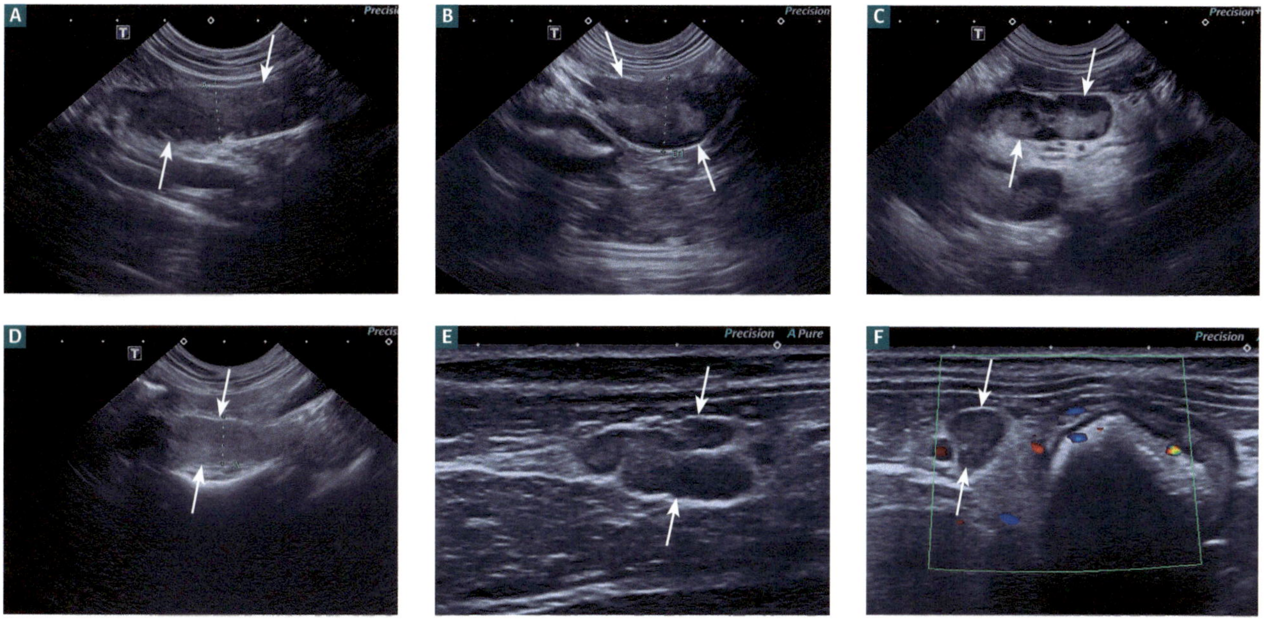

Figure 9. Ultrasound images showing reactive lymphadenopathy involving multiple lymph nodes with different patterns: medial iliac and jejunal lymph nodes in a dog with pyometra (**A**, **B**); mesenteric and medial iliac lymph nodes in a dog with inflammatory bowel disease (**C**, **D**); colic lymph node in a cat with inflammatory colitis (**E**, **F**).

Lymph Node Pathologies

The term **lymphadenopathy** refers to an increase in the size of the lymph nodes. This may be due to benign lesions, for example, reactive hyperplasia or secondary lymphadenitis due to bacterial or fungal infection, or malignant processes, such as a primary or metastatic tumour.

More often than not, the objective of an ultrasonographic examination of the lymph nodes is to be able to determine whether a process is malignant or benign. To this end, there are several ultrasonographic factors that can help with differentiation, although it must be borne in mind that none is pathognomonic and, even if there is a clinical and ultrasonographic suspicion, **cytology or histopathology is always required to obtain a definitive diagnosis.**

Inflammatory Processes

Generally, the abdominal lymph nodes are reactive secondary to an inflammatory or infectious process in the abdominal cavity, or more specifically an organ or a part of the abdomen.

Hyperplastic lymph nodes may be normal in size or slightly enlarged, with an S/L ratio <0.7. The shape and echogenicity of hyperplastic lymph nodes are usually similar to those of normal lymph nodes, although in many cases they have rounded edges and appear hypoechoic and can even have areas of intralesional necrosis that appear as intraparenchymal anechoic structures, with posterior reinforcement (De Swarte et al., 2011). According to Davé et al. (2017), it is rare to identify perinodal inflammation, but in the author's experience, perinodal mesenteric reactions are common, especially in cases of lymphadenitis (Fig. 9).

In **reactive** lymph nodes, an increase in vascularisation in the hilum due to an increase in vascular size and flow (on colour Doppler examination) and low RI and PI (on spectral Doppler) are observed.

A specific case is that of cats with feline infectious peritonitis (FIP), usually in the case of **dry FIP**, in which the lymph nodes can be very variable in shape, echogenicity and size. They may be normal in appearance, or present mild lymphadenopathy with persistence of echogenicity and shape, or show marked lymphadenopathy with rounded and very hypoechoic edges, mimicking a malignant process (Lewis and O'Brien, 2010) (Fig. 10).

Although they are not commonly encountered in Europe, **fungal lesions** should not be discounted, as well as those caused by *Mycobacterium* spp., which can affect the abdominal cavity and abdominal lymph nodes. Examples of infectious causes of lymph node pathologies are histoplasmosis (*Histoplasma* spp.), cryptococcosis (*Cryptococcus neoformans*,

Cryptococcus gatii) and mycobacteriosis (*Mycobacterium tuberculosis*); the latter is common in some areas of Europe. In these cases, generally, the lymph nodes are similar in appearance to those affected by neoplastic processes: they are large, with rounded edges, and are ultrasonographically heterogeneous but mainly hypoechoic, and may even present intralesional dystrophic mineralisation. Therefore, in areas where specific pathogens are endemic, and in the case of animals that have travelled abroad, it is important to take these pathologies into account as possible differential diagnoses (Major et al., 2016; Chávez-Peón et al., 2021; Johnston et al., 2021).

Neoplastic Processes

Staging is a very important factor that must be taken into account in oncology patients. Lymph nodes may be affected by a primary (e.g. lymphoma, histiocytic sarcoma) or secondary and metastatic (e.g. carcinoma, mastocytoma, sarcoma, melanoma) neoplastic process.

Generally, neoplastic processes affect the cortical area of the lymph node and cause an increase in size (>2 cm in diameter), with an S/L ratio >0.7 in the case of deep or abdominal lymph nodes (De Swarte et al., 2011; Nyman, 2007; Llabrés-Díaz, 2004). Neoplastic lymph nodes also show changes in shape, appearing more rounded than normal and with generally irregular edges.

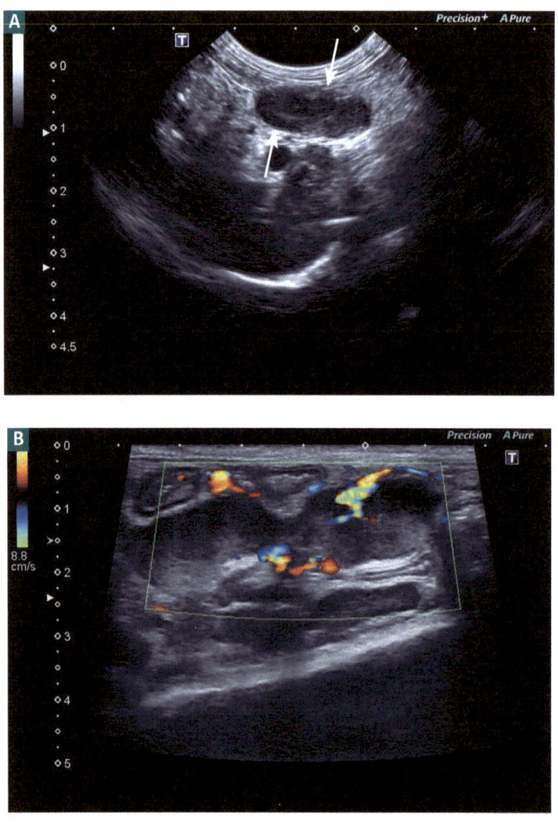

Figure 10. Ultrasound images of a cat with feline infectious peritonitis (**A**, **B**).

It is important to remember that neoplastic lymph nodes may be of normal size; likewise, lymph nodes that are greatly increased in size are not always malignant, and hence sampling is essential to obtain a definitive diagnosis.

The **echogenicity** of lymph nodes affected by neoplastic processes can be very variable, and they can range in appearance from homogeneous to heterogeneous. Although they have been described as heterogeneous in previous studies (Kinns and Mai, 2007; Davé et al., 2017), in the author's experience, most are hypoechoic and present a moderate hyperechoic perinodal reaction, especially in the case of lymphomas (Fig. 11) (Davé et al., 2017). As occurs in the case of lymphadenitis and reactive hyperplasia, neoplastic lymph nodes can contain areas of intraparenchymal necrosis (Llabrés-Díaz, 2004; De Swarte et al., 2011) (Fig. 12).

When colour Doppler is used in these cases, the vascularisation shows a heterogeneous, peripheral pattern, due to the presence of aberrant vessels that have developed as a result of angiogenesis, with a decrease in the tissue definition in the hilum, although the latter can also be observed in benign processes.

As mentioned earlier in the chapter, it has also been determined that a cut off for **RI and PI of 0.67 and 1.02**, respectively **for the medial iliac lymph nodes**, and **RI of 0.76 and PI 1.23 for the mesenteric ones**, can be used to differentiate benign from malignant nodes (Prieto et al., 2009).

In general, the following factors are suggestive of **malignancy**.

1. Increase in size.
2. Rounded shape.
3. Hypoechoic appearance.
4. Perinodal reaction.
5. Irregular vessel diameters, atypical pattern of vascularisation and branching, focal loss of vascularisation, displacement of hilum vessels and presence of subscapular vessels.

Rarely, intralesional mineralisations can be identified, for example, in cases of metastases of prostatic carcinoma or osteosarcoma.

In conclusion, abdominal ultrasonography is a very useful minimally invasive imaging technique that can be used in the veterinary setting to identify pathologies of the abdominal lymph nodes. As described throughout the chapter, there are many factors that should be considered when determining whether a lesion is malignant or benign. However, ultrasonographic findings, the patient's history and clinical signs, changes in laboratory values and, of course, cytology or histopathology of the affected lymph nodes should always be assessed in context and brought together to obtain a definitive diagnosis.

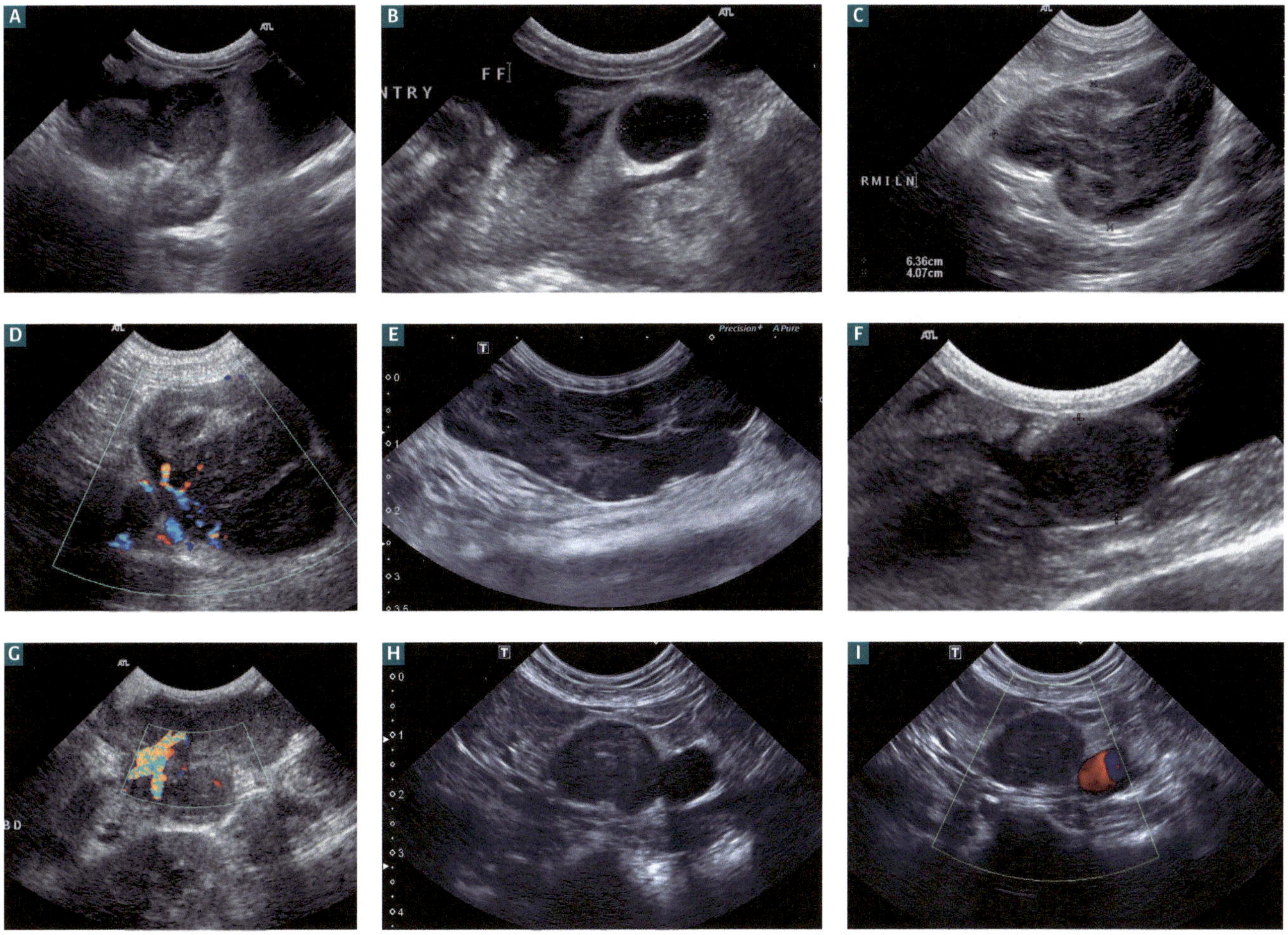

Figure 11. Ultrasound images of lymph nodes in patients with different neoplastic processes: mastocytoma (**A**, **B**), anal lymphoma (**C**, **D**), leukaemia (**E**), intestinal lymphoma (**F**, **G**) and metastasis of prostate carcinoma (**H**, **I**).

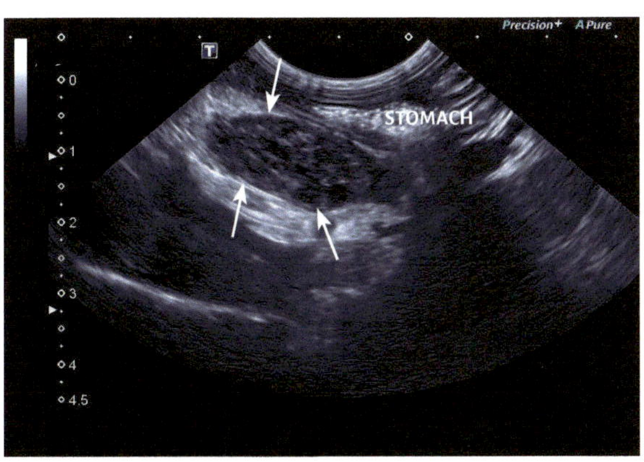

Figure 12. Ultrasound image showing lymphadenopathy with areas of necrosis and perinodal inflammation in a case of metastatic gastric adenocarcinoma (arrows).

Bibliography

- Agthe, P., Caine, A.R., Posch, B., Herrtage, M.E. (2009) Ultrasonographic appearance of jejunal lymph nodes in dogs without clinical signs of gastrointestinal disease. *Vet Radiol Ultrasound*, 50(2):195–200.
- Bezuidebout, A.J. (2012) Regional anatomy of the lymphatic system. In: Evans, H., de Lahunta, A. (eds). *Miller's Anatomy of the Dog*. 4th ed., pp. 550–555. Elsevier.
- Chávez-Peón Berle, E., KuKanich, K., Biller D. (2021) Ultrasonographic findings of gastrointestinal histoplasmosis in dogs. *Vet Radiol Ultrasound*, 62(1):108–115.
- Citi, S., Oranges, M., Arrighi, E., et al. (2020) Sonographic evaluation of medial iliac lymph nodes-to-aorta ratio in dogs. *Vet Sci*, 7(1):22.
- d'Anjou, M. (2008) Abdominal cavity, lymph nodes and great vessels. In: Penninck, D., d'Anjou, M. (eds). *Atlas of Small Animal Ultrasonography*. pp. 445–463. Blackwell Publishing.
- Davé, A.C., Zekas, L.J., Auld, D.M. (2017) Correlation of cytologic and histopathologic findings with perinodal echogenicity of abdominal lymph nodes in dogs and cats. *Vet Radiol Ultrasound*, 58(4):463–470.
- De Swarte, M., Alexander, K., Rannou, B., et al. (2011) Comparison of sonographic features of benign and neoplastic deep lymph nodes in dogs. *Vet Radiol Ultrasound*, 52(4):451–456.
- Johnston, L., Mackay, B., King, T., et al. (2021) Abdominal cryptococcosis in dogs and cats: 38 cases (2000-2018). *J Small Anim Pract*, 62(1):19–27.
- Kinns, J. (2011) Abdomen. In: Barr, F., Gaschen, L. (eds). *BSAVA Manual of Canine and Feline Ultrasonography*. pp. 72–84. BSAVA.
- Kinns, J., Mai, W. (2007) Association between malignancy and sonographic heterogeneity in canine and feline abdominal lymph nodes. *Vet Radiol Ultrasound*, 48(6):565–569.
- Krol, L., O'Brien, R. (2012) Ultrasonographic assessment of abdominal lymph nodes in puppies. *Vet Radiol Ultrasound*, 53(4):455–458.
- Lewis, K.M., O'Brien, R.T. (2010) Abdominal ultrasonographic findings associated with feline infectious peritonitis: a retrospective review of 16 cases. *J Am Anim Hosp Assoc*, 46(3):152–160.
- Llabrés-Díaz, F.J. (2004) Ultrasonography of the medial iliac lymph nodes in the dog. *Vet Radiol Ultrasound*, 45(2):156–165.
- Major, A., Holmes, A., Warren-Smith, C., et al. (2016) Computed tomographic findings in cats with mycobacterial infection. *J Feline Med Surg*, 18(6):510–517.
- Mayer, M.N., Lawson, J.A., Silver, T.I. (2010) Sonographic characteristics of presumptively normal canine medial iliac and superficial inguinal lymph nodes. *Vet Radiol Ultrasound*, 51(6):638–641.
- Nyman, H. (2012) Abdominal lymph nodes. In: O'Brien, R., Barr, F. (eds). *BSAVA Manual of Canine and Feline Abdominal Imaging*. pp. 59–75. BSAVA.
- Nyman, H.T., O'Brien, R. (2007) The sonographic evaluation of lymph nodes. *Clin Tech Small Anim Pract*, 22(3):128–137.
- Nyman, H.T., Lee, M.H., McEvoy, F.J,. et al. (2006) Comparison of B-mode and Doppler ultrasonographic findings with histologic features of benign and malignant superficial lymph nodes in dogs. *Am J Vet Res*, 67(6):978–984.
- Prieto, S., Gomez-Ochoa, P., De Blas, I., et al. (2009) Pathologic correlation of resistive and pulsatility indices in canine abdominal lymph nodes. *Vet Radiol Ultrasound*, 50(5):525–529.
- Pugh, C.R. (1994) Ultrasonographic examination of abdominal lymph nodes in the dog. *Vet Radiol Ultrasound*, 35(2):110–115.
- Schreurs, E., Vermote, K., Barberet, V., et al. (2008) Ultrasonographic anatomy of abdominal lymph nodes in the normal cat. *Vet Radiol Ultrasound*, 49(1):68–72.

Notes

Use of Doppler Techniques to Study Abdominal Pathologies

Abby Caine

THE GREAT VESSELS: AORTA AND CAUDAL VENA CAVA

Ultrasonographic study of the great vessels is important when looking for vascular pathology. It can also be very helpful when locating abdominal organs that are difficult to find because, with a good knowledge of their normal anatomy and location, they can be used as a vascular "map".

Aorta

The aorta (Fig. 1 A) is located in the dorsal retroperitoneal space, slightly to the left of the midline. In most patients, its path can be visualised from the diaphragm to the trifurcation located ventral to the caudal lumbar vertebrae. In many cases it is necessary to scan from the ventral part of the midline or the right side, because the stomach is located on the left side and therefore obscures the view. The clinically relevant anatomical branches of the abdominal aorta, from cranial to caudal, are as follows.

- The most cranial branches of the abdominal aorta are the paired **phrenicoabdominal** and **lumbar arteries**. These may be too small to be visualised ultrasonographically.
- The most cranial abdominal branches of the aorta that can be routinely visualised are two large unpaired arteries that emerge from the aorta in a ventral direction; these are the **coeliac artery**—which emerges more cranially—and the **cranial mesenteric artery**. These vessels supply most of the unpaired abdominal organs, including the liver, spleen and pancreas (which are supplied

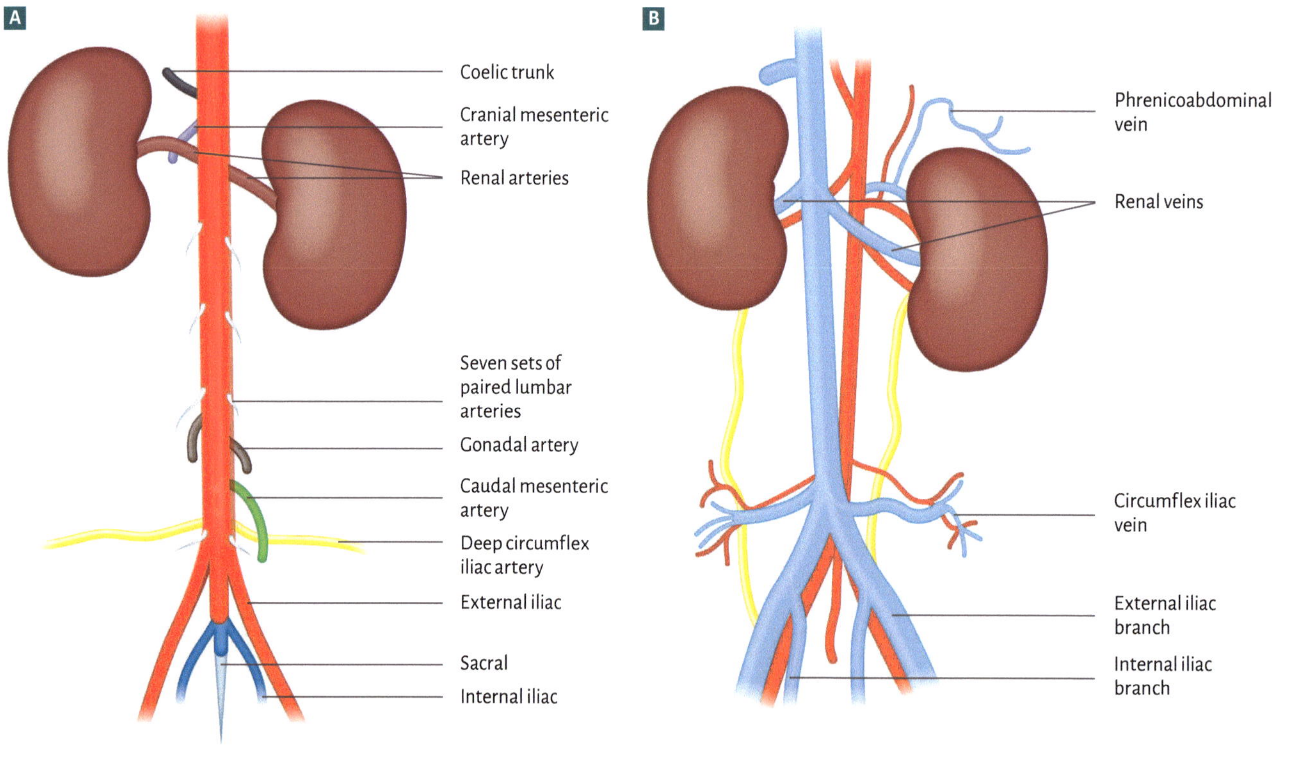

Figure 1. Anatomy of the aorta (**A**) and the caudal vena cava (**B**).

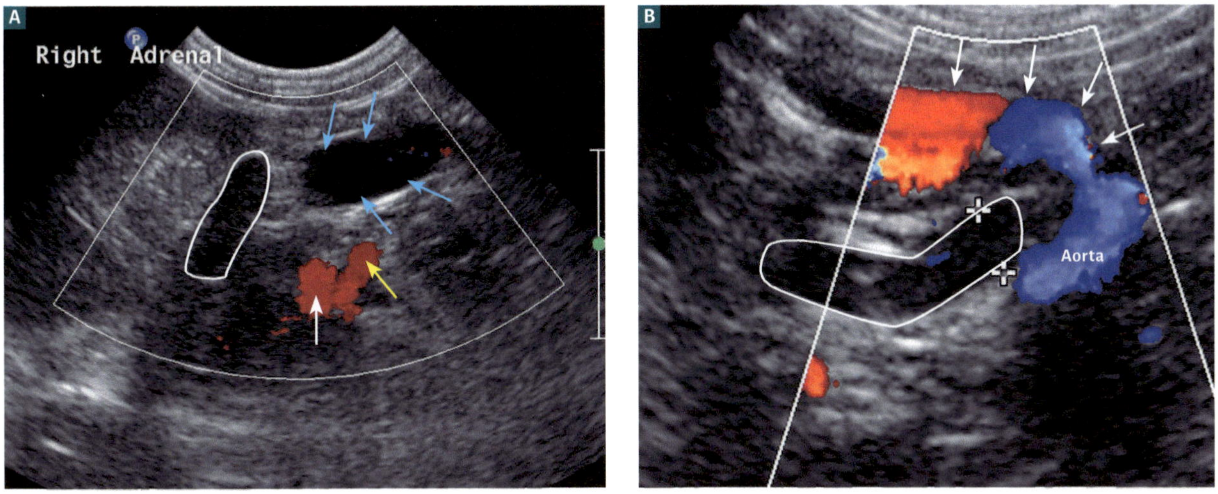

Figure 2. Use of the great vessels as a vascular "map" for locating some of the abdominal organs. **A**. The coeliac artery (white arrow) and cranial mesenteric artery (yellow arrow), which are seen as a pair of vessels in cross section immediately ventral to the aorta that run past the caudal vena cava (CVC; blue arrows), are a landmark for the right adrenal gland (outlined in white). **B**. The hook-shaped left renal artery (white arrows) can be used as a landmark as it curves from the aorta caudal to the left adrenal gland (outlined in white).

by the coeliac artery) and the gastrointestinal tract (which is supplied by the cranial mesenteric artery). It is important to know the location of these vessels and to be able to identify them for two reasons: first so that the coeliac artery is not mistaken for an anomalous vessel in cases where a portosystemic shunt is being investigated, and second because the root of both of these vessels is located close to the adrenal glands, making them a useful landmark to locate the adrenal glands (Fig. 2 A).

- The paired **renal arteries** are usually easily identified. The left renal artery has a characteristic hook shape and curves slightly caudally to the caudal pole of the left adrenal gland; this can serve as another landmark for the left adrenal gland (Fig. 2 B).
- The **gonadal arteries** are not usually identified (however, see the section later in this chapter on acquired portosystemic shunts) and nor are the small paired **lumbar arteries** that emerge from the aorta to each of the seven lumbar vertebrae. However, the paired **deep circumflex iliac arteries**, which are slightly more caudally located, are often identified in large dogs.
- The most caudal branch of the aorta can be seen at the **trifurcation**, where the aorta divides into two **external iliac arteries** and continues as a smaller terminal aorta that gives rise to the **internal iliac arteries**.

Ultrasonographic examination of the aorta is best done with the patient in right lateral recumbency, using a dorsal approach to the left side of the abdomen. However, the branches of the trifurcation and the internal iliac arteries are easier to visualise from the right side. The aortic trifurcation is a good anatomical landmark for identifying the medial iliac lymph nodes, which are located to the left and right of the trifurcation.

Caudal Vena Cava

The **caudal vena cava** (Fig. 1 B) can be visualised in the caudal retroperitoneal space, to the right of the aorta. It can be recognised without the need to use Doppler because it is more compressible than the aorta and also because of its location. It is best examined with a light touch. At the level of the kidneys, the caudal vena cava moves away from the aorta and heads ventrally to pass through the liver and the caval hiatus of the diaphragm, which is located ventrally and to the right of the aortic hiatus. Reviewing the anatomy from cranial to caudal, the abdominal portion of the caudal vena cava receives the three **hepatic veins** while it passes through the liver. From there, no more large veins emptying into the vena cava can be seen with ultrasound until the paired **renal veins**; this is important when investigating a shunt, because if an additional vessel is seen entering the vena cava between these two points it is likely to be anomalous. Usually, the small **gonadal** and **deep circumflex iliac veins** cannot be visualised. The next branch that can be identified when moving caudally is that of the **external iliac branches**, which are considered to be the termination of the caudal vena cava.

Pathologies of the Great Vessels

Ultrasound can detect the following pathologies of the great vessels: vascular invasion by neoplastic tissue, vascular anomalies and thrombi. Vascular thromboembolic disease can develop as a consequence of a triad of pathologies, termed Virchow's triad: hypercoagulability, stasis, endothelial damage

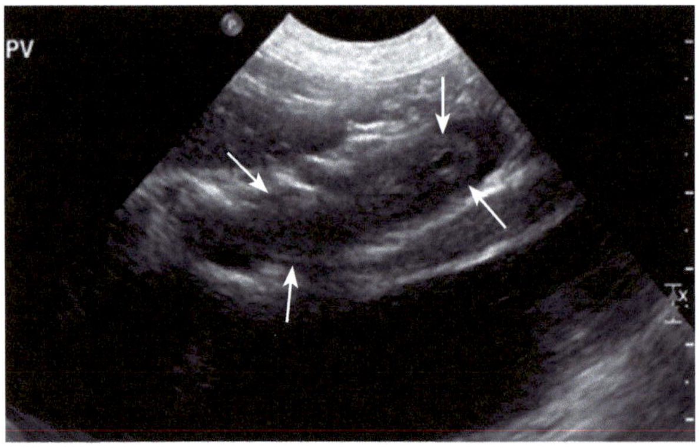

Figure 3. A thrombus at the aortic trifurcation is visualised as a slightly hyperechoic structure (arrows) filling the portal vein, surrounded by anechoic blood.

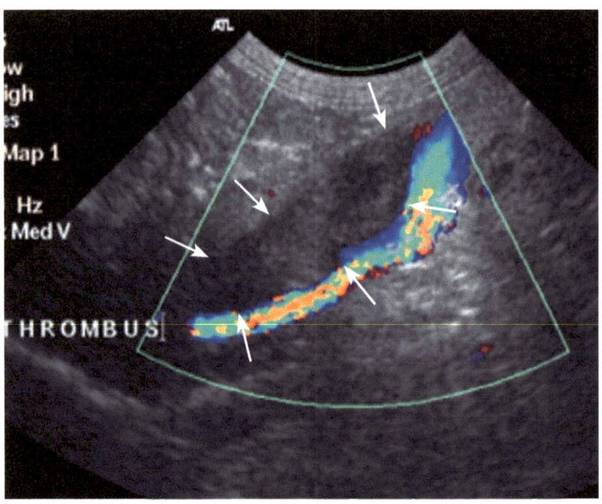

Figure 4. Tumour thrombus (arrows) from a mass in the right adrenal gland invading the caudal vena cava. Turbulent flow can be seen passing around the thrombus.

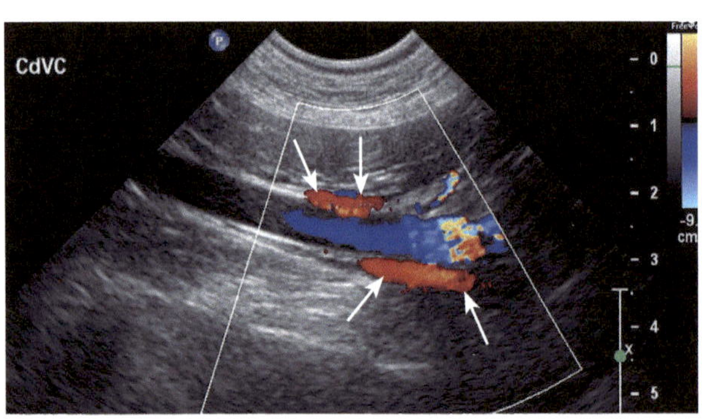

Figure 5. Duplicated caudal segment of the caudal vena cava, which is seen with red Doppler flow (arrows) on either side of the aorta, which has blue Doppler flow.

(cardiac disease, local vascular disease or injury). For this reason, any animal that is in a hypercoagulable state should be carefully examined for thromboemboli, for example, patients with immune-mediated haemolytic anaemia, neoplasia or sepsis, those that have recently undergone surgery or those that have been treated with certain drugs. On two-dimensional (2D) ultrasonographic imaging, a normal vessel should have thin echogenic walls and an anechoic (black) lumen. Colour and spectral Doppler can be used to distinguish arterial from venous blood flow. A thrombus may be seen as an echogenic structure within the vessel (Fig. 3). However, many thrombi are relatively hypoechoic, so Doppler examination can be helpful because the identification of an absence of Doppler signal in a portion of the vessel can indicate the presence of a thrombus. The classic location of a thrombus in feline aortic thromboembolic disease is at the trifurcation, and it may extend into the external iliac arteries (known as the "saddle" thrombus).

Some neoplasms will invade the local vasculature. The surgeon must be aware of this complication before surgery, in order to plan for vascular intervention as necessary. Both adrenal neoplasms (Fig. 4) and renal neoplasms can invade the caudal vena cava via their respective draining veins, so 2D and Doppler examination of the veins in these cases is mandatory.

Congenital vascular anomalies of the aorta are rare. By contrast, anomalies of the vena cava are more frequent, and are estimated to occur in 1% of the canine population, although the majority of these are clinically insignificant. In general, it is important to be able to recognise these anomalies so that they are not misdiagnosed as a more clinically significant vascular anomaly, such as a portosystemic shunt, and to avoid anatomical confusion in cases where the vascular map is incorrect. The most common anomaly of the vena cava identified by ultrasonography is duplication of the most caudal portion of the abdominal caudal vena cava; the caudal vena cava branches either immediately caudal or immediately cranial to the entry point of the renal veins. This is due to a failure of regression of the embryological left caudal vena cava during development, and is a clinically insignificant finding.

Occasionally, there may be aplasia of a more cranial portion of the abdominal caudal vena cava, for example, the segment between the renal and hepatic veins. In this case, the venous return to the heart is carried through an anastomosis to the azygos vein, which runs adjacent to the aorta through the aortic hiatus. In animals in which this occurs, the azygos vein is larger than usual. This clinically insignificant congenital malformation should not be confused with a clinically significant anomalous vessel such as a portoazygos shunt, which can also lead to enlargement of the azygos vein (Fig. 5).

Another congenital anomaly caused by abnormal embryological development of the caudal vena cava is the circumcaval ureter. This anomaly is thought to be due to the persistence of the right posterior cardinal vein (rather than the more typical persistence of the left), which results in the ureter wrapping around the caudal vena cava dorsally. Circumcaval ureter is not infrequently encountered in cats in the general population, and it is believed that there may be a higher prevalence of embryological anomalies of the vena cava in cats than in dogs. Some studies have found a slightly higher incidence of circumcaval ureter in cats with ureteral obstruction compared with cats without this vascular anomaly. It is most commonly associated with ureteral obstruction due to stricture, particularly if it affects the right ureter (Steinhaus et al., 2015). Diagnosis of this embryological anomaly by ultrasound examination is not common unless the ureter is dilated and easy to follow.

The caudal vena cava can become distended if there is an increase in pressure in the venous return system, which may be due to right-sided heart failure or to an obstruction downstream of the heart (a thrombus or mass, which is sometimes termed Budd–Chiari syndrome if the obstruction affects the hepatic veins). This often leads to ascites and oedema/congestion of the cranial abdominal organs. Therefore, if distension of the vena cava is seen, particularly if it is accompanied by ascites, cardiac and thoracic imaging should be performed. There are some breeds of dog in which the caudal vena cava is normally larger than in others (e.g. the sighthounds), so experience is needed to assess the diameter of the caudal vena cava subjectively.

Ultrasonography of the Caudal Vena Cava in Trauma Cases

In human emergency medicine, the caudal vena cava is monitored to provide a reliable estimate of the response to fluid therapy, along with assessment of the volume status and contractility using a right paracostal short-axis view (mushroom view). Published reports have described that the diameter of the caudal vena cava changes with the administration of fluids (Nelson et al., 2010) or with hypovolaemia (Cambournac et al., 2018). To detect these changes, the splenorenal window with a transverse view of the caudal vena cava and aorta is used. One study evaluated the normal variation in caudal vena cava size with breathing movements and established that both a transverse view of the caudal vena cava at the 11th–12th intercostal space and a paracostal view (e.g. the splenorenal view) obtain results that are repeatable between different observers (Darnis et al., 2018) (Fig. 6). In future, the goal should be to use ultrasonography to help calculate the volume of fluid that should be administered, and the rate of fluid administration, to achieve adequate and non-invasive fluid therapy. However, larger-scale studies need to be carried out before this technique can be applied.

Nelson et al. (2010) also used Doppler indices to evaluate the hepatic vein with pulsed-wave (PW) Doppler, and demonstrated that the waveforms changed with the administration of fluids up to the level of overhydration. Again, this technique might be useful in clinical practice in the future.

Portal Vein

The third large vessel of the abdomen that should be examined is the **portal vein** (Fig. 7). This vessel carries blood from the gastrointestinal tract, pancreas and spleen to the liver. It can be visualised in the mid-abdomen among the mesentery

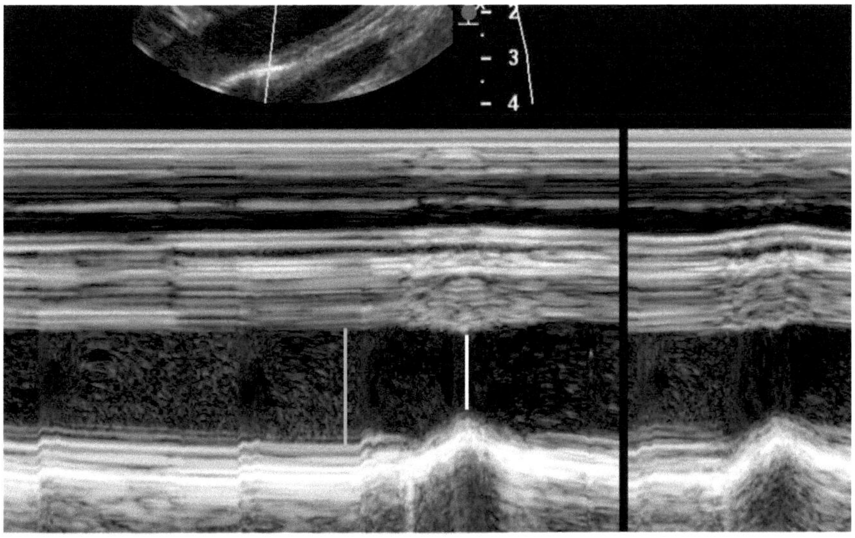

Figure 6. Transverse view of the caudal vena cava showing the variation in diameter during the respiratory cycle documented in M mode. The maximum diameter is marked in blue and the minimum diameter in white; note the difference between them.

as the cranial mesenteric vein. This becomes the portal vein when it joins the caudal mesenteric vein. Before the portal vein enters the liver at the hilum of the liver (porta hepatis), two further tributary veins join it: the splenic vein on the left side, and the gastroduodenal vein on the right. Once in the liver, it divides into left, central (a subdivision of the left) and right branches to supply the liver parenchyma.

The splenic vein is most easily visualised from the ventral or left lateral approach, by following it from the hilum of the spleen to the portal vein. The gastroduodenal vein can be visualised from the pancreatic branch, which lies within the right limb of the pancreas, following it from where it leaves the body of the pancreas to the portal vein, using a ventral or right lateral approach. The porta hepatis can be visualised from a ventral approach or through a dorsal window in the right lateral abdomen, and sometimes also intercostally, although it may be difficult to visualise if there is too much gas in the transverse colon.

When applied to the portal vein, PW Doppler has a uniform or only slightly undulating peak velocity (as opposed to the undulating peak velocity of the caudal vena cava); however, a wide range of velocities are present, giving a "dirty" appearance to the trace (see Fig. 4 in *Doppler Techniques* chapter).

The most common congenital anomalies in the portal system are **portosystemic shunts**. Portosystemic shunts are divided into **intrahepatic** and **extrahepatic** types depending on where the anomalous vessel leaves the portal vein; this distinction is important because it will determine treatment recommendations. Small breeds of dog are more likely to have extrahepatic shunts; large breeds may have either type, although intrahepatic shunts are more commonly identified in large dogs. However in reality, any dog can have any type of shunt, so a thorough examination is necessary to detect any potential anomalies.

The caudal vena cava is the vessel into which shunts most commonly terminate, and all intrahepatic shunts terminate in the caudal vena cava. It is not unusual for an **extrahepatic shunt** to enter the caudal vena cava between the renal vein and the hepatic veins, and a phrenic route for the termination of an extrahepatic shunt is also not uncommon. In this case the shunting vessel enters the vena cava immediately caudal to the diaphragm at the level of the phrenic veins; this location can be difficult to access in some patients. It is also possible for an extrahepatic portosystemic shunt to enter the caudal vena cava at another location (including in its intrathoracic portion or in one of the more caudal tributaries of the caudal vena cava, such as the external iliac veins).

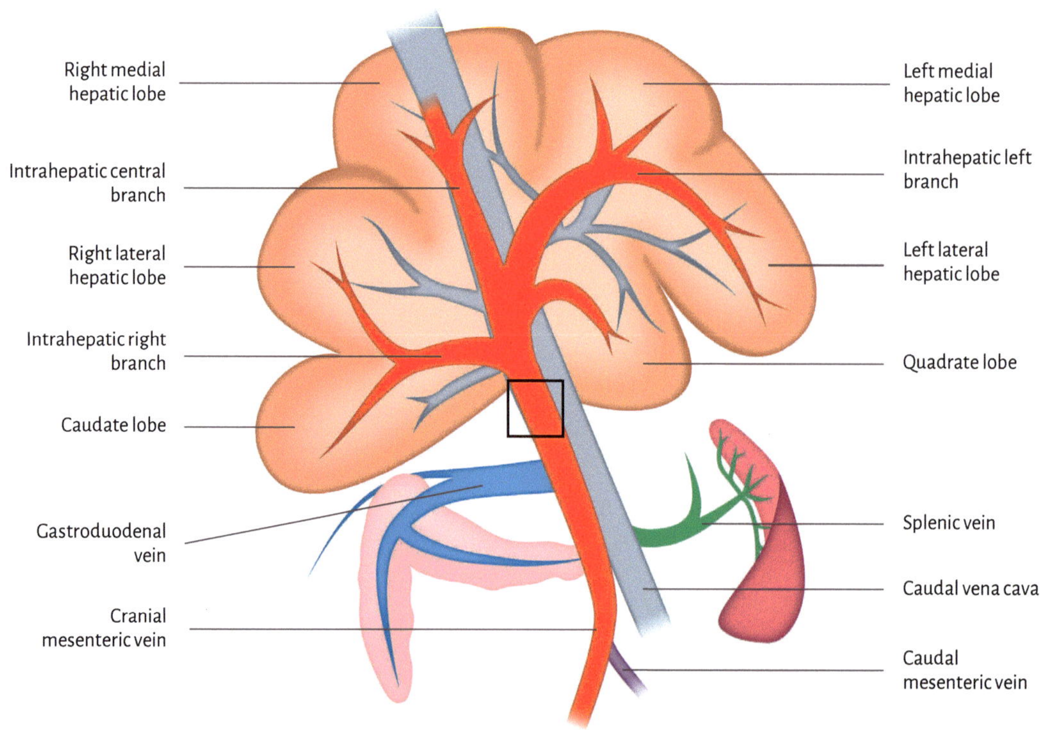

Figure 7. Schematic of the anatomy of the branches of the portal vein, shown from a ventral view. The portal vein is in red, and the porta hepatis is indicated with a black square. The tributary veins of the portal vein are also highlighted (gastroduodenal on the right side, splenic on the left, and the confluence of the cranial and caudal mesenteric veins). The right, central and left intrahepatic branches are shown superimposed on the liver lobes.

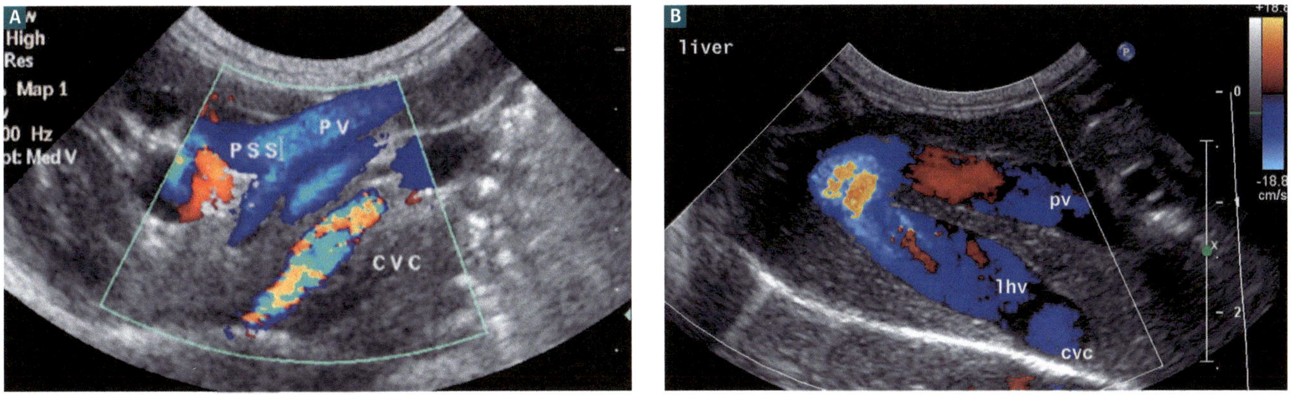

Figure 8. Examples of two congenital portosystemic shunts. **A**. A right-sided extrahepatic portosystemic shunt (PSS) arising from the portal vein (PV) just caudal to the porta hepatis. The portal vein has a reduced diameter cranial to the shunt origin. The caudal vena cava (CVC) is suspected to be the shunt termination as there is evidence of flow turbulence on colour Doppler, although the entrance of the shunt is not visualised. **B**. An intrahepatic portosystemic shunt that emerges from the left intrahepatic portal branch of the portal vein (pv), curves ventrally and enters the caudal vena cava (cvc) via the left hepatic vein (lhv).

An extrahepatic shunt could also drain into another vein, most commonly the azygos vein, although shunt terminations in other vessels, such as the internal thoracic vein, have also been described. The large variety of potential termination sites of an extrahepatic portosystemic shunt is one of the reasons why ultrasonography is not 100% effective for identifying a portosystemic shunt. However, if carried out by an experienced operator, the sensitivity for identification is over 90% (and the specificity is even higher). The accuracy of identification increases if both the termination site and the origin of the shunt are sought. The origin of the shunt will be a vessel that normally starts in the normal anatomical location of one of the portal tributaries (if extrahepatic) or branches (if intrahepatic). The vessel in which the shunt originates is usually larger than normal, and the direction of blood flow in this vessel is away from the portal vein. It is also worth noting that the diameter of the portal vein will decrease cranial to the exit of an extrahepatic portosystemic shunt, because the portal blood will "prefer" to pass through the shunt rather than through the hepatic portal bed, which is at a higher pressure. One study examined the ratio of the diameter of the portal vein at the porta hepatis to the diameter of the aorta at the same level (PV:Ao ratio), and showed that in normal dogs and cats the PV:Ao ratio is between 0.7 and 1.25, whereas in dogs and cats with extrahepatic portosystemic shunts the PV:Ao ratio is 0.65 or smaller because the portal vein is relatively smaller (d'Anjou et al., 2004). However, a reduction in portal vein diameter can also be identified with other pathologies, such as primary portal hypoplasia.

Intrahepatic portosystemic shunts have a variety of conformations. However, they can be broadly divided into a number of categories: left (those that emerge from the left intrahepatic portal branch, also termed patent ductus venosus) and right (those that emerge from the right intrahepatic portal branch). Both left and right intrahepatic shunts usually drain into the caudal vena cava through one of the hepatic veins. A central divisional shunt can also occur, although less frequently, in which the shunt enters the caudal vena cava from the ventral aspect; these shunts sometimes have a wide "window" of communication, which can make them particularly difficult to identify ultrasonographically. Fig. 8 shows examples of extrahepatic and intrahepatic shunts.

In practice, there are a number of locations that should be examined to identify a congenital portosystemic shunt. It is important for examiners to be familiar with the normal ultrasonographic appearance of the vessels, so that they can recognise whether the vessels at each location are normal or abnormal; to gain this familiarity, it is advisable to perform routine examinations of these vessels in patients that do not have portal vascular anomalies. To identify the origin of an extrahepatic portosystemic shunt, a thorough examination of the entire portal tributary system must be performed. To identify the origin of an intrahepatic portosystemic shunt, examination of the intrahepatic portal divisions is necessary. To locate the termination of the anomalous vessel, it is necessary to examine the entire caudal vena cava and azygos vein. It must be taken into account that the azygos vein is not easily identified by ultrasonography. However, the azygos vein is located next to the aorta as it passes through the aortic hiatus, and so the presence of a sizable vein passing though this hiatus should prompt suspicion of a portosystemic shunt terminating in the azygos vein. B mode examination should be used to assess whether the anatomy of the vessels is normal, and colour Doppler examination of the vessels should be performed to look for abnormal flow (particularly turbulence of the flow in the systemic vein into which the shunt deposits blood).

It is important to bear in mind that many dogs with a congenital portosystemic shunt also have a triad of abnormalities in the abdominal organs that can be identified on routine B mode ultrasound. Many of these patients have microhepatica, renomegaly and urolithiasis due to the association of portosystemic shunting with ammonium urate crystalluria.

If a portosystemic shunt cannot be identified in a patient that has clinical signs and blood test results compatible with a shunt, then it may be the case that the examiner did not detect a shunt (and another imaging modality could be considered) or that the patient has primary hypoplasia of the portal vein. This is a congenital underdevelopment of the intrahepatic portal system that cannot be identified by imaging, but can be identified by liver biopsy. On very rare occasions, there is congenital atresia or aplasia of the portal system, in which the main portal vein is usually reduced in size; this can cause portal hypertension.

Another rare congenital anomaly is the arterioportal fistula, in which there is a communication between the hepatic artery and the portal vein. This allows high-pressure arterial flow to be transmitted to the portal system, resulting in portal hypertension, which results in clinical signs of gastrointestinal disturbance and ascites in young animals. In addition to the ascites, a nidus (plexus of tortuous vessels) may be located in the liver at the location of the fistula, and hepatofugal flow might be demonstrated on spectral Doppler evaluation of the portal vein.

Portosystemic shunts can also be acquired secondary to portal hypertension, which in turn can be caused by many chronic liver diseases, including chronic hepatitis, neoplasia or nodular regeneration, or by portal vein diseases, such as arteriovenous fistulae, hypoplasia or thrombosis of the portal vein. The increase in pressure causes collateral vessels to open, allowing the portal system to drain into the central venous system. Multiple small tortuous vessels (varices) are seen; the most common location where these can be detected by ultrasonography is near the left renal and left gonadal veins, as a termination of a larger splenogonadal collateral vessel. Shunts may also be identified in other locations, for example, larger splenophrenic shunts, or as varices around the terminal oesophagus, colon, phrenic vein, duodenum or gallbladder. These patterns of multiple small shunting vessels can be found in relatively consistent locations, so both the different clinical presentations and the imaging findings help differentiate between acquired shunts and a congenital portosystemic shunt (which is usually solitary). However, occasionally a larger collateral vessel (such as a splenogonadal shunt) may be identified, and this can cause confusion. It is essential to be able to distinguish between a congenital shunt and a larger acquired collateral shunt, because surgical attenuation of an acquired shunt will cause marked portal hypertension, which can potentially be fatal. Generally, with acquired portosystemic shunts there is an underlying cause of hepatic or portal disease as well as ascites and reduced portal blood flow (mean flow less than 10 cm/s), although in some cases reduced portal blood flow cannot be demonstrated at the point at which the collateral vessels open. The normal mean portal flow is 10–18 cm/s in the cat and 18 ± 7 cm/s in the dog. To measure the mean portal flow, the spectral PW Doppler gate should be opened wide to include the entire vessel, and flow correction performed if necessary. Some ultrasound machines can calculate the mean flow automatically; however, others cannot, and when using these devices it is necessary to obtain the peak flow with the gate in the centre of the portal vein and then estimate the mean as 0.57 times the peak flow.

In any disease that results in a hypercoagulable state, thrombosis may develop in the portal vein or in one of its tributary veins. Sometimes, this does not cause any clinical signs; however, signs of portal hypertension, such as acquired shunting and ascites, may develop. In some longstanding portal obstructions with a portal thrombus, portoportal collateral vessels develop to bypass the obstruction; these can be in the form of short collateral vessels around the thrombus or longer collateral pathways via the gallbladder, which again can be seen as a collection of small tortuous vessels. In rare cases, portal vein aneurysms can be identified; these have been described to be accompanied by portal vein thrombi and/or collaterals.

Doppler of the Abdominal Organs

The vessels of the parenchymal organs can be interrogated with Doppler. Colour Doppler is a useful technique to observe the presence and distribution of vascular flow within an organ. It has many applications, ranging from locating normal structures, to confirming whether a tubular structure is a vessel or not (e.g. in cases where the tubular structure is a pathological dilation of the biliary tract or a ureter), to identifying whether an organ has adequate vascularisation (e.g. following infarction or trauma). It is also useful when planning an invasive sampling procedure, to verify that there are no blood vessels along the proposed approach to the structure to be sampled. Furthermore, there are data, particularly for lymph nodes, to suggest that an alteration of the normal vascular distribution along the central hilum can help differentiate reactive and neoplastic pathologies.

Power Doppler

Power Doppler is another method for determining the flow within vessels that can be superimposed on a standard 2D

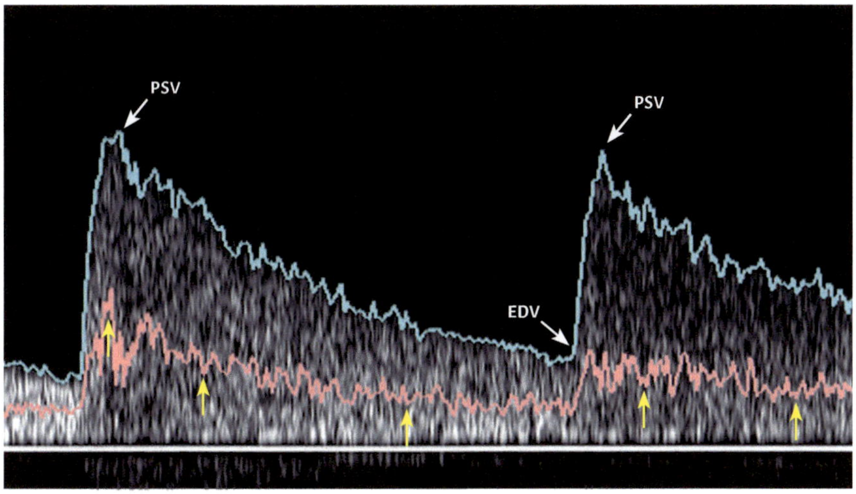

Figure 9. A pulsed-wave Doppler trace of the renal artery, indicating the mean velocity trace from which the time-averaged mean velocity is calculated (yellow arrows), the peak systolic velocity (PSV) and the end-diastolic velocity (EDV).

image; however, this technique has some differences in terms of the underlying physics. It is used to identify vessels that have a very low flow velocity. Standard Doppler requires determination of the velocity and the direction of phase shifts in the returning echo from each gate (from each pixel when superimposed on the 2D image). Power Doppler, by contrast, detects the total amplitude (strength) of all the Doppler signal present, regardless of the frequency shift. This improves sensitivity, at the cost of not having any quantitative information or information on the direction of the blood flow. This makes power Doppler the best technique if there is slow flow. This technique is not greatly affected by the Doppler angle (see Chapter 3), it allows noise from the tissues to be distinguished from blood vessels, and aliasing is not a problem because only the intensity in the shift of frequency of the returning echoes is measured, not their amplitude.

However, power Doppler is more sensitive to the artefactual effects of motion, such as the movement of the patient (including its breathing) and of the transducer. It should be used when the patient is still and there is a need to examine the microvascular architecture of an organ – for example, the distribution of vessels inside a lymph node, or to detect areas of necrosis in a pancreas that has severe acute pancreatitis. Some authors have suggested that it also helps to detect ureteral jets.

Specific Doppler Indices

Using a Doppler waveform, acquired by spectral Doppler from a PW Doppler gate within a vessel, allows calculations to be performed that allow further quantitative assessment of the physiology of the vessel beyond what can be assessed from the overall velocity.

These calculations are based on the factors that influence the waveform of the flow of blood in a vessel:

- **resistance** in the vessel, which is determined by cardiac function and the anatomical location of the vessel
- **variation in pressure** in the vessel, which is determined by its physiological state, which in turn is dependent on the need for blood in the organ that it supplies.

Doppler indices use several points along the waveform to calculate two indices that give an estimation of the physiological function of the "downstream organ" – the **resistive index** (RI) and **pulsatility index** (PI). Both indices are proportions and are not influenced by the Doppler angle, so they can be used on smaller and more tortuous vessels more accurately than a measure of velocity alone. The points on the Doppler waveform that are relevant for calculating the Doppler indices are shown in Fig. 9.

Resistive Index

The RI is a measure of the resistance to flow of the vascular bed downstream from the measured artery (which is actually a combination of vascular resistance and compliance). It is calculated as follows:

$$\mathbf{RI = V_{systole} - V_{diastole} / V_{systole}}$$

Where $V_{systole}$ is the peak systolic velocity and $V_{diastole}$ is the end-diastolic velocity. Using this formula, we can see that:

Resistivity Index	Description
0	Continuous nonpulsatile flow
1	Systolic flow without diastolic flow
>1	Reversed diastolic flow

The RI is widely used in human medicine to assess the umbilical artery, as a measure of placental insufficiency, and is also used to monitor the status of the kidneys, particularly after a kidney transplant. Several uses of the RI have been published in the veterinary field, as detailed in the next section. It is often assessed in combination with the PI.

Pulsatility Index

The PI is, in some ways, a more accurate means of estimating the difference between peak (maximum) and trough (minimum) flow because it also takes into account the mean velocity.

$$PI = V_{systole} - V_{diastole} / V_{mean}$$

Generally, the time averaged mean velocity (V_{mean}) is calculated by the ultrasound machine and superimposed on the Doppler trace.

Veterinary Applications of Doppler Indices

The normal RI and PI of the kidneys have been determined in both dogs and cats. Novellas et al. (2007) recorded normal values for the kidney and eye. It should be noted that several systemic factors have been shown to affect the RI and PI of the kidneys, such as systemic hypotension, a low heart rate, and fluid accumulation in the subcapsular or perirenal area. This study suggested an upper limit of normal interrenal artery RI of 0.72 in unsedated dogs and 0.7 in unsedated cats, and a PI of 1.52 in unsedated dogs and 1.29 in unsedated cats. Values for these indices measured in the eye have been shown to be lower if several anaesthetic agents are used (e.g. butorphanol, medetomidine and ketamine).

Most authors have reported that the left and right kidneys have the same RI. However, a single study (Tipisca et al., 2016) found that in healthy cats the left kidney had a higher RI (0.59 ± 0.08) than the right kidney (0.54 ± 0.07). An increase in RI is a nonspecific finding and has been observed in cases of acute obstruction, acute kidney injury, acute tubular necrosis, perinephric glomerulonephritis, subcapsular fluid accumulation and severe hypotension. One study (Matos et al., 2018) has suggested a cut-off RI value of 0.639 to distinguish between normal cats and cats with chronic kidney disease. A difference in RI between the two kidneys has been suggested to indicate unilateral disease even if both values are within the normal range.

In practice, these indices are used very little in veterinary medicine compared with their use in human medicine. The most frequent application of Doppler indices in the kidney is in the study of ureteral obstruction. An early study (Nyland et al., 2005) in dogs with surgically induced unilateral renal obstruction reported that a measurement of RI above 0.7 was 73% sensitive and 77% specific for obstruction, although the study had only a small number of cases (Fig. 10). It has been proposed that the sensitivity of this technique might be increased if mannitol is administered to induce diuresis.

Doppler indices were also used in the assessment of lymph nodes in the study of Nyman et al. (2005). This study showed that cut-off values of 0.68 for RI and 1.49 for PI were most useful to discriminate between benign (reactive) enlarged superficial lymph nodes and malignant lymph nodes (Fig. 11).

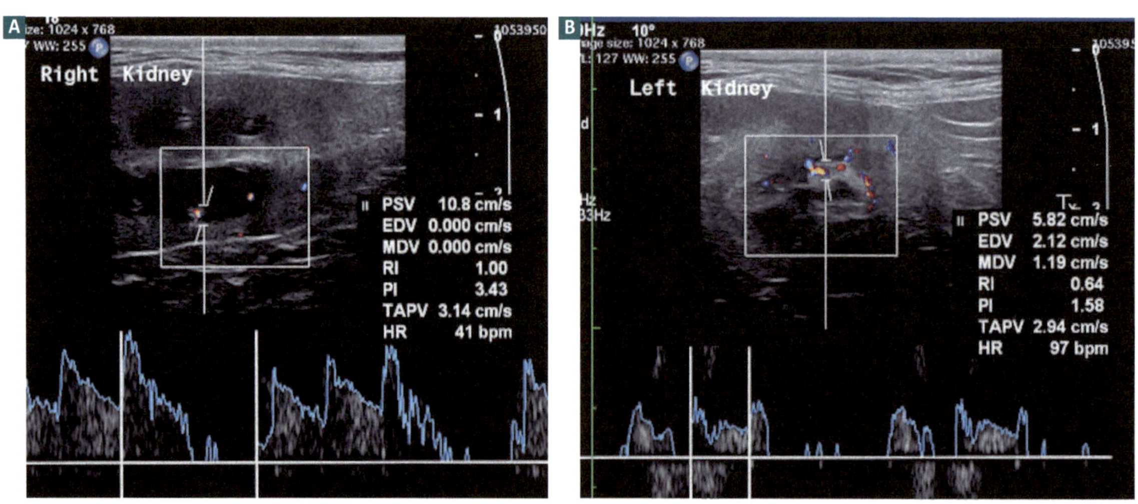

Figure 10. Example of the use of the resistive index (RI) for the kidney (arcuate arteries). This cat had bilateral ureteroliths, with a suspicion of more severe obstruction on the right (since more distension was seen proximal to the ureter and not immediately distal to it). The RI of the right kidney was increased to 1 (**A**), whereas the RI of the left kidney had a normal value of 0.64 (**B**).

These indices were easier to obtain from malignant lymph nodes than normal nodes. There was a classification error of 11% if one of the Doppler indices (PI) was combined with the vascular distribution (malignant nodes did not have vascular flow, only through a central hilar vessel) and the shape of the lymph node (malignant nodes were more rounded, based on the ratio of their short- to long-axis measurements). Although this is not a detailed enough assessment to confirm whether or not a lymph node is malignant, it could help to guide when fine-needle aspirates need to be obtained.

Several other uses of Doppler ultrasound and indices have been described in the veterinary literature; however, these are not currently widely used in everyday clinical practice. These include transcranial Doppler (through fontanelle and temporal windows) of the rostral and caudal cerebral arteries; differences in the values of Doppler indices in the umbilical artery in dogs, as a measure of foetal distress, between normal birth and caesarean delivery; and the increase in RI and PI in the eyes of Beagles with hereditary primary open-angle glaucoma.

Although there are no published studies that show that Doppler indices alone can be used to identify pathologies, they can be used together with other ultrasonographic findings to contribute to an imaging diagnosis.

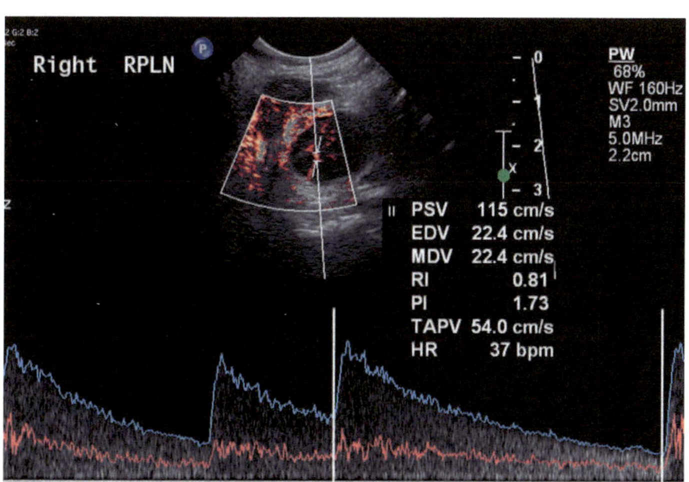

Figure 11. Resistive index (RI) and pulsatility index (PI) above the cut-off values that indicate malignancy in a vessel supplying a lymphomatous lymph node.

Bibliography

Doppler and the Great Vessels

■ Bertolini, G. (2019) Anomalies of the portal venous system in dogs and cats as seen on multidetector-row computed tomography: an overview and systematization proposal. *Vet Sci*, 6(1):10.

■ Cambournac, M., Goy-Thollot, I., Violé, A., Boisvineau, C., Pouzot-Nevoret, C., Barthélemy, A. (2018) Sonographic assessment of volaemia: development and validation of a new method in dogs. *J Small Anim Pract*, 59(3):174–182.

■ d'Anjou, M.A., Penninck, D., Cornejo, L., Pibarot, P. (2004) Ultrasonographic diagnosis of portosystemic shunting in dogs and cats. *Vet Radiol Ultrasound*, 45(5):424–437.

■ Darnis, E., Boysen, S., Merveille, A.C., Desquilbet, L., Chalhoub, S., Gommeren, K. (2018) Establishment of reference values of the caudal vena cava by fast-ultrasonography through different views in healthy dogs. *J Vet Intern Med*; 32(4):1308–1318.

■ Kitrell, D., Berkwitt, L. (2012) Hypercoagulability in dogs: pathophysiology. *Compend Contin Educ Vet*, 34(4):E1–5.

■ Lamb, C. (2005) Doppler ultrasound examination in dogs and cats: 2. Abdominal applications. *In Practice*, 27(5):238–247.

■ Lamb, C., Boswood, A. (2005) Doppler ultrasound examination in dogs and cats: 1. The principles. *In Practice*, 27(4):183–189.

■ Lamb, C.R. (1998) Ultrasonography of portosystemic shunts in dogs and cats. *Vet Clin North Am Small Anim Pract*, 28(4):725–753.

■ Nelson, N.C., Drost, W.T., Lerche, P., Bonagura, J.D. (2010) Noninvasive estimation of central venous pressure in anesthetized dogs by measurement of hepatic venous blood flow velocity and abdominal venous diameter. *Vet Radiol Ultrasound*, 51(3):313–323.

■ Spaulding, K.A. (1997) A review of sonographic identification of abdominal blood vessels and juxtavascular organs. *Vet Radiol Ultrasound*, 38(1):4–23.

■ Specchi, S., d'Anjou, M.A., Carmel, E.N., Bertolini, G. (2014) Computed tomographic characteristics of collateral venous pathways in dogs with caudal vena cava obstruction. *Vet Radiol Ultrasound*, 55(5):531–538.

■ Steinhaus J, Berent, A.C., Weisse, C., Eatroff, A., Donovan, T., Haddad, J., Bagley, D. (2015) Clinical presentation and outcome in cats with circumcaval ureters associated with a ureteral obstruction. *J Vet Intern Med*, 29(1):63–70.

■ White, R.N., Shales, C., Parry, A.T. (2017) New perspectives on the development of extrahepatic portosystemic shunts. *J Small Anim Pract*, 58(12):669–677.

Doppler Indices

■ Gelatt-Nicholson, K.J., Gelatt, K.N., MacKay, E.O., Brooks, D.E., Newell, S.M. (1999) Comparative Doppler imaging of the ophthalmic vasculature in normal beagles and Beagles with inherited primary open-angle glaucoma. *Vet Ophthalmol*, 2(2):97–105.

■ Granata, A., Zanoli, L., Clementi, S., Fatuzzo, P., Di, Nicolò, P., Fiorini, F. (2014) Resistive intrarenal index: myth or reality? *Br J Radiol*, 87(1038):20140004.

■ Matos, I., Azevedo, P., Carreira, L.M. (2018) Pilot study to evaluate the potential use of the renal resistive index as a preliminary diagnostic tool for chronic kidney disease in cats. *J Feline Med Surg*, 20(10):940–947.

■ Novellas, R., Espada, Y., Ruiz de Gopegui, R. (2007) Doppler ultrasonographic estimation of renal and ocular resistive and pulsatility indices in normal dogs and cats. *Vet Radiol Ultrasound*, 48(1):69–73.

■ Nyland, T.G., Fisher, P.E., Doverspike, M., Hornof, W.J., Olander, H.J. (2005) Diagnosis of urinary tract obstruction in dogs using duplex Doppler ultrasonography. *Vet Radiol Ultrasound*, 34(5):348–352.

■ Nyman, H.T., Kristensen, A.T., Skovgaard, I.M., McEvoy, F.J. (2005) Characterisation of normal and abnormal canine superficial lymph nodes using gray scale B mode, colour flow mapping, power and spectral Doppler ultrasonography: a multivariate study. *Vet Radiol Ultrasound*, 46(5):404–410.

■ Tipisca, V., Murino, C., Cortese, L., Mennonna, G., Auletta, L., Vulpe, V., Meomartino, L. (2016) Resistive index for kidney evaluation in normal and diseased cats. *J Feline Med Surg*, 18(6):471–475.

Notes

Thoracic Imaging

Radiography and Computed Tomography of the Thoracic Cavity: Pathologies of the Pulmonary Parenchyma, Pleural Cavity and Thoracic Wall

Vicente Esteve Bernet

Introduction

Thoracic radiography is a very important technique in the diagnosis of thoracic and systemic diseases. It is low cost, fast and available in most veterinary practices. Although it is a widely used technique, thoracic radiographs can sometimes be difficult to interpret, mainly due to overlapping structures, variations among breeds and similarity in the radiographic characteristics of different diseases. Quality radiographs are essential to reduce interpretation-related problems.

When obtaining thoracic radiographs, animals should preferably be sedated or under general anaesthesia. The main problem with the use of sedation is respiratory depression, which causes inhalations with incomplete expansion of the lungs. In cases where greater detail of the pulmonary field is needed, such as when searching for pulmonary metastases, it is recommended to use general anaesthesia and to take radiographs during inspiration when using positive-pressure ventilation. Alternatively, computed tomography (CT) can be performed, and is the recommended option in certain cases.

Radiographic Projections

At least two orthogonal projections should always be taken, preferably right lateral and dorsoventral (DV) or ventrodorsal (VD), and, if possible, three projections (DV or VD, right lateral and left lateral). Radiographs should always be taken during the inspiratory phase.

The sedated animal is positioned more easily in sternal recumbency (for the DV projection) than in dorsal recumbency. In addition, in patients with cardiac disease the DV projection is recommended because the patient remains more stable and the pulmonary vessels are better visualised surrounded by gas in the lungs, although there is a slight magnification effect.

It is important to perform the DV or VD projection first and then the lateral projections to avoid atelectasis, especially in sedated animals that may remain recumbent for long periods of time, and in obese animals.

Positioning and Collimation

The patient should be positioned with the help of sandbags (which should not appear in the collimated area) and foam blocks (Figs. 1 and 2).

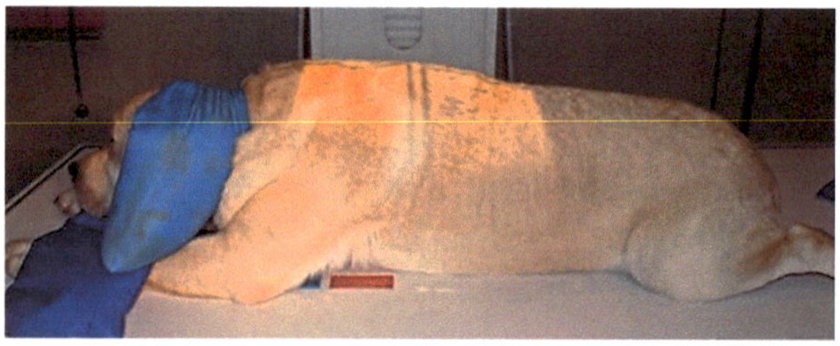

Figure 1. Positioning in sternal recumbency (DV projection) with a support (preferably foam) under the head and a long sandbag over the neck, ensuring that the weight is towards the ends to avoid causing breathing problems. In deep-chested animals, foam wedges attached by straps or sacks laterally to the shoulders can be used to provide greater support.

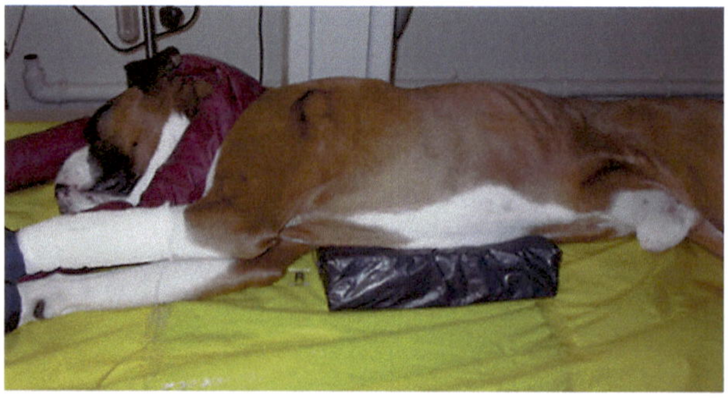

Figure 2. Positioning in right lateral recumbency with long sandbags on the extremities and neck and a foam wedge under the sternum. The forelimbs should be extended. Image courtesy of Alisa Dean, Small Animal Teaching Hospital, University of Liverpool.

When taking lateral projections, a foam wedge should be placed under the animal's sternum to achieve alignment of the spine and sternum. The forelimbs should be extended cranially to avoid overlap of the forelimb muscles with the cranial part of the thorax. The head should be placed on a block of foam and fixed in position with a sandbag surrounding it.

Correct collimation (Fig. 3) is very important and should be **from the shoulder joint to the last rib**. In some cases, with very large animals, dividing the thorax into cranial and caudal parts is necessary, which doubles the number of radiographs to be taken.

Alternative Projections

Horizontal beam radiographs may also be performed in certain cases, particularly in animals with serious respiratory problems that do not tolerate lateral recumbency (in which case the animal is placed in sternal recumbency) or in the case of polytraumatised animals with suspected vertebral fractures (where rotation should be avoided before a diagnosis is made). The horizontal X-ray beam can also be used to detect small volumes of air (pneumothorax) or free fluid (pleural effusion) with the animal placed in lateral recumbency.

Exposure Parameters

In general, for thoracic radiography, a high kilovoltage (kV) and low milliamperage by time (milliampere seconds; mAs) should always be used, with high milliamperage (mA) and a low exposure time (s).

The antiscatter grid should be used for animals with a thorax more than 10 cm thick to reduce the effects of scattered radiation on the radiograph.

Systematic Evaluation of Thoracic Radiography

Once the radiographs have been taken, it is important to use a systematic protocol for their evaluation. There is no single universally established protocol, but it is important to always follow the same protocol on an individual basis. A protocol governed by the anatomical structures is recommended, first assessing the external part of the thorax and then assessing the inside of the thoracic cavity and its structures.

A logical order for evaluation of the structures would be as follows:

- musculoskeletal system (includes the vertebrae, ribs, sternebrae, visible long bones and soft tissue/musculature)
- skin
- visible part of the abdomen and diaphragm
- visible part of the neck
- cardiac silhouette
- lung and pulmonary vessels
- large vessels (aorta and vena cava)
- trachea and bronchi
- remaining part of the mediastinum
- pleurae and pleural space.

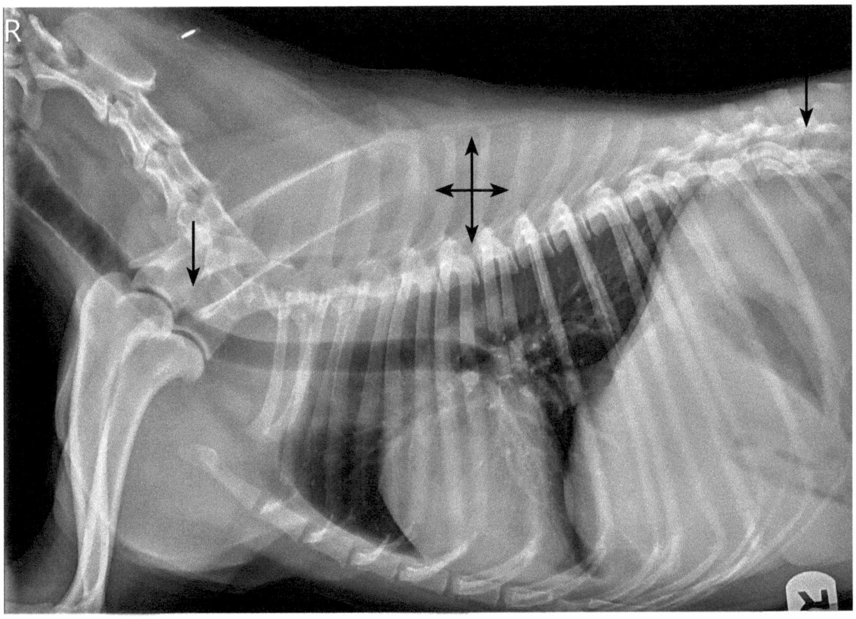

Figure 3. Left lateral thoracic radiograph. The black arrows indicate collimation from the shoulder joint to the last rib. The four-headed arrow indicates the location where the collimation is centred.

Identification of Radiographic Projections

Right Lateral

The right diaphragmatic crus is displaced more cranially than the left crus. The crura usually appear parallel. The continuation of the caudal vena cava with the right crus (caval foramen) (Fig. 4 A) can be seen.

Left Lateral

The left diaphragmatic crus is displaced more cranially than the right crus. The crura are often crossed in a "Y" shape. The caudal vena cava is observed overlapping the left crus (Fig. 4 B).

Dorsoventral

The diaphragmatic dome is observed as the only bulge on this projection. In the stomach, gas is observed in the fundus (Fig. 5 A).

Ventrodorsal

The crura and the dome of the diaphragm are observed as three humps. In the stomach, gas is observed in the body (Fig. 5 B).

In addition, whether the radiograph has been taken in the complete inspiratory phase or not should be evaluated, since the opacity of the lung and the relative cardiac size can vary without being pathological. Among other differences, in the lateral inspiratory projection, the lumbodiaphragmatic recess reaches the level of thoracic vertebra T12. In addition, on this projection the space between the diaphragm and the cardiac silhouette is minimal or nonexistent, and the caudal vena cava follows a horizontal pathway. In the expiratory projection, the lumbodiaphragmatic recess is level with T11. The diaphragm also appears to overlap the cardiac silhouette (left ventricle) and the caudal vena cava follows a caudally ascending pathway. In the DV projection, the diaphragmatic dome

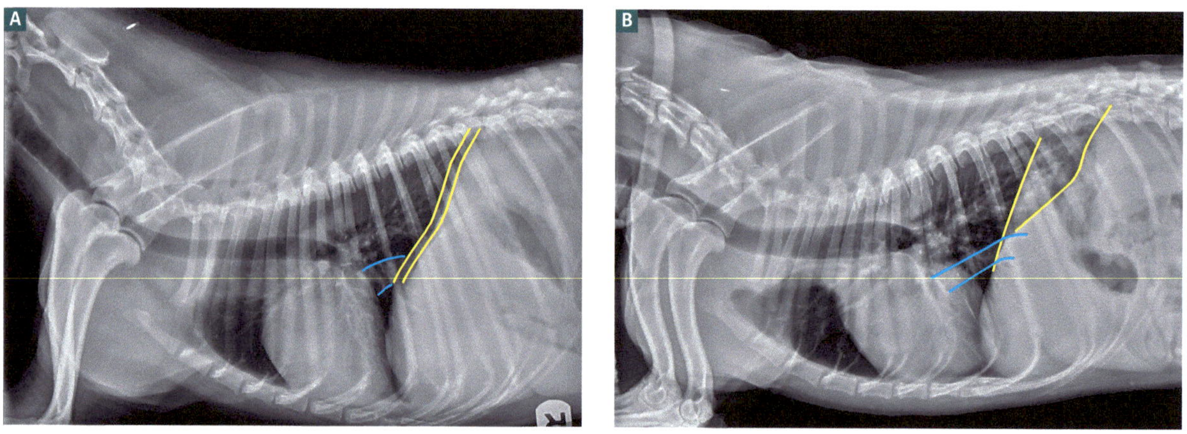

Figure 4. Right lateral (**A**) and left lateral (**B**) radiographs of the thorax of a dog. The diaphragmatic crura are outlined in yellow, the caudal vena cava in turquoise and the gastric fundus in dark blue.

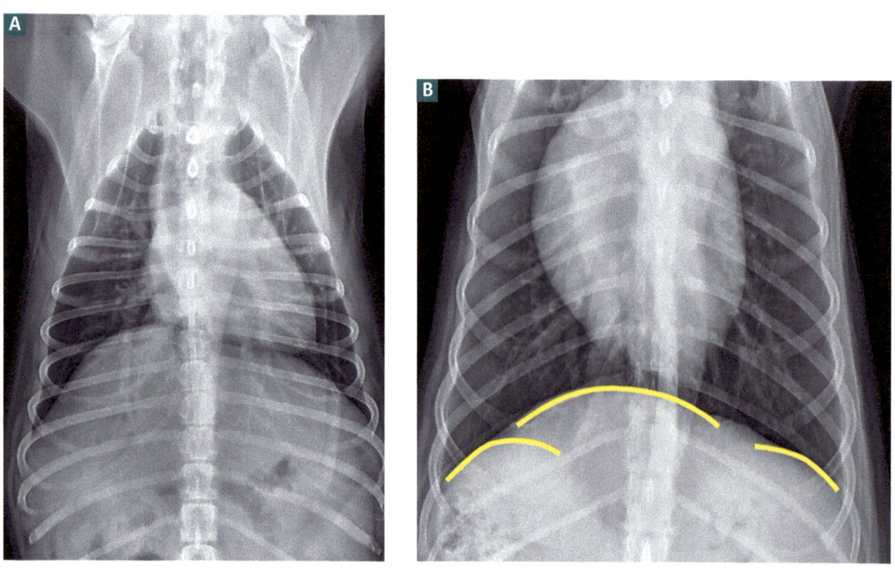

Figure 5. DV (**A**) and VD (**B**) radiographs of the thorax of a dog. The diaphragmatic crura are observed as a single bulge on the DV projection and as three humps (outlined in yellow) on the VD projection. In the DV projection, gas from the stomach is located in the fundus, on the left side of the animal.

is at the level of T8–T10 in the inspiratory phase and T7–T8 in the expiratory phase.

Variations in Radiographic Anatomy

In the **dog** there are many variations in radiographic anatomy. Primarily, this is due to varying thoracic conformation in different breeds: deep-chested breeds, such as Greyhounds or Setters, and wide-chested breeds, such as the English Bulldog or the French Bulldog, have differences in thoracic anatomy. The main differences among breeds are seen in the mediastinum and cardiac silhouette.

There are also breeds that have breed-associated abnormalities such as vertebral malformations, sternal malformations (pectus excavatum) or abnormal costochondral joints, as in the Basset Hound.

Variations can also be found depending on the animal's age. For example, the thymus increases in size up to 4 months of age and then involutes. It can be seen in the cranial mediastinum. Physeal lines can be seen in skeletally immature animals. Elderly animals may present changes such as vertebral degeneration (deforming spondylosis), sternal degeneration and degenerative changes of the costochondral junctions, mineralisation of the bronchial walls and pleural thickening, among others. Geriatric cats may have a cranially sloping cardiac silhouette with an elongated aorta.

Key Concepts of Basic Interpretation

Silhouette Effect (Border Effacement)

The visibility of a structure depends on its opacity and the opacity of the structures around it. Therefore, in the thorax, the cardiac silhouette can be seen more clearly when it is surrounded by the air in the lungs. The silhouette effect refers to the fact that when two structures of the same opacity are in direct contact, their edges become indistinguishable. An example would be a mass with soft tissue opacity in the cranial mediastinum, adjacent to the cardiac silhouette.

Mass Effect

When there is a mass, it tends to displace or compress other organs or structures. This is called the **mass effect**. When this occurs, other structures will appear in an atypical location or have an abnormal shape due to compression. An example is dorsal displacement of the trachea due to a mass in the cranial mediastinum such as a thymic neoplasm.

Mediastinal Shift

The cardiac silhouette and mediastinum may be displaced to the right or left (seen in VD/DV projections) due to a mass effect, for example, if there is a pulmonary mass or, more commonly, due to partial or total collapse of a lung. An example of a pulmonary collapse is pulmonary atelectasis due to prolonged lateral recumbency, especially in animals showing hypoventilation.

Finally, it is worth remembering the six descriptive radiographic characteristics, which are **number**, **size**, **shape**, **opacity**, **location** and **border definition**. These characteristics should be used in the description of lesions visible on radiographs.

Parenchyma and Pulmonary Vessels

Anatomical Conformation and Interpretation of Normal Lung

To correctly interpret pathologies related to the pulmonary parenchyma, first it is important to be familiar with its anatomical conformation (Fig. 6) and its normal radiographic appearance.

In the dog and the cat, the lung is divided into two halves: the right hemithorax, which is in turn divided into four lobes (the cranial, middle, caudal and accessory lobes), and the left hemithorax, which is divided into two lobes (the cranial lobe, which has a cranial segment and a caudal segment, and the caudal lobe). Knowledge of the position of the lung lobes on radiographic images is essential for their proper interpretation.

In lateral projections, owing to the reduction to a two-dimensional image on the radiographs, the pulmonary lobes of the two hemithoraces appear superimposed. Knowledge of the side on which the patient is positioned is also important for understanding the radiographic images, since the side of the chest that is in contact with the table supports the body weight and is therefore less aerated at the time the radiograph is taken. This means that pathologies can be seen better on the side of the chest that is away from the table.

VD projections allow better identification of the hemithorax that is affected by pathology. However, under normal conditions it is not possible to observe the margins of the pulmonary lobes because they all have the same radiopacity.

Normal pulmonary parenchyma (Fig. 7) has a radiolucent appearance, mainly with gas density, within which different soft tissue structures (pulmonary vessels, interstitium, bronchial walls) can be identified; this, in addition to the overlapping of the thoracic walls, means that the pulmonary parenchyma is not completely radiolucent.

Depending on the technology used to acquire the images, these structures can be observed in more or less detail. It is important that this does not lead to the overinterpretation of pulmonary pathologies, which occurs more frequently with direct digital radiography.

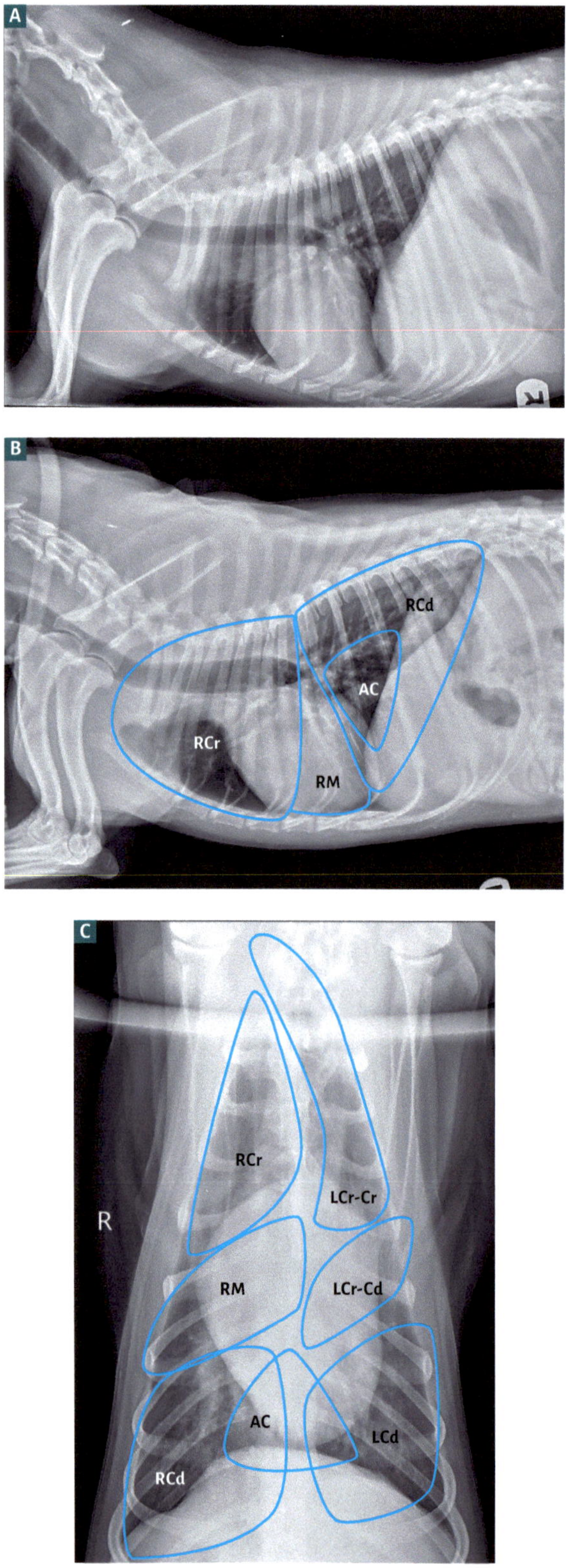

Figure 6. Right lateral (**A**), left lateral (**B**) and VD (**C**) thoracic radiographs. The positions of the right cranial lobe (RCr), cranial segment of the left cranial lobe (LCr-Cr), caudal segment of the left cranial lobe (LCr-Cd), right middle lobe (RM), right caudal lobe (RCd), left caudal lobe (LCd) and accessory lobe (AC) are indicated.

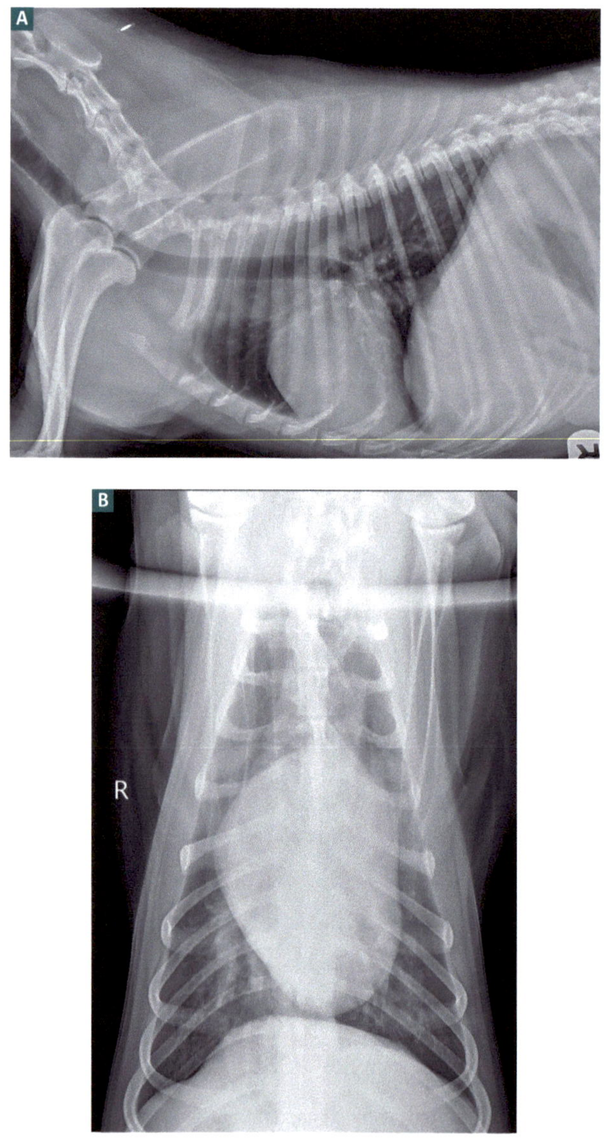

Figure 7. Right lateral (**A**) and VD (**B**) projections of a normal thorax in an adult dog. Under normal conditions, the lung presents a radiolucent appearance of mainly gas density, within which different soft tissue structures (pulmonary vessels, interstitium, bronchial walls) can be seen. This, in addition to the overlapping of the thoracic walls, means that the pulmonary parenchyma is not totally radiolucent.

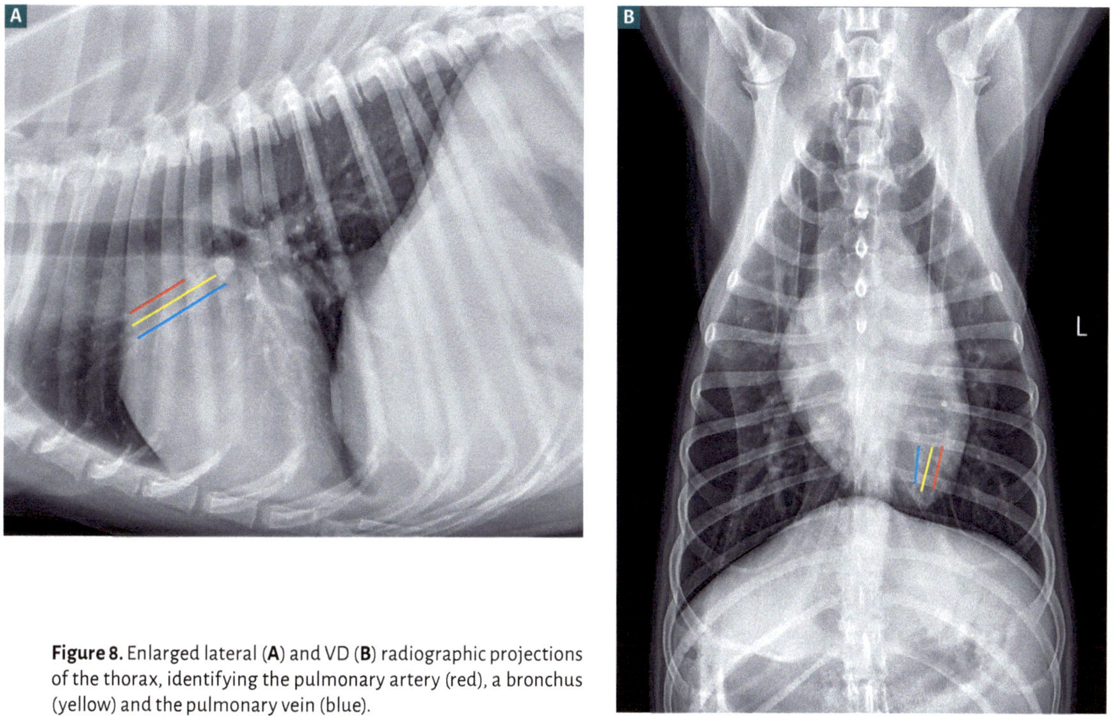

Figure 8. Enlarged lateral (**A**) and VD (**B**) radiographic projections of the thorax, identifying the pulmonary artery (red), a bronchus (yellow) and the pulmonary vein (blue).

In each of the pulmonary lobes it is possible to identify three main structures (Fig. 8): the **pulmonary artery** (dorsal and lateral), the **pulmonary vein** (ventral and medial), which will have a soft tissue radiopacity, and the **bronchus**, which has a gas radiopacity and is located centrally, between the pulmonary artery and vein.

The pulmonary artery and vein originate in the perihilar region and decrease in size as they move away from it. The artery, in its course through the pulmonary field, remains adjacent to the main bronchus, whereas the pulmonary vein can move away from the bronchus in its course through the lung.

Visualisation of the pulmonary field should also take into account the patient's age and body condition. In **puppies**, an increase in pulmonary radiopacity can be observed physiologically due to the presence of a slight amount of fluid in the interstitial space.

In **elderly patients**, the bronchi are usually better visualised, and this is also the case in chondrodystrophic animals due to early mineralisation of the bronchial walls; in both cases this is unrelated to pathological changes. **Obese patients** (Fig. 9) have greater pulmonary radiopacity due to the accumulation of fat subcutaneously, in the muscle layers and intrathoracically. This fat overlapping the lung lobes makes it difficult to visualise the blood vessels and bronchial walls, and should not be confused with a pathological image of the lung parenchyma.

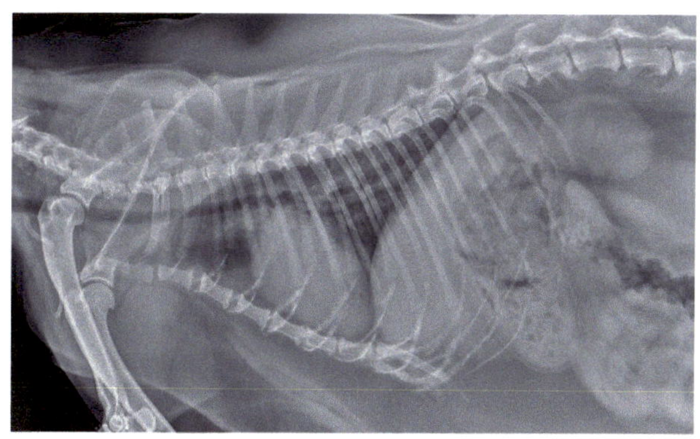

Figure 9. Lateral radiograph of an obese cat demonstrating increased pulmonary radiopacity.

Interpretation of Change in Pulmonary Parenchyma

Visualisation of changes in the pulmonary parenchyma is a significant challenge. The lung is one of the most complex organs to interpret radiographically, due to the overlapping of structures, variations between breeds and individuals, and physiological changes that can be confused with pathological processes. In addition, different pathologies that affect the lung and cause similar radiographic changes also need to be considered.

The main changes that can be observed in the pulmonary parenchyma refer to a large extent to increases in radiopacity and, less frequently, to reductions in radiopacity.

Increased Pulmonary Radiopacity

To interpret an increase in pulmonary radiopacity as pathological, first it is important to try to rule out whether the observed change may be related to physiological changes due to the respiratory phase (expiration) or the animal's age, breed or body condition. Only once these variants have been ruled out can the increase in radiopacity be defined as pathological.

Different lung patterns are used to describe the radiographic appearance of the lungs (Fig. 10), with the intention of relating the radiographic findings produced by the increase in pulmonary radiopacity to the changes that occur morphologically in the lung. These changes can affect the blood vessels, bronchi, alveoli and interstitium.

In most cases it can be seen that the changes found affect more than one component; which makes it difficult to interpret the radiograph and affects the possibility of specifying a list of differential diagnoses. At other times it is obvious that only one component is affected (the alveoli, bronchi, interstitial space or blood vessels); this allows a more specific list of differential diagnoses to be made and a better interpretation of the radiograph.

Interstitial Pattern

The interstitial pattern is described as an increase in pulmonary radiopacity in which the blood vessels remain visible. There is an increase in tissue at the interstitial level, but the contrast created by the air present in the alveoli (gas radiopacity) allows the pulmonary vessels to continue to be visualised.

The interstitial pattern is difficult to assess because, as mentioned above, the physiological changes associated with increases in pulmonary radiopacity produce an image similar to this pattern.

Two types of interstitial pattern can be differentiated: the **structured** or **nodular interstitial pattern** and the **unstructured interstitial pattern** (Boxes 1 and 2). It is important to know the difference between the two presentations because they are associated with different pathologies.

Structured or Nodular Interstitial Pattern

This pattern is characterised by the appearance of well-defined nodules with soft tissue radiopacity, with a size greater than 3–5 mm.

Nodules less than 3 mm in size cannot be visualised radiographically. For their diagnosis, advanced imaging techniques such as CT must be used, to allow the location of small lesions (1–2 mm) that are not visible radiographically or that could be confused with blood vessels.

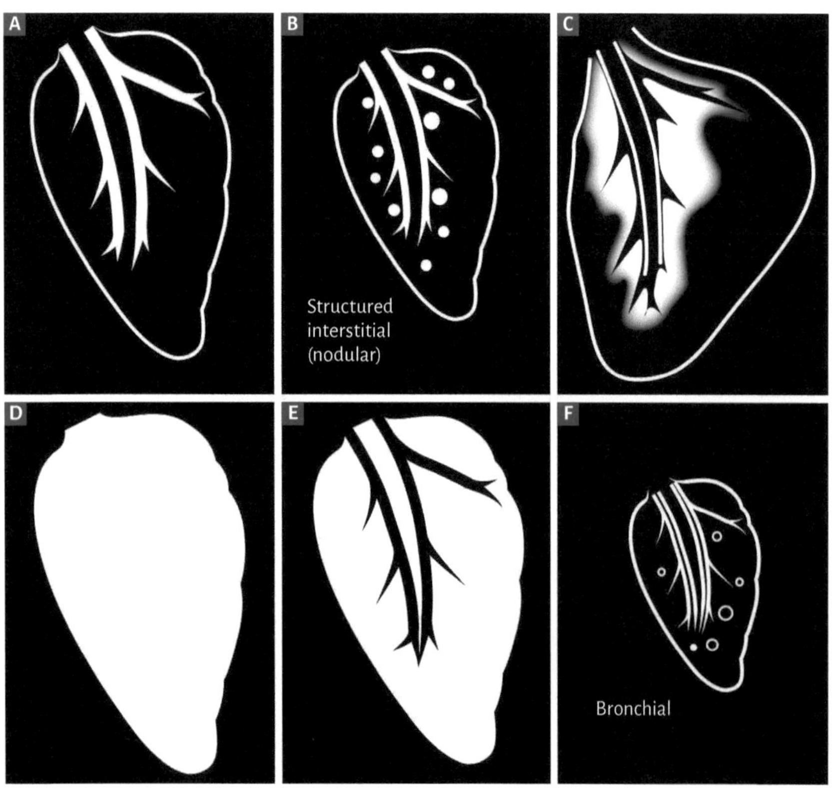

Figure 10. Diagrams showing the different lung patterns that can be identified on radiographs: (**A**) normal lung parenchyma, (**B**) structured interstitial pattern, (**C**) unstructured interstitial pattern, (**D**) alveolar pattern without aerial bronchogram, (**E**) alveolar pattern with aerial bronchogram, (**F**) bronchial pattern.

Box 1. Differential diagnoses for a structured or nodular interstitial pattern

- **Artefactual (nipples, blood vessels in a cross section, costochondral junction, osteomas)**
- **Metastasis**
- **Miliary metastasis**
- **Malignant histiocytosis**
- **Lymphosarcoma**
- **Abscesses**
- **Granulomas**
- **Haematomas**
- **Cysts**
- **Haematogenic pneumonia**
- **Cavitated structures, thin wall (bullae, pneumocoele)**
- **Cavitated structures, irregular wall (neoplastic, abscesses, granulomas).**

Box 2. Differential diagnoses for an unstructured interstitial pattern

- **Physiological (obesity, puppy, geriatric, expiratory radiography)**
- **Mild pneumonia (viral, parasitic, bacterial)**
- **Mild oedema (cardiogenic, noncardiogenic)**
- **Pulmonary fibrosis**
- **Mild bleeding**
- **Eosinophilic bronchopneumonia.**

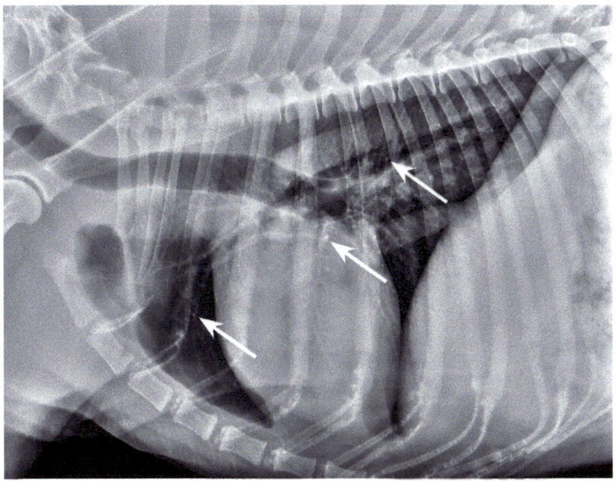

Figure 11. Lateral radiograph of a dog. The arrows point to blood vessels in cross section.

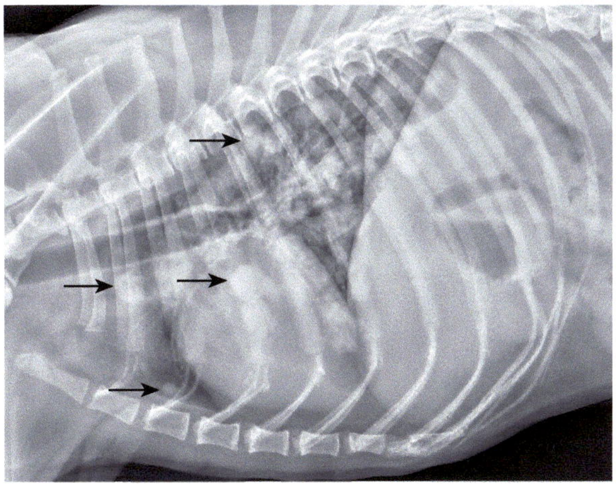

Figure 12. Lateral and VD radiograph of a patient with pulmonary metastasis from mammary carcinoma. Arrows indicate the soft tissue nodules that form the interstitial pattern in this patient.

The nodules that form in the interstitial space should not be confused with osteomas or pleural plaques, which are pulmonary nodules less than 5 mm in size that may be visible because they have a mineral radiopacity. These occur more frequently in adult and geriatric patients and have no associated clinical significance.

Other possible structures that may be confused with a pulmonary nodule on a radiograph are blood vessels in cross section (Fig. 11), costochondral joints or nipples.

If one or more of the patient's nipples are suspected of mimicking a pulmonary nodule, the nipples can be covered with radiopaque contrast agent and radiography repeated. In the event that the observed nodule appears to have metallic radiopacity on the repeat radiographs, it can be deduced that there is actually no pulmonary nodule, but that the structure is a nipple overlapping the pulmonary parenchyma.

The main pathology related to the nodular interstitial pattern is **pulmonary metastasis** (Fig. 12). In this pathology, nodules can be found ranging from solitary to multiple nodules with a multifocal distribution, which is the most frequent presentation.

Other pathologies related to this presentation can be **granulomatous infections** and **primary neoplasms**.

Occasionally, nodules smaller than 3 mm may be visible when a large number of nodules are present, resulting in overlap. This type of presentation is called a **miliary pattern** (Fig. 13) and is mainly associated with lung metastases, lymphosarcoma and haematogenous bronchopneumonia.

This type of interstitial pattern also includes **cavitated pulmonary nodules**, which may have a thin wall and contents of gas density (pulmonary bullae, pneumocoele), or a thick wall with contents of gas and soft tissue density (primary neoplasia, metastasis, abscesses, granulomas).

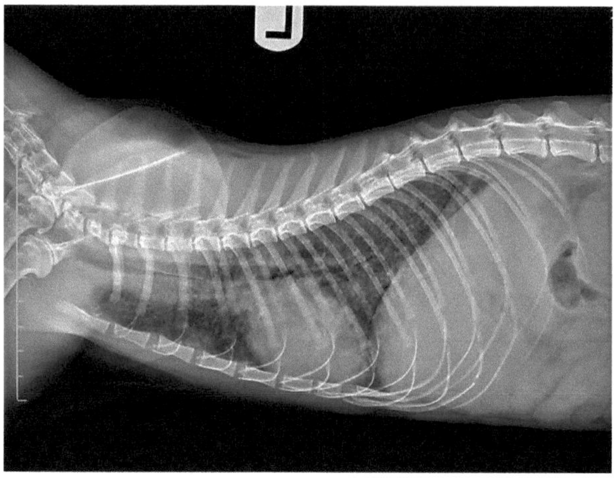

Figure 13. Lateral radiograph of the thorax of a skeletally mature cat, showing a miliary pattern.

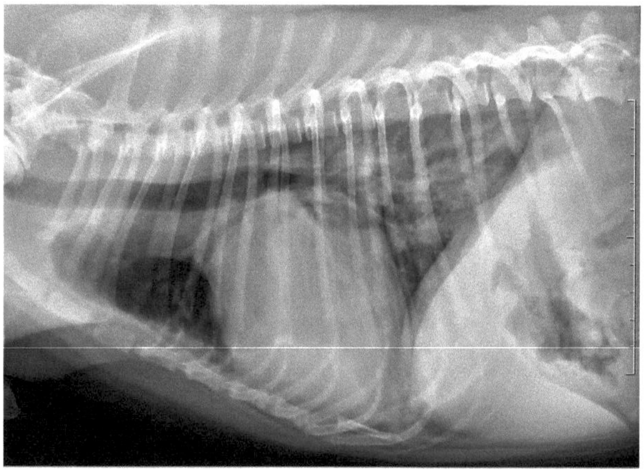

Figure 14. Lateral radiograph of the thorax of a patient with moderate pulmonary oedema, in which an interstitial pattern can be clearly observed.

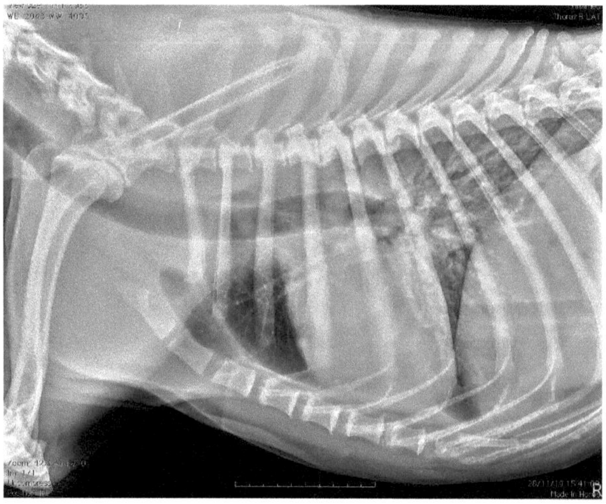

Figure 15. Lateral thoracic radiograph of a patient with a mild interstitial pattern in the projection area of the caudodorsal lobes.

Unstructured Interstitial Pattern

This pattern is characterised by a mild to moderate increase in pulmonary radiopacity (Fig. 14) without the formation of nodules. Visualisation of the blood vessels is difficult, but they do not disappear completely. There are certain pathologies characteristic of this type of pattern:

- **Pulmonary fibrosis** secondary to a chronic or idiopathic respiratory disease, which is most frequently seen in the West Highland White Terrier.
- **Interstitial pneumonia**, mainly of toxic or viral origin, may have an alveolar component in the initial stages or when accompanied by a secondary bacterial infection. When it becomes chronic, it can lead to secondary pulmonary fibrosis.

At other times, this type of pattern is the initial phase or regression phase of pathologies that can trigger an alveolar pattern, such as cardiogenic or noncardiogenic **pulmonary oedema**, **haemorrhage**, **infiltrative neoplasms** (mainly lymphoma) and **parasitic pneumonias**.

To better correlate the pathology present in the animal with the type of interstitial pattern observed radiographically, it is essential to be aware of each type of presentation:

- **caudodorsal locations** (Fig. 15) may be related to pulmonary oedema, whether of cardiac or noncardiac origin
- **cranioventral locations** are related to mild pulmonary oedema
- **ventral** or **cranioventral locations** may be related to pulmonary bleeding and to atelectasis
- **diffuse distributions** (Fig. 16) are related to infiltrative neoplasms, moderate cardiogenic oedema, eosinophilic bronchopneumopathy (mainly of allergic origin) and interstitial pneumonia of mainly viral or toxic origin
- **caudal** and **peripheral distributions** are more commonly related to pneumonias of parasitic origin.

In advanced imaging techniques such as **CT**, the interstitial pattern can be observed as an increase in pulmonary radiopacity with a "ground glass" appearance, which is mainly observed in patients with pulmonary fibrosis.

Bands of soft tissue can also be observed from the pulmonary parenchyma to the pleura, as well as subpleural consolidations.

Alveolar Pattern

The alveolar pattern represents the most serious condition among the changes observed in the pulmonary parenchyma. In many cases it is the evolution of an interstitial pattern (Box 3).

The alveolar pattern is characterised by the absence of air inside the alveoli, due to either compression and removal of the air inside (which results in a reduction in the size of the affected lobe), or replacement of the air in the alveoli by another type of content (liquid, blood, mucus or purulent material).

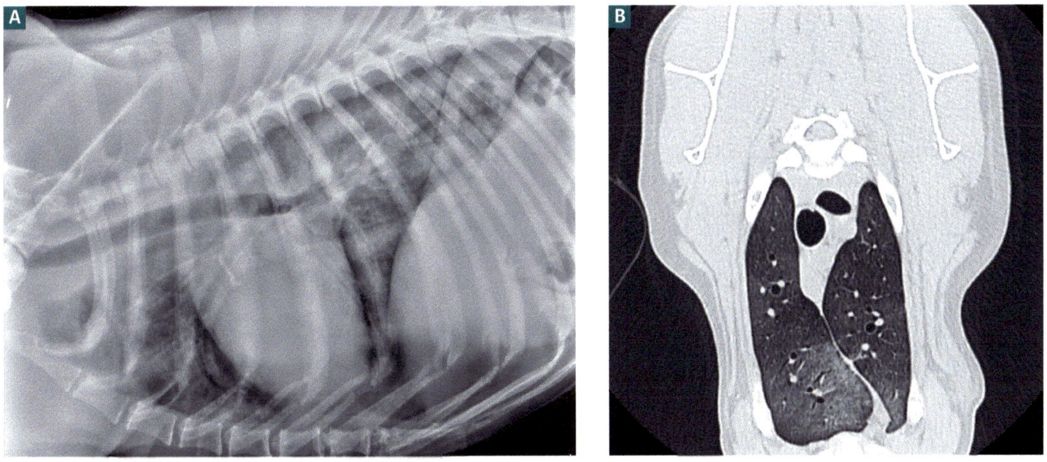

Figure 16. (**A**) Lateral thoracic radiograph of a dog with eosinophilic bronchopneumopathy showing an interstitial pattern affecting all lung lobes. (**B**) CT image of the same patient in an axial section, showing the characteristic "ground glass" appearance in the interstitial pattern.

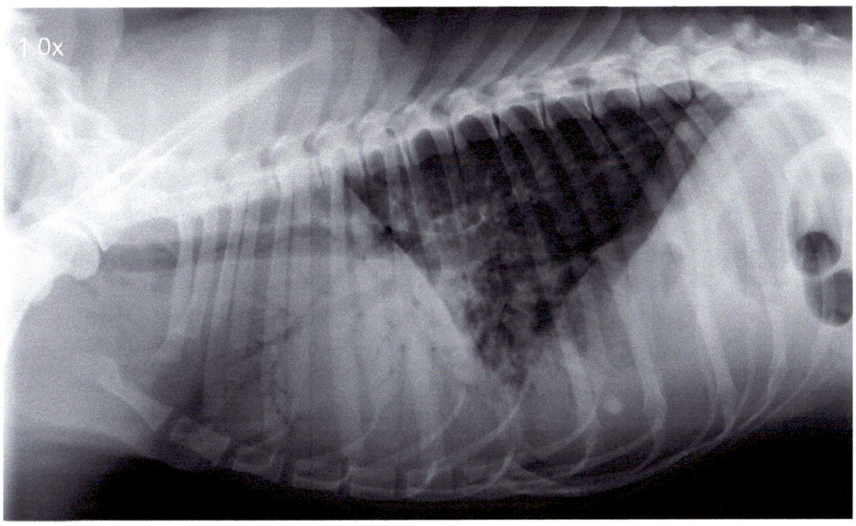

Figure 17. Lateral thoracic radiograph showing an alveolar pattern in the cranial lung lobes.

Box 3. Differential diagnoses for an alveolar pattern

- **Pneumonia (bronchopneumonia, aspiration, parasitic, fungal, foreign body)**
- **Atelectasis**
- **Bleeding (trauma, coagulopathies)**
- **Oedema (cardiogenic, noncardiogenic)**
- **Primary neoplasm**
- **Lobe torsion**
- **Thromboembolism.**

This can cause complete consolidation of the affected lobes or, more frequently, partially affect the alveolar space of one or more lobes. In these cases, the increased radiopacity presents a more heterogeneous soft tissue appearance, with residual aerated areas.

It is important to be aware of a number of **characteristics** presented by alveolar patterns (Fig. 17) to interpret them correctly. Some of these characteristics are pathognomonic of this type of pattern.

- **Increased pulmonary radiopacity** (soft tissue density) with loss of visualisation of blood vessels (Fig. 18).
- **Silhouette sign** (Fig. 19) occurs when the soft tissue radiopacity acquired by the lung overlaps the naturally present soft tissue structures, such as the heart and diaphragm. The loss of visualisation of blood vessels mentioned in the previous point is a type of silhouette sign.
- **Lobar sign** (Fig. 20) occurs when the edge of a fully consolidated pulmonary lobe is observed. This allows it to be differentiated from the adjacent lung lobe that contains radiopaque gas content.
- **Aerial bronchogram** (Fig. 21) refers to when the main bronchus of the affected lobe and its ramifications are observed. This occurs because the bronchus remains aerated with a gas-like radiopacity, whereas the surrounding alveoli present a soft tissue radiopacity, which

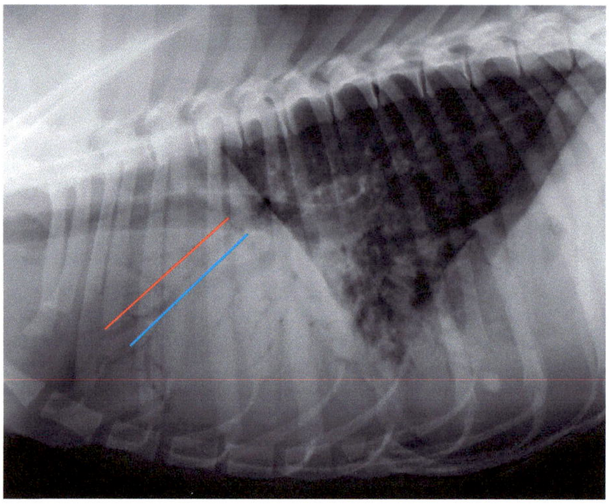

Figure 18. Same radiograph as in Fig. 17, with red and blue lines showing where the blood vessels should be visualised.

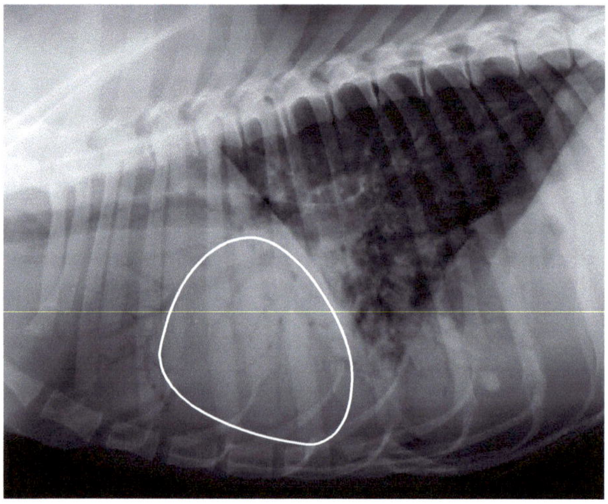

Figure 19. Same radiograph as in Fig. 17, with a white outline showing where the cardiac silhouette should be visible.

produces sufficient radiographic contrast to visualise the bronchus. Under normal conditions it does not occur because both the bronchus and the alveoli are aerated and there is no difference in contrast that allows the bronchus to be fully visualised. This characteristic is pathognomonic of alveolar patterns.

All of these radiographic signs can be seen together in the same patient, or only some of them may be visible on a radiograph. The sign that is usually observed in most cases is loss of visualisation of the blood vessels. In these cases, CT allows better characterisation of the affected lobes, and the characteristics mentioned above can also be observed on CT images (Fig. 22).

The pathology that is most commonly related to alveolar patterns is pneumonia.

- **Bronchopneumonias** are located mainly in the cranioventral lobes; they are usually associated with an aerogenic bacterial infection. Pneumonia of haematogenic origin, whether due to a bacterial, parasitic or fungal cause, will present a different distribution, affecting the entire pulmonary parenchyma in a generalised manner, in which a miliary or nodular pattern can be seen.
- **Aspiration pneumonias** (Fig. 23) are most commonly seen in the cranial lobes and in the right middle lobe, although other lung lobes may be affected depending on the position of the patient at the time aspiration of content occurred.
- **Bronchopneumonias of haematogenic origin** present a multifocal distribution as described for the interstitial pattern.
- **Allergic pneumonias** may also present as an irregular alveolar pattern with a preferentially caudal to diffuse distribution.

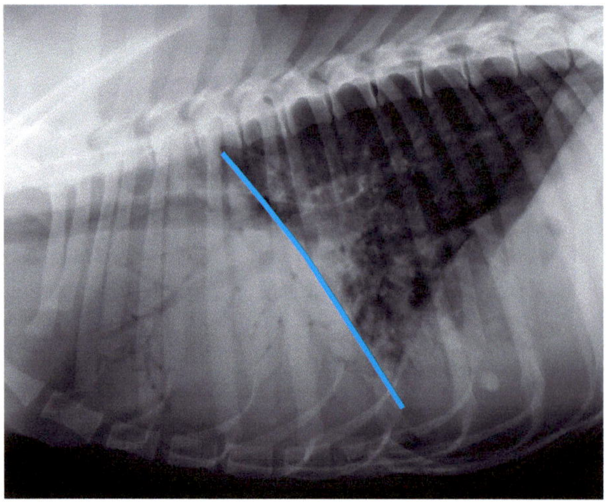

Figure 20. Same radiograph as in Fig. 17, with a blue line showing the radiopaque line that forms the edge of the consolidated lung.

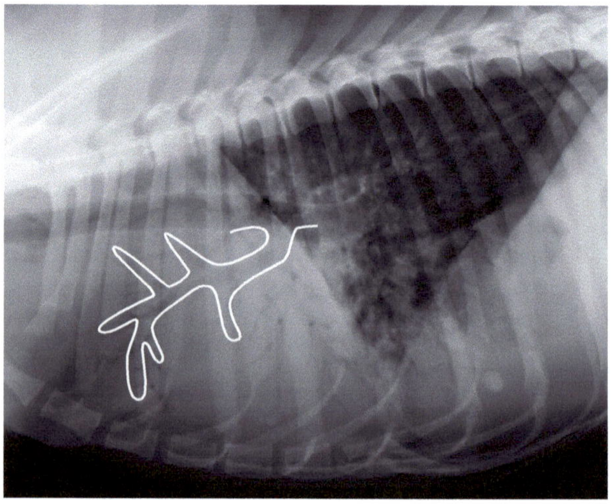

Figure 21. Same radiograph as in Fig. 17, with a white outline showing the path of the visible bronchi as a result of the presence of the alveolar pattern.

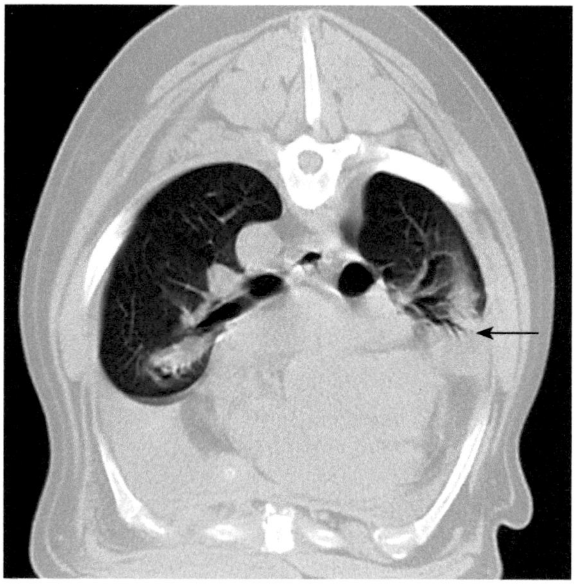

Figure 22. CT image of a patient with bronchopneumonia. An increase in pulmonary radiopacity is observed, with an aerial bronchogram (arrow).

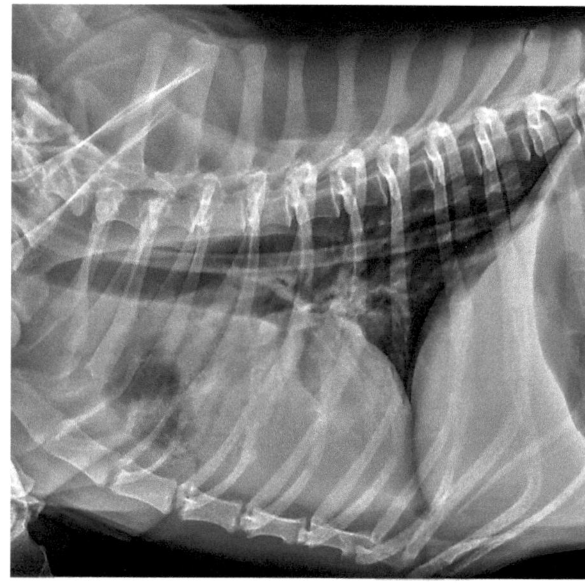

Figure 23. Lateral radiograph of a patient with anorexia in which the presence of an oesophagostomy tube can be seen. Megaoesophagus and an alveolar pattern can be seen in the cranioventral area of the lung. The characteristic signs of this type of pattern can be observed: aerial bronchogram, silhouette sign, lobar sign and loss of visualisation of blood vessels.

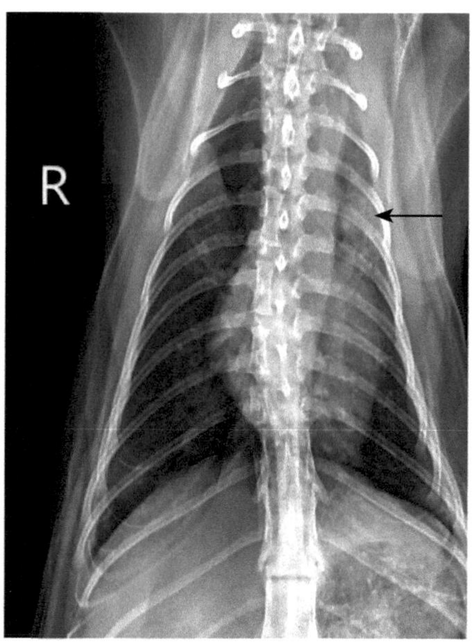

Figure 24. VD radiograph of the thorax of a patient with pulmonary contusion. The arrow indicates the alveolar pattern present in this case. In the right cranial lobe there is a slight pneumothorax as a result of the trauma the patient has suffered.

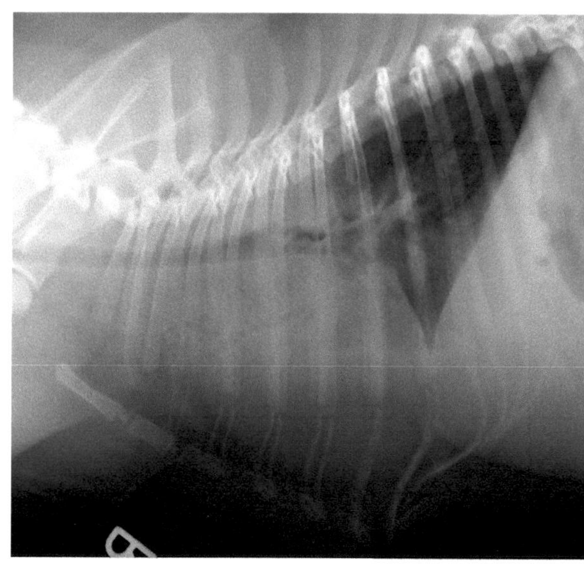

Figure 25. Lateral radiograph of the thorax of a patient with pulmonary torsion, in which a characteristic alveolar pattern with gas vesicles is observed.

Other causes, apart from pneumonia, can also cause an alveolar pattern.

- **Pulmonary haemorrhages** will present an alveolar pattern in their most serious form. Depending on their origin, they may have a cranial to random presentation in the case of coagulopathies. In the case of pulmonary contusions (Fig. 24), the presentation may vary depending on the area where the trauma occurred.
- **Tracheobronchial foreign bodies** may cause obstruction of the affected bronchus and secondary bacterial infection; usually only one affected lung lobe is observed.
- **Pulmonary torsion** (Fig. 25) is a rare condition in companion animals, usually affecting the right middle lobe (in large breeds) or the left cranial lobe (in small breeds).

The pulmonary parenchyma shows an alveolar pattern in the affected lobe, and vesicles of trapped gas may also be seen. There is usually pleural effusion associated with this condition and an abnormal position of the bronchus, which is no longer visualised or sharply reduces in diameter near the carina. The affected lobe may have an increased volume and rounded edges due to associated congestion. In this case, performing a CT scan can help to assess the continuity of the bronchi and blood vessels, which may be difficult to visualise radiographically due to the alveolar pattern or possible pleural effusion.

- **Neoplasia**: the alveolar pattern secondary to a neoplastic process is a chronic process that may be more frequently associated with primary neoplasia (Fig. 26) and metastasis.
  Generally, in cases where a primary neoplasm is present, a single mass can be seen, mainly in the caudodorsal lobes. Sometimes it can affect an entire lung lobe; in these cases it does not usually present an aerial bronchogram and an increase in lung volume can be seen. Involvement of the entire lobe can be caused by the invasion of the neoplasm or by the obstruction of the main bronchus. In cats, a multifocal pattern associated with both primary neoplasia and lung metastasis may also be seen.
  Masses of neoplastic origin may present with cavitations or mineralisation and may be associated with mediastinal lymphadenopathy.
  Other pathologies likely to generate lung masses include:
  - **Granuloma**: usually presents in the form of several nodules, from small to large-sized masses with an irregular edge. Like neoplasms, they can present mineralisation, cavitations and lymphadenopathy.
  - **Abscess**: usually has a thick, irregular wall; the contents can be solid or cavitated, depending on whether or not there is gas inside.
  - **Cyst**: normally appears as a well-defined lesion with soft tissue or gas radiopacity surrounded by a thin wall with a smooth surface.
  - **Pulmonary bulla** (Fig. 27): a lung lesion with gas radiopacity that generally presents a thin, well-defined wall and a rounded shape.
- **Atelectasis** (Fig. 28) is the total or partial collapse of a part of the lung, or of the lung in its entirety. It can occur physiologically (due to prolonged recumbency) or pathologically.
  The most frequent causes of atelectasis secondary to a pathology are usually pneumothorax, tension pneumothorax, pleural effusion, pulmonary masses and bronchial obstruction.
  The affected lobe(s) can be seen to have a reduction in volume; this can generate a mediastinal torsion ipsilateral to the affected lobe, except in cases of tension pneumothorax in which, due to the pressure exerted on the affected hemithorax, mediastinal torsion occurs on the opposite side.

Bronchial Pattern

The bronchial pattern is characterised by an increase in pulmonary radiopacity due to an increase in the radiopacity of the bronchial walls or an increase in the size of the bronchial lumen (Box 4).

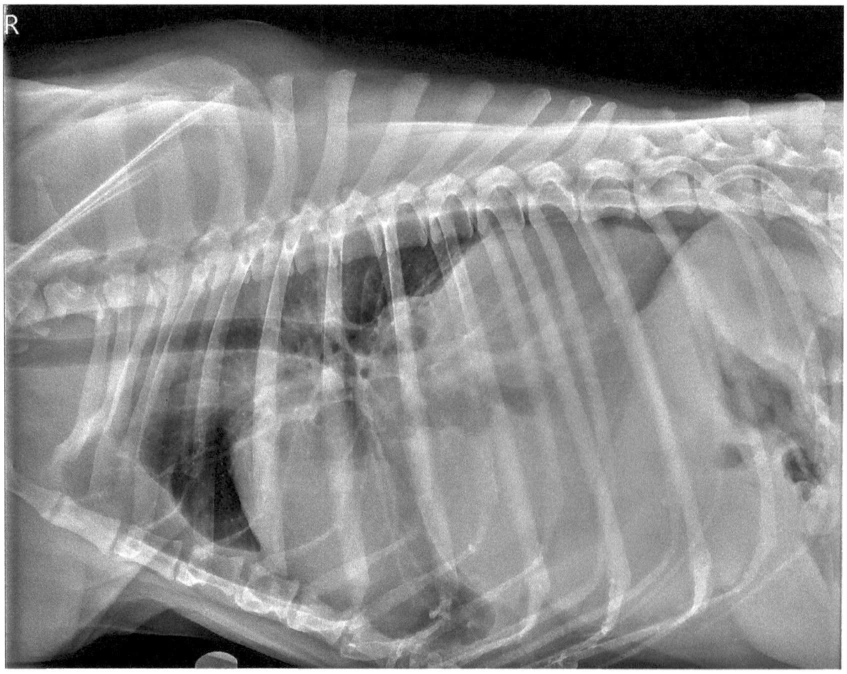

Figure 26. Lateral radiograph of the thorax in which the presence of a mass is affecting a large part of the right caudal lung lobe. The mass is producing a silhouette effect on the diaphragm preventing correct visualisation of the diaphragmatic crura. This appearance should not be confused with a diaphragmatic hernia.

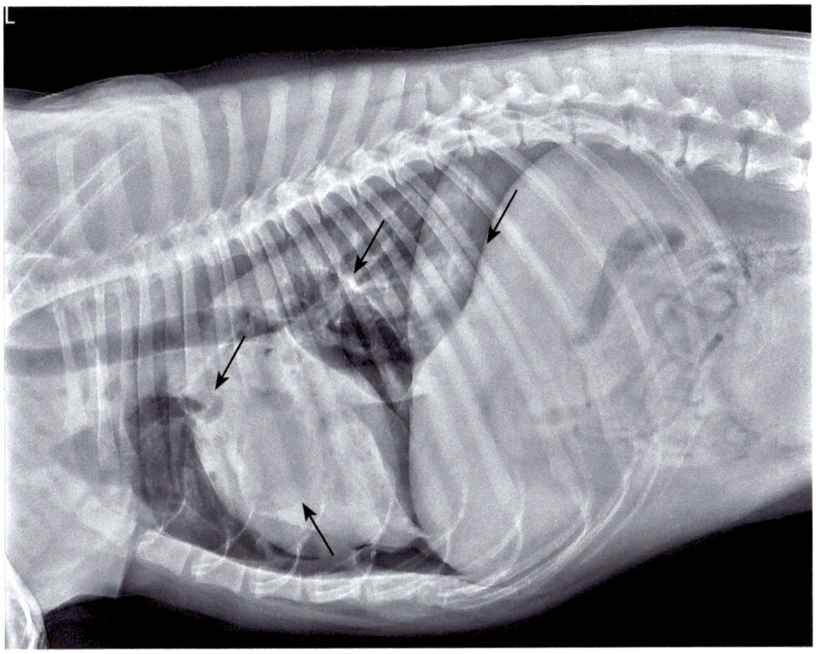

Figure 27. Lateral radiograph of the thorax of a patient presenting with multiple pulmonary bullae (arrows) after thoracic trauma. The patient also presented with pneumothorax and right middle lobe atelectasis.

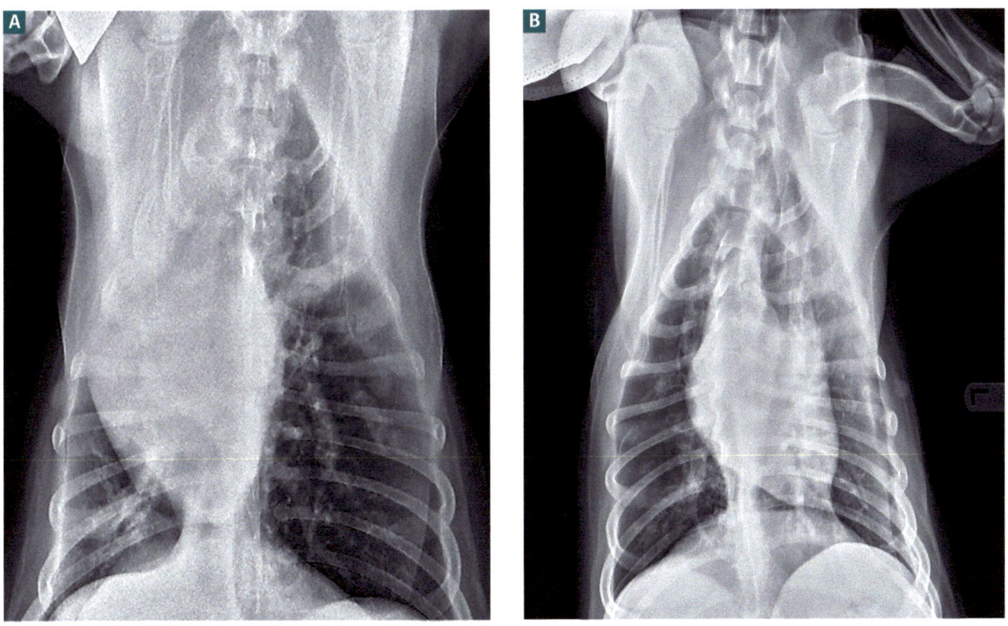

Figure 28. (**A**) Patient with atelectasis in which the right pulmonary lobe can be seen to be reduced in size, the cardiac silhouette is displaced towards the right hemithorax and an alveolar pattern is observed in the right cranial lobe. (**B**) Radiograph of the same patient after intubation and ventilation. The lung can be seen to be more aerated and the heart is in its normal position.

Box 4. Differential diagnoses for a bronchial pattern

- **Normal in geriatric animals**
- **Chronic bronchitis (bacterial, viral, feline asthma)**
- **Neoplasia (bronchogenic carcinoma)**
- **Mineralisation of bronchial walls (hyperadrenocorticism)**
- **Bronchial wall oedema.**

In most cases the bronchial walls become more visible due to an increase in their thickness, with soft tissue density, due to the accumulation of fluid or increased cellularity. On other occasions, the increase in the visibility of the bronchial walls is due to the fact that they present a mineral radiopacity rather than an increase in thickness.

This pattern always presents an added complication when it comes to knowing with certainty whether it is a pathological finding or a consequence of bronchial mineralisation in geriatric patients. This mineralisation can also occur in chondrodystrophic patients at younger ages.

It is essential to relate the radiographic image to the patient's history and clinical signs.

The bronchial pattern (Fig. 29) presents a series of **radiographic characteristics** that aid identification.

- **Circular structures** with thick (soft tissue) or thin (mineral) walls, with a radiolucent centre with gas density, known as "doughnuts". They correspond to visualisation of the bronchi in cross section.
- **Parallel lines**, which can be thick (soft tissue) or thin (mineral) and correspond to visualisation of the bronchi in longitudinal section, are known as "tram lines".

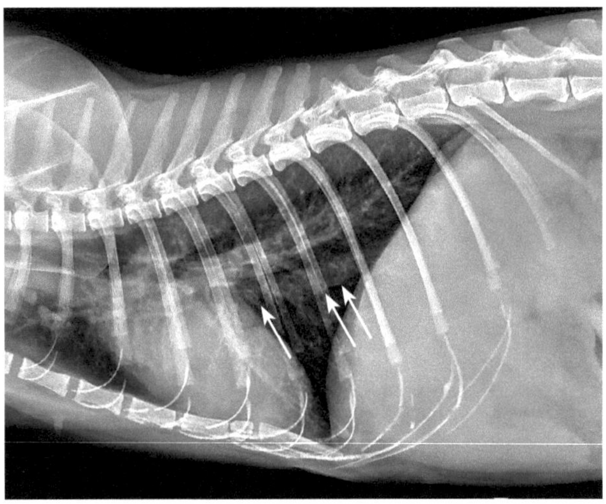

Figure 29. Lateral radiograph of the thorax of a patient with chronic bronchitis; the arrows point to the bronchi in cross section and longitudinally.

The pathology related to this type of pattern is bronchitis.

Chronic Canine Bronchitis

This condition can be caused by multiple pathologies —bacterial, parasitic, viral or irritant— but the main pathology that presents this type of pattern is **allergic** bronchitis. Acute bronchitis, in most cases, is not observed radiographically, but when it is, a bronchial pattern similar to that seen in most chronic cases occurs.

Feline Lower Respiratory Tract Disease

This disease can be caused by multiple different pathologies, the main one being feline **asthma**. In these pathologies a functional obstruction of the bronchi can occur, which is usually reversible. Radiographs may be normal or show a bronchial pattern with peribronchial infiltrations, and in severe cases a mixed pattern may be visible.

Bronchiectasis

Bronchiectasis (Fig. 30) refers to the increase in the diameter of the bronchial lumen, and an irregular bronchial path can also be observed.

Bronchiectasis can be of congenital origin, such as primary ciliary dyskinesia, or acquired, secondary to chronic respiratory processes such as bronchitis. It has also been seen in dogs with tracheal collapse. This is thought to be related to a structural disorder affecting the cartilage.

Other Pathologies

Other pathologies related to bronchial patterns, although less common, are **cardiogenic pulmonary oedema and neoplastic infiltrations**.

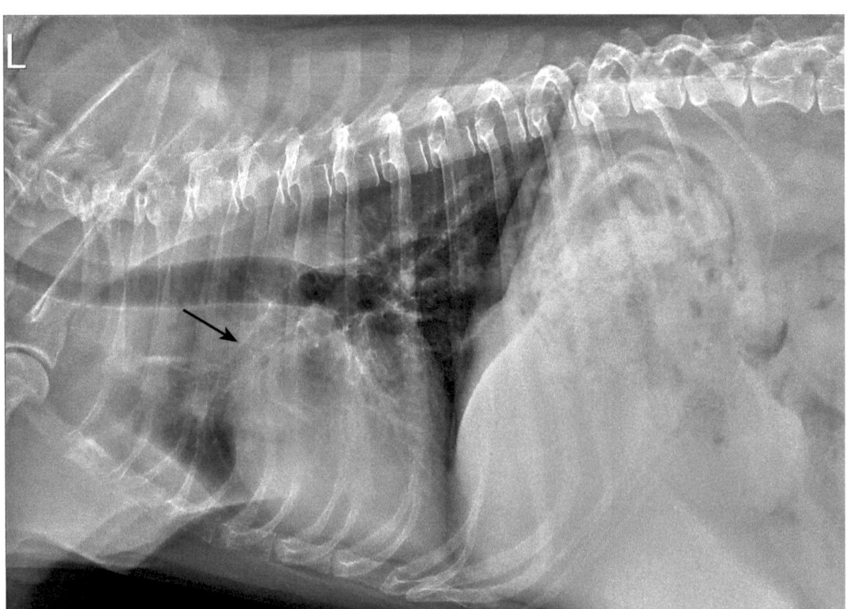

Figure 30. Lateral radiograph of the thorax. The arrow points to a bronchus with a larger than normal diameter.

In relation to bronchial patterns, the collapse of a pulmonary lobe, usually the right middle lobe, due to the accumulation of mucus and exudate from bronchial inflammation, which ends up occupying the bronchial lumen, can be observed. Spontaneous rib fractures (without a traumatic event) and pulmonary hyperinflation can also be seen.

Bronchial mineralisation may be related to hyperadrenocorticism, secondary renal hyperparathyroidism or, less frequently, chronic bronchitis.

Mixed Pattern

In general, it is unusual to observe only one of the lung patterns described above; in most cases pathologies present with radiographic characteristics of two or more patterns. In these situations, the term **mixed pattern** can be used (Fig. 31). In cases where a mixture of radiographic characteristics is observed, the predominant pattern is the one that should be used to make the list of differential diagnoses.

The pathologies that appear most frequently with these types of mixed patterns may be some types of pneumonia.

Parasitic Pneumonia

Parasitic pneumonia is mainly caused by lungworms. An irregular bronchointerstitial pattern with alveolar foci can be observed. Depending on the severity, it can range from a peripheral distribution to a multifocal distribution affecting the entire lung.

Fungal Pneumonia

Fungal pneumonia can present a mixed pattern ranging from bronchointerstitial to alveolar, forming nodules that frequently have a miliary distribution. Tracheobronchial lymphadenopathy can be observed associated with fungal infections. In disseminated fungal infections, together with pulmonary pathology, aggressive polyostotic bone lesions and discospondylitis that usually affect several vertebrae can be seen.

Acute Respiratory Distress Syndrome

Acute respiratory distress syndrome (ARDS) presents with a mixed, bilateral pattern, with an alveolar component with mainly interstitial areas. Changes in the lung parenchyma can also be observed due to the triggering pathology, which may be bronchopneumonia or parasitic or toxic pneumonia, among other pulmonary causes. There are also nonpulmonary causes, such as pancreatitis.

This pathology produces a pattern that worsens over time, and in the final stages pneumothorax and pneumomediastinum can also be observed.

In young dogs less than 1 year of age (predominantly Dalmatians), there is a hereditary component that can trigger ARDS, and it can be associated with renal dysplasia or hydrocephalus.

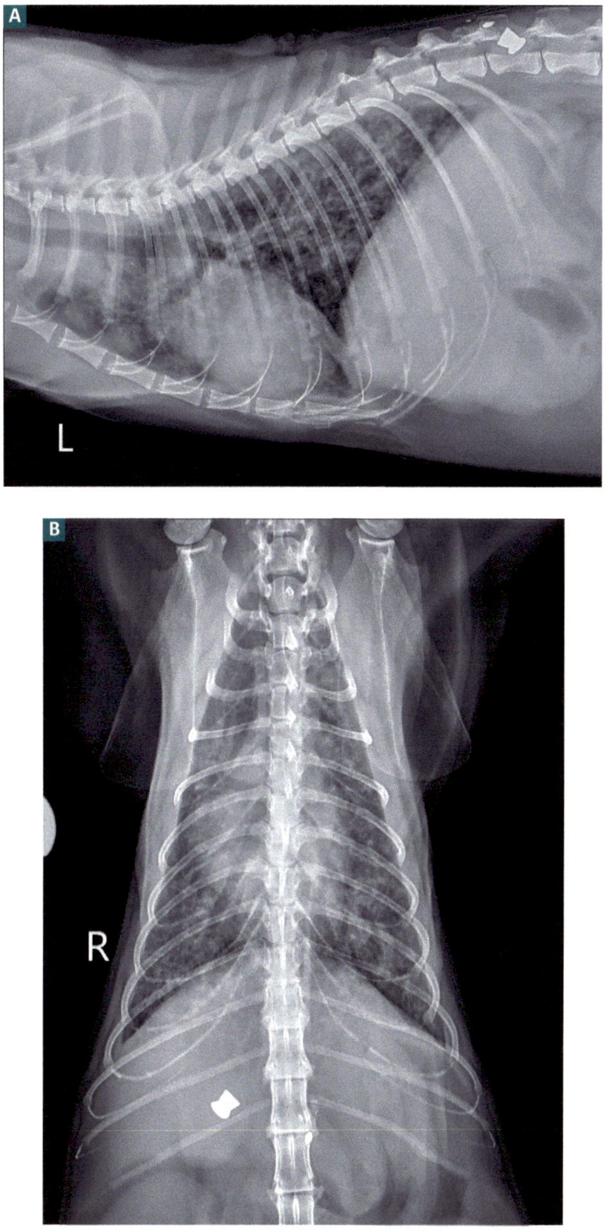

Figure 31. Lateral (**A**) and VD (**B**) thoracic radiographs of a cat with parasitic pneumonia. A mixed pattern is observed, which is mainly bronchointerstitial, with foci showing an alveolar component.

Other Pathologies

Other pathologies related to mixed lung patterns are haemorrhage, bronchopneumonias, allergic pneumonias, infiltrative neoplasms and primary lung neoplasms such as bronchoalveolar carcinoma.

Vascular Pattern

A vascular pattern is defined as a change in the size of the pulmonary blood vessels. Both increases and decreases in the size of the pulmonary veins and arteries can be observed.

These changes in size may be associated with only one type of blood vessel or both.

In some pathologies associated with this change in size, such as dirofilariasis (in which more changes can be seen at the level of the caudal vessels) or thromboembolisms, a change in the normal shape of the vessels can be seen: they can become tortuous and end abruptly.

To assess the changes in size that are apparent radiographically in both veins and arteries, comparisons with vessels that, under normal conditions, should maintain a similar size can be made.

Another way to assess these changes is to compare the blood vessels with other structures that allow the presence of any pathological changes to be assessed.

In lateral views, the pulmonary arteries and veins should not exceed the width of the proximal third of the fourth rib.

In VD or DV views, the image formed by the blood vessels crossing the ninth rib should be similar to a square; if the shape is more like a rectangle, this indicates an increase (Box 5) or decrease in the size of the vessels (Box 6).

- **Increase in the size of the pulmonary arteries** is associated with pulmonary hypertension (increase in size in the perihilar area), thromboembolism, dirofilariasis, left-to-right shunts, angiostrongyliasis or peripheral arteriovenous fistula.
- **Increased pulmonary vein size** is associated with left-sided congestive heart failure and right-to-left shunts.
- **Increase in the size of both veins and arteries** is associated with worsening of the pathologies listed in the previous point; when iatrogenic it can occur due to fluid overdose (Fig. 32).
- **Reduction in the size of pulmonary arteries and veins** is associated with dehydration, shock, hypoadrenocorticism or cardiac tamponade.

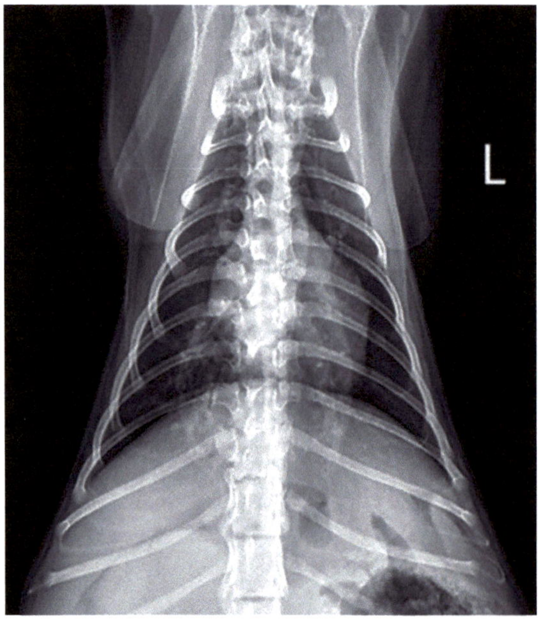

Figure 32. VD radiograph of the thorax of a cat that was overhydrated. An increase in the size of the pulmonary veins and arteries is seen.

Box 5. Differential diagnoses for a vascular pattern due to an increase in the size of the vessels

Pulmonary arteries
- Left-to-right shunts
- Dirofilariasis
- Peripheral arteriovenous fistula
- Pulmonary thromboembolism.

Pulmonary veins
- Left-sided heart failure
- Right-to-left shunts
- Mitral stenosis.

Arteries and veins
- Iatrogenic overhydration
- Worsening of causes of severe venous enlargement (left-sided heart failure, left-to-right shunts).

Box 6. Differential diagnoses for a vascular pattern due to a decrease in the size of the arteries and veins

- Generalised (shock, dehydration, pulmonary overdistension, right-sided heart failure, severe pulmonary stenosis)
- Localised (pulmonary thromboembolism).

Decreased Pulmonary Radiopacity

In patients in which a reduction in pulmonary radiopacity is observed, the pulmonary parenchyma can be seen to become more radiolucent, with blood vessels that are smaller than usual but still visible throughout the lung (Fig. 33). The increase in pulmonary radiolucency should not be confused with a pneumothorax.

Pathologies that cause a greater decrease in radiopacity at the level of the pulmonary lobes are generally associated with increases in lung volume, due to either an obstructive process, lower respiratory tract pathologies that make it difficult to remove air during expiration or pathologies that promote hyperventilation. In these cases, the increase in lung size causes a caudal displacement of the diaphragm, which has a "tent" shape in the VD view. In lateral views, an increase in the size of the lung parenchyma protruding from the ribs and flattening of the diaphragmatic crura are observed (Fig. 33). A decrease in the size of the caudal vena cava and the heart, and a horizontal position of the ribs relative to the spine, can also be seen.

Pathologies related to pulmonary hypoperfusion can also be seen. Radiographically, these cause a decrease in the size of peripheral blood vessels, resulting in more radiolucent areas in the lung, mainly in the outermost regions of the caudal lobes. In these cases, **pulmonary hypertension** or **thromboembolisms** are often the cause.

Pulmonary Emphysema

This is a rare pathology in dogs and cats. An increase in alveolar size occurs due to a break in the walls of the surrounding alveoli. It is mainly the result of obstructive processes that generate entrapment, which usually occurs at the periphery of the pulmonary lobes.

It can be congenital; a rare condition of the bronchial cartilage has been described in breeds such as the Shih Tzu and Jack Russell. It can also be acquired.

Radiographically, an increase in the size of the entire lung parenchyma or the affected lobe, with a decrease in radiopacity, can be seen. Flattening of the diaphragmatic dome and chronic rib fractures can be seen associated with these changes.

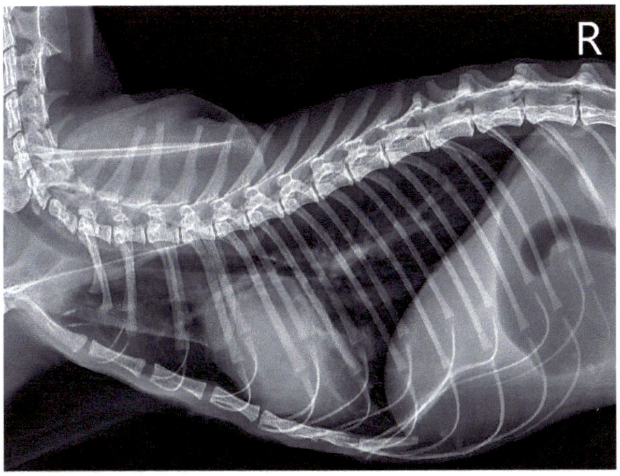

Figure 33. Lateral radiograph of the thorax of a patient with pulmonary hyperinflation. The diaphragmatic dome has a flattened shape, and the pulmonary field is more radiolucent than normal.

Pleural Space

Anatomy and Normal Appearance

The pleural space is defined as the cavity between the parietal and visceral pleurae in each hemithorax. This means that in the dog and cat there are two independent pleural spaces separated in the centre by the mediastinum.

The **parietal pleura** (costal, mediastinal and diaphragmatic) forms the outer layer of the pleural space. The **visceral pleura** (which covers the pulmonary surface and forms the pleural fissures) is the inner layer of the pleural space. Physiologically, there is a small amount of fluid in the space that reduces friction between the layers during breathing (Fig. 34).

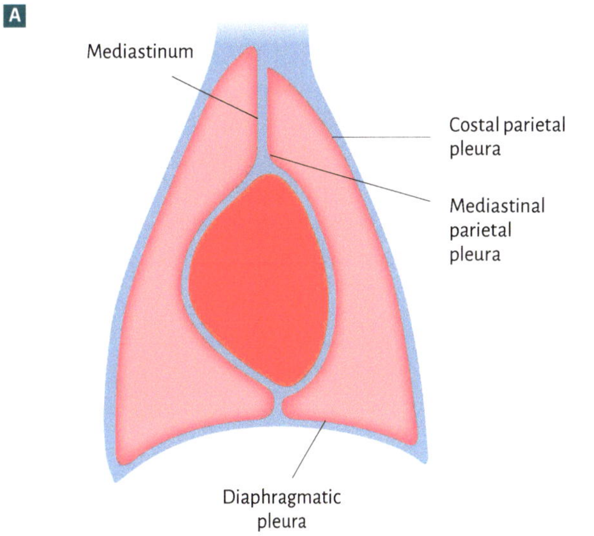

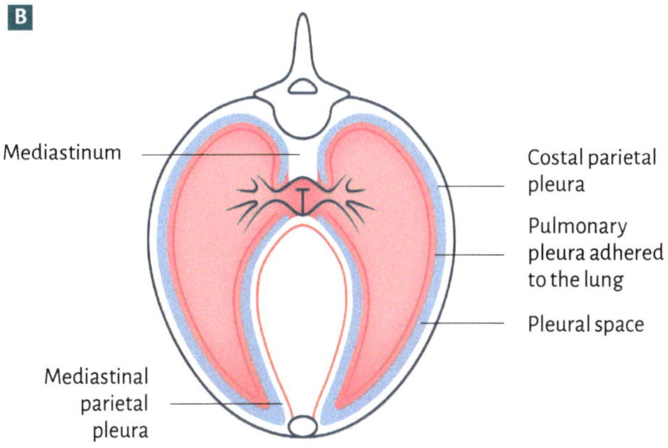

Figure 34. Diagram of the pleural space. In image (**A**), the arrows point to the parietal pleura in contact with the costal wall and the visceral pleura in contact with the pulmonary surface. In image (**B**), the pleural space between the two pleural layers is identified.

Radiographic Appearance

Under normal conditions the pleurae are not observed radiographically because they are extremely thin. Fine lines can be observed between the pulmonary lobes only if the radiographic view crosses the pleurae tangentially. These lines cannot be differentiated from a slight thickening of the pleurae; in both cases the appearance is not usually of clinical significance unless the increase in pleural thickness is more severe (Fig. 35).

In the VD or DV view, a soft tissue line joining the heart and diaphragm can be seen in the left hemithorax. This line is formed by the contact of the visceral and parietal pleurae of the accessory lobe and the left caudal lobe, which causes an accumulation of radiographically visible tissue called the caudal mediastinal recess (Fig. 36).

In the lateral views, a soft tissue line can be seen between the cranial portion of the left cranial lobe and the right caudal lobe; this is called the cranial mediastinal recess (Fig. 37).

Pleural Effusion

Pleural effusion is the accumulation of excessive fluid in the pleural space. This accumulation of fluid is visible radiographically; however, radiographs do not provide information regarding the nature of the fluid (hydrothorax, pyothorax, chylothorax or haemothorax). Fluid in the pleural space is located in the most dependent position in the chest. For this reason, in order to better visualise the cardiac silhouette in patients with moderate pleural effusion, a VD view should be obtained because in the DV view the fluid accumulates around the heart, producing a silhouette effect that prevents correct visualisation. In most cases, pleural effusions are bilateral due to the fenestrations of the pleura. In cases secondary to neoplasia, pleuritis or congenital closure of these fenestrations, a unilateral pleural effusion can occur.

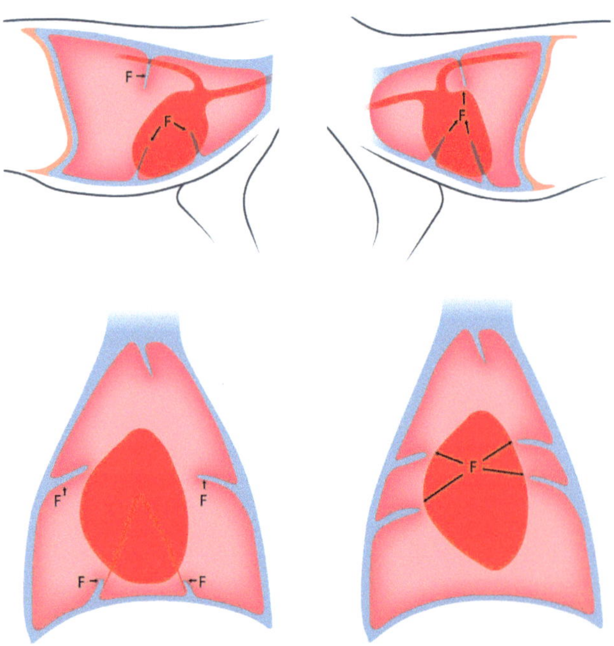

Figure 35. Schematic representation of the location of pleural lines over the pulmonary field. F: pleural fissure.

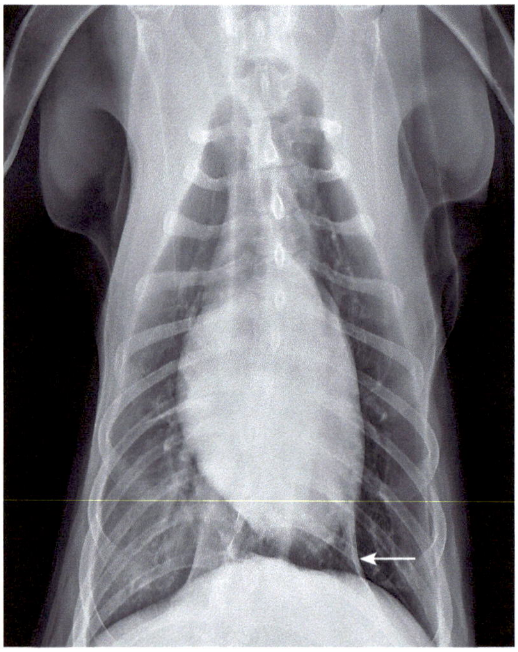

Figure 36. VD radiograph of the thorax of a skeletally mature dog. The arrow points to the caudal mediastinal recess.

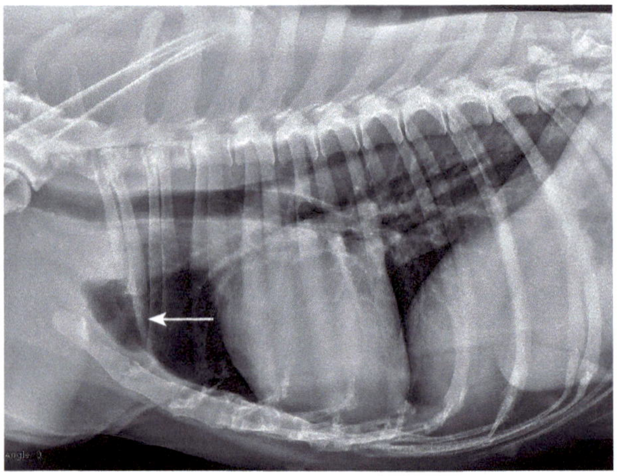

Figure 37. Right lateral radiograph of the thorax of a skeletally mature dog. The arrow points to the cranial mediastinal recess.

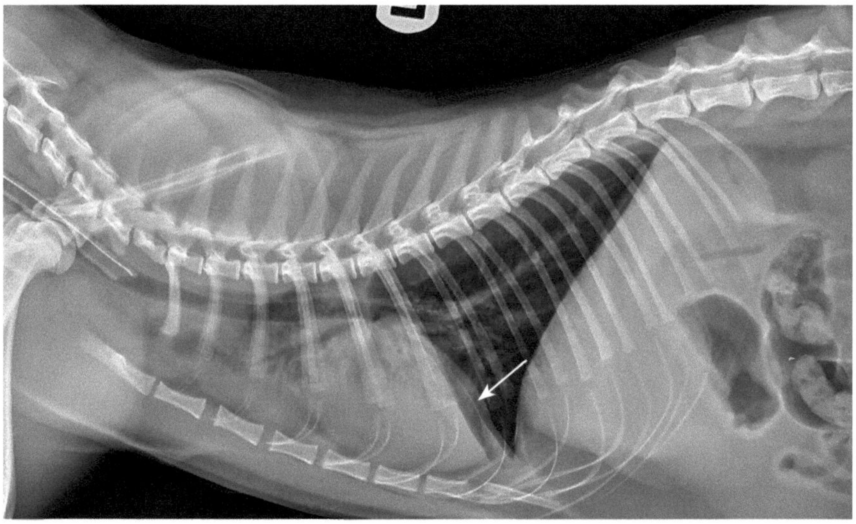

Figure 38. Lateral radiograph of the thorax of a cat with bronchopneumonia and a mild pleural effusion. A pleural line caudal to the cardiac silhouette (arrow) can be seen. In this case, removal of the pleural fluid revealed that it was a pyothorax.

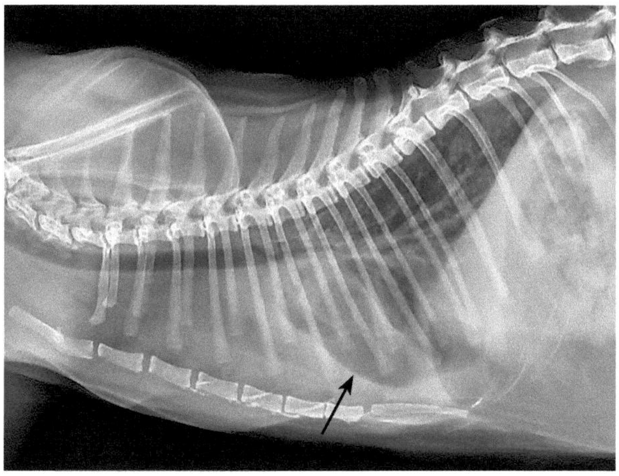

Figure 39. Lateral thoracic radiograph of a cat with a moderate pleural effusion. Retraction of the lung lobes (arrow) can be seen.

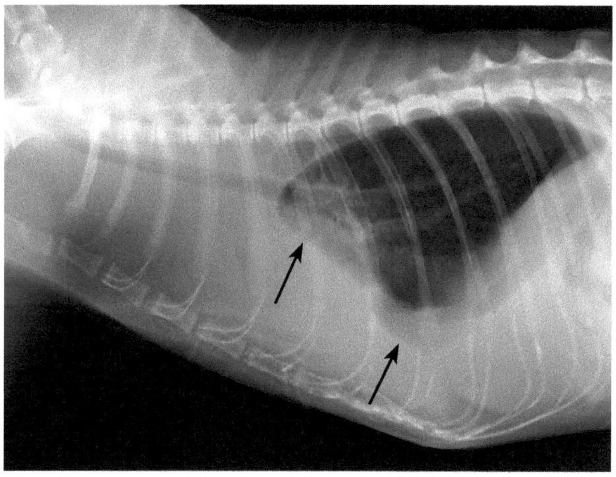

Figure 40. Lateral radiograph of the thorax of a cat with a severe pleural effusion. The lungs are floating in the fluid and appear to be displaced caudally (arrows) and dorsally.

If the volume of fluid is not very large (**mild pleural effusion**), pleural lines can be observed; these are lines with soft tissue density produced by the accumulation of fluid located between two lung lobes (Fig. 38). In these cases, lateral views are the views of choice to detect pleural effusion.

In cases with **moderate pleural effusion** (Fig. 39), pulmonary retraction can be observed, in which the pulmonary lobes separate from the costal wall because the fluid located in the pleural space causes them to retract. This retraction, in most cases, means that the edges of the rounded lung lobes can be visualised. In these cases, it is easier to locate pleural fissures.

In cases of **severe pleural effusion** (Fig. 40), the pulmonary lobes and the trachea move towards a caudodorsal position, and the thorax expands, potentially causing flattening of the diaphragm.

The **causes of pleural effusion** are very varied and largely depend on the type of fluid that the patient presents with. CT can be of great help to detect the underlying cause of pleural effusion, especially in cases of masses, pulmonary lobe torsion or pneumonia, because this imaging modality avoids the overlapping of structures. In some cases, the fluid in the pleural cavity is encapsulated or trapped in a specific area, usually due to fibrosis. In these cases, it is difficult to differentiate the presence of fluid or a mass radiographically. In cases of localised pleural effusions, the use of CT or ultrasonography allows determination of whether or not there is an accumulation of fluid.

Pneumothorax

Pneumothorax is defined as the accumulation of gas in the pleural space.

The views of choice to observe small amounts of free gas in the pleural space are DV and lateral projections, on which gas can be located in the caudodorsal area of the lung. On VD views, the gas is located in the centre of the radiograph, so it is difficult to demonstrate the presence of small amounts of gas on this projection.

When it is possible to perform VD radiographs with the patient in lateral recumbency (with the X-ray beam horizontal), this is the projection of choice because with the patient in this position the air moves to the highest area of the chest and overlap with the lung is avoided.

Pneumothorax can have a traumatic or spontaneous origin (deep-chested breeds are predisposed).

The accumulation of gas is usually bilateral, causing retraction of the pulmonary borders, which maintain their sharp-edged shape (Fig. 41). The space generated by the separation of the lung from the costal wall is evidenced by the lack of vascular structures in the space.

Pulmonary retraction means that the affected lobes do not expand properly, causing atelectasis. This results in an increase in pulmonary radiopacity, depending on the severity of the pneumothorax, and this can generate an interstitial or alveolar pattern.

The most characteristic sign of pneumothorax is the ipsilateral displacement of the heart towards the hemithorax where the most severe pulmonary retraction occurs; this causes the heart to separate from the sternum, and in lateral views the heart appears elevated relative to its normal position.

In more severe cases, where the pressure in the pleural space exceeds atmospheric pressure, a **tension pneumothorax** occurs. This develops because during inspiration the pleural space fills with air that cannot be released during expiration.

The positive pressure that is created in the pleural space causes the lung lobes to collapse and they are located next to the mediastinum. The thoracic cavity is more radiolucent than normal. The diaphragm can also be seen to flatten due to overdistension of the thorax, and the ribs can be seen to be perpendicular to the vertebrae. In cases of unilateral tension pneumothorax, there is a mediastinal deviation contralateral to the affected hemithorax.

CT can be useful to detect small amounts of gas, and it can also be useful to detect the cause of pneumothorax and can even detect small bullae that are not visible radiographically.

Pleuritis

Pleuritis is the inflammation of the pleural membranes. This inflammation results in thickening of the pleurae, making them visible on radiographs.

The origin of pleuritis may be secondary to reactive pleural effusions, feline infectious peritonitis (the most common

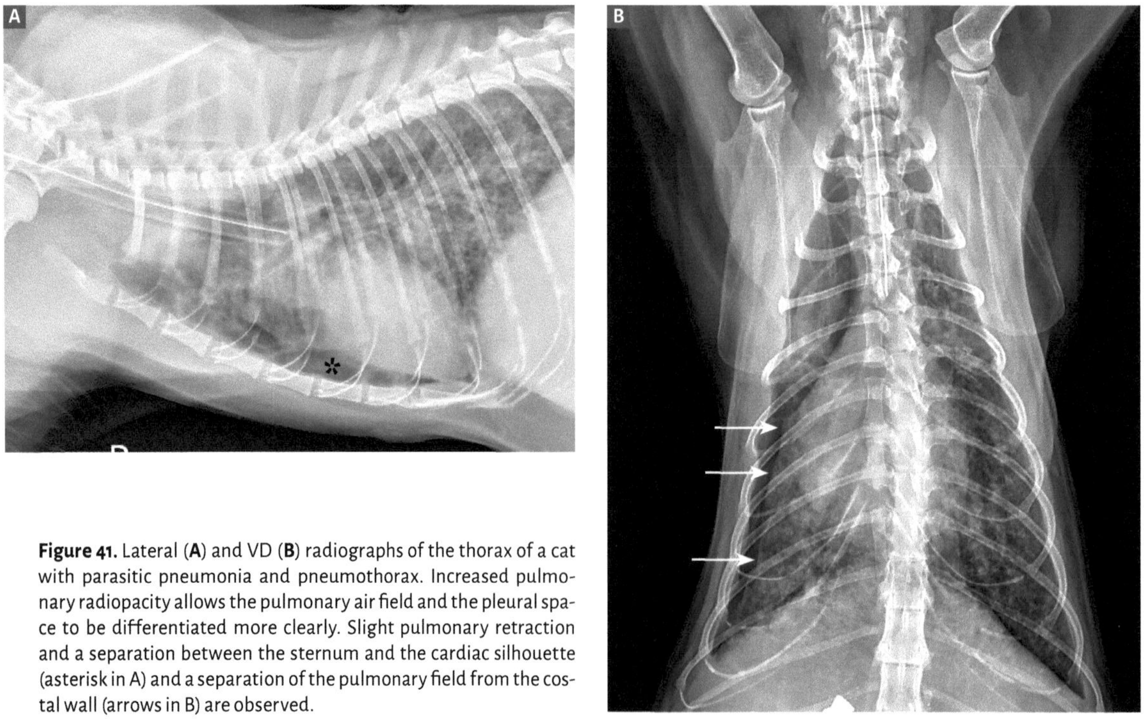

Figure 41. Lateral (**A**) and VD (**B**) radiographs of the thorax of a cat with parasitic pneumonia and pneumothorax. Increased pulmonary radiopacity allows the pulmonary air field and the pleural space to be differentiated more clearly. Slight pulmonary retraction and a separation between the sternum and the cardiac silhouette (asterisk in A) and a separation of the pulmonary field from the costal wall (arrows in B) are observed.

cause in cats), pulmonary pathologies (bronchopneumonia, neoplasia) or systemic pathologies (sepsis).

In both dogs and cats, pleuritis can be identified with the presence of thickened pleural lines or fissures between the pulmonary lobes. In very severe cases, these lines can be seen surrounding the entire pulmonary lobe.

The radiographic presentation of this condition may be confused with small amounts of pleural effusion or, in geriatric patients, with pleural thickening, which may be accompanied by calcifications (osteomas).

In more severe cases, pleuritis can result in an exudative process; in these cases the pleural effusion is secondary to the pleuritis.

Restrictive pleuritis can also occur; these are serious and/or chronic cases where the pleuritis does not resolve even when the pathology that caused it is no longer present. It causes adhesions, preventing the re-expansion of the pulmonary lobes.

Pleural Masses

Pleural masses may have their origin in haematomas, abscessed diaphragmatic hernias or neoplasms, among other pathologies.

The only primary neoplasms of the pleura are **mesotheliomas**, which occur in a disseminated manner and usually generate large amounts of pleural fluid.

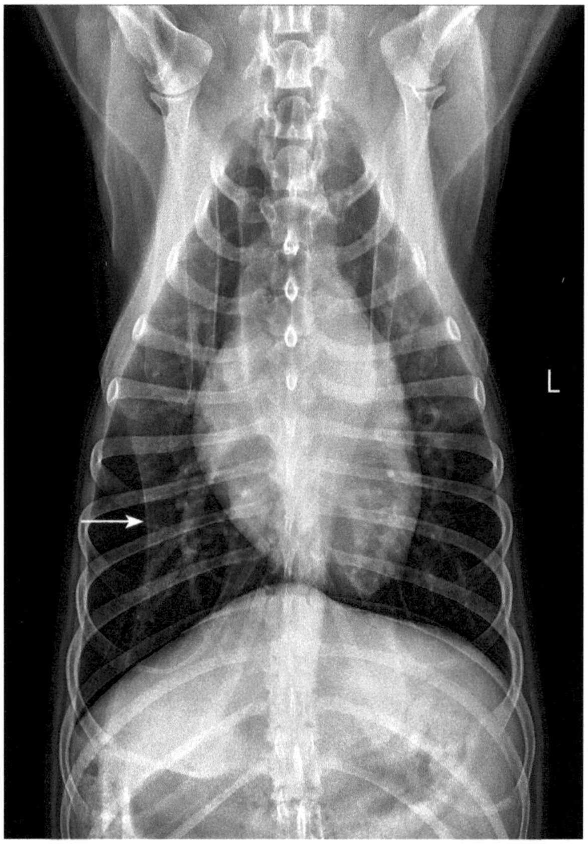

Figure 42. VD radiograph of the thorax of a dog, showing a skin fold protruding from the edges of the thorax (arrow).

Costal Wall

The costal wall refers to the structures surrounding the pleura, lungs and the rest of the viscera of the thoracic cavity. It is formed mainly by the ribs and the soft tissue that covers them, and these structures form the lateral limits of the thorax. The ventral limit is formed by the sternum where the ribs converge, joining through the costal cartilage. Dorsally, the thorax borders the thoracic vertebrae. The caudal border is the diaphragm.

The main function of these structures is to protect the organs inside and allow breathing. During the inspiratory phase the diaphragm contracts and the ribs rotate externally, and during expiration the diaphragm relaxes and the ribs return to their initial position.

When assessing thoracic radiographs, it is important to take into account that there is some overlap of the costal wall with the pulmonary parenchyma. For example, the abundant skin folds of certain breeds of dog can generate lines on thoracic radiographs that mimic pulmonary or pleural pathologies. To differentiate these lines from possible pathologies, the direction and length of the skin folds must be assessed, since they protrude beyond the edges of the thoracic cavity (Fig. 42). By contrast, pleural lines or pulmonary pathologies are seen only within the thoracic cavity.

There are also pathologies affecting the costal wall that can cause an increase or decrease in the radiopacity of the thorax, which can lead to false diagnoses of pulmonary pathologies.

Subcutaneous emphysema, which is the accumulation of air in the subcutaneous tissue, usually as a result of skin lacerations, oesophageal ruptures, or tracheal or pulmonary perforations, can lead to an accumulation of gas that will cause an apparent decrease in radiopacity in the thoracic cavity and can mimic lung lesions.

Subcutaneous oedema can produce a mottled pattern overlapping the chest that will increase the pulmonary radiopacity.

This pattern can also be generated by dirt on the skin or hair, and may also be seen in patients that undergo radiography while their hair coat is wet, for example, soon after an ultrasound examination.

To ensure that these pathologies do not lead to false diagnoses, it is necessary to obtain several views (at least two), and the changes at the level of the costal wall should be carefully examined (Fig. 43).

Costal wall tumours, although not very common, are another type of pathology that must be considered when interpreting thoracic radiographs. They can originate both at the level of the ribs and in the soft tissues that line the chest.

Among the costal wall tumours, the most common are **chondrosarcoma** and **osteosarcoma**; other tumours can also be found. In most cases they will cause inflammation of the soft tissues and bone destruction that is usually monostatic. Benign tumours can also be found, mainly **osteochondromas**, which originate in flat bones and cause a cauliflower-shaped growth with abundant bone formation. Primary tumours, both benign and malignant, usually originate in the distal third of the ribs, at the costochondral joint.

Radiographically, these tumours have a typical appearance of extrapleural masses, which are characteristic as they are surrounded by pleura, which causes them to have smooth edges, a wide base and a convex surface towards the inside of the thoracic cavity.

Unlike primary tumours, **metastases** that occur in the ribs are usually polyostotic, small in size and located in the proximal third of the ribs.

There are other tumours that do not originate in bone structures, but in soft tissues; the most common of these is **fibrosarcoma**, but **lipomas** or **liposarcomas** can also be found.

Diaphragmatic pathologies can be confused with pulmonary pathologies. Any defect in the diaphragm, whether in the form of a diaphragmatic rupture or a diaphragmatic hernia, will cause increases in the pulmonary or mediastinal radiopacity due to the presence of displaced abdominal organs in the thoracic cavity (Fig. 44).

Another diaphragmatic pathology that can cause changes on thoracic radiographs is **hemiparalysis of the phrenic nerve**, which will prevent the affected diaphragmatic crus from moving; it will be displaced cranially on radiographs. In these cases, inspiratory and expiratory radiographs should be taken to assess the changes in the position of the diaphragm in each of the phases of breathing.

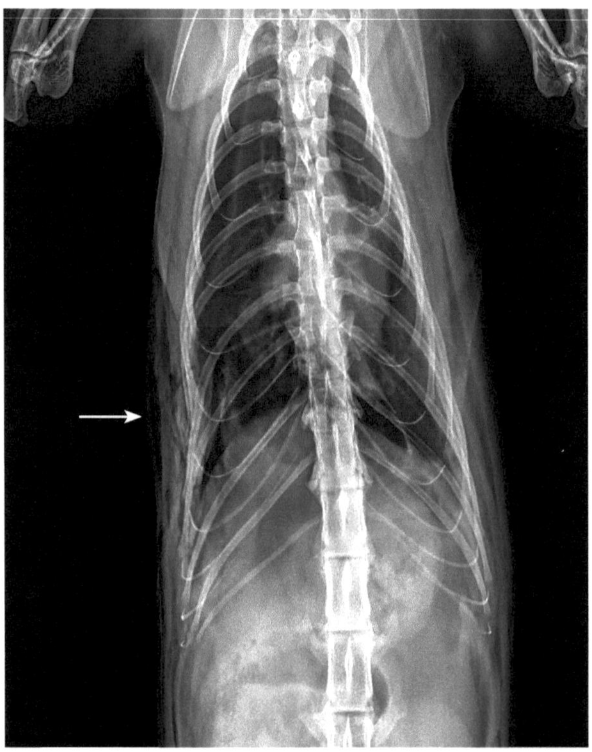

Figure 43. VD radiograph of the thorax of a patient with subcutaneous emphysema (arrow). In lateral radiographs, the costal wall lesion overlaps the lung, and the VD view is necessary to show that the lesion is extrapulmonary.

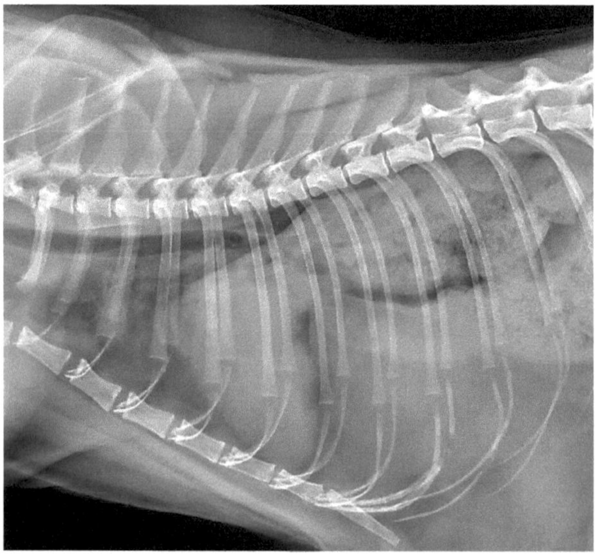

Figure 44. Lateral radiograph of the thorax of a cat with a diaphragmatic hernia. An increase in radiopacity is observed in the thorax, which should not be confused with pulmonary pathology.

Bibliography

- Agut, A. (2014) *Diagnóstico por Imagen en Pequeños Animales.* 1st ed. Multimédica Ediciones Veterinarias.
- d'Anjou, M.A., Tidwell, A.S., et al. (2005) Radiographic diagnosis of lung lobe torsion. *Vet Radiol Ultrasound,* 46(11):478–484.
- Forrest, L.J., Graybush, C.A. (1998) Radiographic patterns of pulmonary metastasis in 25 cats. *Vet Radiol Ultrasound,* 39(1):4–8.
- Hawkins, E.C., Basseches, J., Berry, C.R., et al. (2003) Demographic, clinical, and radiographic features of bronchiectasis in dogs: 316 cases (1988–2000). *J Am Vet Med Assoc,* 223(11):1628–1635.
- Hyun, C. (2004) Radiographic diagnosis of diaphragmatic hernia: review of 60 cases in dogs and cats. *J Vet Sci,* 5(2):157–162.
- Kogan, D.A., Johnson, L.R., Jandrey, K.E., et al. (2008) Clinical, clinicopathologic, and radiographic findings in dogs with aspiration pneumonia: 88 cases (2004–2006). *J Am Vet Med Assoc,* 233(11):1742–1747.
- Lamb, C.R., Withlock, J., Foster-Yeow, A.T.L. (2019) Prevalence of pulmonary nodules in dogs with malignant neoplasia as determined by CT. *Vet Radiol Ultrasound,* 60(3):300–305.
- Lobetti, R., Milner, R.J., Lane, E.P. (2001) Chronic idiopathic pulmonary fibrosis in five dogs. *J Am Anim Hosp Assoc,* 37(2):119–127.
- Lynch, K.C., Oliveira, C.R., Matheson, J.S., et al. (2012) Detection of pneumothorax and pleural effusion with horizontal beam radiography. *Vet Radiol Ultrasound,* 53(1):38–43.
- Schwarz, T., Johnson, V. (eds) (2008) *BSAVA Manual of Canine and Feline Thoracic Imaging,* 1st ed. BSAVA.
- Johnson, E.G., Wisner, E.R. (2007) Advances in respiratory imaging. *Vet Clin North Am Small Anim Pract,* 37(5):879–900.

Thrall, D.E. (ed) (2018) *Textbook of Veterinary Diagnostic Radiology.* 7th ed. Elsevier.

Radiography and Computed Tomography of the Thoracic Cavity: The Cardiovascular System and Mediastinum

Patricia Laborda Vidal

Introduction

This chapter covers the radiographic anatomy and the most frequent pathologies of the thoracic cardiovascular system and the mediastinum in dogs and cats.

Cardiovascular System

Radiographic Cardiac Anatomy

The cardiac silhouette is located in the central mediastinum, between the third and sixth intercostal spaces in lateral radiographic projections (Fig. 1).

The term **cardiac silhouette** is used instead of heart because the heart cannot be differentiated radiographically from the pericardium, pericardial fat or fluid, the small coronary vessels, or the exit and entry of the large vessels into the cardiac chambers. The cardiac silhouette is oval in shape, with the base located dorsally and the apex ventrally. In lateral views, the cardiac silhouette is tilted craniodorsally, with the apex in a more caudal position. In the dorsoventral (DV) and ventrodorsal (VD) views, the apex points to the left of the thorax.

Cardiac Chambers and the Clock Analogy

A good way to understand the position of the cardiac chambers is by viewing an angiocardiogram. Angiocardiography is a method of imaging in which radiographs are taken while the cardiac chambers are filled with contrast medium. On left-sided angiocardiography (Fig. 2 A), the left ventricle,

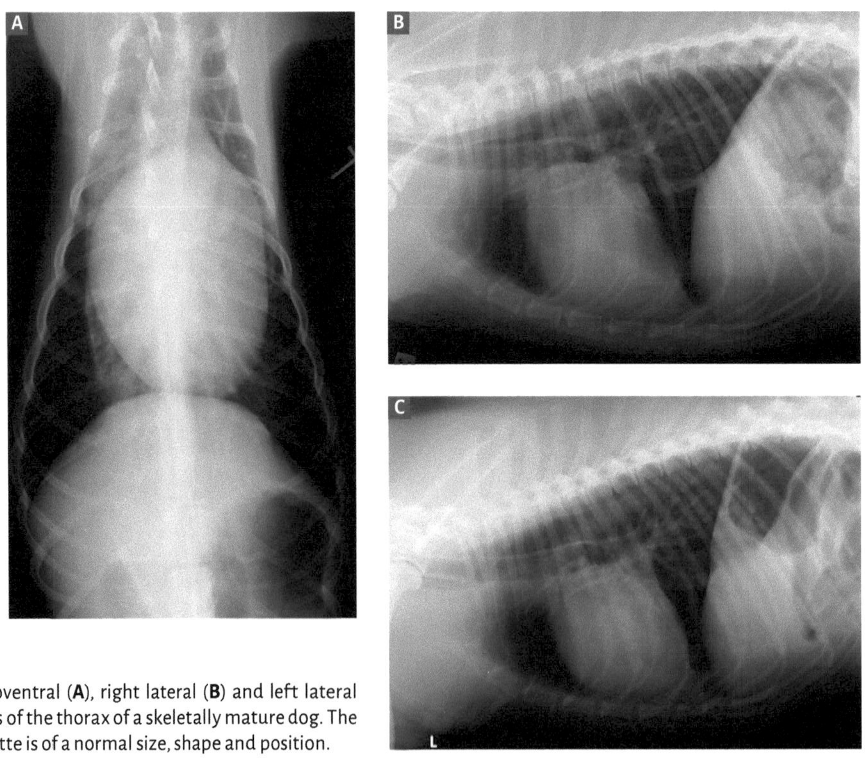

Figure 1. Dorsoventral (**A**), right lateral (**B**) and left lateral (**C**) radiographs of the thorax of a skeletally mature dog. The cardiac silhouette is of a normal size, shape and position.

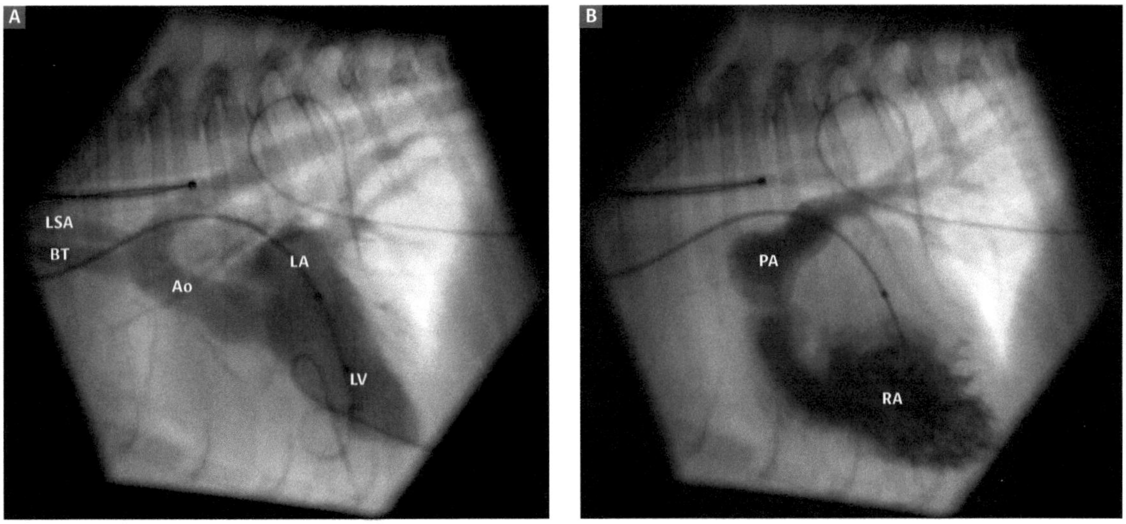

Figure 2. Left-sided (**A**) and right-sided (**B**) angiocardiograms of a dog with pulmonary stenosis. Poststenotic dilation is observed in the main pulmonary artery. LA: left atrium, LV: left ventricle, Ao: aorta, BT: brachiocephalic trunk, LSA: left subclavian artery, RV: right ventricle, PA: main pulmonary artery.

sometimes the left atrium, the aortic valve, the ascending aorta, the brachiocephalic trunk and the left subclavian artery can be seen. On right-sided angiocardiography (Fig. 2 B), contrast fills the right ventricle, the pulmonary valve, and the main pulmonary artery and its right and left branches.

Based on knowledge of the angiocardiographic appearance, it is then easier to imagine the position of the cardiac chambers when viewing a radiograph without contrast. The left-sided chambers are to the left and caudal, and the right-sided chambers are on the right and cranial. The cardiac apex can serve as a point of separation between the right and left sides.

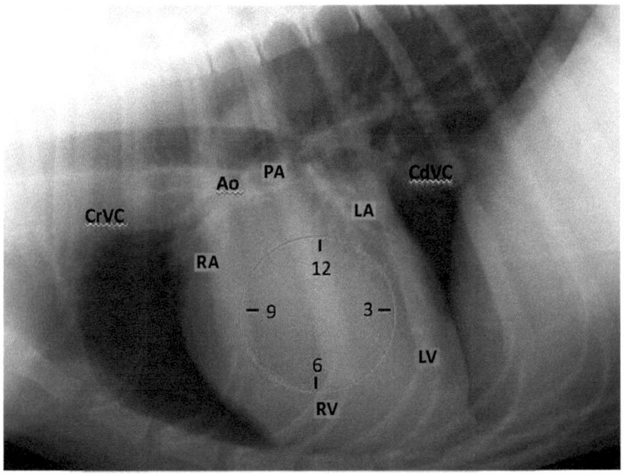

Figure 3. Representation of the clock analogy on a lateral radiograph of the thorax of a dog. LA: left atrium, LV: left ventricle, RA: right atrium, RV: right ventricle, Ao: aorta, PA: pulmonary arteries, CrVC: cranial vena cava.

The atria are located dorsally to the position of the caudal vena cava in a lateral view (the right cranially, the left caudally). The dorsal and caudodorsal borders of the left atrium, which are in a caudodorsal position in the lateral view, cannot be clearly delimited under normal conditions because they coincide with the entrance of the pulmonary veins and overlap with the exit of the right pulmonary artery.

To identify the location of the cardiac chambers and large vessels on a radiograph, the **clock analogy model** can be followed. This model is described in Figure 3 and Table 1.

Table 1. Description of the cardiovascular anatomy according to the clock analogy.

Lateral view	12–2 o'clock	Left atrium
	2–5 o'clock	Left ventricle
	5–9 o'clock	Right ventricle
	9–10 o'clock	Right atrial appendage and main pulmonary artery
	10–11 o'clock	Aortic arch
Dorsoventral view	11–1 o'clock	Aortic arch
	1–2 o'clock	Main pulmonary artery
	2–3 o'clock	Left atrial appendage
	3–5 o'clock	Left ventricle
	5–9 o'clock	Right ventricle
	9–11 o'clock	Right atrium

In dogs, when the left atrium is enlarged it is located between 5 and 7 o'clock according to the clock analogy (between the main caudal bronchi). In cats, it has a more cranial location, between 1 and 2 o'clock. This explains the shape of the well-known "Valentine's heart" when there is an increase in the size of the left atrium (and sometimes also of the right atrium) (Oura et al., 2015).

Cardiac Size

It is important to correctly measure the cardiac size on radiographs, but it should be noted that radiographic measurements and evaluations are imprecise for the identification of cardiomegaly; echocardiography and magnetic resonance imaging are the most appropriate diagnostic methods for this.

Table 2. Summary of objective assessment of heart size.

Evaluation	Dog	Cat
Right lateral view · Heart height · Intercostal spaces · Position of trachea	· 70% · 2.5–3.5 · Angle depends on breed	2.0–2.5
VD/DV view · Heart width	· 60–65%	
Vertebral heart score (VHS)	· 8.7-10.7	6.9–8.1

Table 3. Breed variations of the vertebral heart score (VHS) (Lamb et al., 2001; Bavegems et al., 2005; Marin et al., 2007; Kraetschmer et al., 2008; Jepsen Grant et al., 2013).

Breed	Vertebral heart score (VHS) (measured on vertebral bodies)
Boxer	11.6 ± 0.8
Cavalier King Charles Spaniel	10.6 ± 0.5
Dobermann	10.0 ± 0.6
German Shepherd	9.7± 0.7
Whippet	11.0 ± 0.5
Greyhound	10.5 ± 0.1
Labrador Retriever	10.8 ± 0.6
Yorkshire Terrier	9.7 ± 0.5; 9.9 ± 0.6
Boston Terrier	11.7 ± 1.4
Bulldog	12.7 ± 1.7
Pug	10.7 ± 0.9
Pomeranian	10.5 ± 0.9

There are various methods for measuring heart size, which will be explained in this chapter. These are forms of objective measurements. Objective measurements are just as important as the subjective assessment of heart size. It is important to remember that there are many variations in normal heart size.

In a right lateral view (Table 2):

- the **height of the heart** (from base to apex) should not exceed 70% of the height of the thoracic cavity;
- the **width of the cardiac silhouette** in dogs should measure 2.5–3.5 intercostal spaces, depending on whether the animal is of a deep-chested or wide-chested breed; and
- in cats, the width of the cardiac silhouette should measure 2.0–2.5 intercostal spaces.

In a DV view (Table 2):

- the width of the cardiac silhouette should measure 60–65% of the width of the thoracic cavity.

The **vertebral heart score** (VHS) was proposed in 1995 to eliminate variations inherent in the breed and chest conformation of dogs. Subsequently, breed variations have been observed, many of which have been detailed (Table 3). Therefore, the VHS should never replace a subjective evaluation, but it can be of great help for inexperienced personnel and in the sequential evaluation of the heart size of the same individual animal. To measure cardiac size using the VHS, a line is drawn from the ventral part of the carina/cardiac base to the cardiac apex in a well-positioned right lateral view, and measured. A second line is drawn perpendicular to the first in the widest area of the cardiac silhouette. The two measurements are then superimposed on the thoracic spine from T4 (Fig. 4). The number of vertebrae equivalent to each of these measurements is counted, and the two numbers are added up to give the VHS.

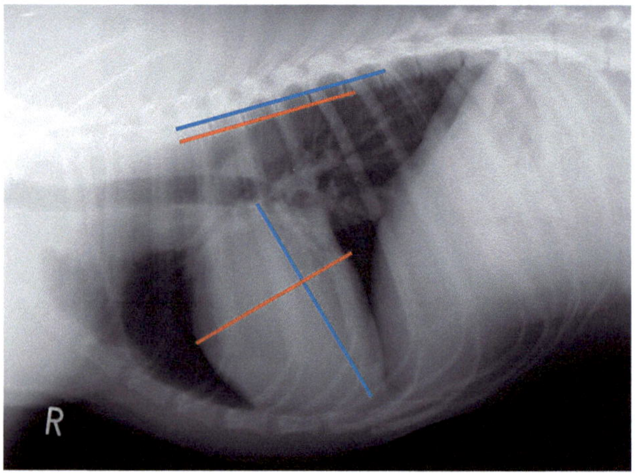

Figure 4. Right lateral radiograph of a dog. Red and blue lines indicate the measurements made for determining the vertebral heart score.

According to this system, in dogs the cardiac size should be 9.7 $\pm$ 0.5 (8.7–10.7), and in cats it should be 7.5 $\pm$ 0.3 (6.9–8.1).

Another indicator of cardiomegaly is the position of the trachea. Under normal conditions, in a lateral view, the position of the trachea diverges from that of the thoracic spine. The angle that is formed between these structures is quite consistent among cat breeds but can vary among dog breeds, being greater in deep-chested breeds and almost disappearing in barrel-chested breeds.

Microcardia usually appears as a narrow cardiac silhouette with a pointed apex in lateral radiographic views (Fig. 5). The apex may lose its contact with the sternum. The pulmonary vessels may be reduced in size and the lung may be hyperlucent without being hyperinflated. The caudal vena cava may also be reduced in size.

Factors Affecting Cardiac Size and Shape

Factors such as the animal's breed, amount of pericardial fat, age, position and respiratory phase affect cardiac size and shape.

Breed-related variations have been explained in the previous section.

Pericardial Fat

A large amount of pericardial fat can lead to a misdiagnosis of cardiomegaly (Fig. 6). It is important to distinguish between the fatty opacity of the pericardial space and the soft tissue opacity of the heart. The cardiac silhouette of obese animals may have less well-defined margins than that of a lean animal.

Age

Skeletally immature dogs appear to have an increased cardiac size. This is due to the smaller size of the rib cage compared with an adult dog. In general, VHS reference values in dogs are also applicable in puppies. In puppies, it is especially important to examine the shape of the cardiac silhouette for possible congenital heart disease.

Geriatric cats usually have a cranially inclined cardiac silhouette, presenting an increase in sternal contact. They may also have a redundant aortic arch. The causes of these changes with age are unknown.

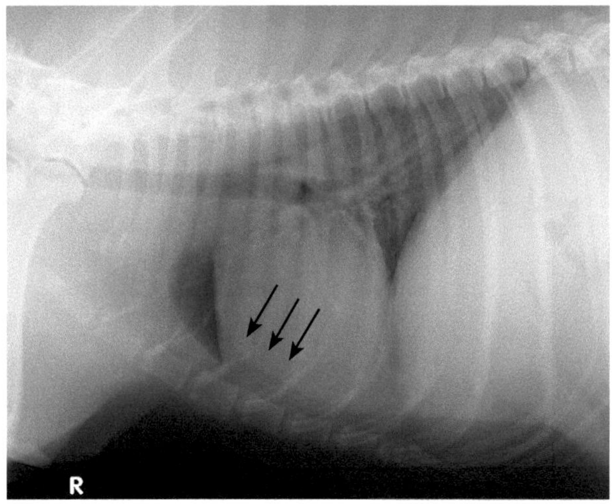

Figure 6. Lateral thoracic radiograph of a dog with a moderate amount of pericardial fat. Arrows indicate the pericardial fat.

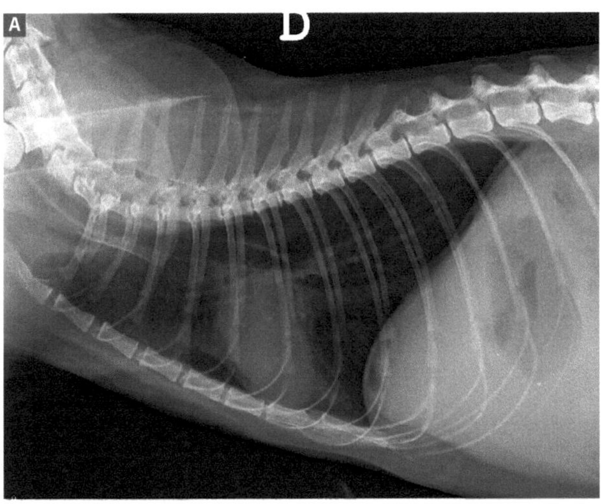

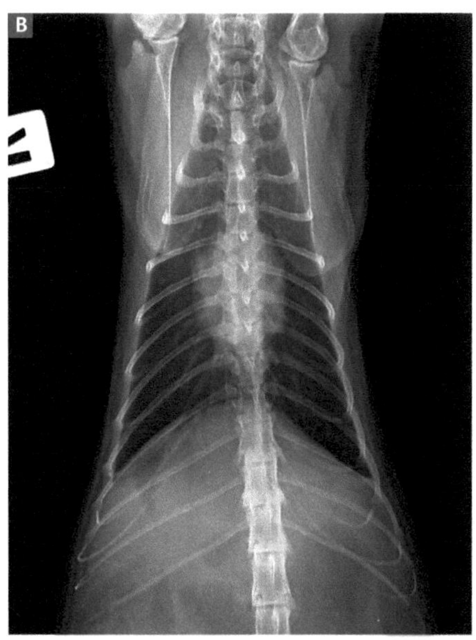

Figure 5. Right lateral (**A**) and dorsoventral (**B**) radiographs of the thorax of a cat with microcardia and a hypovascular lung pattern (see Chapter 13).

Body Position

Body position can cause variations in the size of the cardiac silhouette. For standardised heart size measurements, DV and right lateral views are always recommended.

Respiratory Phase (Fig. 7)

The cardiac silhouette may appear enlarged during expiration, due to the smaller size of the rib cage and the smaller volume of the lungs. In addition, during expiration, the margins of the cardiac silhouette may be more difficult to differentiate due to overlap with the diaphragm, mediastinal fat and increased lung opacity. These changes are more evident in barrel-chested dogs and obese animals.

Radiographic Anatomy of Large Vessels and Pulmonary Vessels

Aorta

The aortic arch and descending thoracic aorta can be identified on lateral and DV/VD radiographs, as seen in Figure 8. The diameter of the aorta should be similar to the height of an adjacent thoracic vertebral body, and is not affected by hypovolaemia or congestion, unlike the caudal vena cava. The aorta passes into the abdominal cavity (retroperitoneal space) through the aortic hiatus.

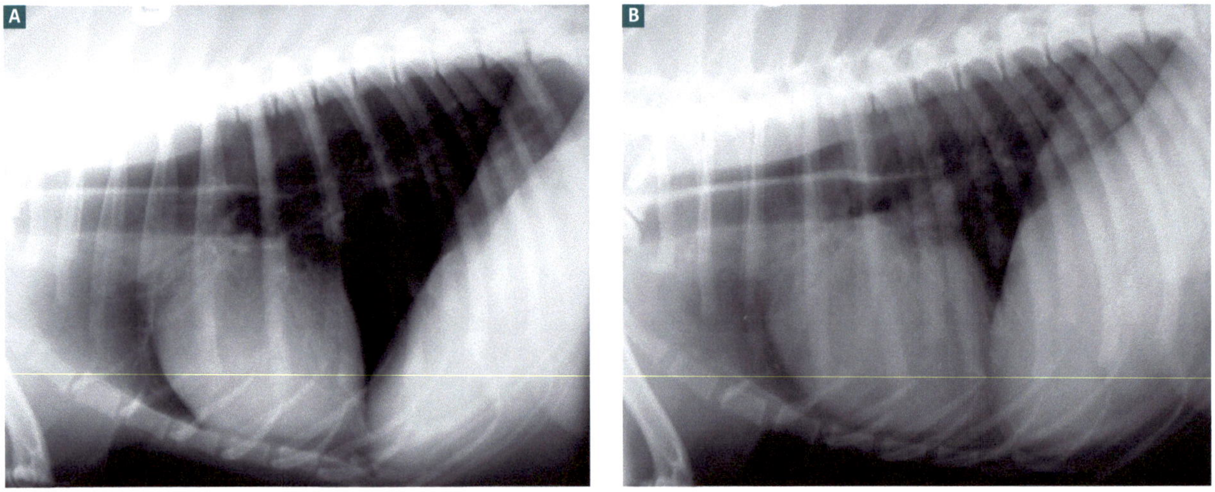

Figure 7. Lateral radiographs of the thorax of a dog on inspiration (**A**) and on expiration (**B**).

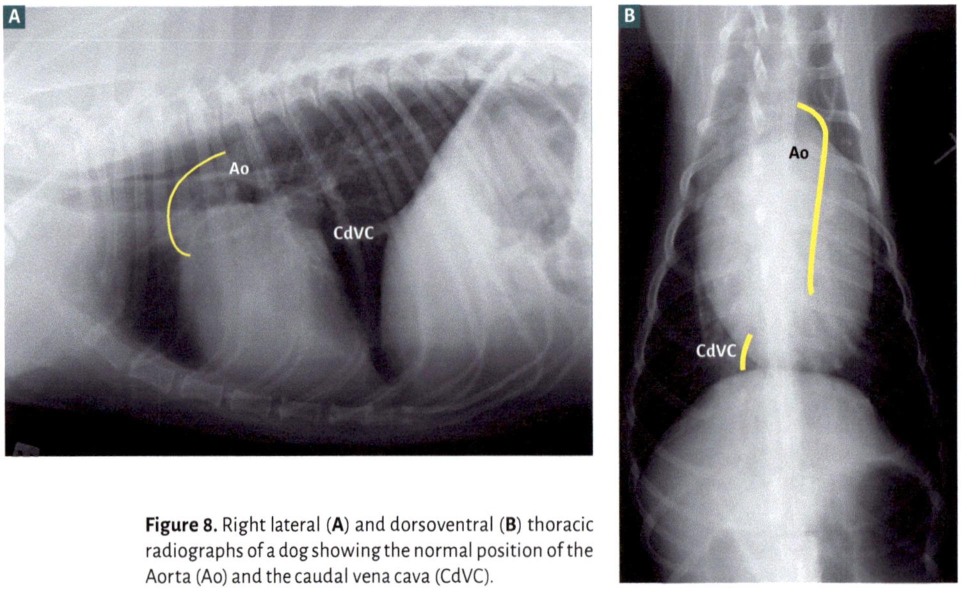

Figure 8. Right lateral (**A**) and dorsoventral (**B**) thoracic radiographs of a dog showing the normal position of the Aorta (Ao) and the caudal vena cava (CdVC).

Vena Cava

The caudal vena cava reaches the thorax from the abdomen through the hiatus or plica venae cavae, on the right side of the diaphragm. Its caudal portion can be seen, before it overlaps the cardiac silhouette (Fig. 8).

The cranial vena cava and its tributaries (right and left brachiocephalic veins) are located in the cranial mediastinum and can be identified radiographically only if there is a pneumomediastinum.

Pulmonary Arteries and Veins

The main pulmonary artery is not usually identifiable on plain radiographs because it overlaps the cardiac silhouette. In some animals it may appear in the VD view as a small bulge at 1–2 o'clock according to the clock analogy. The right and left main arteries and the lobar arteries can be identified (see Chapter 13).

Cardiovascular Diseases: Radiographic Signs

Generalised Cardiomegaly

Comparing radiographs from the same patient and measuring the VHS on each radiograph is very useful to detect initial or mild generalised cardiomegaly.

Dilated cardiomyopathy is one of the most common causes of generalised cardiomegaly. Radiographically, generalised cardiomegaly can be confused with a pericardial effusion. In pericardial effusion, the edge of the cardiac silhouette appears better defined than in generalised cardiomegaly, the shape is usually rounded or globoid, and the lungs usually appear hypoperfused due to cardiac tamponade (unlike in generalised cardiomegaly, where the pulmonary veins are usually congested/distended). The best method to differentiate generalised cardiomegaly from pericardial effusion is ultrasonography, with which an accumulation of anechoic fluid in the pericardial space can be observed.

It is important to remember that there are many diseases affecting the heart that may not result in an increase in cardiac size on radiographs. Among these are:

- endocarditis
- concentric ventricular hypertrophies: hypertrophic cardiomyopathy, aortic stenosis, pulmonary stenosis
- acute rupture of the chordae tendineae
- small defects in the atrial wall, ventricular wall, or small persistent arterial ducts
- constrictive pericarditis
- arrhythmias
- other heart diseases: acute myocardial failure, mild myocarditis, myocardial neoplasia.

Enlargement of a Specific Cardiac Chamber

Left Atrium

Left atrial enlargement is the most frequent cardiac chamber enlargement and is usually due to myxomatous degenerative disease of the mitral valve, as described below.

In the **lateral view**, it appears as a bulge at 12–2 o'clock, according to the clock analogy. Instead of curving in the direction of the tracheal carina, the caudodorsal part of the cardiac silhouette extends in a dorsal or caudodorsal direction, producing a straightening or even slightly concave aspect to the caudal margin. The appearance is also described as a loss of the caudal "waist" of the heart or as a higher caudodorsal cardiac border. In addition, dorsal displacement or compression of the left main bronchus may occur. Pulmonary veins may be congested and are seen as nodules with soft tissue opacity in the left atrial region (Fig. 9).

In the **DV view**, the left atrium is projected on to the cardiac silhouette at 5–7 o'clock according to the clock analogy, in a centred position between the main bronchi, which it displaces laterally. The main bronchi create a "bow-legged cowboy" shape. The double wall or double opacity sign is also usually observed, which is produced by the overlapping and summation effect of two soft tissue structures corresponding to the left atrium and the left ventricle.

Sometimes it is also possible to observe an increase in size of the left atrial appendage at 2–3 o'clock according to the clock analogy.

In the cat, the more cranial position of the left atrium causes the bulge to be seen on the left cranial edge of the cardiac silhouette in the DV view and may be difficult to locate on the lateral view. A widening of the base of the heart is usually seen in this view. When atrial dilation is marked, a so-called "Valentine's heart" can be observed (Fig. 10). This "Valentine's heart" can be observed with or without concurrent dilation of the right atrium. Occasionally, the dilated left atrium displaces the interatrial septum and the right atrium to the right.

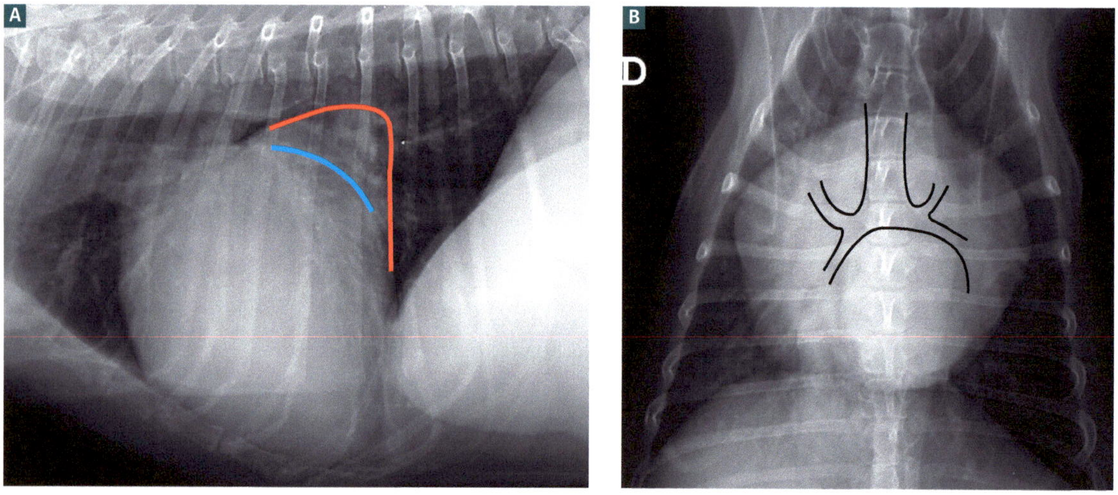

Figure 9. Right lateral (**A**) and dorsoventral (**B**) thoracic radiographs of a dog with a severe increase in left atrial size, dorsal displacement of the trachea, and compression of the carina and left main bronchus (B). In the lateral view, the red line marks the dimensions of the left atrium and the blue line indicates the margins of the normal atrium.

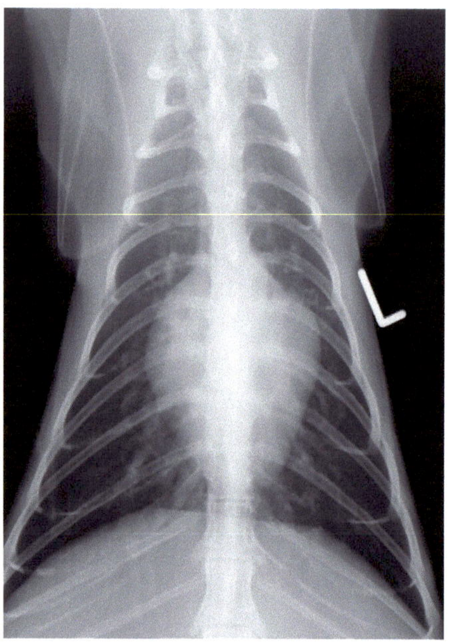

Figure 10. Dorsoventral thoracic radiograph of a cat with hypertrophic cardiomyopathy and dilation of the left atrium, showing the so-called "Valentine's heart".

Left Ventricle

As mentioned above, only eccentric ventricular hypertrophies (associated with an increase in volume, as in mitral insufficiency) can be distinguished radiographically, because concentric hypertrophies (associated with an increase in pressure, as in aortic stenosis) can occur with radiographically normal cardiac silhouettes.

In the **lateral view**, a dorsal displacement of the trachea is observed, with loss of the terminal curvature of the trachea.

In the **DV view**, a slightly rounded apex and a slightly elongated cardiac silhouette can be seen. The apex may be slightly displaced to the left hemithorax.

Right Atrium

An isolated enlargement of the right atrium is uncommon in dogs and cats and may not be seen on radiographs until it is very marked. It can be seen in some cases of tricuspid valve dysplasia.

In the **lateral view**, a bulge can be seen at the craniodorsal border of the cardiac silhouette, although this bulge is also observed when there is dilation of the aortic arch and the main pulmonary artery. If dilation is marked or there is a mass in the right atrium, dorsal displacement of the terminal trachea, cranially to the carina, may occur.

In the **DV view**, a bulge can be observed between 9 and 11 o'clock according to the clock analogy.

Right Ventricle

Right ventricular enlargement is usually caused by hypertrophy associated with pulmonary stenosis or pulmonary hypertension (e.g. filariasis).

Right ventricular enlargement tends to be overdiagnosed by radiography in barrel-chested dog breeds, due to increased

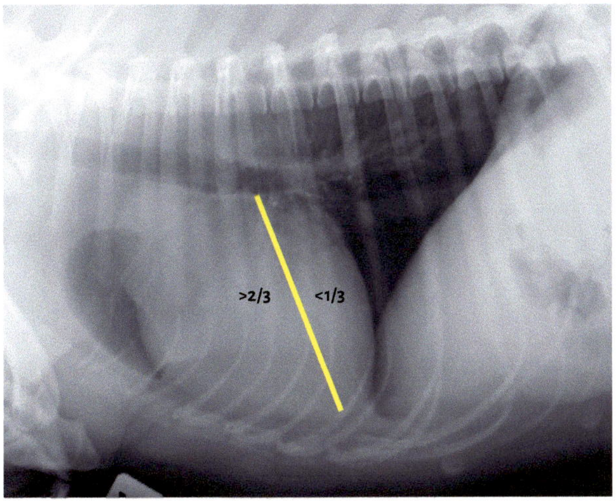

Figure 11. Right lateral radiograph of a dog with right-sided cardiomegaly.

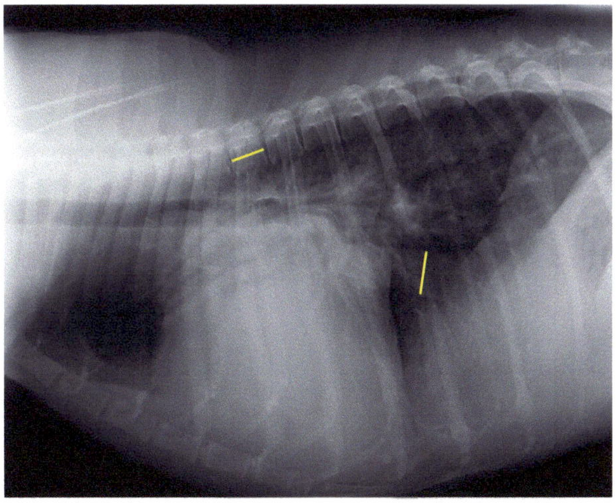

Figure 12. Right lateral radiograph of a dog with generalised cardiomegaly and congestive heart failure, showing dilation of the caudal vena cava and a hypervascular pulmonary pattern (enlarged pulmonary arteries and veins).

sternal contact in the lateral view compared with deep-chested breeds.

In the **lateral view**, the size of the right ventricle is assessed by drawing a line from the carina to the cardiac apex. Under normal conditions, two-thirds of the cardiac silhouette should be cranial to this line and one-third caudal to it. The cranial part corresponds to the right side of the heart (Fig. 11). An increase in the cranial component indicates an increase in the size of the right side of the heart.

In the **DV view**, a dilated right ventricle appears rounded and occupies a greater than normal proportion of the right hemithorax. The cardiac silhouette acquires an inverted D shape (Fig. 14). The cardiac apex may be displaced to the left hemithorax. It is important not to overinterpret the inverted D shape as right-sided cardiomegaly, especially in barrel-chested breeds, as the right ventricle is more rounded than the left ventricle in all dogs.

Microcardia

The radiographic characteristics of microcardia have been outlined previously (Fig. 5).

Differential diagnoses for microcardia include:

- hypovolaemia, shock and dehydration
- Addison's disease
- emaciation
- myopathies
- artefactual: pneumothorax, deep-chested dogs, deep inspiration.

Changes in the Main Vessels

Caudal Vena Cava

The diameter of the caudal vena cava may vary depending on the respiratory phase and cardiac cycle. If its diameter is greater than the length of the fifth or sixth thoracic vertebra, or if it is greater than 1.5 times the diameter of the aorta, it can be considered dilated (Lehmkuhl et al., 1997) (Fig. 12).

The caudal vena cava may be dilated if central venous pressure is increased. It may indicate right-sided heart disease but should be accompanied by other findings.

Aorta

If the aortic arch is dilated, a bulge is observed in the craniodorsal part of the cardiac silhouette in the lateral view, as well as a bulge at 11–1 o'clock (according to the clock analogy) in the DV view (Fig. 13).

Congenital cardiovascular diseases

This chapter will cover the most common congenital cardiovascular anomalies in dogs and cats.

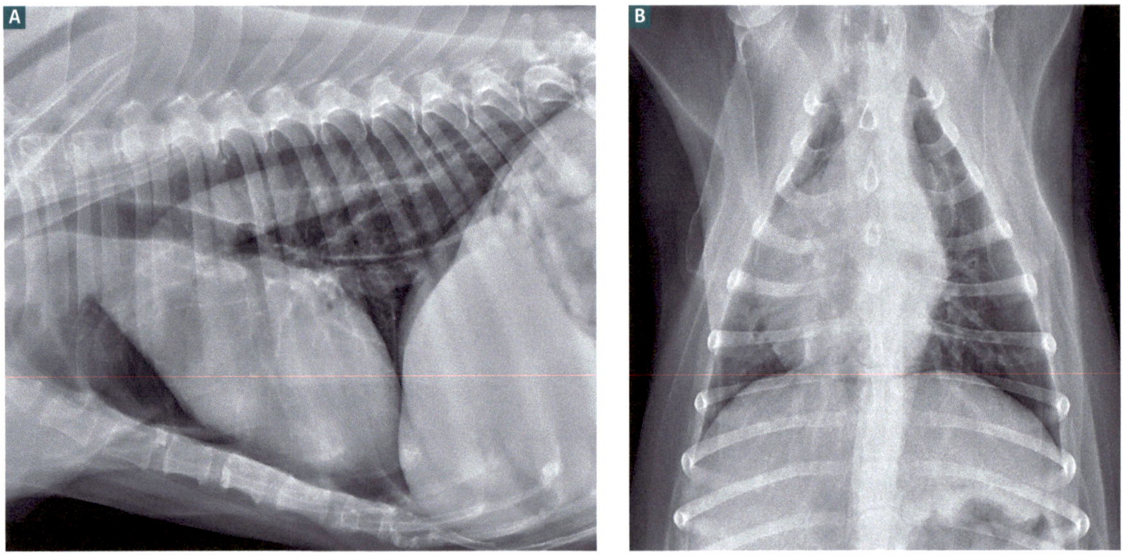

Figure 13. Right lateral (**A**) and dorsoventral (**B**) radiographs of a dog with a dilated aortic arch.

Pulmonary Stenosis

Pulmonary stenosis is one of the most common congenital heart diseases in dogs (Oliveira et al., 2011), but is rare in cats. Boxers and English Bulldogs are the breeds most frequently affected, but it has also been described in other breeds, usually small or medium sized.

Radiographic features include:

- right-sided cardiomegaly (increased sternal contact in the lateral view and an inverted D shape in the DV view) (Fig. 14);
- bulging in the area of the main pulmonary artery (poststenotic dilation) in the DV view (1–2 o'clock), and possibly in the lateral view, superimposed on the trachea (hat sign) (Fig. 15); and
- a pulmonary vascular pattern with reduction of pulmonary vessel size in severe cases (Fig. 11).

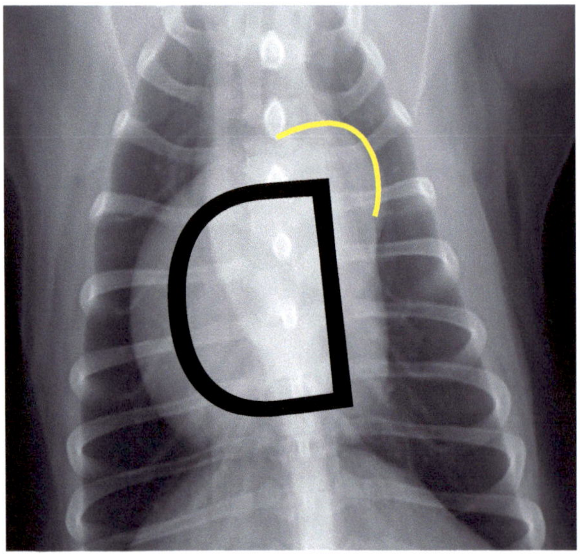

Figure 14. Dorsoventral thoracic radiograph of a dog with pulmonary stenosis and right-sided cardiomegaly. The reverse D sign and a bulge in the projection area of the main pulmonary artery (indicated with the yellow line, at 1–2 o'clock according to the clock analogy) are observed.

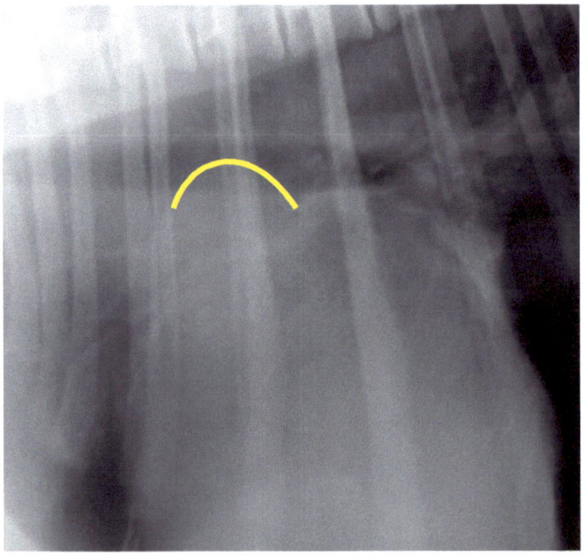

Figure 15. Detail of a right lateral thoracic radiograph of a dog with pulmonary stenosis, where the hat sign (shown by the yellow line) is observed.

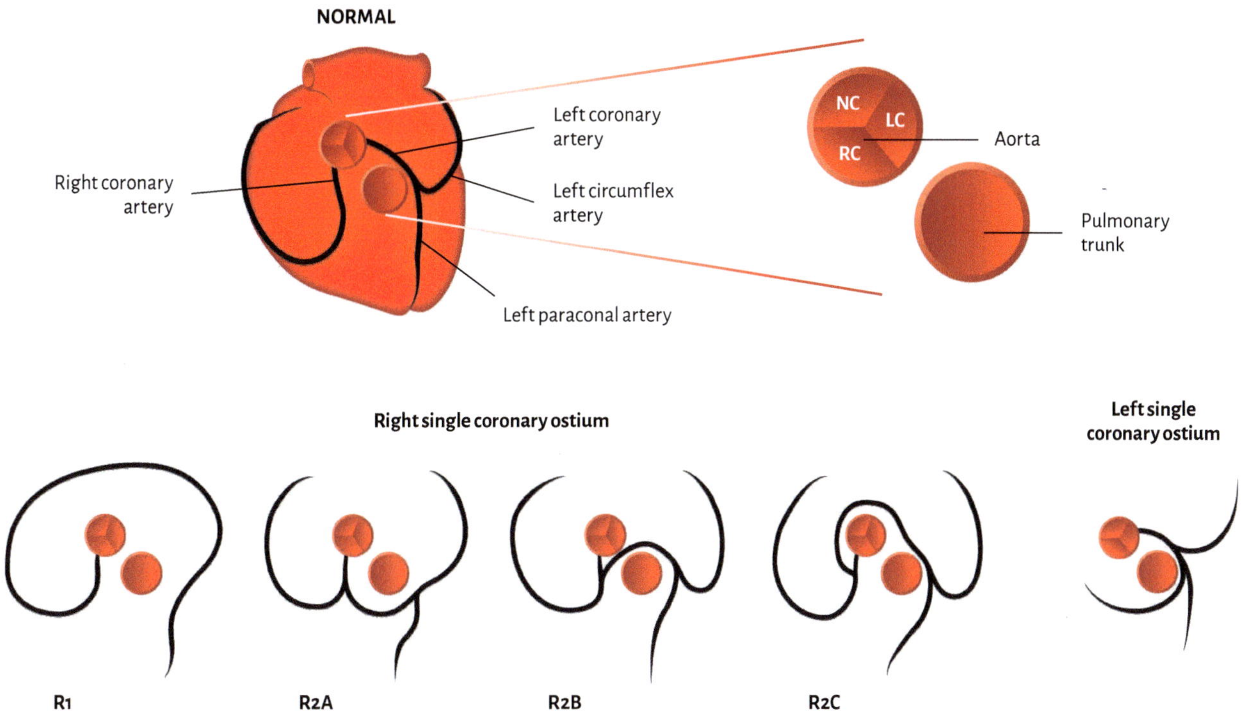

Figure 16. Schematic representation of coronary artery location and coronary abnormality patterns with a single right coronary ostium (with its variants: R1, R2A, R2B, R2C) and a single left coronary ostium. The R2A variant of the single right coronary ostium and the single coronary left ostium have an aberrant coronary artery surrounding the pulmonary trunk. These variants have been described by Buchanan (1990) and Visser et al. (2013), respectively. LC: left cusp, NC: non-coronary cusp, RC: right cusp.

The stenosis can be valvular, subvalvular or supravalvular, and echocardiography allows a definitive diagnosis to be made. In Boxers and English Bulldogs, the R2A-type coronary anomaly has been described, in which there is a single right coronary ostium (Buchanan, 1990) (Fig. 16). Subsequently, an aberrant right coronary artery with a single left coronary ostium has also been described (Visser et al., 2013). In these breeds, detection of these abnormalities prior to balloon valvuloplasty treatment is vital to avoid a reduction in coronary flow, or a coronary avulsion during the procedure, which can result in the death of the patient. The use of cardiac computed tomography (CT) has recently been described in patients with pulmonary stenosis (Laborda-Vidal et al., 2016; Gunther-Harrington et al., 2019). It allows visualisation of the pulmonary annulus, pulmonary valves, pulmonary arteries and cardiac chambers, and evaluation of the coronary arteries in a more precise manner than in selective coronary angiography (due to the absence of overlap) (Fig. 17).

Patent Ductus Arteriosus

Patent ductus arteriosus (PDA) is another of the most common congenital heart diseases in dogs. The German Shepherd and some small breeds (Bichon Frise, Poodle, Chihuahua, Pomeranian, Maltese, Shetland Sheepdog) are predisposed. It is uncommon in cats.

Communication between the pulmonary artery and the descending aortic artery through the ductus arteriosus is normal in the foetal circulation. However, the ductus should close at between 7 and 10 days postpartum, and the arterial ligament remains. When it remains open after that period, communication between the pulmonary and systemic circulation is maintained.

Radiographically, the following can be seen (Fig. 18):

- left-sided cardiomegaly or sometimes generalised cardiomegaly
- an increase in aortic arch size due to turbulent flow
- increased size of the main pulmonary artery due to increased pressure and flow
- an increase in size of the left atrium due to increased flow
- an increase in left ventricular size
- a hypervascular pulmonary pattern due to pressure and flow overload
- in the DV view, all three bulges (corresponding to the aortic arch, pulmonary trunk and left atrial appendage) can be observed at 11–1 o'clock, 1–2 o'clock and 2–3 o'clock, respectively. These three bulges are pathognomonic for PDA but are seen in only approximately 20–25% of dogs.

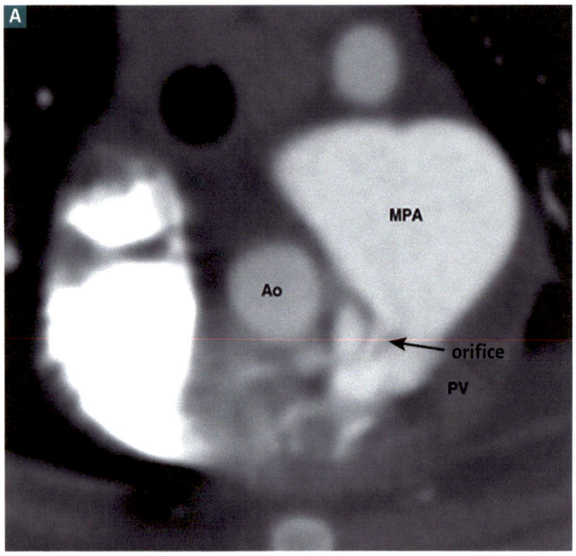

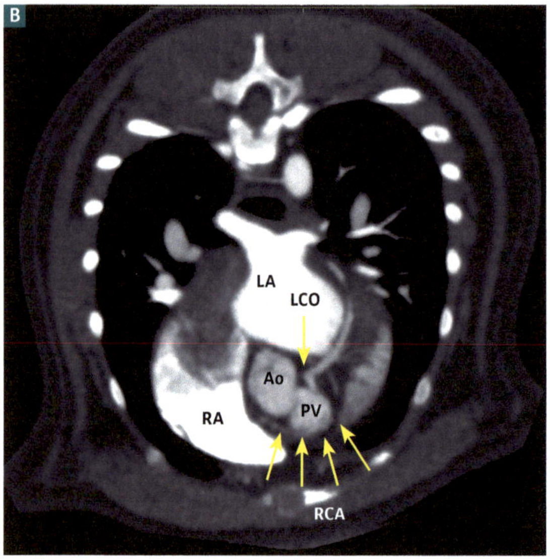

Figure 17. Cardiac CT of a dog with pulmonary stenosis and aberrant coronary artery. Multiplanar reconstructions showing (**A**) pulmonary valve (PV) stenosis and the exit orifice, the main pulmonary artery (MPA) with severe poststenotic dilation, and the Aorta (Ao); and (**B**) a single left coronary ostium (LCO), from which the aberrant right coronary artery (RCA) exits and surrounds the main pulmonary artery at the height of the pulmonary valve (PV). Ao: Aorta, LA: left atrium, RA: right atrium.

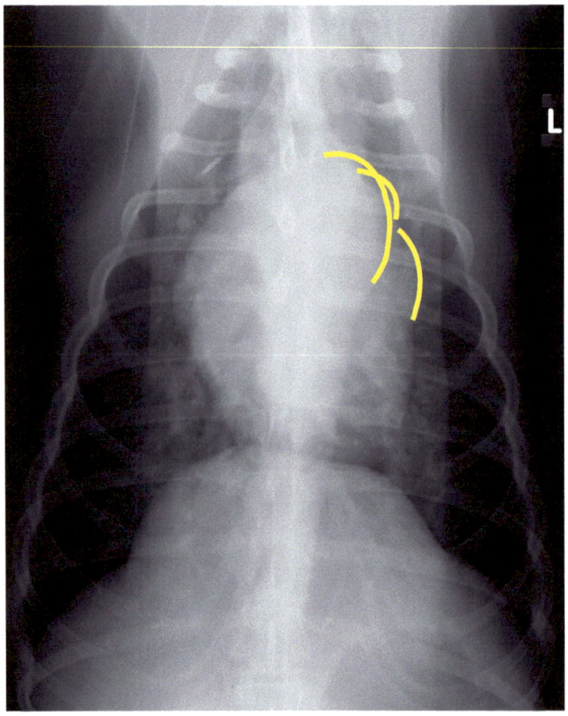

Figure 18. Dorsoventral thoracic radiograph of a dog with patent ductus arteriosus. Three bulges (indicated with yellow lines) can be seen corresponding to the aortic arch, pulmonary trunk and left atrial appendage. In addition, there is a hypervascular lung pattern with dilation of tortuous pulmonary arteries.

PDA morphology has been described using angiography and has been classified into three main types (Miller et al., 2006). Subsequently, abnormalities of the thoracic aorta, including PDA, have also been described using CT (Henjes et al., 2011). PDAs have been classified as follows (Fig. 19).

- I: the diameter of the ductus gradually decreases from the aorta to the main pulmonary artery.
- IIA: the walls of the ductus are parallel until its diameter is abruptly reduced in the area of insertion into the main pulmonary artery.
- IIB: the ductus has a funnel shape, narrowing towards the main pulmonary artery. This is the most frequent presentation. Flow is from left to right.
- III: a cylindrical ductus, without final narrowing, is the least common type. This presentation is associated with postnatal pulmonary hypertension and a bidirectional or right-to-left shunt (Eisenmenger syndrome), also known as reverse PDA. It is the only case in which there is a hypovascular lung pattern.

Aortic Stenosis

Among the breeds of dog predisposed to this anomaly are the Boxer, Golden Retriever, German Shepherd, Pointer, Rottweiler, Bulldog, Bull Terrier and Newfoundland. In mild cases of aortic stenosis, radiographs are usually normal, as occurs with other congenital diseases (Lamb et al., 2001). In severe cases (Fig. 20), the radiographic changes that are observed are:

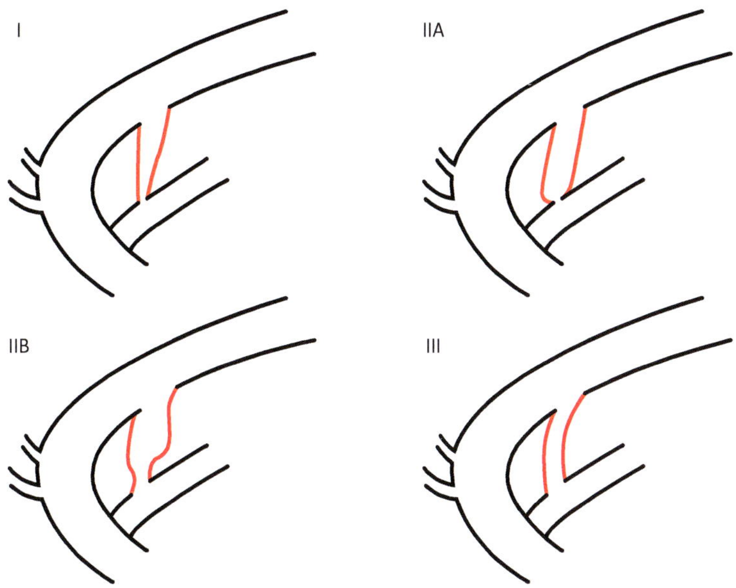

Figure 19. Representation of the four types of patent ductus arteriosus described using aortic angiography. I: the diameter of the ductus gradually decreases. IIA: the walls of the ductus are parallel until it narrows in the insertion zone in the pulmonary artery. IIB: the ductus is funnel shaped, narrowing towards the main pulmonary artery. III: the ductus is cylindrical, without final narrowing. Adapted from Miller et al. (2006).

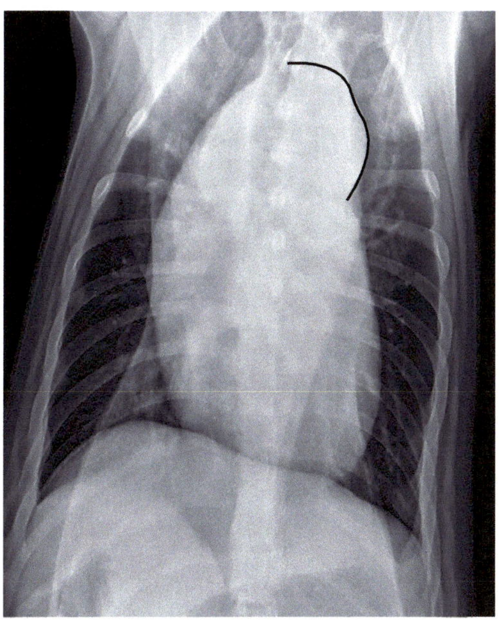

Figure 20. Dorsoventral thoracic radiograph of a dog with severe aortic stenosis. A marked bulge is observed in the projection area of the aorta (indicated with the black line, at 11–1 o'clock according to the clock analogy), as well as a rounded left ventricle.

- an increase in aortic arch size due to turbulent flow;
- left ventricular enlargement (hypertrophy);
- left atrial dilation may be present, especially if there is mitral regurgitation; and
- normal pulmonary vessels if there is no left-sided heart failure.

Ventricular Septal Defect

Ventricular septal defect (VSD) is a common congenital defect in both dogs and cats. Predisposed breeds of dog include the Springer Spaniel, Border Collie and West Highland White Terrier.

During systole, due to the pressure difference between the right and left sides and the position of the defect, blood is channelled from the left ventricle to the outflow tract of the right ventricle or the pulmonary arteries. This causes the following radiographic characteristics:

- normal radiographs when the VSD is small
- slight hypertrophy of the right ventricle due to pressure and volume overload
- a hypervascular pulmonary pattern due to pulmonary overcirculation
- an increase in the size of the atrium and left ventricle due to eccentric hypertrophy, in cases of large defects.

Atrial septal defects are uncommon in the dog and cat and therefore will not be addressed in this chapter.

Mitral Dysplasia

This is the most common congenital heart disease in cats. In dogs, predisposed breeds include the Great Dane, English Bulldog, Bullmastiff, Bull Terrier, German Shepherd, Golden Retriever and Newfoundland.

The radiographic characteristics are similar to those described in mitral regurgitation due to degenerative mitral valve disease:

- atrial and left ventricular enlargement (eccentric hypertrophy due to volume overload)
- pulmonary vein dilation
- left-sided congestive heart failure: pulmonary oedema (and possible pleural effusion in cats) in severe cases.

Tricuspid Dysplasia

This disease is more common in dogs than in cats. One of the most predisposed breeds is the Labrador Retriever.

The radiographic features are those of right-sided cardiomegaly:
- increases in right atrial and ventricular size (dilation)
- left shift of the apex in the DV view
- dilation of the caudal vena cava, hepatomegaly and ascites in cases of right-sided congestive failure.

Persistence of the Fourth Right Aortic Arch

Persistence of the fourth right aortic arch (P4RAA) is the most common vascular ring anomaly in dogs; predisposed breeds include the German Shepherd, Irish Setter and Greyhounds. It is usually identified in young animals presenting with megaoesophagus and associated problems.

The radiographic characteristics are:
- oesophageal dilation cranial to the cardiac base;
- focal curvature of the trachea to the left in the DV view cranial to the cardiac silhouette. This is a pathognomonic finding of P4RAA in young animals presenting with compatible symptomatology (Buchanan, 2004) (Fig. 21);
- ventral displacement of the trachea cranial to the cardiac base;
- the left margin of the descending aorta is not visible; and
- a ventral lobar alveolar pattern if aspiration pneumonia is present.

Acquired Valvular Diseases

Myxomatous Degenerative Valve Disease

This disease can occur in the mitral or tricuspid valve. It is the most common acquired valve disease in small and medium-sized breeds of dog, with a predisposition in certain breeds such as the King Charles Cavalier Spaniel, Poodle and Chihuahua. It is uncommon in cats.

Radiographic signs are variable, depending on the severity of the disease. Depending on whether the mitral or tricuspid valve is affected, the following signs can be observed:
- increase in left atrial size (mitral). This is one of the most consistent signs and has an early onset (Figs. 9 and 22)
- increase in left ventricular size (mitral) (Fig. 22)
- increase in right atrial and ventricular size (tricuspid)
- left-sided congestive heart failure, with pulmonary venous congestion and/or cardiogenic (mitral) pulmonary oedema
- right-sided congestive heart failure (tricuspid).

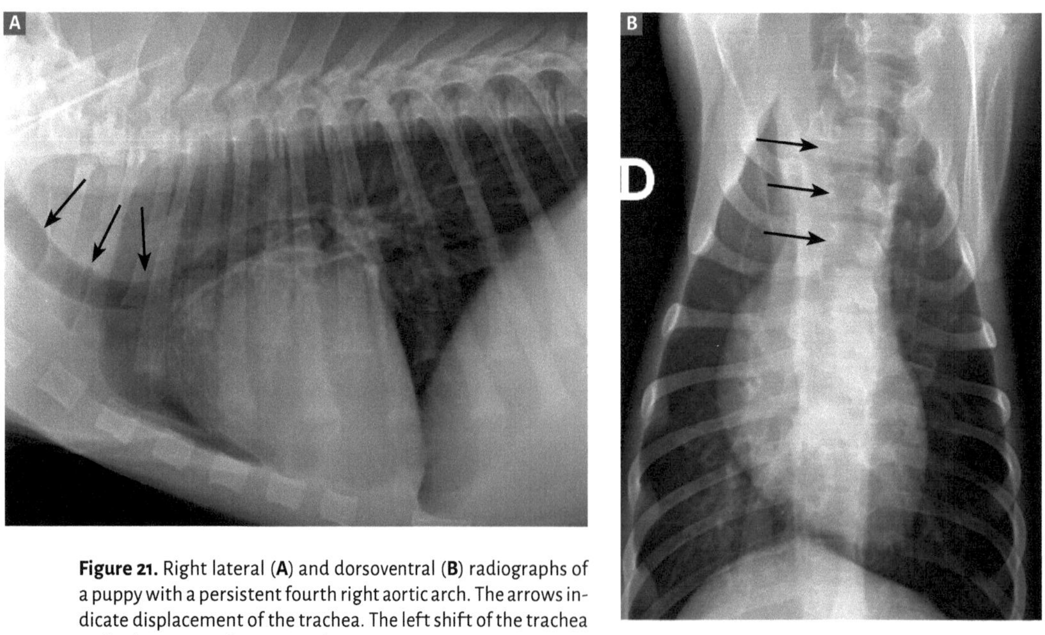

Figure 21. Right lateral (**A**) and dorsoventral (**B**) radiographs of a puppy with a persistent fourth right aortic arch. The arrows indicate displacement of the trachea. The left shift of the trachea in the dorsoventral view is pathognomonic.

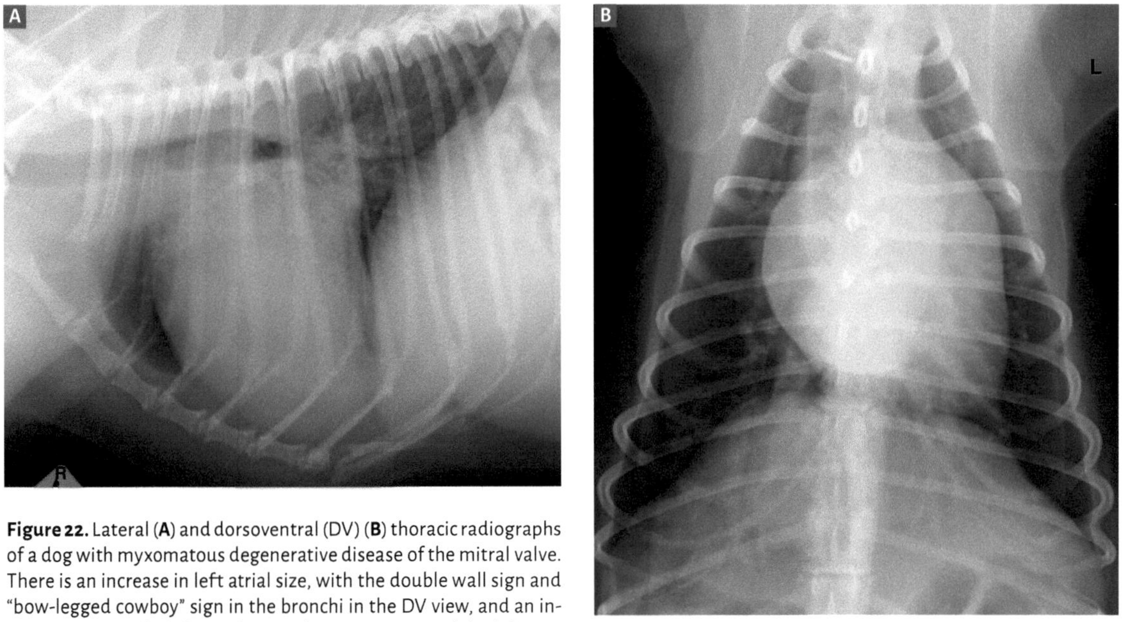

Figure 22. Lateral (**A**) and dorsoventral (DV) (**B**) thoracic radiographs of a dog with myxomatous degenerative disease of the mitral valve. There is an increase in left atrial size, with the double wall sign and "bow-legged cowboy" sign in the bronchi in the DV view, and an increase in size in the left atrial appendage (DV view) and the left ventricle, without congestive disease.

Echocardiography allows a diagnosis to be made. Studies on the quantification of left atrial size using radiographs in dogs with degenerative myxomatous mitral disease have been published (Malcolm et al., 2018; Lam et al., 2021).

Acute rupture of chordae tendineae or papillary muscles can occur as a result of acute trauma. The radiographic characteristics are very variable; in cases of left-sided ruptures, acute pulmonary oedema usually occurs.

Other acquired valve diseases such as **aortic** or **pulmonary insufficiency** or **bacterial endocarditis** are usually diagnosed by echocardiography without presenting radiographic alterations in the initial phases of the disease.

Myocardial Diseases

In general, it is not possible to differentiate between cardiomyopathies radiographically. Myocardial diseases can be of primary origin or secondary to other pathologies, such as hyperthyroidism or hypothyroidism, hypertension, acromegaly and pulmonary pathologies, among others. The most common ones are described in this chapter.

Dilated Cardiomyopathy

Breeds of dog that are predisposed mainly include the Dobermann, Great Dane, Newfoundland, Saint Bernard, Irish Wolfhound and Spaniels. Animals usually present due to the onset of congestive heart failure or to rule out disease prior to breeding. Dilated cardiomyopathy is difficult to detect on radiographs in animals in the preclinical phase.

Radiographic characteristics include (Fig. 23):

- left atrial and ventricular enlargement due to dilation (sometimes dilation of all four cardiac chambers);
- congestive heart failure, usually left-sided; and
- extremely well-defined cardiac borders in advanced cases due to systolic dysfunction.

Arrhythmogenic Right Ventricular Cardiomyopathy

This is a hereditary disease in Boxers. It has also been seen in cats. Boxers may present with the typical features of dilated cardiomyopathy, or there may be no structural changes despite the presence of severe ventricular arrhythmias.

Hypertrophic Cardiomyopathy

This is the most common myocardial disease in cats (especially in the Maine Coon and Persian breeds; Baty, 2004) and is rare in dogs. Autosomal dominant genetic transmission has been demonstrated in Maine Coons (Meurs et al., 2005). It is characterised by thickening or concentric hypertrophy of the left ventricular wall. Cats frequently show signs of acute left-sided congestive heart failure.

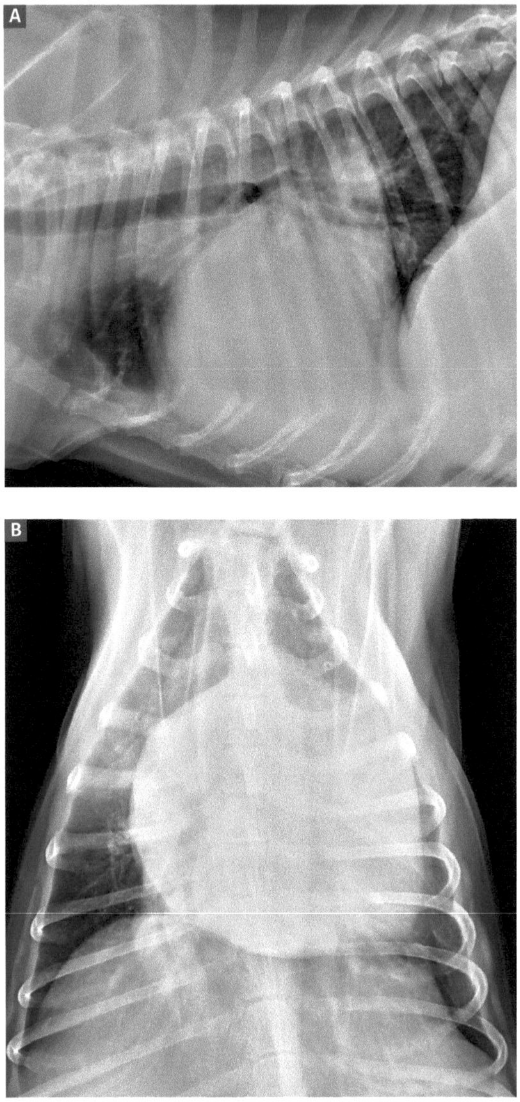

Figure 23. Right lateral (**A**) and dorsoventral (**B**) radiographs of a dog with severe dilated cardiomyopathy and congestive heart failure. There is a hypervascular lung pattern. Several interlobar fissure lines are observed.

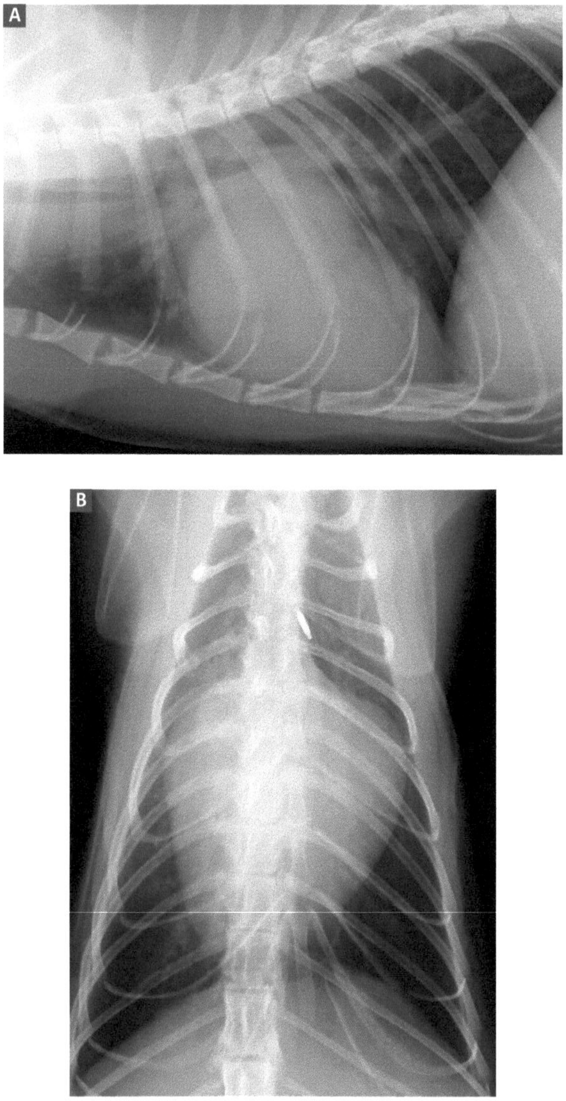

Figure 24. Right lateral (**A**) and dorsoventral (**B**) thoracic radiographs of a cat with hypertrophic cardiomyopathy. There is a marked increase in the size of the left atrium and atrial appendage, which in the dorsoventral view results in the "Valentine's heart" appearance.

Radiographically, an increase in left atrial size, dilation of the pulmonary veins, and interstitial or alveolar pulmonary oedema can be seen, and there may also be pleural effusion (Fig. 24). The "Valentine's heart" shape is sometimes seen on the DV view. In animals that are not showing clinical signs, the cardiac silhouette may be normal.

Feline Restrictive Cardiomyopathy

The radiographic characteristics of feline restrictive cardiomyopathy are the same as those of hypertrophic cardiomyopathy. Radiographic alterations are not usually seen in animals that are not showing clinical signs. Cats with clinical signs usually present with severe left atrial dilation (which can give the appearance of biatrial dilation) and signs of congestive heart failure or thromboembolic complications.

Feline Dilated Cardiomyopathy

This condition is rare in cats. Left ventricular dilation may be a consequence of a primary or secondary cardiomyopathy in the cat, such as hypertrophic cardiomyopathy or thyrotoxic cardiomyopathy.

Radiographically, pleural effusion, generalised cardiomegaly and a rounded cardiac apex can be observed. It is not possible to distinguish this disease radiographically from other cardiomyopathies.

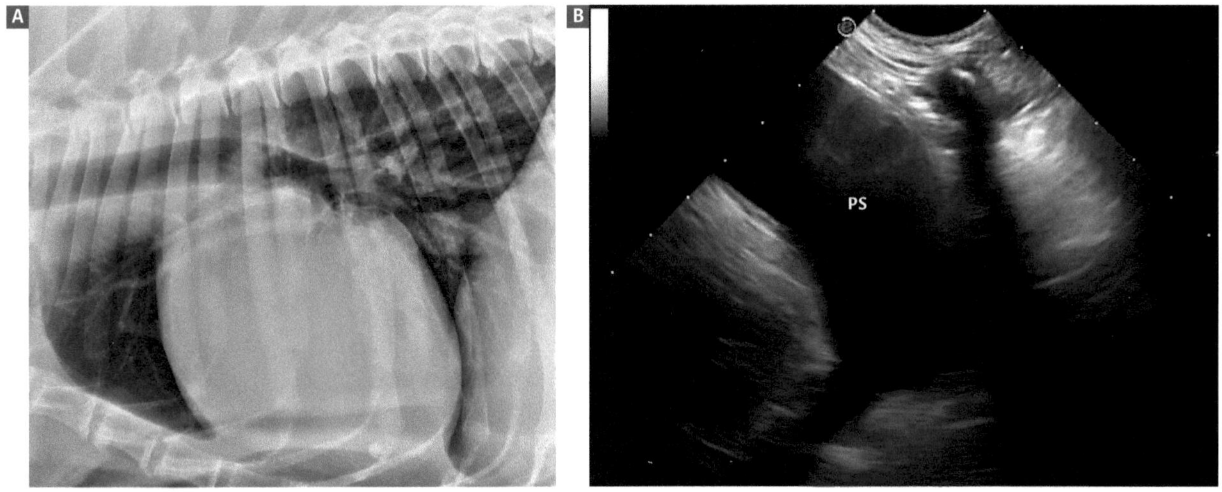

Figure 25. (**A**) Right lateral radiograph of the thorax of a dog with a pericardial effusion associated with a bleeding mass (haemangiosarcoma) in the right atrium. The cardiac silhouette is globoid in shape and very well defined. (**B**) Ultrasonographic image showing a large accumulation of anechoic fluid in the pericardial space (PS).

Pericardial Disease

Pericardial Effusion and Cardiac Tamponade

This is the most common pericardial alteration in small animals. The origin of the effusion may be systemic, pericardial or cardiac. Depending on the characteristics of the pericardial fluid, it can be classified as noninflammatory, inflammatory, neoplastic or haemorrhagic. Cardiac tamponade occurs when the heart is compressed by an excessive accumulation of pericardial fluid.

Animals present with nonspecific signs (anorexia, lethargy, dyspnoea), collapse and abdominal distension. Heart sounds are muffled and there are signs of right-sided heart failure.

The most frequent causes are:

- cardiac haemangiosarcoma (Fig. 25)
- idiopathic pericardial effusion
- cardiac base neoplasia
- mesothelioma
- congestive heart failure
- feline infectious peritonitis
- lymphoma (usually in cats).

As previously described, in pericardial effusion, the edge of the cardiac silhouette usually appears well defined due to reduced cardiac contractility, the shape is usually rounded or globoid, and the lungs usually appear hypoperfused due to cardiac tamponade. On ultrasonography, a variable amount of anechoic or hypoechoic fluid is observed in the pericardial space. It is important to perform echocardiography before draining a pericardial effusion to maximise the possibility of observing small masses.

Peritoneopericardial Diaphragmatic Hernia

This congenital defect is often accompanied by abnormalities in the sternum and umbilical hernias. The defect is usually seen in adult animals despite being a congenital disease.

Radiographically, an enlarged cardiac silhouette is observed, with heterogeneous content (Fig. 26). The content may be gaseous due to the presence of intestinal loops or part of the stomach, have soft tissue opacity due to hepatic lobes, gallbladder or spleen, or fatty opacity due to mesenteric or falciform fat.

Other rare pericardial abnormalities are cysts and pseudocysts, pericardial defects and pneumopericardium.

Cardiac Neoplasms

Right Atrial Haemangiosarcoma

Haemangiosarcoma is the most common neoplasm in the right atrium and in the heart in general (Treggiari et al., 2015). It can be primary or metastatic. Breeds of dog that are predisposed include the German Shepherd and the Golden Retriever. Metastasis is usually present at the time of diagnosis, so primarily the lung, liver and spleen should be thoroughly examined. It is usually associated with pericardial bleeding, usually due to rupture of the mass.

The radiographic features are pericardial effusion; a mass or enlargement associated with the right atrium is not usually observed. There are usually miliary metastases in the lungs

(Fig. 27) and hepatosplenomegaly, due to either right-sided congestive heart failure or metastasis.

Cardiac Base Neoplasms

The most frequent neoplasms in the cardiac base are chemodectomas, tumours of neuroendocrine origin. They may be associated with pericardial effusion. Brachycephalic dogs are predisposed.

These tumours, when small in size, may go unnoticed on radiographic images. If they are large, they can cause displacement of the trachea cranially to the carina, dorsally in the lateral view and laterally in the DV view (Fig. 28).

These masses are easy to detect on CT with contrast. They appear as well-defined masses originating around the ascending aorta (Fig. 29).

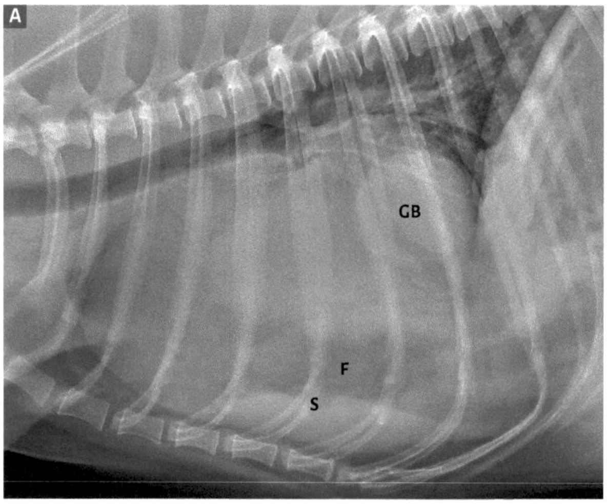

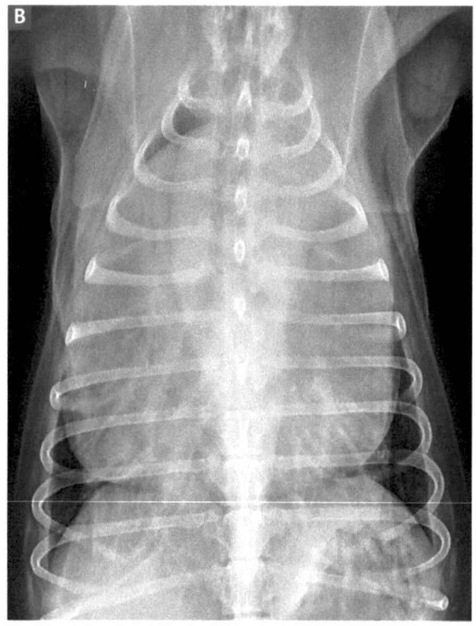

Figure 26. Right lateral (**A**) and dorsoventral (**B**) thoracic radiographs of a dog with a peritoneopericardial diaphragmatic hernia. The diaphragmatic defect is very large, approximately 50% of its height, and the cardiac silhouette is severely enlarged, nearly occupying the entire thorax. Inside, there is a rounded structure of soft tissue opacity (gallbladder), an elongated organ of soft tissue opacity (spleen), and a large amount of mesenteric and falciform fat. GB: gallbladder, S: spleen, F: fat.

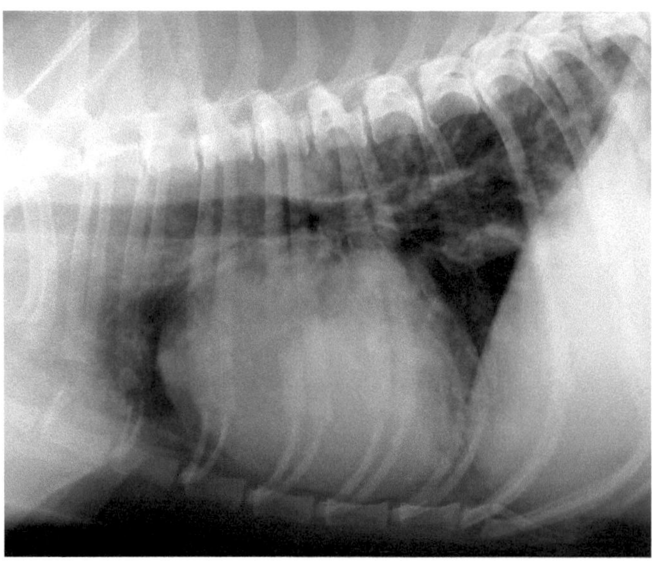

Figure 27. Right lateral radiograph of the thorax of a dog with a haemangiosarcoma in the right atrium, with miliary and nodular pulmonary metastases. In this case, right-sided cardiomegaly is observed, with a marked increase in the size of the right atrium.

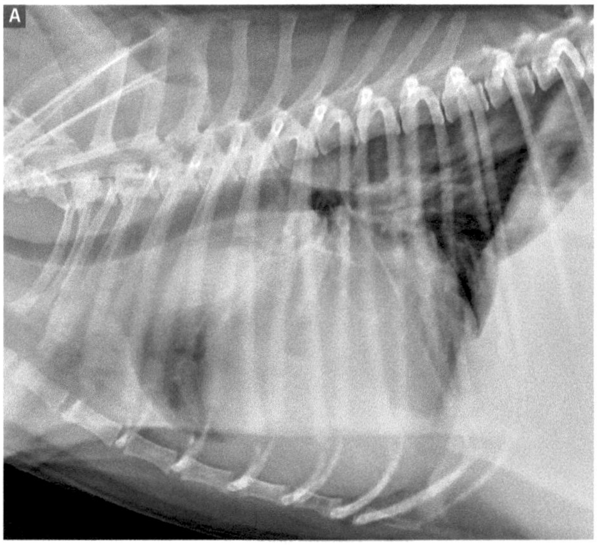

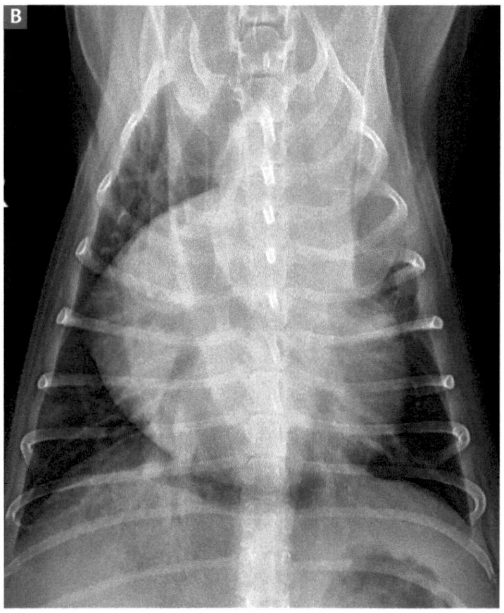

Figure 28. Right lateral (**A**) and dorsoventral (**B**) radiographs of the thorax of a dog with pericardial effusion and a cardiac base neoplasm that surrounds the base of the aorta and the pulmonary trunk, causing displacement of the trachea cranially to the carina. There is slight pleural effusion and moderate tracheal collapse at the thoracic inlet.

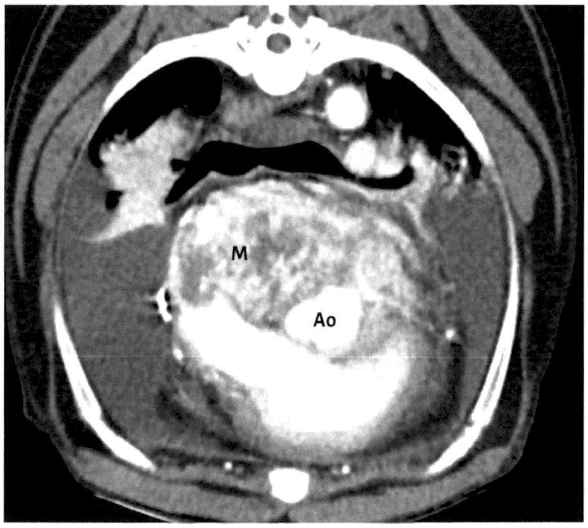

Figure 29. Cross-sectional multiplanar CT reconstruction at the level of the cardiac base where a large mass is observed, with heterogeneous contrast uptake, surrounding the base of the aorta. M: mass, Ao: aorta.

Lymphoma

Lymphoma is the most common cardiac neoplasm in cats. It usually presents as a disseminated disease in the myocardium, causing thickening. There is usually associated pericardial effusion and a diagnosis is usually reached after analysis of the effusion.

The Noncardiac Mediastinum

Anatomy

The mediastinum is the space between the right and left pleural cavities. It is defined by the mediastinal pleura, which is formed by the reflection of the parietal pleura at the thoracic inlet and diaphragm. The mediastinum communicates cranially with the fasciae of the neck through the thoracic inlet and caudally with the retroperitoneal space through the aortic hiatus. Structures located in the mediastinum include the trachea, oesophagus, heart and great vessels, thoracic duct, nerves, lymph nodes (LNs) and thymus. Except for the trachea, and sometimes the oesophagus, all the structures are of soft tissue opacity and cannot be differentiated on radiographs.

It is important to be aware that there are three mediastinal reflections (Fig. 30).

- Cranioventral: originates due to displacement of the mediastinum by the right cranial lung lobe. It can be seen in the two orthogonal views.
- Caudoventral: originates from the displacement of the mediastinum to the left by the accessory lung lobe. It can be seen in the VD view (where it is seen better than in a DV view).
- Plica venae cavae: surrounds the caudal vena cava. It is not visible radiographically as an individual structure.

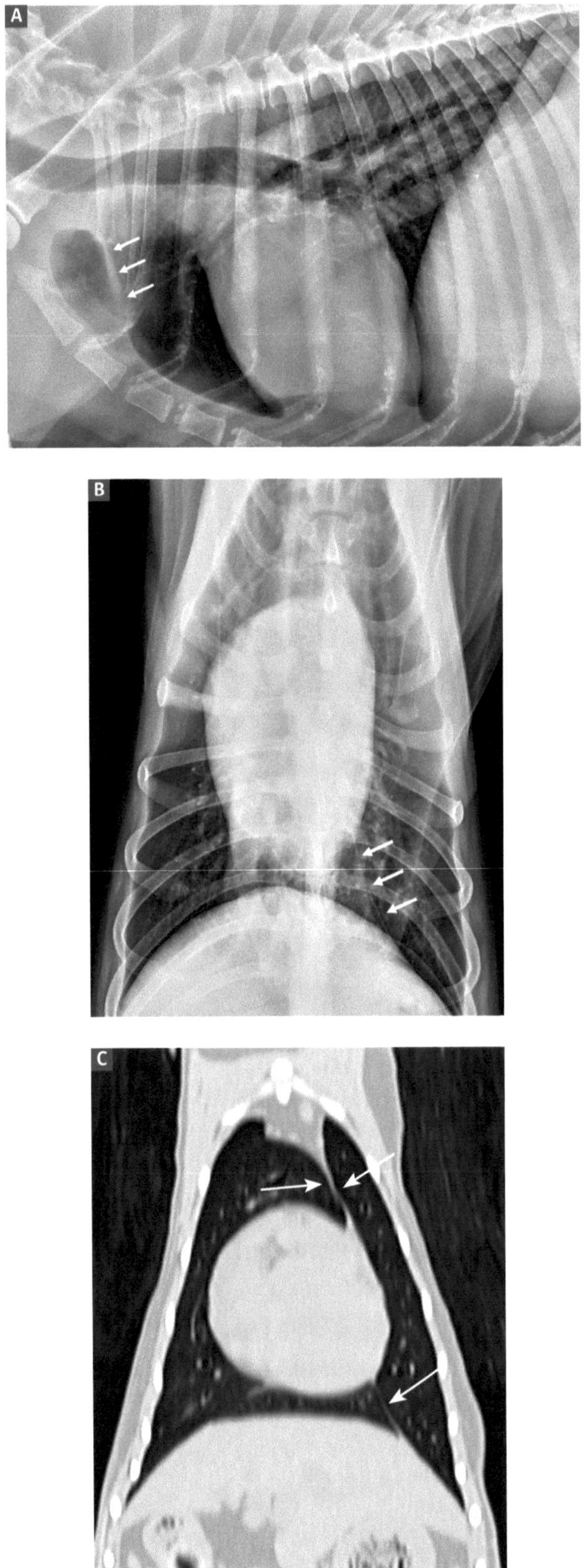

Figure 30. Cranioventral and caudoventral mediastinal reflections (arrows) in lateral (**A**) and dorsoventral (**B**) thoracic radiographs and in a multiplanar CT reconstruction (**C**).

The mediastinum can be divided into three parts in order to examine it: the cranial mediastinum, middle mediastinum and caudal mediastinum. The structures found in the mediastinum and their visualisation on radiographs are detailed in Table 4.

Table 4. Structures of the cranial, middle and caudal mediastinum. Only structures marked in bold are visible radiographically.

Cranial mediastinum	Middle mediastinum	Caudal mediastinum
Trachea	**Trachea, bifurcation**	
Oesophagus	**Oesophagus**	**Oesophagus**
Thymus	**Aorta**	**Aorta**
Cranial vena cava	Caudal vena cava	**Caudal vena cava**
Brachiocephalic trunk	Azygos vein	Azygos vein
Left subclavian artery	Pulmonary trunk	
Cranial mediastinal lymph nodes	(Distal) pulmonary vein	
Sternal lymph nodes	Tracheobronchial lymph nodes	
Vagus nerve	Vagus nerve	Vagus nerve
Recurrent laryngeal nerve	Recurrent laryngeal nerve	Recurrent laryngeal nerve
Phrenic nerve	Phrenic nerve	Phrenic nerve
Thoracic duct	Thoracic duct	Thoracic duct
	Heart, pericardium*	**Heart, pericardium***

*In radiography the term cardiac silhouette is used, which refers to both the heart and the pericardium.

In the DV or VD view, the cranial mediastinum usually measures 1.5–2.0 times the width of the vertebral bodies and has smooth, well-defined borders. Brachycephalic dogs and/or obese animals may accumulate fat in the mediastinum, causing increases in cranial mediastinal size above these values.

In cats, the width of the mediastinum should not exceed the width of the vertebral bodies.

Lymph Nodes

There are usually two sternal LNs; these are located dorsally to the second sternebra in dogs and slightly more caudally in cats. They drain the chest wall and the cranial abdomen.

Cranial mediastinal LNs vary in number and are located in the cranial and dorsal mediastinum, adjacent to the cranial vena cava, the brachiocephalic trunk, the left subclavian vein and the trachea (Fig. 31).

The bronchial LNs consist of pulmonary (often absent in small animals) and tracheobronchial LNs. There are three tracheobronchial LNs: two lateral, located laterally to the main bronchi, and one medial, located caudal and dorsal to the carina.

An increase in size of the sternal LNs is observed as a soft tissue opacity with a broad base, located over the second sternebra, creating an extrapleural sign.

An increase in cranial mediastinal LN size is observed as a mass in the cranial/craniodorsal mediastinum and a widening of the cranial mediastinum in the DV/VD view.

An increase in tracheobronchial LN size is observed as a soft tissue opacity with poorly defined edges in the perihilar region. The medial tracheobronchial LN causes ventral displacement and/or compression of the carina (lateral view), and lateral and ventral displacement of the main bronchi (lateral and DV/VD views). The lateral tracheobronchial LNs cause ventral displacement and/or compression of the trachea cranially to the carina (lateral view), and lateral displacement and/or compression of the cranial lobar bronchi (DV/VD view).

Thymus

The thymus reaches its maximum size at 4 months of age and subsequently involutes during the first year of life.

The thymus is seen as a soft tissue opacity on the left side of the chest in the DV/VD view and is identifiable by the thymic candle sign (usually visible in dogs). In the lateral view it is seen as an elongated structure with soft tissue opacity parallel to the cranial edge of the cardiac silhouette (usually visible in cats) (Fig. 32). In adult animals, a thymic remnant is occasionally seen.

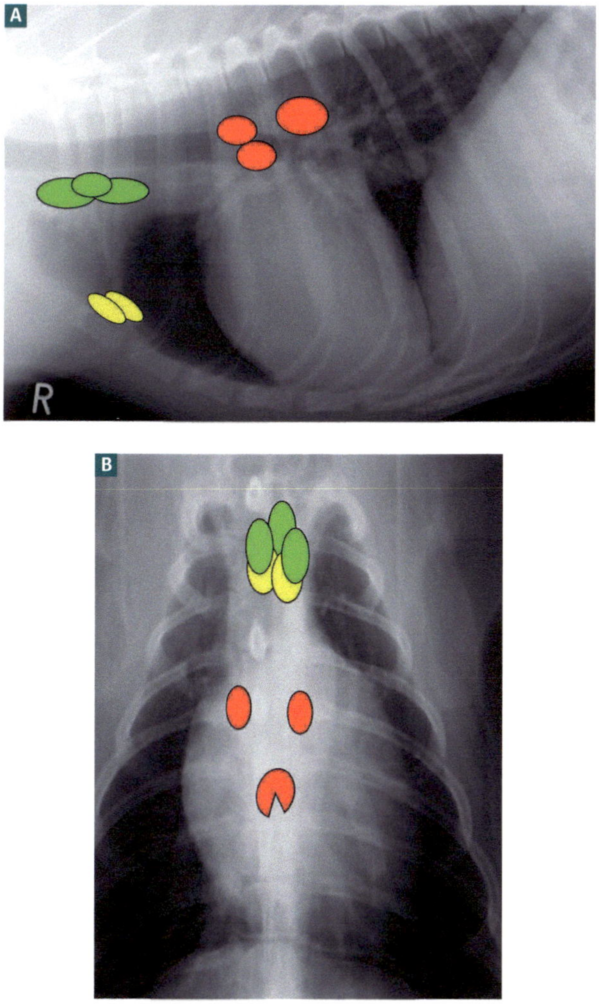

Figure 31. Lateral (**A**) and dorsoventral (**B**) thoracic radiographs with the anatomical position of the cranial (green), sternal (yellow) and tracheobronchial (red) mediastinal lymph nodes marked.

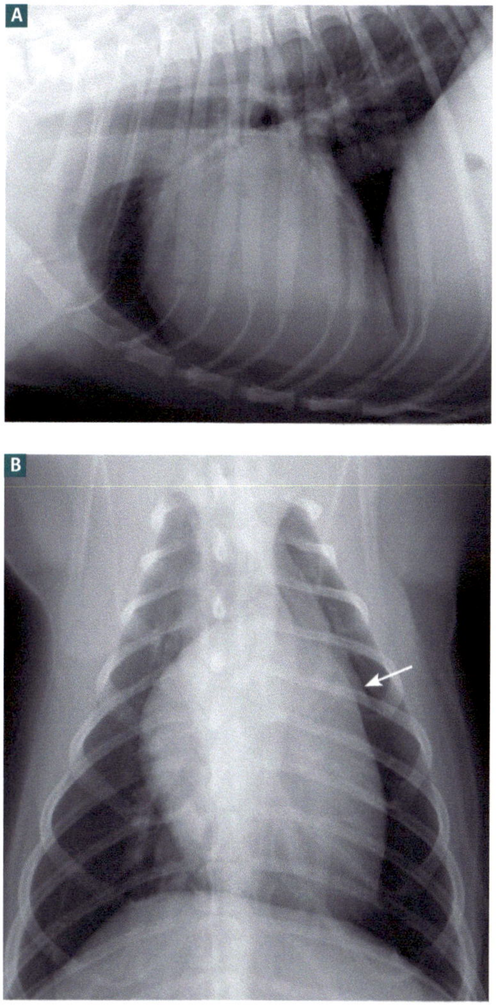

Figure 32. Right lateral (**A**) and dorsoventral (**B**) thoracic radiographs of a young dog, showing (A) an elongated structure with soft tissue opacity parallel to the cranial edge of the heart, compatible with the thymus, and (B) the thymic candle sign (arrow).

Diseases of the Mediastinum

The most common diseases affecting the mediastinum are mediastinal masses, mediastinal cysts, pneumomediastinum, mediastinal effusion and mediastinitis.

Mediastinal Masses

The location of mediastinal masses usually determines their organ of origin. Common locations are the cranioventral mediastinum and the perihilar region. The associated clinical signs are usually cough, dyspnoea and exercise intolerance. When the nerves are compressed, symptoms can include Horner's syndrome, change in the tone of the bark (in dogs) and laryngeal paralysis. If the vessels (cranial vena cava) or lymphatics are compressed, there may be oedema of the head, neck and forelimbs, or ascites if the caudal vena cava is compressed.

Cranioventral Location (Figs. 33 and 34)

One of the most important radiographic signs of cranioventral mediastinal masses is the displacement of the carina caudally into the sixth intercostal space, and of the trachea dorsally into the cranial mediastinum.

Other radiographic signs are thickening of the cranial mediastinum in the DV and VD views; these views also facilitate the differentiation between a lung mass and a mediastinal mass. The cranial lung lobes are usually displaced caudally. The increase in size of the masses with or without associated pleural effusion produces a silhouette effect with the cardiac silhouette.

Craniodorsal Location (Fig. 35)

With craniodorsal masses, the trachea is usually displaced ventrally and to the right. There may be vertebral alterations or an increase in size of the intervertebral foramen.

Perihilar location (Fig. 36)

An increase in undefined soft tissue opacity is usually observed in the perihilar region. There is usually ventral displacement and/or compression of the carina. There may be compression or displacement of the main bronchi.

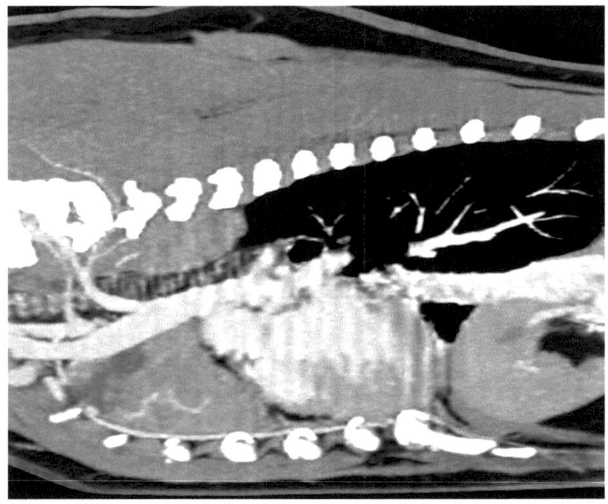

Figure 34. Maximum intensity projection of the thorax of a dog with a cranioventral mediastinal mass. The diagnosis was a thymoma.

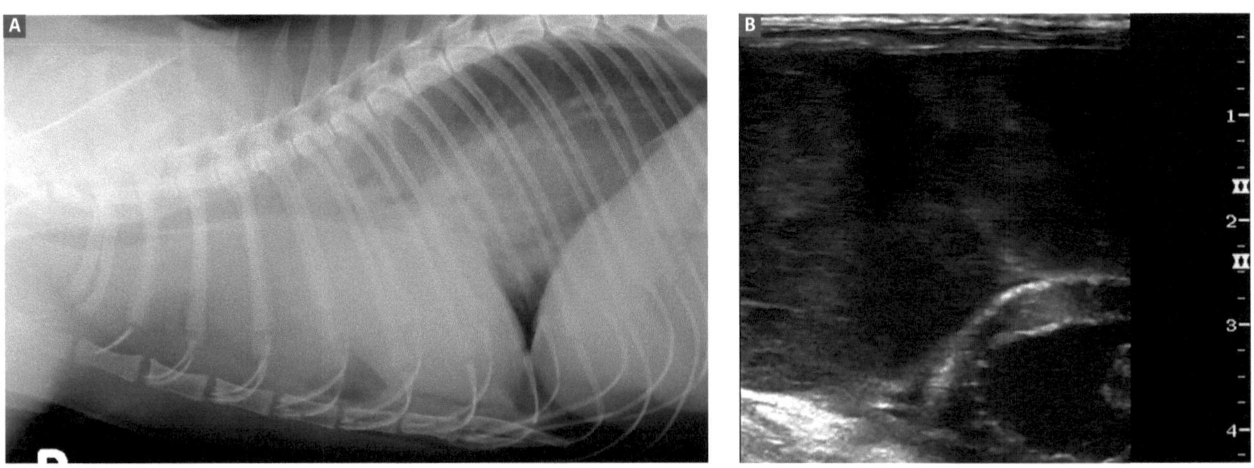

Figure 33. (**A**) Right lateral thoracic radiograph of a cat with a large cranioventral mediastinal mass. There is a silhouette effect with the cardiac silhouette and a mass over the trachea, which is displaced dorsally, in addition to associated pleural effusion. (**B**) Ultrasonographic image of the chest of a cat with a cranioventral mediastinal mass. The mass is hypoechogenic, heterogeneous and large in size. The diagnosis was mediastinal lymphoma.

CAUDODORSAL AND CAUDOVENTRAL LOCATION (FIG. 37)

A silhouette effect is usually observed with the diaphragm and/or with the cardiac silhouette. The oesophagus or caudal vena cava may be displaced or compressed.

The possible origins or causes of mediastinal masses are listed in Table 5.

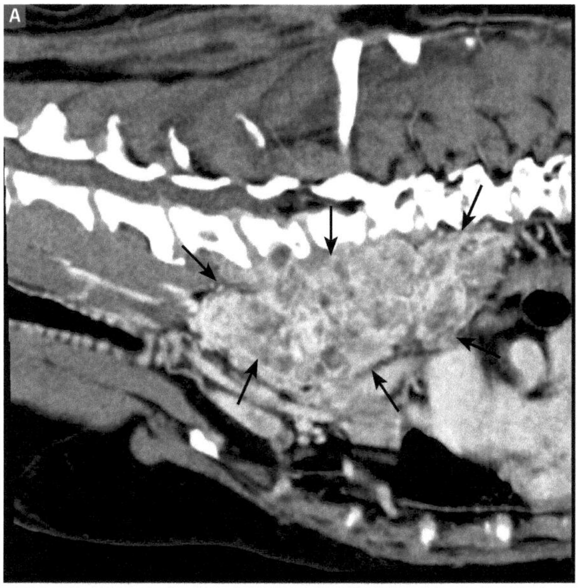

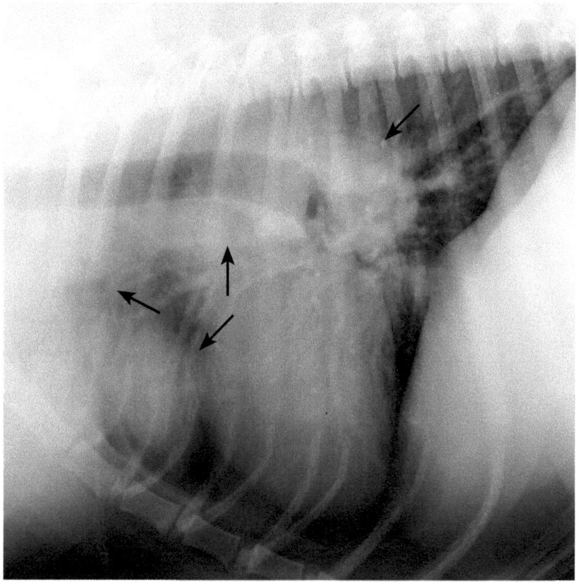

Figure 36. Right lateral radiograph of the thorax of a dog with mediastinal lymphadenopathy (cranial mediastinal, sternal and tracheobronchial LNs). Masses with soft tissue opacity and poorly defined margins are observed in the location of the LNs (arrows). There is dorsal deviation of the trachea dorsally to the cardiac base and ventral deviation of the carina and main bronchi. In addition, there is moderate bronchiectasis.

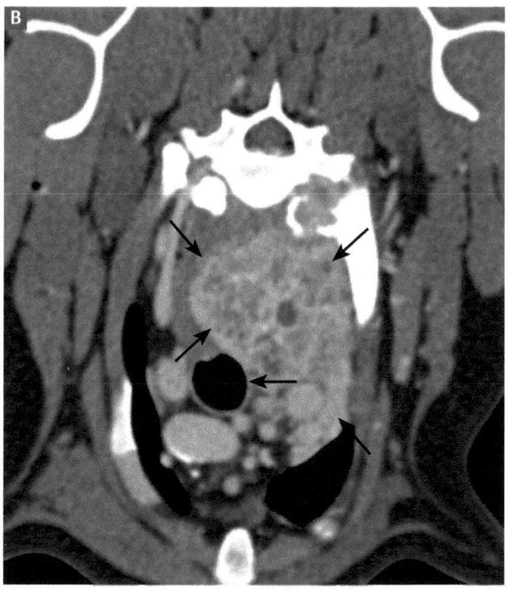

Figure 35. Multiplanar CT reconstructions of the thoracic inlet region of a dog. (A) A large mass (arrows) is observed with strong contrast uptake located in the craniodorsal mediastinum. (B) There is right ventrolateral displacement of the trachea and the rest of the mediastinal structures. In addition, the mass has invaded and produced osteolysis in the costal head on the left side.

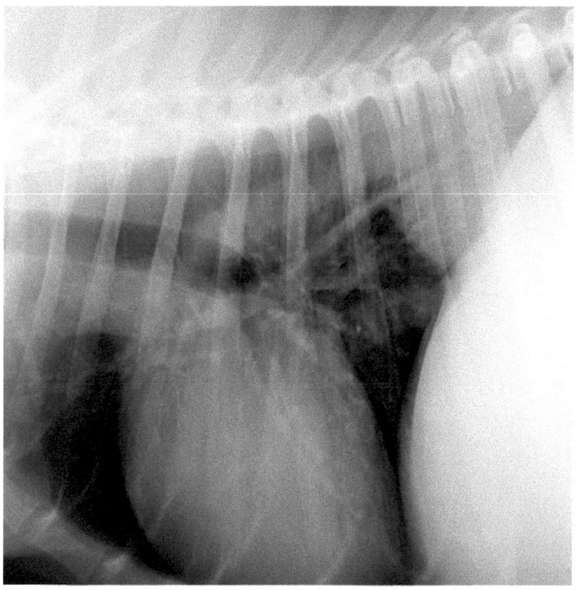

Figure 37. Left lateral radiograph of the thorax of a dog with a mass with soft tissue opacity located in the caudodorsal mediastinum. The mass has well-defined, rounded borders superimposed and with a slight silhouette effect with the aorta and diaphragm. This mass was not seen in the right lateral or dorsoventral views. The diagnosis was a sliding hiatal hernia.

Table 5. Most frequent causes of mediastinal masses according to their location.

Cranioventral	Craniodorsal
· Lymphoma · Thymic disease (neoplasia, hyperplasia, haematoma, amyloidosis, branchial cysts) · Sternal lymphadenopathy · Mediastinal cyst · Pericardial cyst · Ectopic thyroid and parathyroid neoplasms · Mediastinal haemorrhage	· Oesophageal lesions · Neoplasms of neural or neuroendocrine origin · Vertebral or paravertebral neoplasms · Aortic aneurysm
Perihilar	**Caudodorsal and caudoventral**
· Chemodectoma · Other heart base neoplasms · Tracheobronchial lymphadenopathy (lymphosarcoma, metastasis, fungal disease, tuberculosis) · Bronchogenic cysts · Oesophageal foreign bodies	· Oesophageal lesions · Neoplasms of neural origin · Hiatal hernia · Peritoneopericardial diaphragmatic hernia · Migratory foreign bodies · Diaphragmatic lesion (hernia, neoplasm, abscess, haematoma) · Traumatic diaphragmatic rupture · Pericardial (ventral) cysts

Other lesions
Abscesses, granulomas, haematomas, primary mediastinal neoplasms, bronchial neoplasms

CT with contrast makes visualisation of the mass possible, in order to study its margins and vascularisation, and to investigate the origin of the lesion and the invasion of the vascularisation of the mediastinum and other adjacent structures. In addition, it allows CT-guided punctures and biopsies to be performed.

Mediastinal Cysts

Mediastinal cysts are common in older cats and rare in dogs. They are usually incidental findings unless their size causes compression of or damage to adjacent structures, resulting in chronic mediastinitis (Zekas and Adams, 2002).

Although most cysts are benign, it should be kept in mind that the origin of the cysts can be varied, including neoplastic, thymic, lymphatic, bronchogenic, branchial and pleural.

The radiographic signs include rounded structures with soft tissue opacity, frequently located in the cranioventral mediastinum (Fig. 38 A). Ultrasonographically and on CT images, they are observed as cystic, round, well-defined structures with a thin membrane that surrounds them (Figs. 38 B and C).

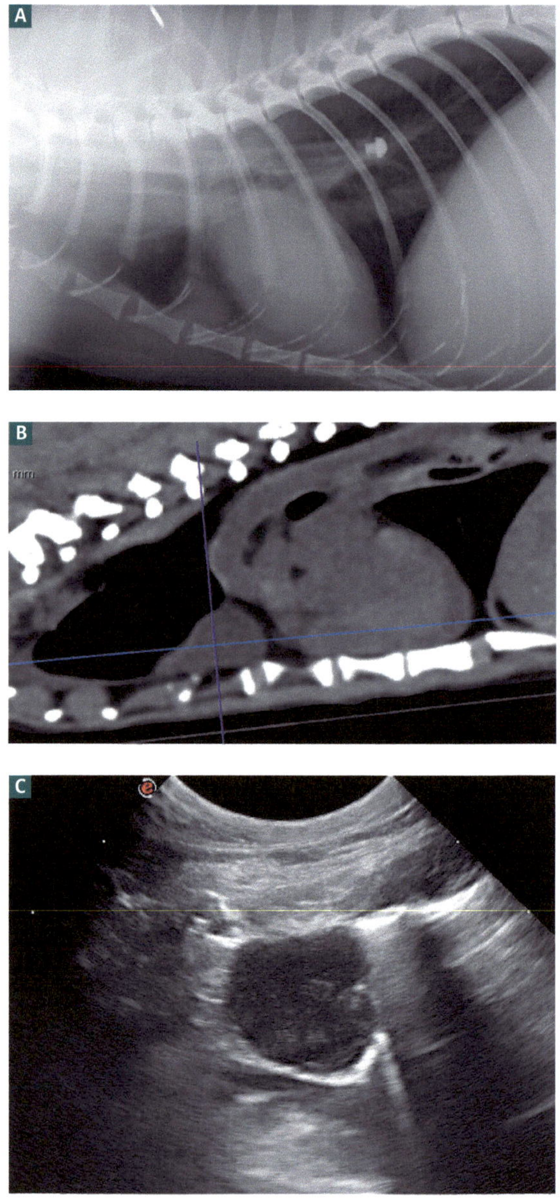

Figure 38. (**A**) Right lateral thoracic radiograph of a cat with a small oval mass in the cranioventral mediastinum, dorsal to the fourth and fifth sternebrae. (**B**). Multiplanar CT reconstruction (without contrast) of the thorax of the same cat; the mass is observed to have liquid attenuation, consistent with a mediastinal cyst. (**C**) Ultrasonographic image of a cat with a mediastinal cyst. The cyst is thin walled and has anechoic to slightly hypoechoic content.

Pneumomediastinum

Pneumomediastinum is the presence of gas in the mediastinal space. It is important to determine the cause. It can occur in isolation (and usually resolves spontaneously) or be associated with subcutaneous emphysema, pneumothorax and/or pneumoretroperitoneum. Clinical signs are dyspnoea and tachypnoea in the case of pneumothorax or discomfort in emphysema. It is important to remember that in the presence of

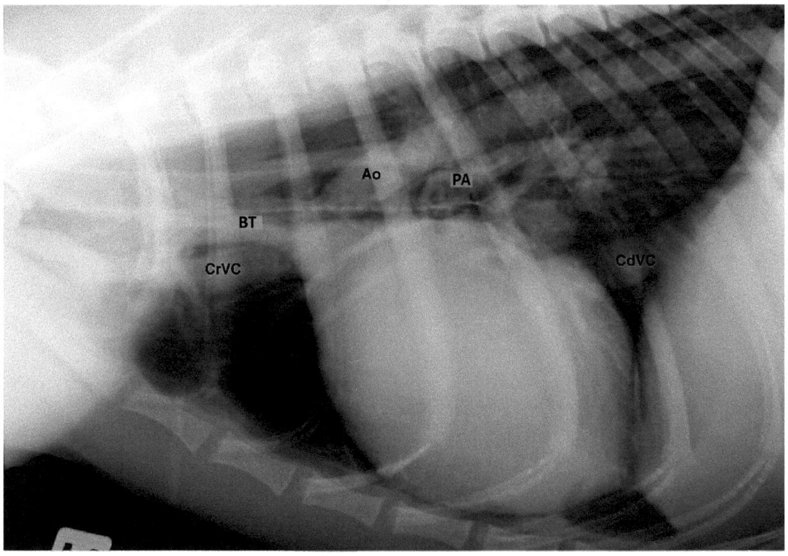

Figure 39. Right lateral radiograph of the thorax of a dog with pneumomediastinum. The main vessels that run through the mediastinum can be distinguished. Ao: aorta, PA: pulmonary arteries, BT: brachiocephalic trunk, CrVC: cranial vena cava, CdVC: caudal vena cava.

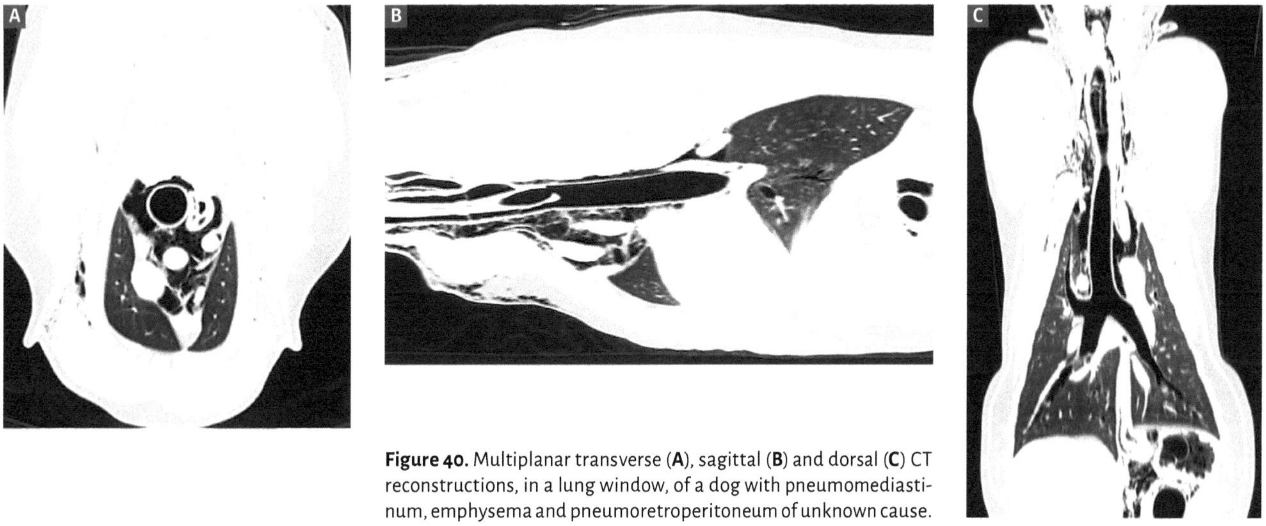

Figure 40. Multiplanar transverse (**A**), sagittal (**B**) and dorsal (**C**) CT reconstructions, in a lung window, of a dog with pneumomediastinum, emphysema and pneumoretroperitoneum of unknown cause.

simultaneous pneumomediastinum and pneumothorax, it is the pneumomediastinum that occurs initially and gives rise to pneumothorax, and never the other way around. The cause is frequently a tracheal, oesophageal or thoracic tear/perforation or a penetrating lesion in the cervical region. Spontaneous pneumomediastinum can occur after a persistent cough or due to poisoning by the herbicide paraquat.

Radiographically, gas is observed in the mediastinal space, delimiting the soft tissue structures that are not seen in normal radiographs (Van den Broek, 1986) (Fig. 39). If there is associated emphysema, gas bubbles in the fascia can make the assessment of the mediastinum difficult. If oesophageal perforation has occurred, there is usually free fluid in the mediastinum and mediastinitis is present. If pneumothorax occurs, it can make it difficult to visualise the air in the mediastinum.

CT can facilitate the identification of pneumomediastinum and its cause (Fig. 40). Alternatively, 5–10 ml of nonionic iodinated contrast medium can be introduced into the oesophagus or trachea to find the lesion.

Mediastinitis

Mediastinitis can be of primary origin, due to a chronic fungal or bacterial infection, or of secondary origin, as a result of perforation of the trachea or oesophagus or by extension of inflammation or infection from the cervical region, the pericardium, the lung or the pleural space. It is usually associated with pneumomediastinum if the origin is a tracheal or oesophageal perforation (Fig. 41). Small amounts of fluid not visible radiographically can be detected by CT.

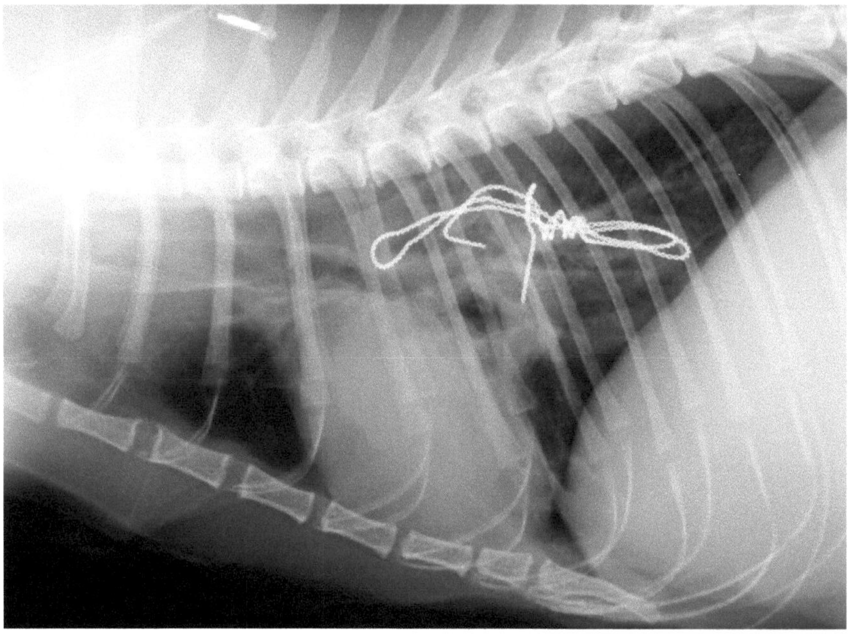

Figure 41. Right lateral radiograph of a dog with a penetrating oesophageal foreign body and secondary mediastinitis. A loss of definition of the mediastinal structures is observed in the caudal third of the thorax due to the accumulation of mediastinal fluid and gas.

Oesophageal Injuries

Redundant Oesophagus

This is usually an incidental finding. It is seen as a small deviation of the oesophagus ventrally or laterally. Brachycephalic breeds are predisposed.

Megaoesophagus

The causes of megaoesophagus are very varied. They are rarely congenital, and there is a familial predisposition in certain breeds of dog (Irish Setter, Great Dane and Labrador Retriever, among others). They are frequently acquired, secondary to neuromuscular disease (myasthenia gravis, polymyositis/polymyopathies or systemic lupus erythematosus, among others), secondary to an oesophageal obstruction (due to neoplasia, a foreign body, constrictions or vascular ring abnormality), of toxic origin (lead and organophosphates) or secondary to other diseases, such as hypoadrenocorticism, thymoma (megaoesophagus due to paraneoplastic myasthenia gravis), hiatal hernia, or oesophagitis due to reflux or gastric dilatation and volvulus. Animals usually present with regurgitation and/or cough associated with aspiration pneumonia.

It is important to remember that animals that are sedated or anaesthetised, that have an oesophageal tube, or that are showing dyspnoea and aerophagia may present with transient dilation of the oesophagus with gas.

Radiographic signs include (Fig. 42):

- focal or generalised oesophageal dilation (with gas or with ingested material);
- the tracheo-oesophageal band sign (the dorsal wall of the trachea is observed overlapping the oesophagus, which contains air);
- displacement of the trachea ventrally and to the right; and
- compression of the cardiac silhouette ventrally in severe cases.

Oesophagitis

No radiographic changes are usually observed, except for focal or generalised oesophageal dilation. After administration of barium contrast (provided there is no suspicion of perforation or risk of aspiration), thickening of the oesophageal walls, irregularities in the mucosa and ulcerations may be observed.

Oesophageal Constrictions

Generally, oesophageal constrictions are intraluminal and are secondary to severe trauma or inflammation. As in oesophagitis, radiographs usually have a normal appearance except for a dilation of the oesophagus cranial to the area of constriction. Barium contrast studies typically confirm the diagnosis of oesophageal constriction. Preferably, contrast-enhanced oesophagograms are performed using fluoroscopy (Fig. 43).

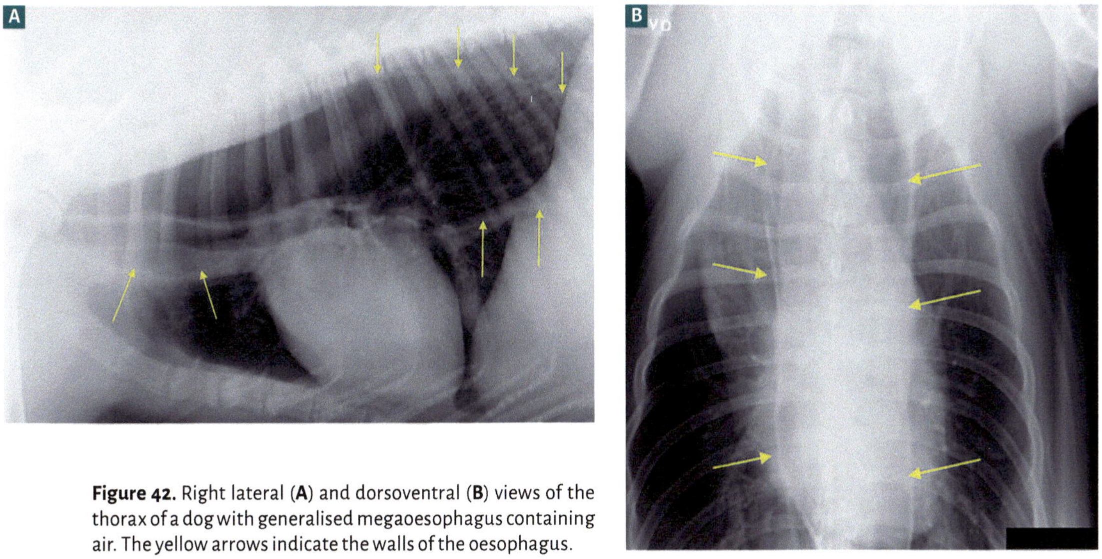

Figure 42. Right lateral (**A**) and dorsoventral (**B**) views of the thorax of a dog with generalised megaoesophagus containing air. The yellow arrows indicate the walls of the oesophagus.

Oesophageal Diverticula

These are sacculations of the oesophageal wall. They can be congenital or acquired. They should not be confused with redundant oesophagus.

Radiographically, an oesophageal sacculation can be observed with air or ingested material inside it (Fig. 44). The accumulation of ingested material can cause oesophagitis, obstructions or alterations in motility.

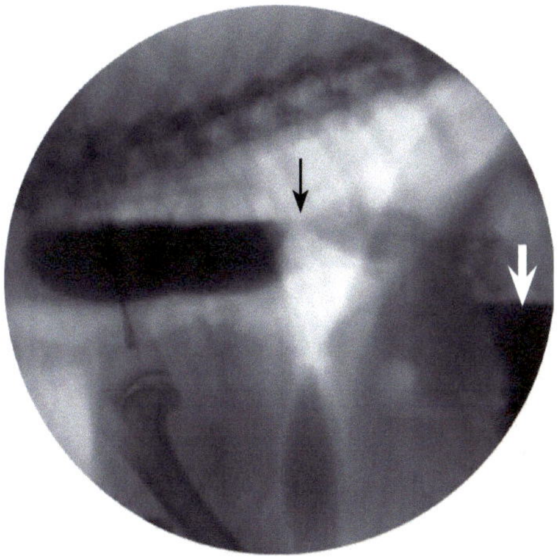

Figure 43. Fluoroscopic image of a constriction (black arrow) in the caudal part of the thoracic oesophagus during a barium transit study. Oesophageal dilation is observed with the accumulation of contrast and gas immediately cranial to the constriction; in the stomach there is a fluid line and a gas–liquid interface (white arrow).

Foreign Bodies

Radiographically, radiopaque foreign bodies and oesophageal dilation cranial to the obstruction can be observed (Figs. 45 and 46). Signs of complications include aspiration pneumonia and oesophageal perforation, with mediastinitis, pleuritis and associated effusion.

When contrast is administered to visualise radiolucent foreign bodies, a nonionic iodinated contrast medium should always be chosen if perforation is suspected.

Neoplasia

The most frequent neoplasms are fibrosarcoma and osteosarcoma as a malignant transformation of *Spirocerca lupi* granulomas. Other oesophageal neoplasms are very rare in dogs and cats, so they will not be discussed further in this chapter.

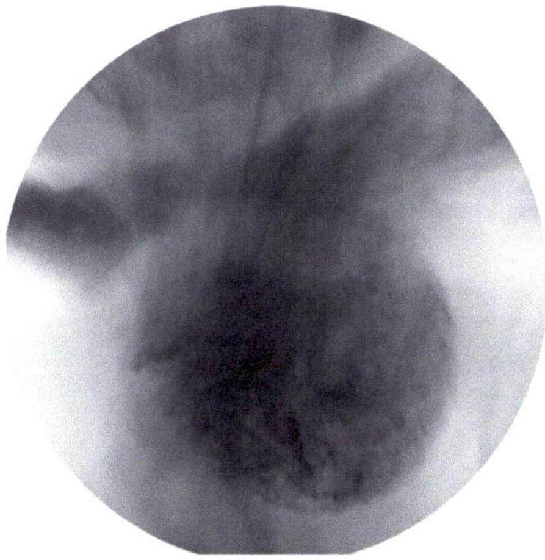

Figure 44. Fluoroscopic image of a large oesophageal diverticulum during a barium transit study.

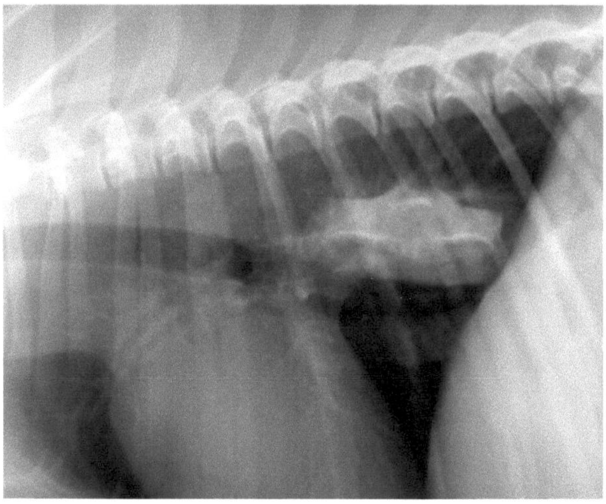

Figure 45. Right lateral view of the thorax of a dog. A well-defined foreign body with mineral opacity is observed in the caudal portion of the oesophagus.

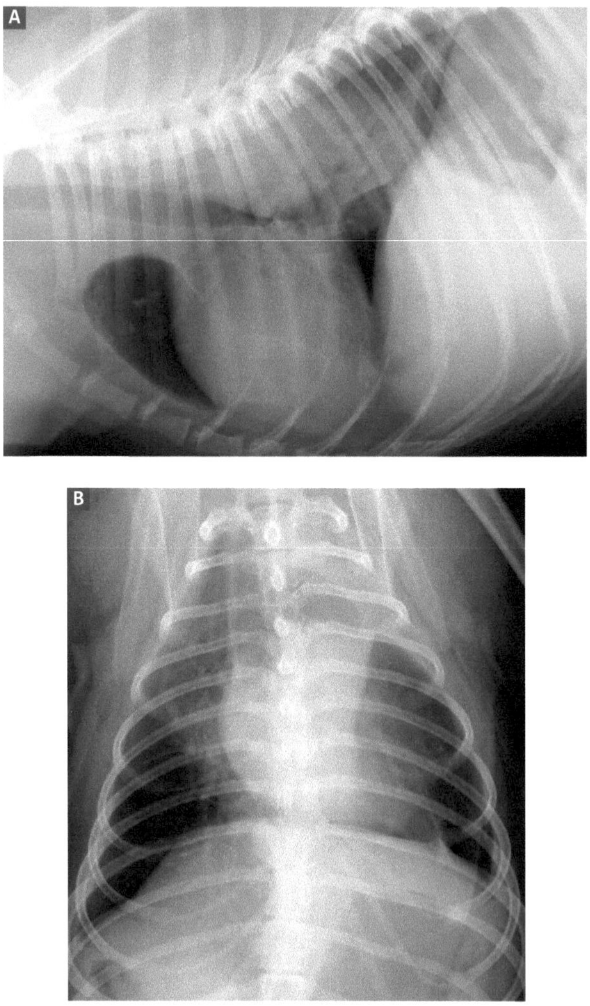

Figure 46. Right lateral (**A**) and dorsoventral (**B**) radiographs of the thorax of a dog with a large oesophageal foreign body, which has soft tissue opacity and appears to partially overlap with the carina.

Spirocercosis

Spirocercosis is a granulomatous disease caused by the nematode *Spirocerca lupi*. It is endemic in certain tropical and subtropical countries, and very rare in other regions. Granulomas can undergo neoplastic transformation (Kirberger et al., 2013, 2015).

Radiographic signs include:

- a mass in the caudal oesophagus, with possible mineralised foci
- oesophageal dilation cranial to the mass
- ventral displacement of the caudal vena cava
- spondylitis in caudal thoracic vertebrae (pathognomonic sign)
- periosteal reactions in the ribs
- hypertrophic osteopathy
- pulmonary metastases
- aortic aneurysm.

CT allows the detection of incipient mineralisation of the mass, which is indicative of neoplastic transformation, aortic mineralisation, initial spondylitis and small lung metastases.

Gastro-oesophageal Intussusception

This is a rare condition. It consists of invagination of the stomach (and possibly other abdominal viscera such as the spleen or pancreas) in the caudal portion of the oesophagus. Clinical signs include vomiting and regurgitation. If the intussusception is of a large part of the stomach or includes other viscera, it may be a surgical emergency.

Radiographic signs include:

- a mass with soft tissue opacity in the caudal part of the oesophagus
- visualisation of gastric folds inside the dilated oesophagus
- megaoesophagus
- gastric silhouette absent in the cranial abdomen.

Given the possible complications and the need for emergency surgery, the administration of contrast, especially barium, is contraindicated.

CT allows visualisation of the stomach inside the caudal oesophagus.

Tracheal Lesions

Tracheal Hypoplasia

Tracheal hypoplasia is a congenital condition in which there is a narrowing of the trachea by at least 50%. English Bulldogs and Mastiffs are predisposed. Tracheal hypoplasia is one of the four components of brachycephalic obstructive airway syndrome (BOAS). Clinical signs are usually dyspnoea, exercise intolerance and cough.

Radiographic signs include a uniformly narrowed trachea. The diameter of the trachea can be measured, and the ratio of its diameter to the height of the thoracic inlet calculated (Fig. 47). Normal values have been established as:

- 0.21 ± 0.03 in normal nonbrachycephalic dogs
- 0.16 ± 0.03 in brachycephalic dogs
- 0.11 ± 0.03 in the English Bulldog (Fig. 48).

Tracheal Collapse

Tracheal collapse is a degenerative condition affecting the tracheal rings. A flattening of the trachea occurs due to deformation of the tracheal rings and redundancy of the membrane and tracheal muscle. Tracheoscopy can be used to classify the degree of collapse, based on the approximate percentage reduction of the tracheal diameter, as mild (25%), moderate (50%), severe (75%) or complete (100%). Small and miniature breeds of dog are predisposed, as are elderly animals.

The typical clinical sign is cough exacerbated by compression of the trachea. Many animals do not show clinical signs when the condition is mild.

Radiographic signs may be inconsistent when dealing with dynamic tracheal collapse. During inspiration there is usually tracheal collapse in the neck and at the thoracic inlet, and during expiration in the intrathoracic trachea (Fig. 49). Sometimes fluoroscopy or repeated views on inspiration and expiration must be obtained to confirm tracheal collapse.

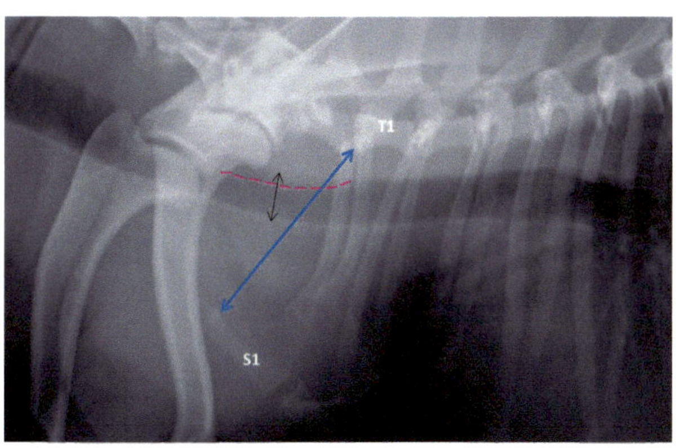

Figure 47. Detail of a lateral thoracic radiograph of a dog where the diameter of the trachea is measured (indicated by the black double-headed arrow) and compared with the height of the thoracic inlet (between the first sternebra [S1] and the first thoracic vertebra [T1]). The pink line indicates redundancy of the dorsal tracheal membrane due to slight tracheal collapse.

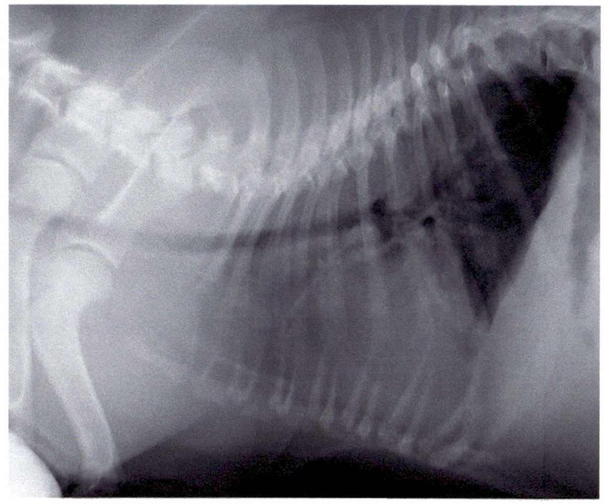

Figure 48. Right lateral thoracic radiograph of an English Bulldog with tracheal hypoplasia and noncardiogenic pulmonary oedema.

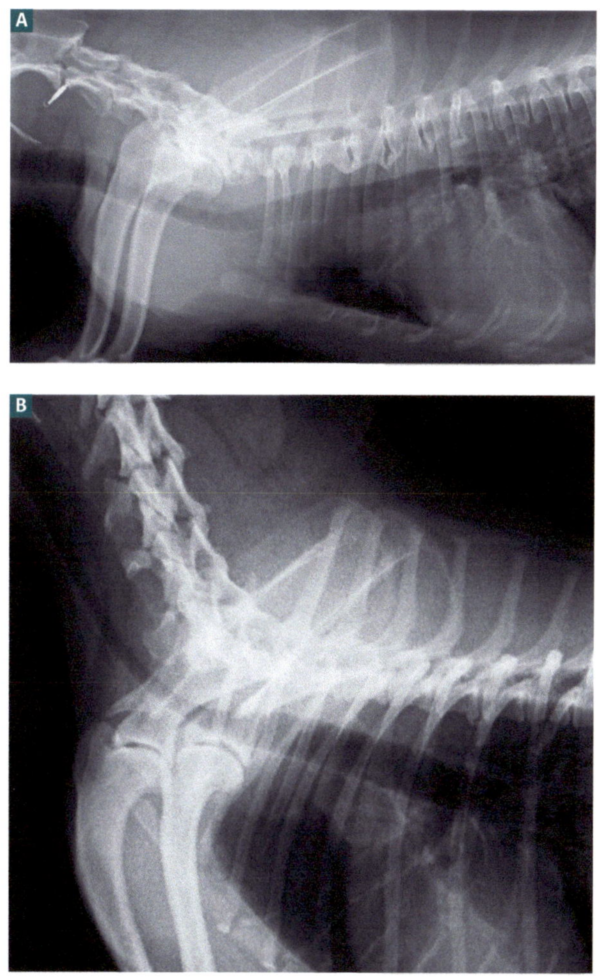

Figure 49. Lateral radiographs of the neck and thorax of two dogs with moderate (**A**) and severe (**B**) tracheal collapse in the cervical trachea and at the thoracic inlet (collapse of approximately 50% and 75% of the tracheal diameter, respectively).

The tangential view of the thoracic inlet has been found to be more reliable for detecting tracheal collapse than the lateral view of the thorax.

CT has demonstrated advantages over other techniques for performing measurements of tracheal diameter. One study showed its importance especially in the diagnosis of axial rotation of the trachea (Heng et al., 2018), which could be misdiagnosed as a foreign body or tracheal neoplasm.

Tracheal Neoplasia

Tracheal neoplasia is rare, and sometimes animals do not show clinical signs until complications such as a tracheal obstruction or perforation and a pneumomediastinum occur.

The primary radiographic sign is a structure with soft tissue opacity partially obstructing the radiolucent lumen of the trachea (Fig. 50). If the mass is intrathoracic, a hyperinflated lung field can be seen. If the mass is cervical, the lung will be poorly expanded due to the obstruction preventing air from entering.

CT allows the location and extent of the mass to be determined (Figs. 50 B and C).

Tracheal Haemorrhage

Tracheal haemorrhage can occur focally secondary to trauma or in a more generalised manner associated with coagulation abnormalities, for example, after rodenticide poisoning. Blocker and Roberts (1999) described the first case of acute tracheal obstruction associated with rodenticide poisoning in a dog. After poisoning, diffuse bleeding occurs in the tracheal submucosa and usually at other sites in the body, such as the mediastinum and lung.

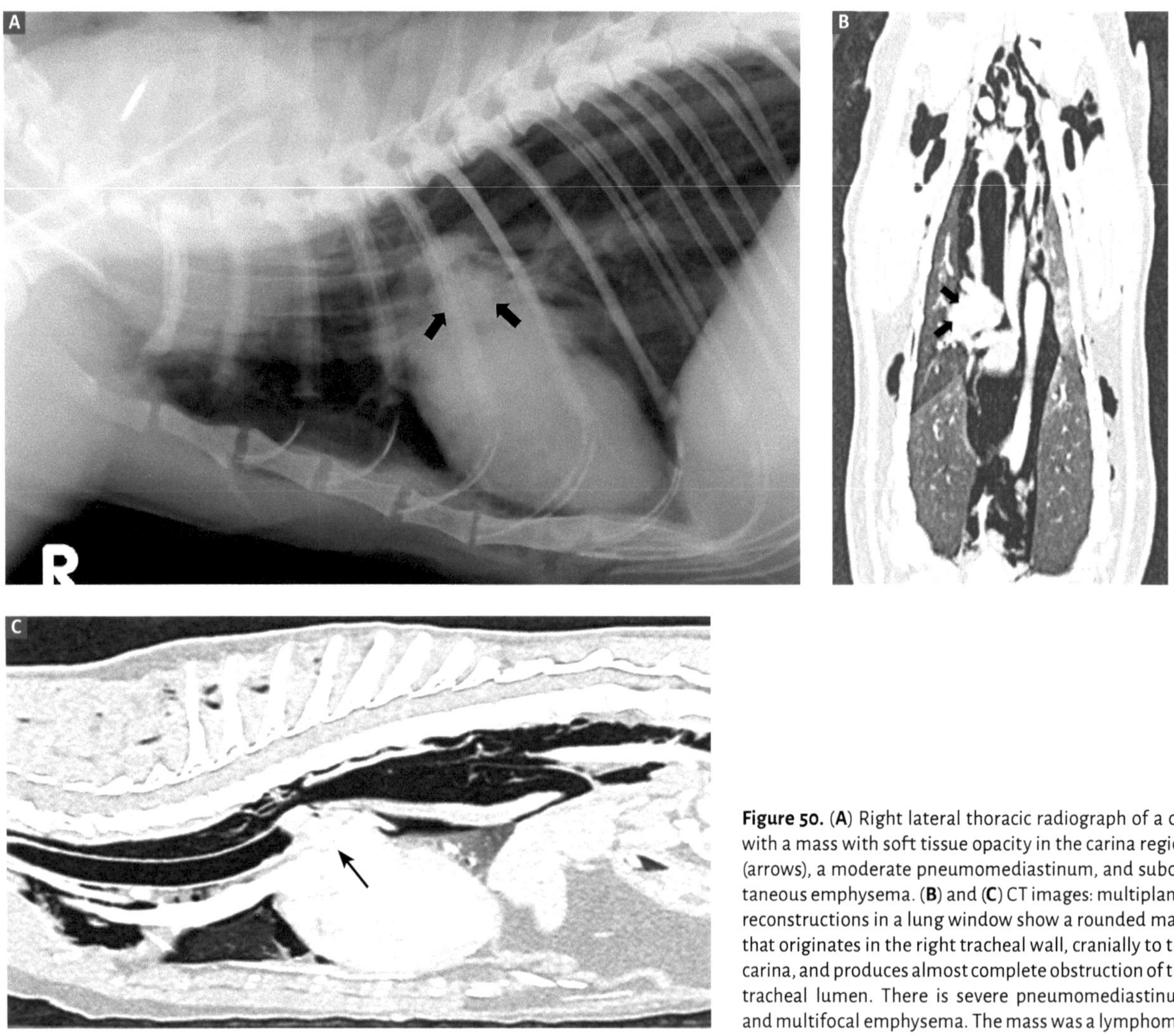

Figure 50. (**A**) Right lateral thoracic radiograph of a cat with a mass with soft tissue opacity in the carina region (arrows), a moderate pneumomediastinum, and subcutaneous emphysema. (**B**) and (**C**) CT images: multiplanar reconstructions in a lung window show a rounded mass that originates in the right tracheal wall, cranially to the carina, and produces almost complete obstruction of the tracheal lumen. There is severe pneumomediastinum and multifocal emphysema. The mass was a lymphoma.

Bibliography

- Baty, C.J. (2004) Feline hypertrophic cardiomyopathy: an update. *Vet Clin North Am Small Anim Pract*, 34(5):1227–1234.
- Bavegems, V., Van Caelenberg, A., Duchateau, L., et al. (2005) Vertebral heart size ranges specific for whippets. *Vet Radiol Ultrasound*, 46(5):400–403.
- Blocker, T.L., Roberts, B.K. (1999) Acute tracheal obstruction associated with anticoagulant rodenticide intoxication in a dog. *J Small Anim Pract*. 40(12):577–580.
- Buchanan, J.W. (1990) Pulmonic stenosis caused by single coronary artery in dogs: four cases (1965-1984). *J Am Vet Med Assoc*, 196(1):115–120.
- Buchanan, J.W. (2004) Tracheal signs and associated vascular anomalies in dogs with persistent right aortic arch. *J Vet Intern Med*, 18(4):510–514.
- Buchanan, J.W., Bücheler, J. (1995) Vertebral scale system to measure heart size in radiographs. *J Am Vet Med Assoc*, 206(2):194–99.
- Dennis, R., Kirberger, R.M. (eds) (2010) *Manual of Small Animal Radiology and Ultrasound. Techniques and Differential Diagnosis*. 2nd ed. Elsevier.
- Gunther-Harrington, C.T., Phillips, K.L., Visser, L.C., et al. (2019) Non-electrocardiographic-gated computed tomographic angiography can be used to diagnose coronary artery anomalies in Bulldogs with pulmonary valve stenosis. *Vet Radiol Ultrasound*, 60(1):38–46.
- Heng, H.G., Lim, C.K., Gutierrez-Crespo, B., et al. (2018) Radiographic and computed tomographic appearance of tracheal collapse with axial rotation in four dogs. *J Small Anim Pract*, 59(1):53–58.
- Henjes, C.R., Nolte, I., Wefstaedt, P. (2011) Multidetector-row computed tomography of thoracic aortic anomalies in dogs and cats: patent ductus arteriosus and vascular rings. *BMC Vet Res*, 7:57.
- Jepsen-Grant, K., Pollard, R.E., Johnson, L.R. (2013) Vertebral heart scores in eight dog breeds. *Vet Radiol Ultrasound*, 54(1):3–8.
- Kirberger, R.M., Cassel, N., Stander, N., et al. (2015) Triple phase dynamic computed tomographic perfusion characteristics of spirocercosis induced esophageal nodules in non-neoplastic versus neoplastic canine cases. *Vet Radiol Ultrasound*, 56(3):257–263.
- Kirberger, R.M., Stander, N., Cassel, N., et al. (2013) Computed tomographic and radiographic characteristics of aortic lesions in 42 dogs with spirocercosis. *Vet Radiol Ultrasound*, 54(3):212–222.
- Kraetschmer, S., Ludwig, K., Meneses, F., et al. (2008) Vertebral heart scale in the beagle dog. *J Small Anim Pract*, 49(5):240–243.
- Laborda-Vidal, P., Pedro, B., Baker, M., et al. (2016) Use of ECG-gated computed tomography, echocardiography and selective angiography in five dogs with pulmonic stenosis and one dog with pulmonic stenosis and aberrant coronary arteries. *J Vet Cardiol*, 18(4):418–426.
- Lam, C., Gavaghan, B.J., Meyers, F.E. (2021) Radiographic quantification of left atrial size in dogs with myxomatous mitral valve disease. *J Vet Intern Med*, 35(2):747–754.
- Lamb, C.R., Wikeley, H., Boswood, A., et al. (2001) Use of breed-specific ranges for the vertebral heart scale as an aid to the radiographic diagnosis of cardiac disease in dogs. *Vet Rec*, 148(23):707–11.
- Lehmkuhl, L.B., Bonagura, J.D., Biller, D.S., et al. (1997) Radiographic evaluation of caudal vena cava size in dogs. *Vet Radiol Ultrasound*, 38(2):94–100.
- Malcolm, E.L., Visser, L.C., Phillips, K.L., et al. (2018) Diagnostic value of vertebral left atrial size as determined from thoracic radiographs for assessment of left atrial size in dogs with myxomatous mitral valve disease. *J Am Vet Med Assoc*, 253(8):1038–1045.
- Marin, L.M., Brown, J., McBrien, C., et al. (2007) Vertebral heart size in retired racing Greyhounds. *Vet Radiol Ultrasound*, 48(4):332–34.
- Meurs, K., Sanchez, X., David, R.M., et al. (2005) A cardiac myosin binding protein C mutation in the Maine Coon cat with familial hypertrophic cardiomyopathy. *Hum Mol Genet*, 14(23):3587–3593.
- Miller, M.W., Gordon, S.G., Saunders, A.B., et al. (2006) Angiographic classification of patent ductus arteriosus morphology in the dog. *J Vet Cardiol*, 8(2):109–114.
- Oliveira, P., Domenech, O., Silva, J., et al. (2011) Retrospective review of congenital heart disease in 976 dogs. *J Vet Intern Med*, 25(3):477–483.
- Oura, T.J., Young, A.N., Keene, B.W., et al. (2015) A valentine-shaped cardiac silhouette in feline thoracic radiographs is primarily due to left atrial enlargement. *Vet Radiol Ultrasound*, 56(3):245–250.
- Schwarz, T., Johnson, V. (eds) (2008) *BSAVA Manual of Canine and Feline Thoracic Imaging*. 1st ed. BSAVA.
- Thrall, D.E. (ed) (2018) *Textbook of Veterinary Diagnostic Radiology*. 7th ed. Elsevier.
- Treggiari, E., Pedro, B., Dukes-McEwan, J., et al. (2017) A descriptive review of cardiac tumours in dogs and cats. *Vet Comp Oncol*, 15(2):273–288.
- van den Broek, A.V.D. (1986) Pneumomediastinum in seventeen dogs: aetiology and radiographic signs. *J Small Anim Pract*, 27(11):747–757.
- Visser, L.C., Scansen, B.A., Schober, K.E. (2013) Single left coronary ostium and an anomalous prepulmonic right coronary artery in 2 dogs with congenital pulmonary valve stenosis. *J Vet Cardiol*, 15(2):161–169.
- Wisner, E.R., Zwingenberger, A.L. (eds) (2015) *Atlas of Small Animal CT and MRI*. John Wiley & Sons.
- Zekas, W., Adams. W.M. (2002) Cranial mediastinal cysts in nine cats. *Vet Radiol Ultrasound*, 43(5):413–418.

Echocardiographic Imaging Modes and Echocardiographic Examination Protocol

M. Josefa Fernández del Palacio

Transthoracic echocardiography is the main imaging technique used for examination of the heart and great vessels. It is noninvasive and has no known side effects. It uses ultrasound to image the heart in motion, and provides information on both cardiac anatomy and functionality. It is a technology that is fully integrated into cardiovascular medicine and is, in most cases, the definitive diagnostic tool. This is because ultrasound examination is innocuous, almost universally available, relatively inexpensive, can be performed on an outpatient basis and also in intensive care, and provides valuable clinical and prognostic information (Solomon, 2007).

The results of the echocardiographic examination must be considered in the clinical context of the patient, together with the clinical history, physical examination and other examination techniques, so that the clinician can make a clinical and aetiological diagnosis that is as accurate as possible and establish and monitor treatment (Fernández del Palacio, 2014).

Indications for Echocardiographic Examination

Echocardiographic examination is indicated in patients with clinical signs and physical examination findings compatible with cardiorespiratory conditions, in many cases allowing a diagnosis to be established. Thus, ultrasonography should be considered an indispensable technique in the following clinical situations (Armstrong and Ryan, 2010; Fernandez del Palacio, 2014).

- **Examination of patients with symptoms potentially due to cardiopathies.**
- **Evaluation of suspected congenital heart disease, in both young and adult animals.**
- **Initial evaluation of murmurs in patients with reasonable suspicion of valvulopathy or structural heart disease.**
- **Initial evaluation for suspected endocarditis with positive blood culture or new murmurs.**
- **Evaluation of cardiac masses (suspected tumour or thrombus).**
- **Evaluation of pericardial pathologies: pericardial effusion and constrictive pericarditis.**
- **Initial evaluation for known or suspected cardiomyopathy.**
- **Monitoring of patients after a diagnosis or during treatment of heart disease.**

Echocardiographic Imaging Modes

Ultrasonography is the result of a combination of physics, engineering, anatomy and physiology. As it is a very operator-dependent technique, knowledge of the basis of the discipline is necessary, in order to obtain good-quality diagnostic images and interpret them adequately, in the context of the clinical case (Gómez et al., 2012).

Echocardiography is based on the reflection of ultrasound waves (frequency >20 Hz) in cardiovascular tissues. As the ultrasound waves progress, part is reflected and part is refracted, enabling examination of deeper tissues. Subsequently, through specialised processing of the signals that return to the transducer (i.e. are reflected), they are transformed and reproduced in visual or audible formats on the ultrasound machine's monitor (Armstrong and Ryan, 2010).

The main modes used in practice are:

- two-dimensional, B mode or 2D echocardiography
- time-motion, M mode or TM echocardiography
- Doppler echocardiography.

Two-Dimensional or B Mode Echocardiography

Two-dimensional (2D) echocardiography allows the heart to be examined in a specific plane and obtains a 2D image (Fig. 1). This method makes evaluation of the anatomy and movement of cardiac structures possible, and allows specific measurements used in the study of cardiac functionality to be made. In addition, it constitutes a guide for the use of the other echocardiographic modes (Armstrong and Ryan, 2010).

Time-Motion or M Mode Echocardiography

Time-motion (TM) mode allows examination of the heart by means of a single ultrasound beam, obtaining a one-dimensional image (Armstrong and Ryan, 2010). The ordinate (Y axis) shows the depth of the cardiac structures and the abscissa (X axis) shows time, that is, the movement of the structures during the cardiac cycle (Fig. 2). The main use for M mode is to obtain quantitative data on the size of the cardiac chambers, walls and great vessels, as well as on the movement of cardiac structures.

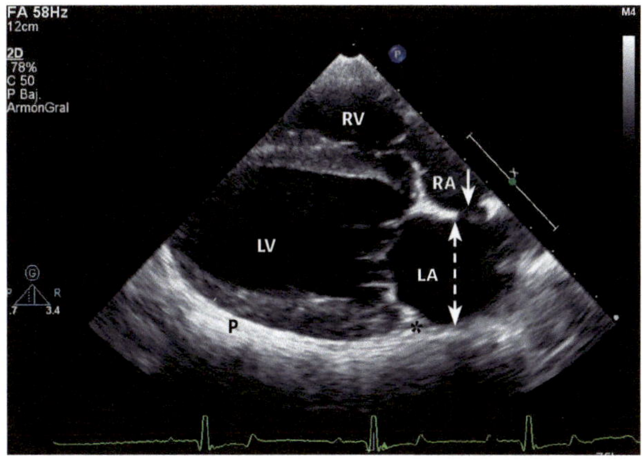

Figure 1. 2D echocardiogram of a normal dog, obtained using a right long-axis parasternal access. Four-chamber view: the left-sided chambers appear larger than the right-sided ones and the atrioventricular valves are located between the atria and the ventricles. Note the lack of echoes in the interatrial septum corresponding to the fossa ovalis (arrow). The pericardium (P) is seen as a hyperechoic line surrounding the heart. Note the measurement site of the left atrium (LA) parallel to the mitral annulus. The asterisk indicates the position of the coronary sinus. LV: left ventricle; RA: right atrium; RV: right ventricle.

Doppler Echocardiography

Doppler echocardiography allows the evaluation of normal flow within the cardiac and vascular structures, as well as detection of the presence of abnormal flow due to changes in its direction and speed. In addition, it can provide information on the presence of valve lesions (stenosis or insufficiencies) and abnormal cardiac communications (Bonagura et al., 1998a; Armstrong and Ryan, 2010; Boon, 2011).

Doppler technology is based on the changes in frequency undergone by sound waves when they are reflected by a moving object. When an object moves towards the observer, the frequency increases relative to the original frequency; when the object moves away from the observer, the frequency decreases. In the case of echocardiography, the change in frequency of the ultrasound waves occurs over the blood cells, which are the moving object(s). Ultrasound waves are emitted from the transducer with a certain frequency, so that, when they come into contact with the moving red blood cells, the return frequency differs from that of the original emission. The difference between the emitted and the reflected frequencies is proportional to the speed of the object against which the ultrasound wave has "collided", in this case, the blood cells. This phenomenon is known as the **Doppler effect** because it was described by the Austrian physician and astronomer Johann Christian Doppler (Armstrong and Ryan, 2010).

Under normal conditions, blood flows through cardiovascular structures forming laminar flows, that is, layers of ordered red blood cells in suspension, moving in the same direction and at very similar speeds. However, when anomalous flows exist, the layers of red blood cells tend to become disordered, forming eddies and thus changing direction and speed abruptly, causing the appearance of turbulent flow patterns. Doppler is used in echocardiographic studies to detect flow, to classify flow as normal or turbulent, and to quantify the velocity and pressure gradient.

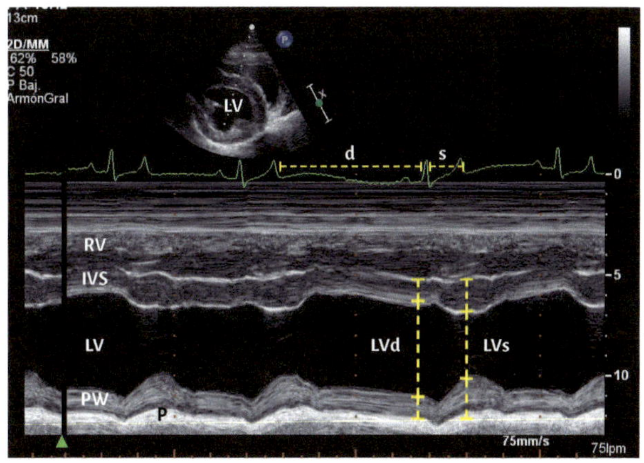

Figure 2. M mode echocardiogram, at the level of the left ventricle, obtained using a right short-axis parasternal access, in a normal dog. At the top of the image, the short axis of the left ventricle (LV) can be seen by 2D echocardiography, which serves as a guide to position the cursor and obtain the corresponding M mode view. Echocardiography can be used to easily identify the phases of the cardiac cycle, systole (s) and diastole (d). Note that the interventricular septum (IVS) and the posterior wall (PW) of the left ventricle (LV) approximate in systole and separate in diastole; the diastolic measurements are made at the level of the Q wave on the electrocardiogram and the systolic measurements are made where the IVS is lower, in both cases from the upper edge to the upper edge. P: pericardium; RV: right ventricle.

There are two main modes of Doppler ultrasound:

- spectral Doppler, which in turn can be:
  - pulsed Doppler
  - continuous Doppler
- colour Doppler.

Spectral Doppler

In spectral Doppler, the Doppler signal or spectrum collected by the transducer is arranged along an axis on which time is represented horizontally, while the speed (cm/s or m/s) is represented on the vertical axis. Therefore, the baseline is 0 m/s; above are the "positive" velocities of the flows that move towards the transducer, and below are the "negative" ones, that is, those that move away from the transducer (Bonagura et al., 1998a).

Pulsed Doppler

Pulsed Doppler uses a single piezoelectric crystal that acts as both an emitter and a receiver of the ultrasound waves. The transducer emits a pulse with a certain interval and the next pulse is not sent until the reflection of the previous one has returned. This type of Doppler allows measurements to be made in a specific area. The sample volume to be interrogated with pulsed Doppler is shown on an image in 2D mode. If a colour Doppler study has previously been carried out, areas of abnormal flow can be identified quickly and the sample volume of the pulsed Doppler can be imposed on the anomalous colour Doppler image (Fig. 3).

This type of Doppler has speed limits, since it cannot detect large changes in frequency, which are those that generally occur at speeds above 2 m/s. When the difference exceeds the maximum speed, a phenomenon called aliasing occurs, which causes artefacts and errors in the speed and direction of blood flow. The limit at which aliasing occurs is called the Nyquist limit, and it depends on the frequency of ultrasound emission, the distance at which the point of interest is located and the speed of the blood flow at that point. Continuous Doppler can be used to measure these abnormally high speeds (Bonagura et al., 1998a; Armstrong and Ryan, 2010).

Continuous Doppler

The continuous Doppler system employs two piezoelectric crystals: one emits ultrasound and the other receives the echoes that are reflected. This mode complements pulsed Doppler because it allows high speeds to be measured that produce aliasing with pulsed Doppler. Continuous Doppler is guided with a cursor, not with a sample volume, and therefore does not allow a specific area to be selected: it examines the flow along the entire ultrasound beam (Fig. 4). As it does not depend on a repetition pulse, it is not affected by the Nyquist limit and therefore the aliasing artefact does not occur (Bonagura et al., 1998a; Armstrong and Ryan, 2010).

From the measurement of the blood flow velocities (V), a haemodynamic study can be carried out, calculating the pressure gradient (PG) by using the simplified Bernoulli equation:

$$\textbf{PG Doppler (mmHg)} = 4 \times V2$$

Equation for the determination of V:

$$V = C \times f_d / 2\,(f_o) \times \cos \Theta$$

C: constant corresponding to the speed of ultrasound in the tissues (about 1540 m/s)
f_d: detected frequency variation between the emitted and received frequencies
f_o: emission frequency
cos Θ: cosine of the angle between the ultrasound beam and the blood flow

It is critical for the operator to consider the scan angle, so that the ultrasound beam is aligned as closely as possible with the direction of blood flow to obtain its maximum velocity.

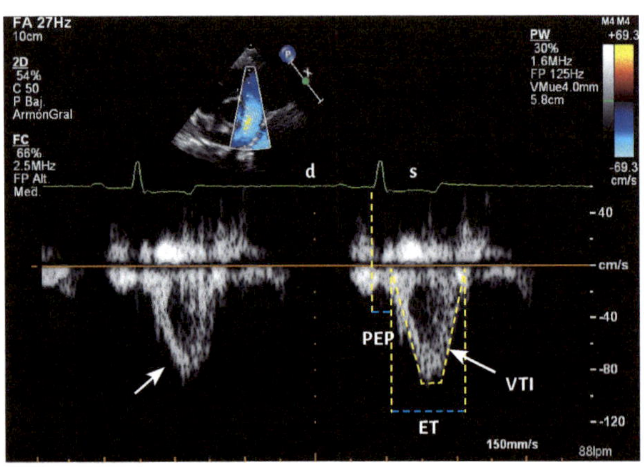

Figure 3. Pulsed Doppler echocardiogram of pulmonary flow (arrows) in a normal dog, obtained using a right short-axis parasternal access. On the right side, a scale corresponding to the speed range can be seen. ET: ejection time; PEP: pre-ejection time; VTI: velocity time integral.

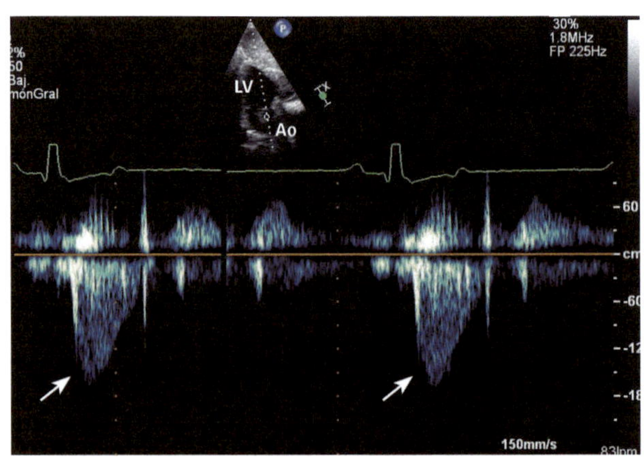

Figure 4. Continuous Doppler echocardiogram of aortic flow (arrows) in a normal dog, obtained using a subcostal access, in which the liver acts as a window for the passage of ultrasound waves. Ao: ascending aorta; LV: left ventricle.

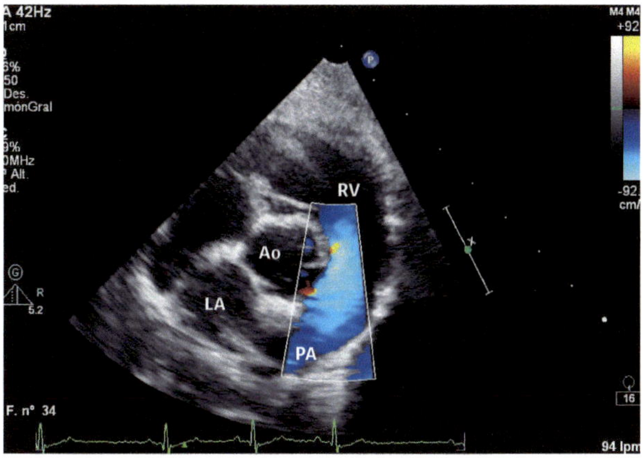

Figure 5. Colour Doppler echocardiogram of pulmonary flow in a normal dog, obtained through a right transaortic short-axis parasternal access. Blue represents blood flow moving away from the transducer, from the right ventricle (RV) into the pulmonary artery (PA). On the right side of the image, a colour scale is observed, with numbering correlating with the pulse repetition frequency that shows the speed of the flow being measured. Ao: aorta; LA: left atrium.

As the angle increases, the calculated velocity decreases. This is because the equation uses the cosine of the angle between the Doppler cursor and the blood flow; as the angle increases, the cosine value decreases and gets closer to zero.

Another important parameter is **distance**: when using a pulsed Doppler measurement, the greater the distance to the measurement point, the lower the maximum speed that can be measured.

Likewise, the **transducer frequency** influences the Doppler measurement: lower frequencies allow higher speeds to be measured.

The examination of blood flow by **Doppler ultrasound** requires a **synchronous electrocardiogram** (**ECG**) with the echocardiographic images, which allows measurement of the phase of the cardiac cycle in which the different Doppler spectra are obtained, as well as the presence of arrhythmias during the echocardiographic examination.

Colour Doppler

Colour Doppler **uses the two ultrasound modes**, combining 2D imaging and the movement of the blood flow (Fig. 5). It uses the same technology as pulsed Doppler, but differs in that it **uses multiple sample volumes** along the multiple ultrasound beams scanning a given area (Bonagura and Miller, 1998b; Armstrong and Ryan, 2010).

Differences in flow velocity and direction are colour coded, with **red showing flow approaching** the transducer and **blue showing flow moving away**. The **brighter the colour, the higher the flow velocity**.

As this modality uses **pulsed Doppler**, it can also be subject to aliasing effects, which are observed as colour inversions (turbulence patterns or a colour mosaic) when flow speeds exceed the preset limits. When using colour Doppler, the size of the window to be examined can also be selected. The larger the size of the window, the more likely it is there will be errors, so **the window should be adjusted to the area to be evaluated**.

Colour Doppler should be used as the first option and, if abnormal flow is observed, it should be studied and quantified using spectral Doppler.

Echocardiographic Examination Protocol

The echocardiographic examination is an interactive procedure involving the clinician, the ultrasound team and the animal. The optimal interaction between these three components is the key to obtaining images and echocardiographic signals that can be useful in diagnosing or monitoring heart disease.

The clinician performing the examination should be aware of the following (Armstrong and Ryan, 2010; Boon, 2011):

- ultrasound and the basics of ultrasound physics
- the anatomy and physiology of the cardiovascular system
- the haemodynamic effects of different heart diseases.

Ultrasound equipment should include:

- 2D, M and spectral Doppler (pulsed and continuous) modes, and colour flow Doppler;
- video and image recording system;
- specific software for the measurement of cardiac structures and blood flow velocities;
- phased-array sectoral transducers of a frequency appropriate for the size of the animal. Conventionally, high frequencies are used for small dogs and cats, and lower frequencies for medium-sized and large dogs (Fig. 6). The frequency affects the ultrasound penetration depth and image resolution (a higher frequency provides lower penetration and better resolution; lower frequencies achieve deeper penetration but with poorer resolution). The animal's body condition should also be

considered: transducers with lower frequencies should be used for obese animals. Doppler ultrasound requires low-frequency transducers, which allow the pulse repetition frequency to be increased and higher speeds to be obtained without the presence of aliasing; and

– synchronous ECG, in order to obtain the ECG trace and display it simultaneously with the echocardiographic image (Fernández del Palacio, 2014). This enables the operator to recognise the phase of the cardiac cycle to which each image corresponds (especially important for making measurements or evaluating Doppler spectra). To do this, three electrodes are attached to the limbs by means of paediatric adhesive discs (and then covered with cohesive bandage) or with crocodile clips (Fig. 7).

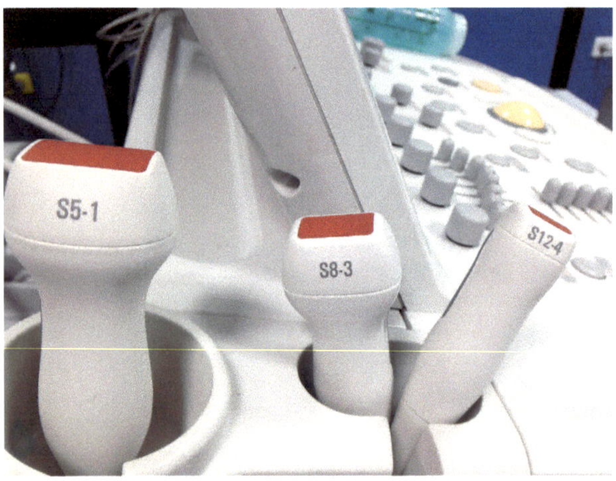

Figure 6. Sectorial phased-array transducers, of different frequencies, used by the author for echocardiographic examination of dogs and cats of different sizes: 5–1 MHz for large dogs and Doppler, 8–3 MHz for small to medium-sized dogs and 12–4 MHz for very small dogs and cats.

Preparation and Positioning of Animals

Preparation

Echocardiographic examination is generally **well tolerated** by most animals, but for puppies, some unruly animals and animals that are stressed, **sedation** may be necessary. However, it must be taken into account that most of the sedative agents or combinations of drugs used cause cardiovascular side effects (modifying sympathetic tone, changing the blood pressure or altering ventricular function) and therefore sedation should be avoided where possible (Seiler et al., 2008). The most commonly used options for sedation are as follows.

- In dogs: the combination of acepromazine (0.03 mg/kg) and buprenorphine (0.005–0.0075 mg/kg) IM or IV.
- In cats: the combination of acepromazine (0.1 mg/kg) and butorphanol (0.25 mg/kg) IM. In difficult-to-handle and uncooperative cats, an intramuscular injection of midazolam (0.2 mg/kg) and ketamine (5 mg/kg), in the same syringe, can be given.
- **In most animals requiring sedation, the author uses only butorphanol (0.25 mg/kg) IM**. In this way, it is possible to eliminate the patient's anxiety for long enough for a standard scan and to record the diagnostic videos and images. Quantitative data can subsequently be obtained offline.

To improve the quality of the images, **clipping the hair from the cardiac area**, from the third to sixth intercostal spaces, on both sides of the thorax and in the subxiphoid region, is recommended; the skin should then be cleaned with an alcohol-based solution.

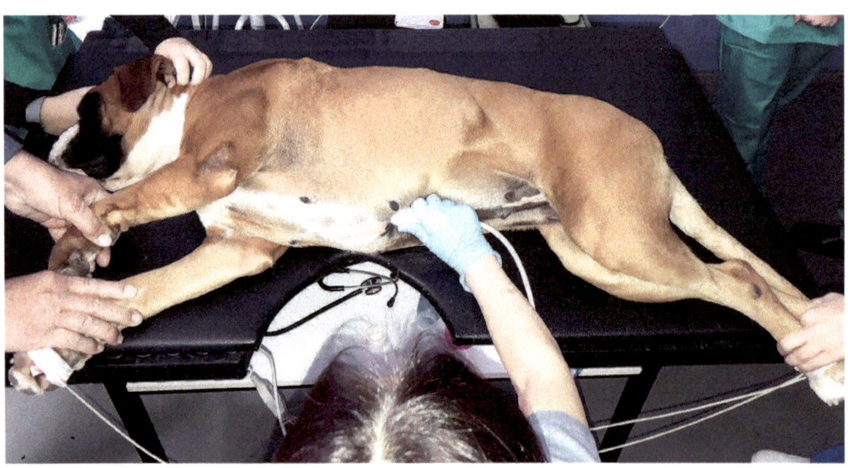

Figure 7. Positioning of a dog in right lateral recumbency for an echocardiographic examination; the placement of the transducer for subcostal access and the electrodes located on the pads for simultaneous ECG recording with the echocardiographic images are observed.

Positioning

To begin the examination, the animal is placed in **lateral recumbency** (Fig. 7) **on a notched table**, which is lined up with the cardiac area, to facilitate positioning of the transducer underneath and expand the access window to the heart (Thomas et al., 1993). When this position is not well tolerated, especially in **dyspnoeic animals**, a rapid echocardiographic examination can be performed with the **animal standing (dogs)** or in **sternal recumbency (cats)** to determine the cardiac cause of the clinical signs and guide emergency treatment.

Basic Ultrasound Equipment Controls

Once the animal is ready and the ultrasound machine is turned on, some **basic controls should be adjusted** on the ultrasound equipment to obtain an adequate 2D ultrasound image (Boon, 2011).

- **Field depth**: the image of the cardiac structures to be visualised must occupy most of the sector of the 2D image. A scale indicating the depth will appear on the sides of the sector, and the distance between two points corresponds to 1 cm.
- **Gain**: this is used to control the signal intensity in the whole sector. Very high gains produce a very white image, whereas very low gains will result in a weak signal and a poor-quality image. The ideal gain allows the cardiac structures to be clearly visualised without superimposed echoes.
- **Time gain compensation**: this consists of increasing the gain at different depths, so that a good-quality image can be obtained without losing information in near or deep fields.
- **Sector size**: the sector width can be adjusted from approximately 120° to 45°; reduction implies a better resolution of the image by increasing the number of images per second. Setting the sector size is also recommended when using Doppler mode.

Obtaining Standard Echocardiographic Images

Animal Position: Right Lateral Recumbency

With the animal in this position, the transducer should be placed below, over the fourth to fifth intercostal space at a variable distance from the sternum to the costochondral junction (1–5 cm from the sternal edge). Plenty of ultrasound gel should be applied, in order to optimise the passage of the ultrasound waves through the skin (Thomas et al., 1993; Seiler et al., 2008; Fernández del Palacio, 2014).

Once the cardiac structures have been located, the transducer should be oriented to obtain standardised images from the different projections.

Right Parasternal Projection, Long Axis

With the transducer mark pointing towards the most dorsal part of the scapula, images should be obtained that correspond to two main sections.

a. **Four-chamber view** (atria and ventricles) (Fig. 1). The proportions of the four-chamber view should be observed, with the largest size corresponding to the left-sided chambers. The atrioventricular valves separate the atria and ventricles. The hyperechogenic line surrounding the heart corresponds to the pericardium. Specifically, the following features should be evaluated (Seiler et al., 2008; Boon, 2011).
   - The appearance, opening and closure of the tricuspid and mitral valves (valve prolapse may be observed in dogs with chronic degenerative mitral disease).
   - The ventricular and atrial septa; the latter deserves special attention because, in the four-chamber image, the area corresponding to the oval fossa can simulate an atrial septal defect (Fig. 1).
   - The coronary sinus located in the coronary sulcus. This appears dilated in patients with significant pressure/volume overload in the right atrium and also in cases of abnormal venous drainage (persistent left cranial vena cava, azygos vein) (Fig. 1).
   - Measurement of the left ventricle (LV) systolic (VOLs) and diastolic (VOLd) volumes using the modified Simpson method, optimising the image for the complete visualisation of the LV, including the apex (Fig. 8 A). From the volumes, the ejection fraction (EF) can be determined using the formula EF (%) = VOLd – VOLs / VOLd. The normal EF is approximately 50%.
   - The long (L) and short (S) axes of the LV in diastole to determine the sphericity index (SI) according to the formula SI = L / S; normal SI is >1.7 (Seiler et al., 2008). The short axis can also be measured in M mode at the transventricular level.
   - The size of the right pulmonary vein (PV) and pulmonary artery (PA). These are important in patients with pulmonary hypertension, and can be measured by optimising the image to visualise the cardiac base. In normal dogs, these vessels are of equivalent sizes (Birettoni et al., 2016) (Fig. 8 B). In a recent study in healthy cats, the PVmax/PAmax and PVmin/PAmin ratios were 0.67 and 0.51, respectively; these indices have made it possible to discriminate between cats with cardiomyopathy with and without congestive heart failure (Patata et al., 2020).
   - Measurement of the largest diameter of the left atrium (LA) in systole, parallel to the mitral valve annulus (Fig. 1).

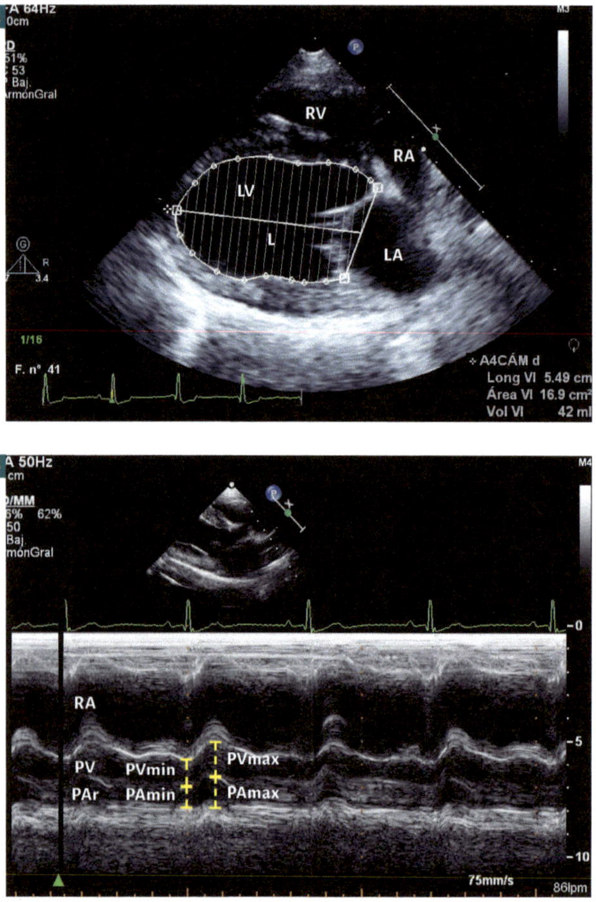

Figure 8. 2D (A) and M mode (B) echocardiograms of a normal dog, obtained using a right long-axis parasternal access; four-chamber view. **A**. The trace for measurement of left ventricle (LV) volume is shown, as well as the measurement of the ventricular long axis (L). **B**. The trace and measurement of the diameter of the pulmonary vein (PV) and right pulmonary artery (PAr) are shown. LA: left atrium; RA: right atrium; RV: right ventricle.

- Transvalvular flows using colour Doppler, to determine whether there are abnormal flows of valve insufficiency or stenosis.
- The atrial and ventricular septa, when a possible septal defect is suspected, can be investigated using colour Doppler.

b. **Five-chamber view**. This can be obtained from the four-chamber view, rotating the transducer 10° anticlockwise, towards the head of the animal. The LV outflow tract and ascending aorta can be visualised, with the apex to the left of the image, as well as the right-sided chambers and the LA, which is smaller in size (Fig. 9).

Specifically, the following features should be evaluated.

- The appearance of the LV outflow tract and ascending aorta, paying special attention to the appearance and movement of the aortic valve cusps, the most basal interventricular septum for the detection of subvalvular stenosis or ventricular septal defects (VSDs), and the movement of the anterior leaflet of the mitral valve (especially in cats with obstructive hypertrophic cardiomyopathy).
- Measurement of the diameter of the aortic annulus (Fig. 9) and the ascending aorta at several levels.
- The flow through the LV outflow tract and ascending aorta using colour Doppler, determining whether there is abnormal flow due to valve insufficiency or valvular stenosis and, if so, at what level.
- Measurement of the ventricular septum and LV free wall in diastole (Fig. 10), in cats with suspected LV hypertrophy (normal range <6 mm).
- The interventricular septum, when a possible septal defect is suspected, using colour Doppler, especially in the most basal part where most membranous-type VSDs are located.

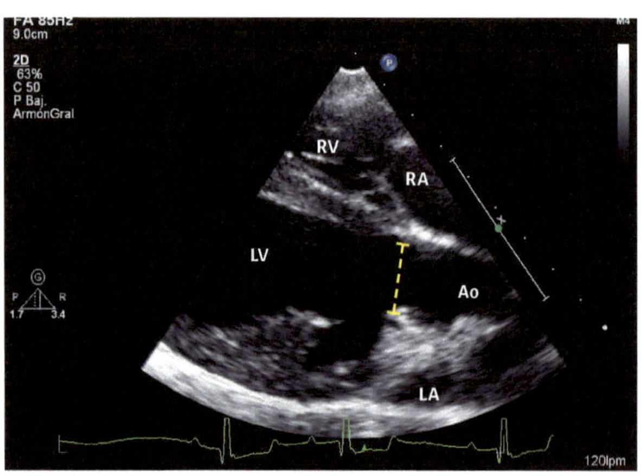

Figure 9. 2D echocardiogram of a normal dog, right long-axis parasternal access; five-chamber view at the level of the left ventricular (LV) outflow tract and ascending aorta (Ao). Measurement of the aortic annulus can be seen with the aortic valve open (systole). LA: left atrium; RA: right atrium; RV: right ventricle.

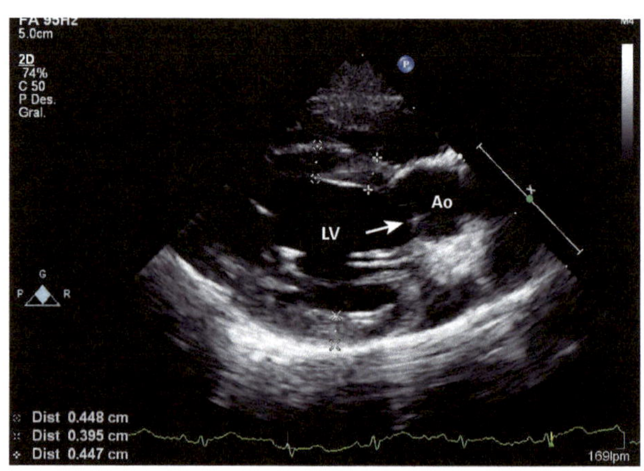

Figure 10. 2D echocardiogram of a normal cat, right long-axis parasternal access; five-chamber view in which the measurement of the ventricular septum and the free wall of the left ventricle (LV) are observed during diastole. Two of the cusps of the closed aortic valve are also observed (arrow). Ao: ascending aorta.

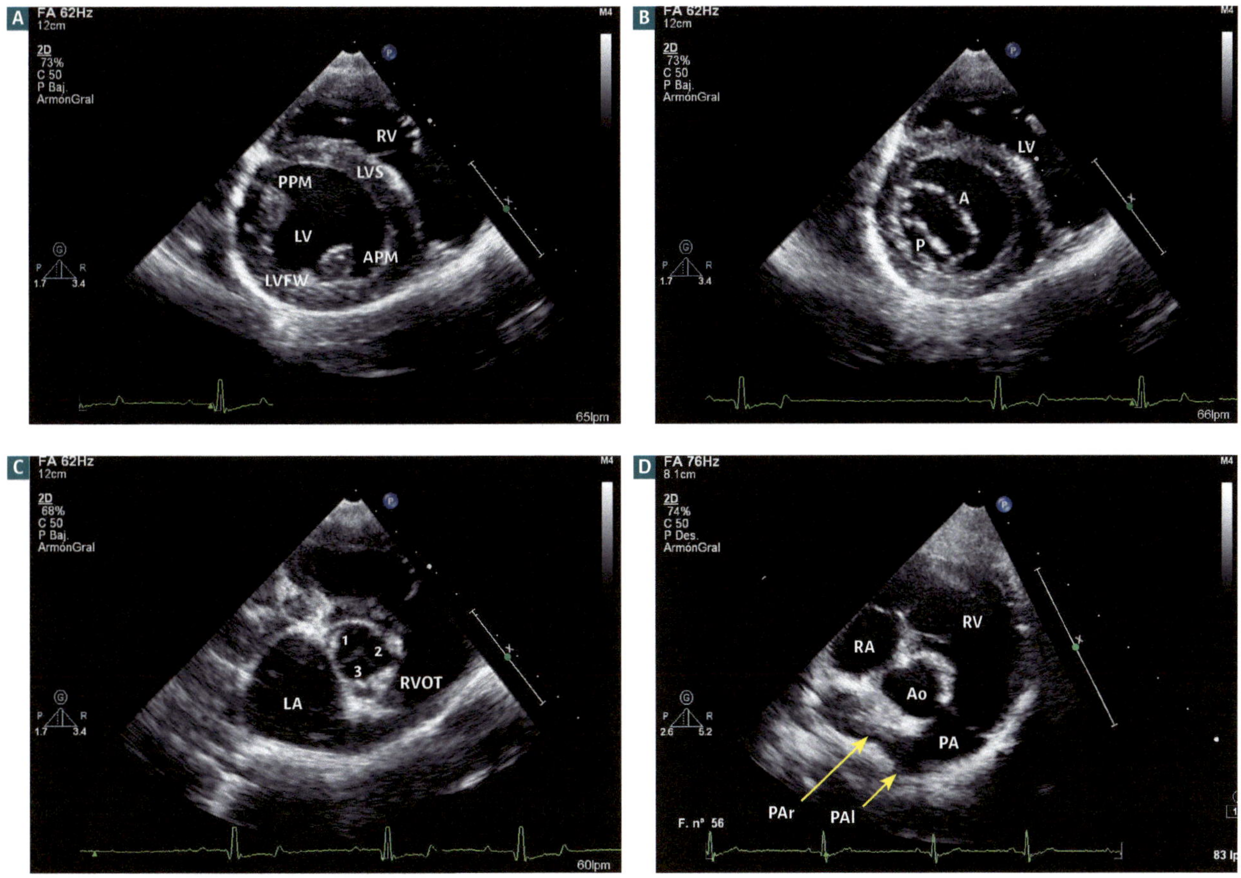

Figure 11. 2D echocardiograms, right short-axis parasternal access at different levels. **A**. Transventricular level: the left ventricle (LV) is observed with the papillary muscles (APM: anterior papillary muscle; PPM: posterior papillary muscle; LVFW: left ventricular free wall; LVS: left ventricular septum) protruding towards the lumen, and the right ventricle (RV) as the crescent shape at the top of the image. **B**. Transmitral level: the mitral valve is observed as an oval shape (A: anterior leaflet; P: posterior leaflet). **C**. Transaortic level: the aorta is seen in the centre of the image, surrounded by the left atrium (LA), right atrium and right ventricular outflow tract (RVOT); the closed aortic valve appears similar to the "Mercedes" symbol (1: noncoronary cusp; 2: right coronary cusp; 3: left coronary cusp). **D**. Transaortic level, more basal: the aorta (Ao) is observed in the centre of the image, and the pulmonary artery (PA) with its bifurcation (PAr: right pulmonary artery; PAl: left pulmonary artery).

Right Parasternal Projection, Short Axis

From the position where long-axis images are obtained, the transducer is rotated 90° anticlockwise, and cross-sectional images of the heart are obtained from the apex to the cardiac base, passing through the LV papillary muscles, the chordae tendineae, the mitral valve and the great vessels (Thomas et al., 1993; Luis Fuentes 2010; Boon, 2011).

- **Image at the transventricular level** (chordae tendineae) (Fig. 11 A): the LV can be seen to have a circular shape, and the right ventricle, which is smaller in size, can be seen as a crescent shape in the upper part of the image; the papillary muscles appear to protrude towards the LV cavity.
- **Image at the transmitral level** (Fig. 11 B): the mitral valve leaflets are observed in systole as two parallel lines in the centre of the ventricular cavity and are oval in shape when the valve is open, during diastole.
- **Image at the transaortic level and of the LA** (Fig. 11 C): the aorta is observed in the centre of the image with the cusps of the aortic valve showing a similar shape to the "Mercedes" symbol during diastole; the diameters of the LA and the aorta (Ao) (with the valve closed) are measured to obtain the LA/Ao ratio. Normal LA/Ao values are <1.6 in dogs and <1.3 in cats (Fig. 12).
- **Image at the transasortic level including the pulmonary artery**: two of the leaflets of the pulmonary valve are observed, as well as the main pulmonary artery and its bifurcation. In this view, the diameter of the main pulmonary annulus (d) is measured in dogs with suspected pulmonary stenosis (Fig. 11 D). Flow through the pulmonary artery is evaluated using colour Doppler (Fig. 5) and its velocity (V) is then measured using pulsed Doppler, placing the sample volume behind the pulmonary valve (normal V = 0.8–1.6 m/s) (Boon, 2011) (Fig. 3). If the flow is turbulent, as occurs in dogs with pulmonary stenosis, it should be evaluated using continuous Doppler. In addition, ventricular pre-ejection (PEP)

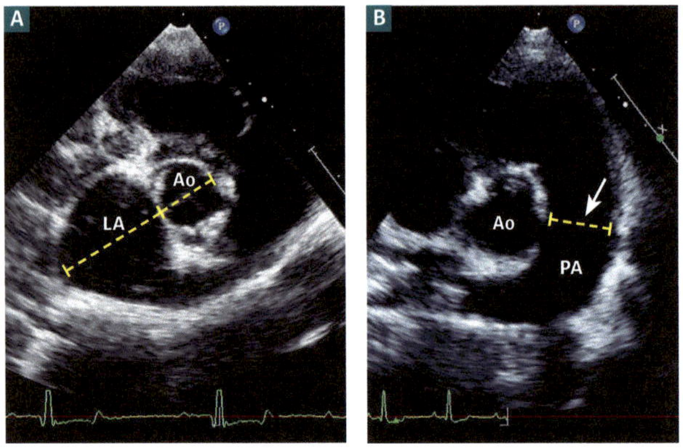

Figure 12. 2D echocardiograms, right short-axis parasternal access. **A**. Transaortic level: the measurement of the left atrium (LA) and aorta (Ao) is shown, from which the LA/Ao ratio is obtained. **B**. Aorta (Ao) and pulmonary artery (PA) level, showing measurement of the pulmonary annulus (arrow) with the leaflets open (systole).

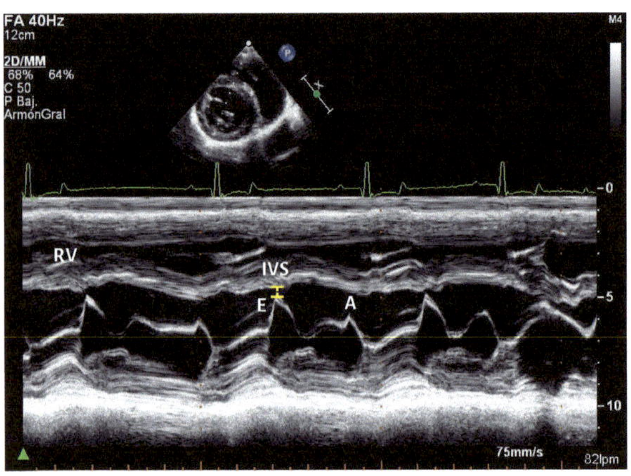

Figure 13. M mode echocardiogram, at the transmitral level, obtained using a right parasternal access, where the image of the anterior leaflet (with an "M" shape) and the posterior leaflet (with a "W" shape) is observed. The measurement is shown from the point of maximum excursion from the mitral valve (E) to the interventricular septum (IVS). RV: right ventricle; E and A are the names of the two pics of the mitral valve when it is opened.

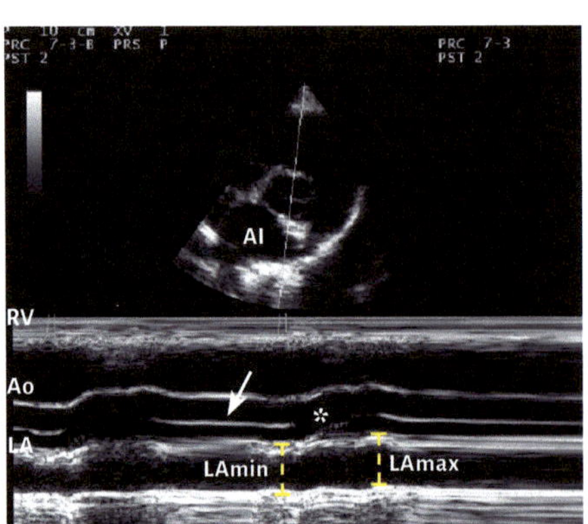

Figure 14. M mode echocardiogram, at the transaortic level, showing the measurement of the maximum (LAmax) and minimum (LAmin) size of the left atrium (LA) to determine the fractional shortening. Ao: aorta; RV: right ventricle.

and ejection (ET) times are measured, as well as the velocity time integral (VTI). From the VTI and the pulmonary annulus diameter measurement (d) made in the 2D image, the systolic ejection volume (EV) can be determined using the following formula: EV (ml) = π (d / 2) × VTI (Armstrong and Ryan, 2010).

From the cross sections described above and by placing the M mode cursor on the 2D images, standardised sections are obtained from which **direct measurements** of cardiac structures (walls, chambers and great vessels) can be made (Tables 1 and 2) (Cornell et al., 2004; Luis Fuentes, 2010; Boon, 2011; Häggström et al., 2016; Schober et al., 2017):

- Transventricular level (chordae tendineae): the septal and parietal thicknesses and ventricular chambers are measured in both systole (LVs) and diastole (LVd) (Fig. 2). Standard measurements are taken from the upper edge to the upper edge of each cardiac structure, following recommendations made by the American Society of Echocardiography (Sahn et al., 1978). Owing to the large variability in heart rate in dogs (sinus arrhythmia), performing at least three measurements in consecutive cardiac cycles is recommended.
  From the direct measurements, the fractional shortening (FS), an index of LV functionality, can be obtained: FS (%) = (LVd – LVs / LVd) × 100.
  - In dogs: FS = 24–44%.
  - In cats: FS = 30–50%.
- Transmitral level (Fig. 13): the mitral valve is observed inside the ventricular cavity. The anterior leaflet is "M" shaped and the posterior leaflet is "W" shaped during diastole (when the valve is open), and the valve is seen as two parallel lines that are joined during systole (when the valve is closed). The measurement to be made in this image is the distance between the point of maximum opening of the mitral valve (E) and the interventricular septum (IVS): normal E–IVS is <7 mm.
- Transaortic level (Fig. 14): this image shows the aortic valve as having a "box" shape during systole and as a hyperechogenic line in the centre of the vessel during diastole. Although the size of the aorta (at the end of diastole) and the LA (at the end of systole) can be measured, in dogs these measurements are obtained using 2D images because in M mode the cursor passes through the LA appendage and not through the atrium (Rishniw and Erb, 2000; Hansson et al., 2002). In addition, this image is used to determine the left atrial fractional shortening (LAFS) from the maximum (LAmax) and minimum (LAmin) dimensions of the LA, using the formula: LAFS (%) = (LAmax – LAmin / LAmax) × 100 (normal value in cats = 25–40). This index has been shown to be a good indicator of atrial functionality in cats with hypertrophic cardiomyopathy (Abbott and MacLean, 2006; Baron Toaldo et al., 2020).

Table 1. Measurements (in M mode) of the left ventricle, the interventricular septum and the posterior wall in dogs according to body weight (Cornell et al., 2004).

Body weight (kg)	LVd (cm)	LVs (cm)	PWd (cm)	IVSd (cm)
3	2.1 (1.8–2.6)	1.3 (1.0–1.8)	0.5 (0.4–0.8)	0.5 (0.4–0.8)
6	2.6 (2.2–3.1)	1.7 (1.2–2.2)	0.6 (0.4–0.9)	0.6 (0.4–0.9)
9	2.9 (2.4–3.4)	1.9 (1.4–2.5)	0.7 (0.5–1.0)	0.7 (0.5–1.0)
15	3.4 (2.8–4.1)	2.2 (1.7–3.0)	0.8 (0.5–1.1)	0.8 (0.6–1.1)
20	3.7 (3.1–4.5)	2.4 (1.8–3.2)	0.8 (0.6–1.2)	0.8 (0.6–1.2)
30	4.2 (3.5–5.0)	2.8 (2.1–3.7)	0.9 (0.6–1.3)	0.9 (0.7–1.3)
40	4.5 (3.8–5.5)	3.0 (2.3–4.0)	1.0 (0.7–1.4)	1.0 (0.7–1.4)
50	4.8 (4.0–5.8)	3.3 (2.4–4.3)	1.1 (0.7–1.5)	1.1 (0.7–1.5)
60	5.1 (4.2–6.2)	3.5 (2.6–4.6)	1.1 (0.7–1.6)	1.1 (0.8–1.6)
70	5.3 (4.4–6.5)	3.6 (2.7–4.8)	1.1 (0.8–1.6)	1.1 (0.8–1.6)

Table 2. Measurements (in M mode) of the left ventricle, the interventricular septum and the posterior wall in cats (Luis Fuentes, 2010; Schober et al., 2017).

Parameter	Measurement
Body weight (kg)	2–8.0
HR (beats/min)	145–267
IVSd (mm)	4.2–5.1
LVd (mm)	12.3–16.3
PWd (mm)	3.3–4.4
IVSs (mm)	4.4–10.1
LVs (mm)	7.6–10.9
PWs (mm)	5.6–9.5

Traditionally, in dogs, direct measurements of cardiac structures have been considered based on the animal's body weight and surface area. Recent publications have also shown that body weight influences the dimensions of the cardiac structures in cats (Häggström et al., 2016; Schober et al., 2017).

Subxiphoid or Subcostal Projection

This projection is used for the measurement of aortic flow velocity in dogs, especially those with suspected congenital stenosis of the LV outflow tract. With the animal in right lateral recumbency, a low-frequency transducer (2–2.5 MHz) is used; by placing the transducer parallel to the longitudinal axis of the animal and with the mark oriented towards the spine, the LV outflow tract and the ascending aorta can be examined, obtaining a good alignment between the Doppler ultrasound beam and blood flow, and therefore the greatest velocity (V) of the aortic flow (important in dogs with aortic stenosis) (V = 1.7–2.35 m/s) (Abbott and MacLean, 2003) (Fig. 4).

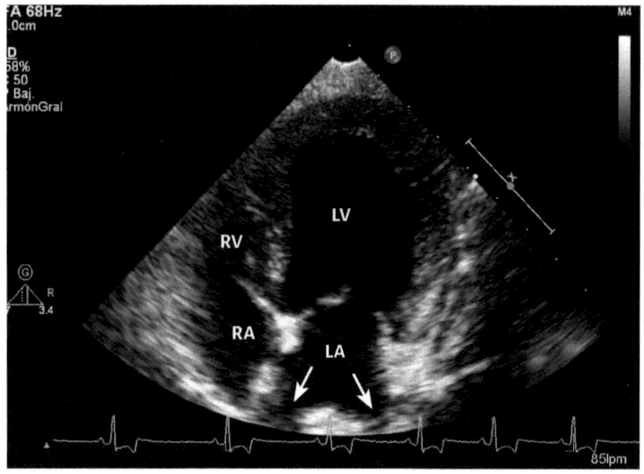

Figure 15. 2D echocardiogram obtained using a left apical parasternal four-chamber access in a normal dog. The left-sided chambers are larger than the right-sided ones and the entrance points of the pulmonary veins (arrows) ventrally into the left atrium (LA) are observed. LV: left ventricle; RA: right atrium; RV: right ventricle.

The use of continuous Doppler is recommended as obtaining the aortic spectrum is easier with this mode. From the Doppler spectrum, the pre-ejection and ejection times and the VTI are also measured, in the same way as mentioned above in the case of pulmonary artery flow, for the calculation of the systolic ejection volume (EV) and cardiac output (CO): CO = EV × HR (HR: heart rate).

Animal Position: Left Lateral Recumbency

Diagnostic images are obtained by placing the transducer in two main positions, caudal and cranial (Thomas et al., 1993; Gómez et al., 2012).

Left Caudal or Apical Parasternal Projection

The transducer is placed over the fifth to seventh left intercostal spaces, pointing dorsally towards the cardiac base (Boon, 2011).

- **Four-chamber image**. The two atria and the two ventricles are observed, with the apex at the top of the image (Fig. 15). The left-sided chambers appear larger than the right ones. From this image, the movement of the septal mitral annulus can be obtained using M mode (Fig. 16); this is indicative of the apex–base movement of the LV.
- From the 2D image of the four chambers, transmitral flow can be evaluated, first using colour Doppler and then using pulsed Doppler. Placing the sample volume just after the mitral valve, in the LV, two peaks of transmitral flow are obtained, E (normal V_{max} = 0.5–1 m/s) and A (normal V_{max} = 0.3–0.6 m/s) (Fig. 17). In patients with atrial fibrillation, only peak E is observed.
- Likewise, using pulsed Doppler and placing the sample

volume inside the pulmonary veins, information about the flow in these vessels can be obtained. It consists of three peaks, systolic, diastolic and reverse (Fig. 17 C), and measurement of this flow is useful for the evaluation of LV diastolic function (Schober et al., 1998).

– By optimising the image to better visualise the right-sided chambers, the morphology of the tricuspid valve and transvalvular flow can be evaluated with both colour Doppler and pulsed Doppler (Fig. 18). This flow also consists of two peaks, E and A, with slightly lower velocities than transmitral flow. Placing the M mode cursor over the lateral annulus of the tricuspid valve shows its trace (tricuspid annular plane systolic excursion; TAPSE) (Visser et al., 2015; Caivano et al., 2018), which is used for indirect evaluation of right ventricular function (Fig. 19). Likewise, right ventricular function can be evaluated by determining the area of shortening of the chamber of the right ventricle both in this image and in the left cranial projection.

– **Three-/five-chamber image**. In this position, the inflow and outflow tracts of the LV and part of the right-sided chambers are observed. It is used to obtain the aortic flow velocity in cats and also in dogs when it is not possible to measure it using subcostal access. It allows the morphology and nature of the flow of the LV outflow tract to be evaluated—that is, if it is laminar or turbulent—first by means of colour Doppler and then with pulsed Doppler, placing the sample volume just after the aortic valve, in the ascending aorta (V_{max} = 0.8–1.7 m/s) (Fig. 20).

– **Two-chamber image**. This is obtained from the apical position and with the ultrasound beam parallel to the long axis of the heart. The LV, LA and appendage are observed, separated by the mitral valve (Fig. 21). This image allows visualisation of the appendage, which is important in cats with suspected thromboembolism (Côté et al., 2011).

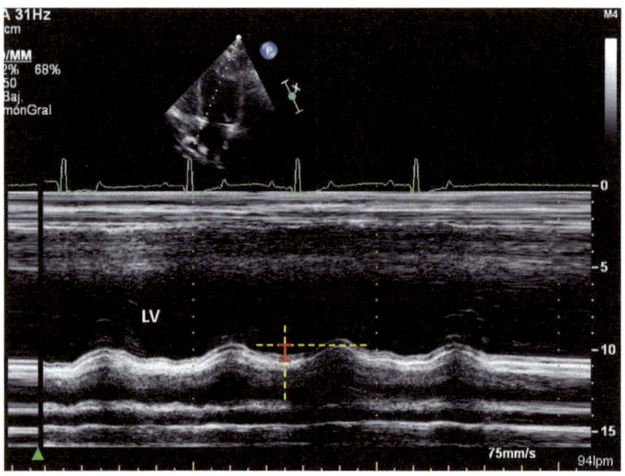

Figure 16. M mode echocardiogram obtained using a left apical parasternal four-chamber access in a normal dog. By placing the M mode cursor over the septal mitral annulus, its movement is obtained in the form of a hyperechoic line in the centre of the image. Likewise, the position of the measurement of this movement during systole is shown (red line). LV: left ventricle.

Left Cranial Parasternal Projection

From the caudal or apical position, the transducer is advanced to a more cranial position, over the third to fourth intercostal space, to obtain long- and short-axis cardiac images.

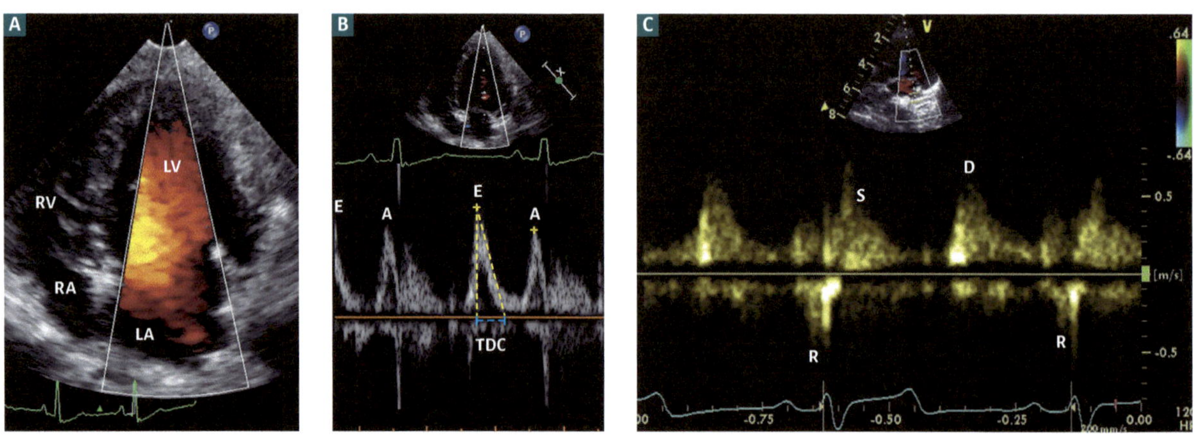

Figure 17. Colour Doppler (A) and pulsed Doppler (B and C) echocardiograms obtained using a left apical parasternal four-chamber access in a normal dog. **A**. This image shows the transmitral flow from the left atrium (LA) to the left ventricle (LV); the flow is red because it is moving towards the transducer. **B**. The transmitral flow spectrum is visualised: peak E corresponds to the initial phase of diastole and peak A, which is of lower velocity, to the final phase or atrial systole. The callipers (+) correspond to the location of measurement of the velocities of both peaks. TDC represents the time of deceleration of peak E, which is useful for the evaluation of LV diastolic function. **C**. Pulmonary vein systolic (S), diastolic (D) and reverse (R) flow is shown.

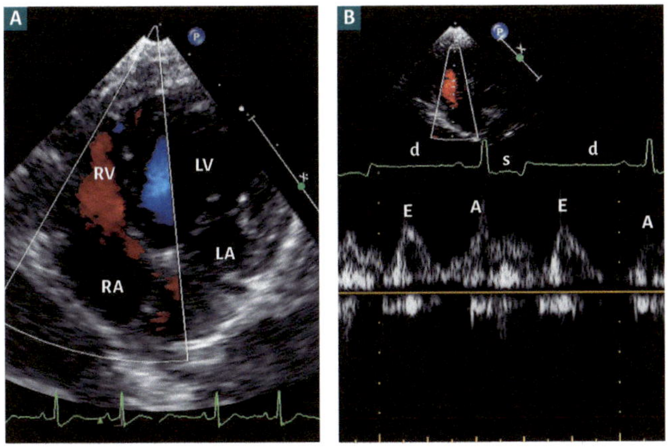

Figure 18. Colour Doppler (A) and pulsed Doppler (B) echocardiograms obtained using a left apical parasternal four-chamber access in a normal dog. **A**. Laminar-type flow is observed through the tricuspid valve from the atrium (RA) to the right ventricle (RV); the flow is red as it is moving towards the transducer. **B**. The transtricuspid flow spectrum is displayed; peak E corresponds to the initial phase of diastole and peak A, which is of lower velocity, compared to the final phase or atrial systole.

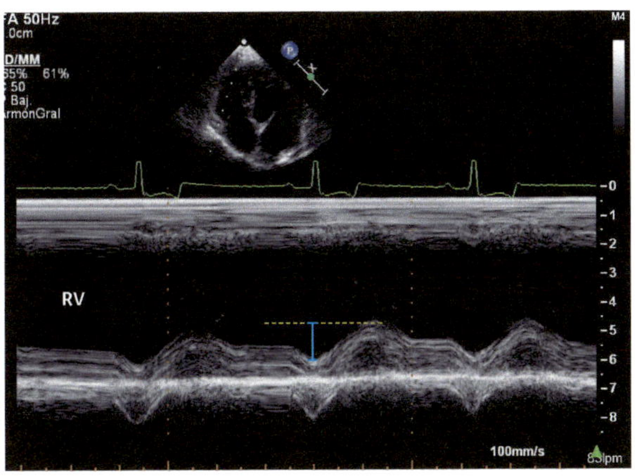

Figure 19. M mode echocardiogram obtained using a left apical parasternal four-chamber access in a normal dog. By placing the M mode cursor on the lateral annulus of the tricuspid valve, the tricuspid annular plane systolic excursion (TAPSE) is obtained; the location of the measurement of this excursion is shown (blue line). RV: right ventricle.

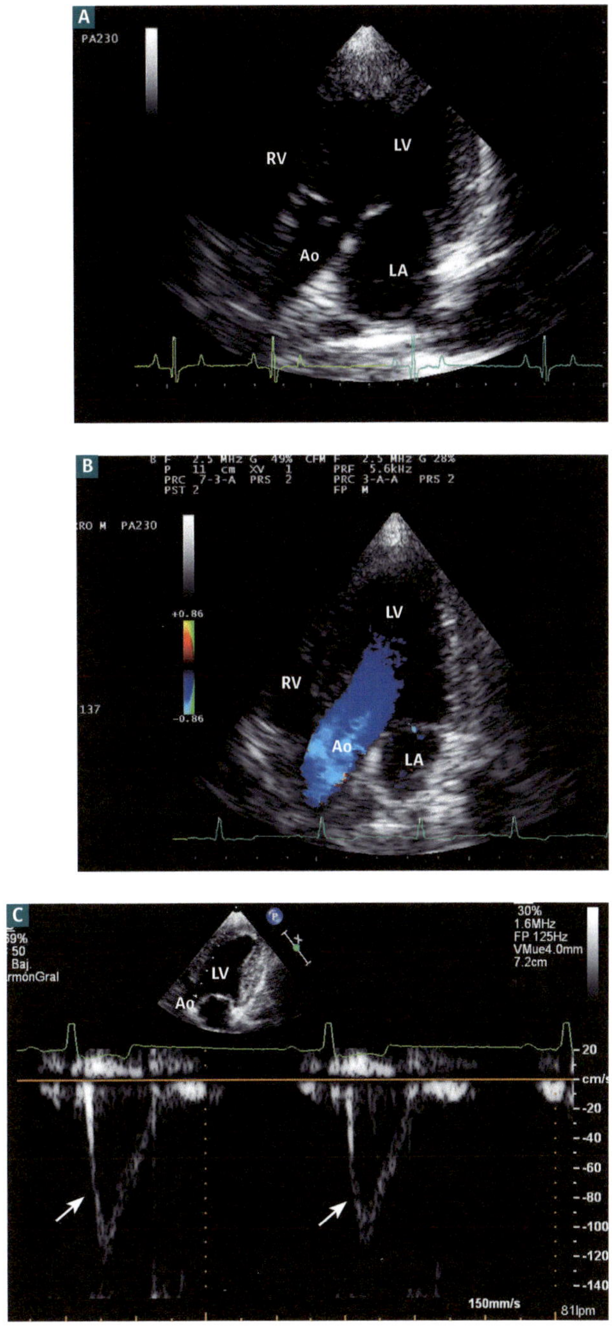

Figure 20. 2D (A), colour Doppler (B) and pulsed Doppler (C) echocardiograms obtained using a left apical parasternal three-/five-chamber access in a normal dog. **A**. The inlet and outflow tracts of the left ventricle (LV) can be seen. **B**. The flow through the ventricular outflow tract is visualised as blue as the flow is moving away from the transducer. **C**. The spectrum of the aortic flow is shown below the baseline, corresponding to a flow that goes from the LV to the ascending aorta (Ao). LA: left atrium; RV: right ventricle.

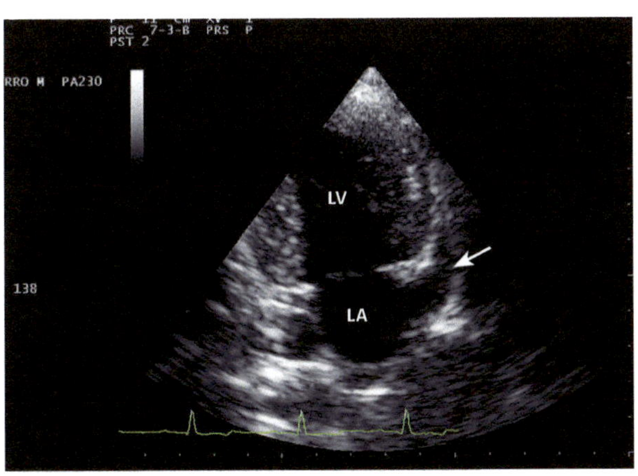

Figure 21. 2D echocardiogram obtained using a right apical parasternal two-chamber projection; the left ventricle (LV), left atrium (LA) and the appendage (arrow) are observed.

Long-Axis Images

These images are obtained by rotating the transducer 90° clockwise so that the mark on the transducer is towards the head. The main images obtained are as follows.

- **Image of the LV outflow tract, aortic valve and ascending aorta** (Fig. 22 A). This image is suitable for evaluation of the LV outflow tract, especially in dogs with aortic or subaortic stenosis, and of the entire ascending aorta.
- **Oblique image of the LV, right atrium, caudal vena cava inlet, tricuspid valve, and right ventricular inlet tract with the atrial appendage**. This view is important for the visualisation of neoplasms such as haemangiosarcoma in dogs with pericardial effusion (Fig. 22 B).
- **Image of the left and right ventricular outflow tracts, pulmonary valve and main pulmonary artery**. This image is useful for the evaluation of pulmonary artery flow and for the visualisation and measurement of persistent ductus arteriosus (Fig. 22 C) (Fernández del Palacio, 2014).

Short-Axis Images

From the long-axis images, a short-axis image is obtained by rotating the transducer 90° anticlockwise. In this image, the aorta is in the centre, surrounded by the structures of the right side of the heart (right atrium, tricuspid valve, right ventricular outflow tract and main pulmonary artery with its bifurcation) (Fig. 23). From this image, flow through the tricuspid valve and pulmonary flow can be evaluated.

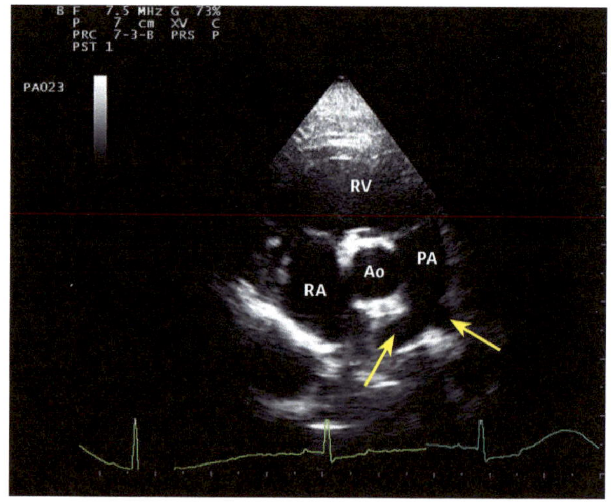

Figure 23. 2D echocardiogram obtained from a left cranial short-axis parasternal location. The aorta (Ao) is observed in the centre of the image and, surrounding it, the right atrium (RA) and right ventricle (RV) on the left and the main pulmonary artery (PA) with the bifurcation (arrows) to the right of the image.

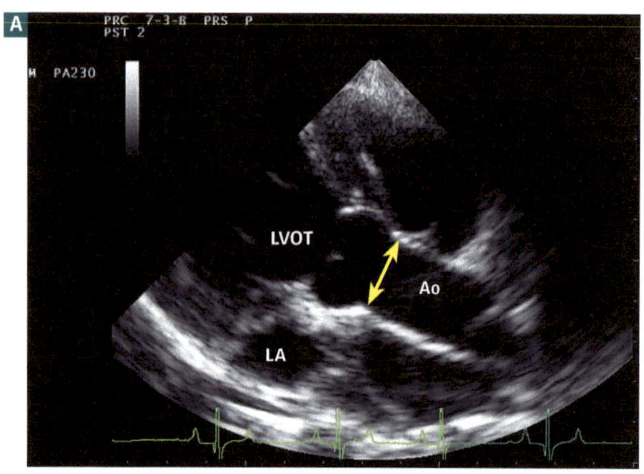

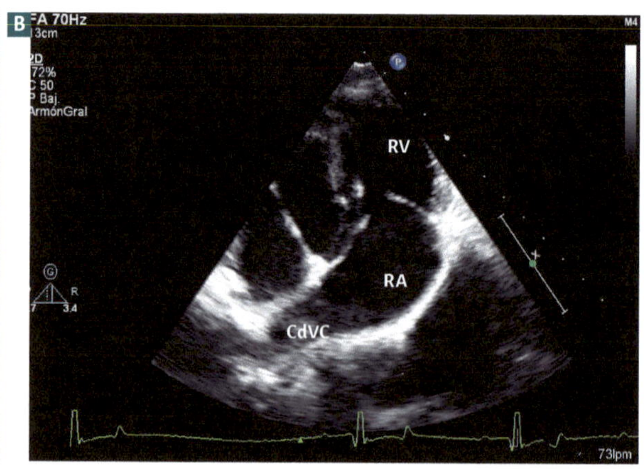

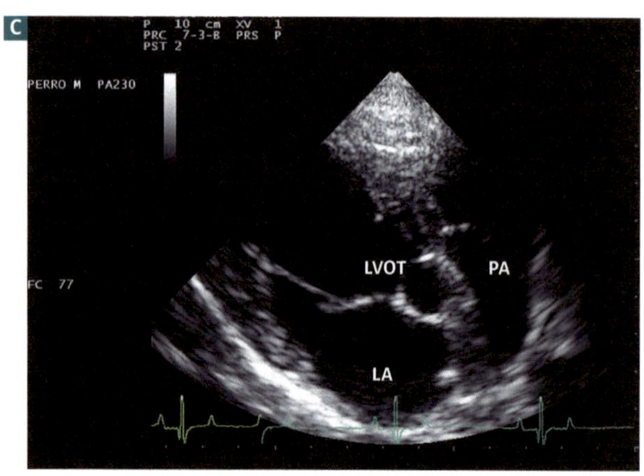

Figure 22. 2D echocardiograms obtained from a left cranial long-axis parasternal location. **A**. The left ventricular outflow tract (LVOT), left atrium (LA) and aorta (Ao) are observed, as well as the aortic valve leaflets. **B**. The right ventricle (RV), tricuspid valve, right atrium (RA) and caudal vena cava inlet (CdVC) are observed. **C**. The LVOT, LA and pulmonary artery (PA) are observed.

Main Parameters and Indices Indicative of Ventricular Functionality Measured Using 2D Echocardiography, M Mode and Spectral Doppler

Systolic Function

- LV fractional shortening
- LV ejection fraction
- distance between the point of maximum opening of the mitral valve and the interventricular septum (E–IVS)
- ventricular volumes
- ventricular dimensions.

Diastolic Function

- left atrial dimensions
- isovolumic relaxation time
- E/A ratio
- A wave duration
- pulmonary veins: systolic/diastolic (S/D) ratio
- pulmonary veins: reverse (R) peak flow (velocity and duration).

Echocardiographic Report

The echocardiographic report is the means by which both the descriptive results of the echocardiographic examination and the clinical implications and diagnostic considerations are conveyed, all within the clinical context of the patient.

A report should include:

- animal's details: age, breed, sex, body condition
- summary of echocardiographic examination of the patient
- qualitative description of the cardiac structures from an anatomical point of view, highlighting abnormalities
- quantitative data on the size of the cardiac structures and great vessels, as well as indices of ventricular systolic and diastolic function
- Doppler haemodynamic data, indicating the qualitative and quantitative characteristics of transvalvular flows and possible pathological communications
- summary and conclusions from a diagnostic and therapeutic point of view.

Bibliography

- Abbott, J.A., MacLean, H.N. (2003) Comparison of Doppler-derived peak aortic velocities obtained from subcostal and apical transducer sites in healthy dogs. *Vet Radiol Ultrasound*, 44(6):695–698.
- Abbott, J.A., MacLean, H.N. (2006) Two-dimensional echocardiographic assessment of the feline left atrium. *J Vet Intern Med*, 20(1):111–119.
- Armstrong, W.F., Ryan, T. (2010) *Feigenbaum's Echocardiography*. 7th ed. Lippincott Williams & Wilkins.
- Baron Toaldo, M., Pollesel, M., Diana, A. (2020) Effect of pimobendan on left atrial function: an echocardiographic pilot study in 11 healthy cats. *J Vet Cardiol*, 28:37–47.
- Birettoni, F., Caivano, D., Patata ,V., et al. (2016) Canine pulmonary vein-to-pulmonary artery ratio: echocardiographic technique and reference intervals. *J Vet Cardiol*, 18(4):326–335.
- Bonagura, J.D., Miller, M.W., Darke, P.G.G. (1998a) Doppler echocardiography I. Pulsed-wave and continuous-wave examinations. *Vet Clin North Am Small Anim Pract*, 28(6):1325–1359.
- Bonagura, J.D., Miller, M.W. (1998b) Doppler echocardiography II. Color Doppler imaging. *Vet Clin North Am Small Anim Pract* 28(6):1361–1389.
- Boon, J.A. (2011) *Veterinary Echocardiography*. 2nd ed. Wiley-Blackwell.
- Caivano, D., Dickson. D., Pariaut, R., et al. (2018) Tricuspid annular plane systolic excursion-to-aortic ratio provides a bodyweight-independent measure of right ventricular systolic function in dogs. *J Vet Cardiol*, 20(2):79–91.
- Cornell, C.C., Kittleson, M.D., Della Torre, P., et al. (2004) Allometric scaling of M-mode cardiac measurements in normal adult dogs. *J Vet Intern Med*, 18(3):311–321.
- Côté, E., MacDonald, K.A., Meurs, K.M., Sleeper, M.M. (eds.). (2011) *Feline Cardiology*. Wiley-Blackwell.
- Fernández del Palacio, M.J. (2014) Ecocardiografía: modalidades de imagen y protocolo de examen. In: Agut, A. (ed). *Diagnóstico por Imagen en Pequeños Animales*, pp. 493–509. Multimédica Ediciones Veterinarias.
- Gómez, A., Fernández del Palacio, J., Latorre, R., et al. (2012) Plastinated heart slices aid echocardiographic interpretation in the dog. *Vet Radiol Ultrasound*, 53(2):197–203.
- Häggström, J., Andersson, Å.O., Falk, T., et al. (2016) Effect of body weight on echocardiographic measurements in 19,866 pure-bred cats with or without heart disease. *J Vet Intern Med*, 30(5):1601–1611.
- Hansson, K., Häggström, J., Kvart, C., et al. (2002) Left atrial to aortic root indices using two-dimensional and M-mode echocardiography in Cavalier King Charles Spaniels with and without left atrial enlargement. *Vet Radiol Ultrasound*, 43(6):568–575.
- Luis Fuentes, V. (2010) Echocardiography. In: Luis Fuentes, V., Johnson, L.R., Denis, S. (eds). *BSAVA Manual of Canine and Feline Cardiorespiratory Medicine*. 2nd ed, pp. 79–97. BSAVA.
- Patata, V., Caivano, D., Porciello, F. et al. (2020) Pulmonary vein to pulmonary artery ratio in healthy and cardiomyopathic cats. *J Vet Cardiol*, 27:23–33.
- Rishniw, M., Erb, H.N. (2000) Evaluation of four 2-dimensional echocardiographic methods of assessing left atrial size in dogs. *J Vet Intern Med*, 14(4):429–435.
- Sahn, D.J., DeMaria, S., Kisslo, J., et al. (1978) Recommendations regarding quantitation in M-mode echocardiography: results of a survey of echocardiographic measurements. *Circulation*, 58(67):1072–1083.
- Schober, K., Luis Fuentes, V., Dukes-McEwan, J., et al. (1998) Pulmonary venous flow characteristics as assessed by transthoracic pulsed Doppler echocardiography in normal dogs. *Vet Radiol Ultrasound*, 39(1):33–41.
- Schober, K., Savino, S., Yildiz, V. (2017) Reference intervals and allometric scaling of two-dimensional echocardiographic measurements in 150 healthy cats. *J Vet Med Sci*, 79(11):1764–1771.
- Seiler, G., Dukes-McEwan, J., Gaschen, L. (2008) Basics of thoracic ultrasonography. In: Evan-Schwarz, T., Johnson, V. (eds). *BSAVA Manual of Canine and Feline Thoracic Imaging*. pp. 20–65. BSAVA.
- Solomon, S.D. (2007) Echocardiographic Instrumentation and principles of Doppler echocardiography. In: Solomon, S.D. (ed). *Essential Echocardiography*. pp. 3–17. Humana Press.
- Thomas, W.P., Gaber, C.E., Jacobs, G.J., et al. (1993) Recommendations for standards in transthoracic two-dimensional echocardiography in the dog and cat. *J Vet Intern Med*, 7(4):247–252.
- Visser, L.C., Scansen, B.A., Schober, K.E., Bonagura, J.D. (2015) Echocardiographic assessment of right ventricular systolic function in conscious healthy dogs: repeatability and reference intervals. *J Vet Cardiol*, 17(2):83–96.

Notes

Echocardiography in the Evaluation of Major Congenital and Acquired Heart Diseases

M. Josefa Fernández del Palacio

Introduction

The diagnosis and management of heart disease is an important part of day-to-day practice in small animals. Although heart disease can be detected through the clinical history and physical examination, definitive diagnosis and evaluation of its severity requires the use of echocardiography. This technique allows evaluation of the cardiac anatomy and functionality in a noninvasive manner. In addition, it is repeatable in expert hands and safe for both the patient and the operator (Boon, 2011). However, the findings of echocardiographic examination should be considered in the patient's clinical context along with electrocardiographic data, thoracic radiographs and laboratory tests, among others.

This chapter will address both the qualitative and quantitative results of echocardiographic examination in dogs and cats with congenital and acquired cardiac conditions.

Congenital Cardiopathies

Congenital cardiopathies (CCs) are cardiac anomalies that are present at birth and may be hereditary or acquired during foetal development. Although most CCs are detected by auscultation of a heart murmur, echocardiographic examination is necessary not only to determine the diagnosis but also to determine its severity and identify any coexisting abnormalities that might modify the prognosis and therapeutic plan (Bonagura et al., 1998; Oyama and Sisson, 2001). Echocardiography has largely supplanted cardiac catheterisation and angiocardiography, which are generally reserved for use in interventional therapy procedures and when abnormal vascular connections are suspected.

The main congenital anomalies that are diagnosed in small animal practice can be classified as follows.

- **Valvular malformations: aortic/subaortic stenosis, pulmonary stenosis and atrioventricular valve dysplasia.**
- **Shunts: patent ductus arteriosus and atrial and ventricular septal defects.**
- **Vascular abnormalities: persistent left cranial vena cava.**
- **Complex anomalies: tetralogy of Fallot.**

Valvular Malformations

Subaortic Stenosis

Left ventricular outflow tract (LVOT) stenosis is one of the most common CCs in large-breed dogs (Boxer, Golden Retriever, Rottweiler, Newfoundland and Samoyed, among others) (Oliveira et al., 2011). It is less common in cats.

LVOT obstructions can be found in three locations.

- **Supravalvular**: a crest of tissue located distal to the aortic valve, at the sinotubular junction. It is very rare in both dogs and cats.
- **Valvular**: varying degrees of thickening or fusion of the aortic valve leaflets; the bicuspid aortic valve can also cause stenosis.
- **Subvalvular (subaortic)**: consists of varying degrees of LVOT stenosis below the aortic valve leaflets. It is the most frequent form of LVOT obstruction in the dog. Generally, this defect is absent at birth and develops in the postnatal period, so that the most severe forms are found in animals older than 6–12 months of age (Pyle et al., 1976). This anomaly has been classified into several types according to the degree of severity (obstruction), which are still used today.
    - Type 1: small nodules of fibrous tissue protruding from the endocardium in the ventricular septum below the aortic valve.
    - Type 2: an endocardial subvalvular fibrous ring.
    - Type 3: a fibromuscular tunnel over the endocardium, completely surrounding the LVOT.

In addition to fixed types of LVOT obstruction, in which the degree of obstruction during systole does not change, a dynamic form can also be observed (in which the degree of obstruction is variable during systole) which, in some dogs, can coexist with the fixed form.

LVOT obstructions may be associated with mitral valve dysplasia in some animals (Fernández del Palacio et al., 1998), pulmonary stenosis and, less frequently, ventricular septal defects or patent ductus arteriosus.

2D and M Mode

- **Direct signs**: in two-dimensional (2D) mode, using right parasternal access (long axis, five-chamber view) and left apical five-chamber and left cranial long-axis views, the types and degrees of obstruction described above (Fig. 1) can be observed (Bussadori et al., 2000). Moderate and severe forms are easily identifiable, whereas mild type 1 lesions can be difficult to visualise. In the dynamic forms, the systolic anterior motion of the anterior leaflet of the mitral valve towards the ventricular septum is observed during systole in both 2D and M mode (Fernández del Palacio et al., 1998). Valvular stenosis can be seen as thickening of the leaflets (Fig. 2) or as an opening deficit.
- **Indirect signs**: varying degrees of concentric hypertrophy of the left ventricular walls and papillary muscles are observed due to the pressure overload to which they are subjected during ventricular systole (Fig. 1). In severe forms, hyperechoic papillary muscles can be observed due to fibrosis and mineralisation (Fernández del Palacio et al., 1998). Poststenotic dilation of the ascending aorta may also be seen in some dogs. In some dog breeds, such as Boxers, the LVOT may appear smaller in size compared with other breeds of the same weight (Menegazzo et al., 2012).
- **Functionality indices**: the fractional shortening (FS) may be normal or increased; in cases of major obstruction and advanced stages in which there is inadequate hypertrophy (afterload mismatch), signs of myocardial failure may be observed, such as dilation of the left-sided chambers, thinning of the left ventricular walls, decreased FS and mitral regurgitation. Diastolic dysfunction is common in patients with moderate to severe obstruction (Boon, 2011).

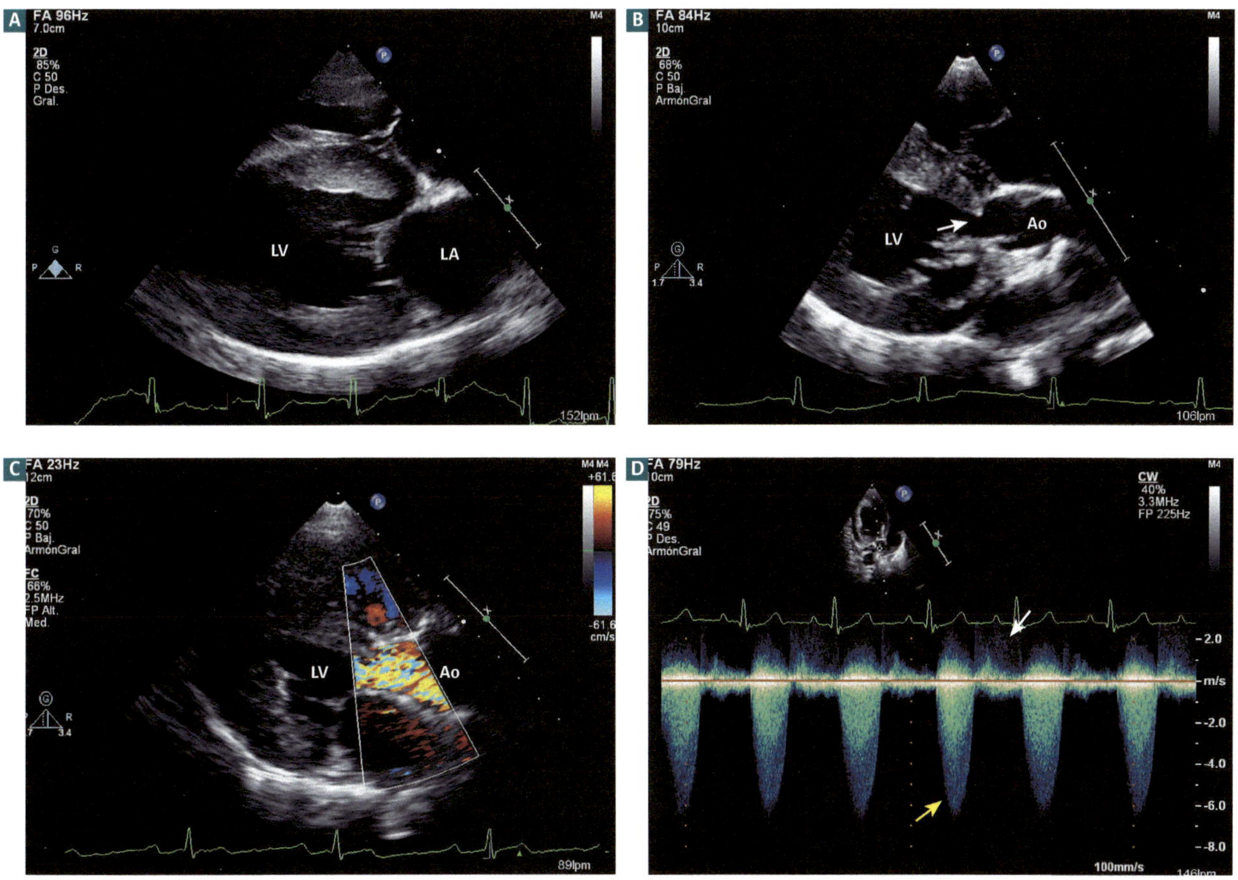

Figure 1. Echocardiograms of a dog with severe subvalvular stenosis. **A.** 2D echocardiogram, right long-axis parasternal access, four-chamber view showing concentric left ventricular (LV) hypertrophy. **B, C.** 2D and colour Doppler echocardiograms showing a type 2 subvalvular stenosis lesion (B) and turbulent flow in the LV outflow tract and ascending aorta (Ao) (C). **D.** Continuous Doppler echocardiogram (subcostal access) showing a high-velocity turbulent flow in systole characteristic of severe stenosis (yellow arrow) and insufficiency (white arrow). LA: left atrium.

Colour and Spectral Flow Doppler

Turbulent flow (visualised as a mosaic image) is observed in the LVOT and ascending aorta using **colour Doppler** (Fig. 1). Using **spectral Doppler**, the aortic flow velocity can be measured using the subcostal (subxiphoid) view in dogs and the left apical five-chamber parasternal view in cats (Fig. 1). Because aortic flow velocity can be influenced by many factors, it is difficult to use this parameter in isolation for the diagnosis of mild stenosis (which is difficult to visualise in 2D mode). In most dogs, when calm and in the absence of a patent ductus arteriosus, ventricular septal defect, systemic arterial hypertension or hyperdynamic states, obtaining maximum aortic flow velocities greater than 2.25–2.5 m/s on a subcostal view indicates LVOT obstruction. The diagnosis of dynamic stenosis is made and characterised by continuous Doppler, based on the fact that a "dagger"-shaped spectrum is obtained, because the degree of obstruction is maximum at the end of systole.

Based on the Doppler pressure gradient (DPG) across the stenosis, obstruction of the LVOT is classified as:

- mild: DPG 20–49 mmHg
- moderate: DPG 50–80 mmHg
- severe: DPG >80 mmHg (Bussadori et al., 2000).

Pulmonary Stenosis

Pulmonary stenosis is a common CC in English and French Bulldogs, the Beagle, West Highland White Terrier, Chihuahua, Cocker Spaniel, Bull Mastiff and Boykin Spaniel. It is also diagnosed with some frequency in cats.

Several forms of right ventricular outflow tract obstruction (RVOT) have been described.

- **Subvalvular**: may appear as infundibular stenosis, a double-chambered right ventricle and the presence of an abnormal coronary artery type R2A surrounding the pulmonary trunk (in the English Bulldog and Boxer).
- **Supravalvular**: distal to the pulmonary valve leaflets.
- **Valvular**: the most common form of RVOT obstruction in dogs. Two types (and their combinations) have been described.
  - Type A: characterised by a pulmonary artery with a normal-sized annulus and fusion of the valve leaflets.
  - Type B: characterised by a hypoplastic annulus and thickened, fused valve leaflets.
- **Pulmonary artery atresia**: the most severe form of RVOT obstruction.

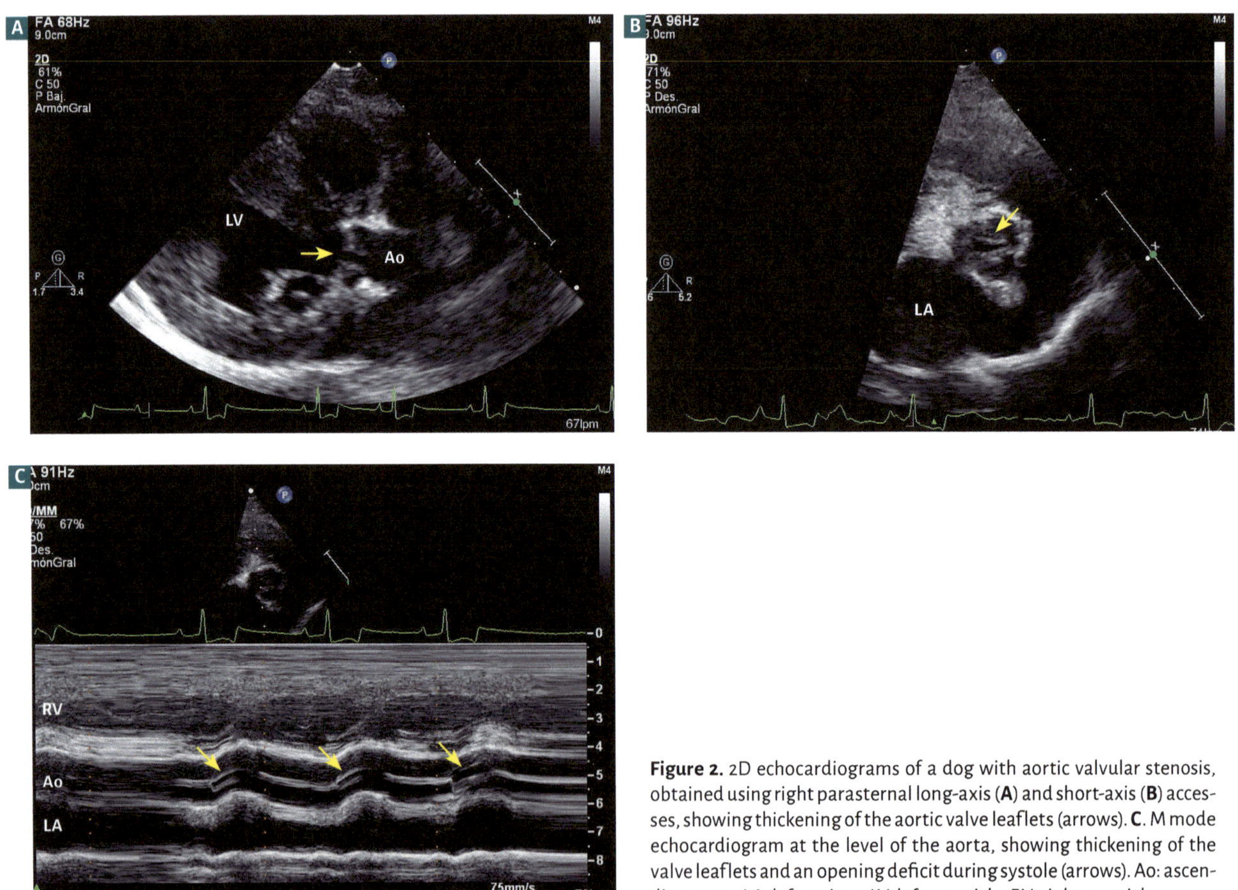

Figure 2. 2D echocardiograms of a dog with aortic valvular stenosis, obtained using right parasternal long-axis (**A**) and short-axis (**B**) accesses, showing thickening of the aortic valve leaflets (arrows). **C.** M mode echocardiogram at the level of the aorta, showing thickening of the valve leaflets and an opening deficit during systole (arrows). Ao: ascending aorta; LA: left atrium; LV: left ventricle; RV: right ventricle.

2D and M Mode

- **Direct signs**: the right and left short-axis parasternal accesses together with the left cranial long-axis parasternal access allow the best visualisation of the RVOT and the pulmonary artery (Fig. 3). With the **type A** valvular form, the valve leaflets appear slightly thickened and the commissures are fused, presenting a dome-shaped image in systole (Fig. 3). The diameter of the pulmonary annulus is normal compared with the aortic annulus (aortic annulus: pulmonary annulus ratio ≤1.2), with frequent poststenotic dilation. In **type B** stenosis, the valve leaflets appear markedly thickened, there is a hypoplastic pulmonary annulus (aortic annulus:pulmonary annulus ratio >1.2) and infundibular hypertrophy; poststenotic dilation is rarely present in this type (Fig. 3).
- **Indirect signs**: in the moderate and severe forms, hypertrophy of the right ventricular free wall is observed (Visser et al., 2019), as well as a flat interventricular septum and, sometimes, paradoxical movement during systole (due to elevated pressure of the right ventricle) and a reduction in the size of the left-sided chambers (Fig. 4). In M mode, the degree of thickness of the right ventricular free wall can be quantified (in normal animals, the thickness of the right ventricular free wall should be one-third of that of the posterior left ventricular wall). In severe forms, dilation of the right atrium due to secondary tricuspid regurgitation can also be observed.

Colour and Spectral Flow Doppler

Colour Doppler shows turbulent flow in the pulmonary artery during systole and, in most cases, in diastole (pulmonary insufficiency) (Fig. 3). In severe forms, or when tricuspid valve abnormalities are present, varying degrees of tricuspid regurgitation may be observed. Pulmonary artery velocities greater than 1.6–1.8 m/s are obtained using **spectral Doppler** in the absence of other causes responsible for right ventricular volume overload (Fig. 3).

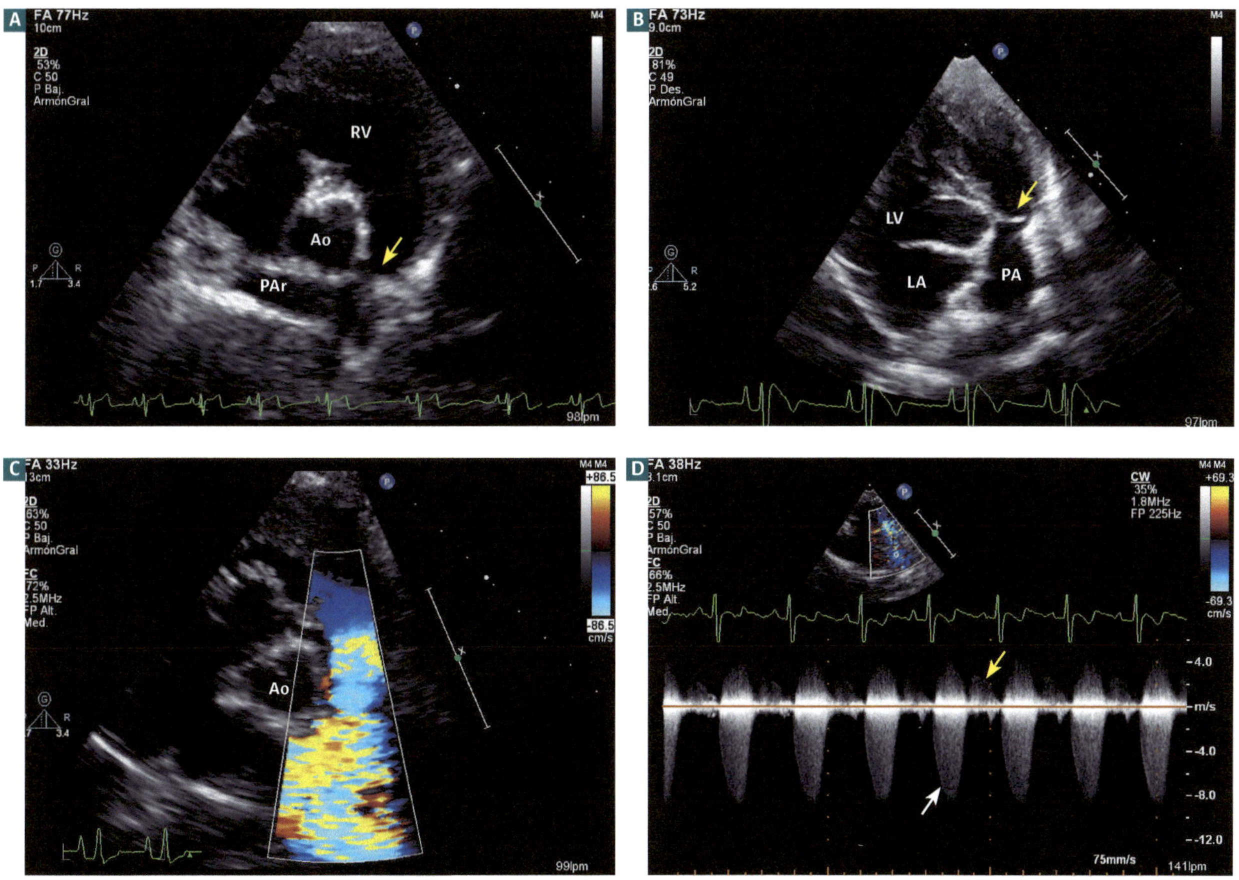

Figure 3. Echocardiograms of two dogs with congenital pulmonary stenosis. **A**. Right short-axis parasternal access, showing type B stenosis, with thickening of the pulmonary valve leaflets and reduced pulmonary annulus size (arrow). **B**. Left cranial parasternal access, showing the dome-shaped leaflets in systole (arrow), characteristic of type A stenosis. **C**. Colour Doppler echocardiogram, obtained with a right short-axis parasternal access, showing a mosaic image indicating high-velocity turbulent flow due to stenosis. **D**. Continuous Doppler echocardiogram, obtained with a left cranial parasternal access, showing high-velocity flow (8 m/s and DPG = 256 mmHg) during systole (white arrow) and insufficiency (yellow arrow). Ao: aorta; LA: left atrium; LV, left ventricle; PA: main pulmonary artery; PAr: right pulmonary artery; RV: right ventricle.

Pulmonary stenosis is classified according to the DPG as:

- mild: DPG 20–49 mmHg
- moderate: DPG 50–80 mmHg
- severe: DPG >80 mmHg (Bussadori et al., 2000, Nishimura et al., 2018).

Atrioventricular Valve Dysplasia

Atrioventricular valve dysplasia includes a broad spectrum of valve malformations affecting the papillary leaflets, chordae tendineae and/or muscles, such as thickened or split

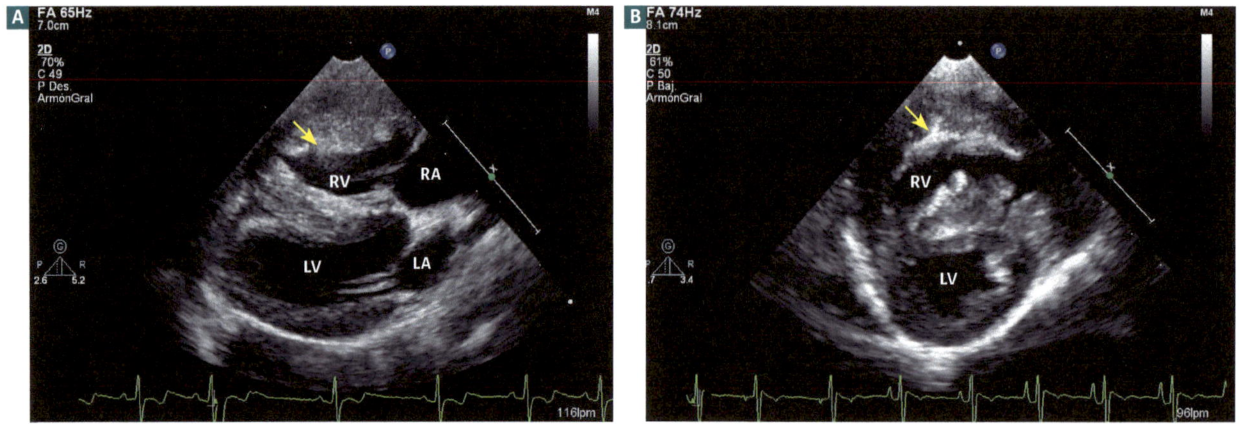

Figure 4. 2D echocardiograms of a dog with pulmonary stenosis. Right long-axis parasternal access showing a four-chamber view (**A**) and short ventricular axis (**B**) showing severe hypertrophy of the right ventricular (RV) free wall (arrow) and the left-sided chambers, which are reduced in size. LA: left atrium; LV: left ventricle; RA: right atrium.

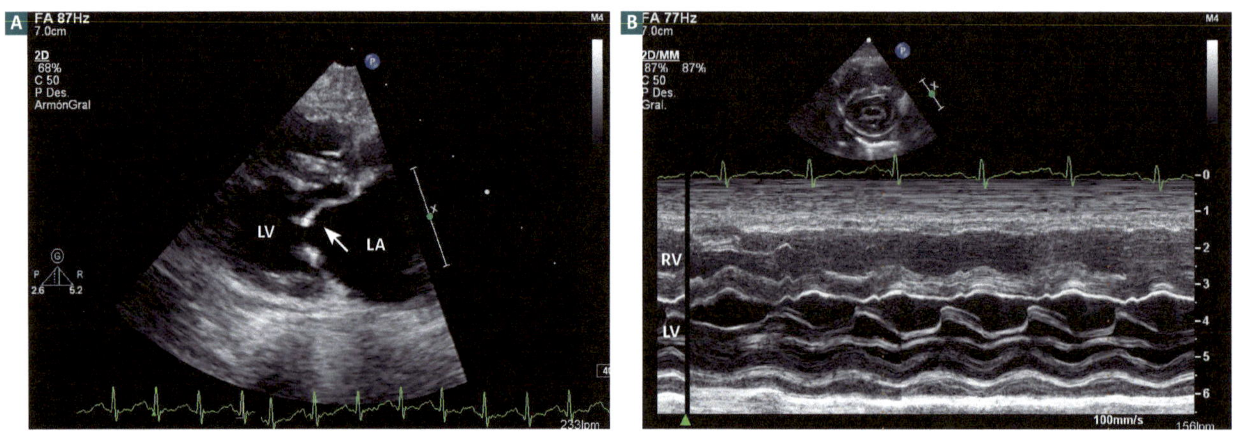

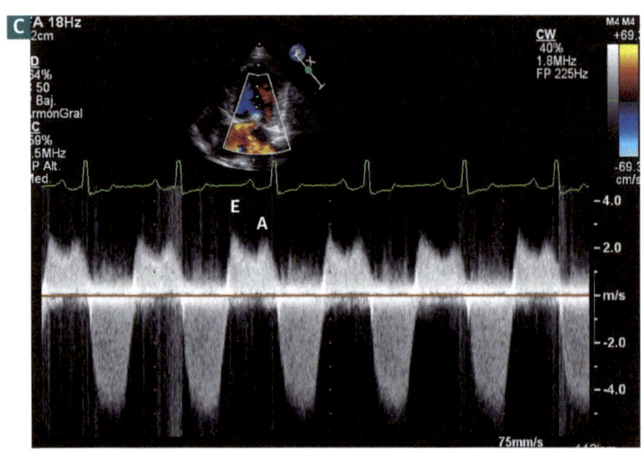

Figure 5. Echocardiograms of a cat with mitral stenosis. **A**. 2D long-axis parasternal access, four-chamber view, showing deficient, dome-shaped mitral valve opening (arrow) and dilation of the left atrium (LA). **B**. M mode, right short transmitral axis parasternal access, showing an opening deficit of the anterior leaflet and movement of the posterior leaflet towards the anterior leaflet during diastole, characteristic of mitral stenosis. **C**. Doppler showing high-velocity flow during systole due to mitral regurgitation. Transmitral flow during diastole exhibits elevated velocity at peaks E and A; despite the elevated heart rate, peak E shows increased hemipressure time, characteristic of stenosis. LV: left ventricle; RV: right ventricle.

valve cusps, fusion and thickening or elongation of chordae tendineae, direct insertion of the cusps into the papillary muscles, atrophy or hypertrophy of papillary muscles, or misalignment of them (Boon, 2011; Navarro-Cubas et al., 2017). Apical displacement of the tricuspid valve insertion is called Ebstein's anomaly. Atrioventricular valve dysplasia usually occurs with insufficiency, although stenosis may be observed in some cases.

Atrioventricular valve dysplasias are the most common congenital forms, along with septal defects.

The dog breeds most commonly affected are (Oliveira et al., 2011):

- **mitral valve dysplasia**: Great Dane, German Shepherd Dog, Bull Terrier, Golden Retriever, Newfoundland, Dalmatian, Mastiff
- **tricuspid valve dysplasia**: Old English Sheepdog, German Shepherd Dog, Weimaraner, Labrador Retriever.

2D and M Mode

- **Direct signs**: the valve modifications described above can be seen affecting the annulus, leaflets, chordae tendineae or papillary muscles, as well as causing their dysfunction (Figs. 5 and 6). In the case of tricuspid valve dysplasia, valve displacement can be observed apically; this presentation is called Ebstein's anomaly (Navarro-Cubas et al., 2017).
- **Indirect signs**: volume overload of the corresponding atrium and ventricle (Fig. 6). In cases of valvular stenosis, severe dilation of the corresponding atrium is observed. Persistence of the foramen ovale may be observed in some cases, with dysplasia of the tricuspid valve.

Colour and Spectral Flow Doppler

A regurgitant flow from the ventricle to the atrium is revealed by **colour Doppler**, and regurgitant flow velocities are obtained by **spectral Doppler**: transmitral maximum velocity (V_{max}) = 5–6 m/s (Fig. 5); transtricuspid <2.7 m/s (Boon, 2011) (Fig. 6).

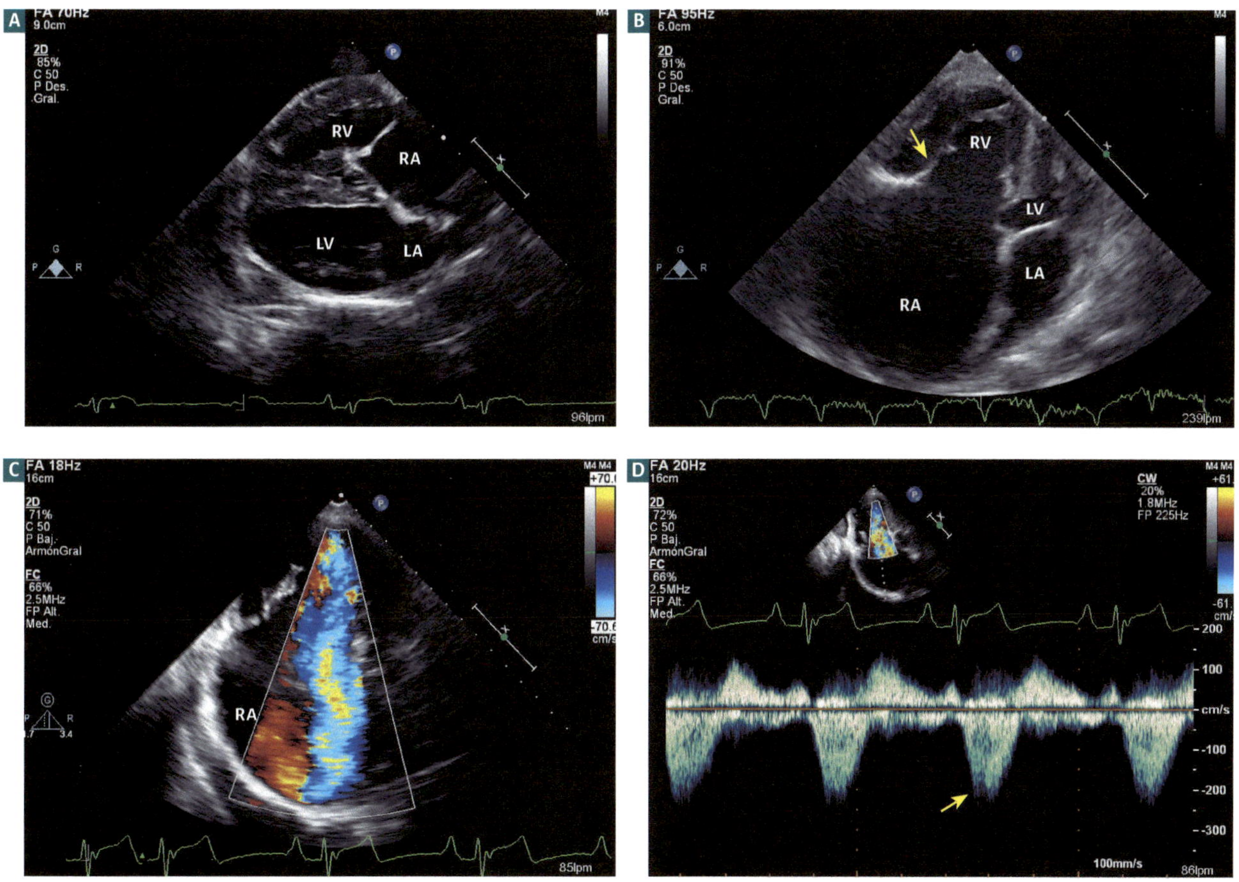

Figure 6. Echocardiograms of a cat and a dog with tricuspid dysplasia. **A**. 2D right long-axis parasternal access, four-chamber view, showing dilation of the right-sided chambers and insertion of the tricuspid valve leaflets into the papillary muscles with very short chordae tendineae. **B**. 2D left apical parasternal access showing an anomalous tricuspid valve (arrow) and severe dilation of the right atrium (RA). **C**. Colour Doppler, left apical view, showing turbulent, high-velocity flow in the RA due to tricuspid regurgitation. **D**. Continuous Doppler, where a regurgitation flow of 2 m/s and DPG of 16 mmHg is observed during systole (arrow). LA: left atrium; LV: left ventricle; RV: right ventricle.

When valve malformation occurs with stenosis, a convergent diastolic flow can be observed at the atrial level using colour Doppler. Spectral Doppler shows high velocity of the E and A waves during transmitral flow (even the velocity of the A wave is >1.5 m/s due to atrial contraction) as well as an increase in the mean pressure half-time (PHT) of the E wave (Fig. 5). The PHT is the time required for the DPG to halve (normal range: 0.025–0.045 s) (Boon, 2011).

Shunts

Patent Ductus Arteriosus

Patent ductus arteriosus is one of the most common congenital malformations in dogs. It is rare in cats. It consists of the persistence after birth of the foetal communication between the pulmonary artery and the descending aorta (Buchanan, 2001). As the pressure is greater in the aorta than in the pulmonary artery, in both systole and diastole, there is a continuous diversion of blood to the pulmonary artery, causing volume overload of the left-sided chambers and, in some cases, congestive heart failure. In some animals, excess blood flow to the lungs can cause hypertrophic lesions in their arteries so that the lumen is obstructed; this increases the pressure in the arteries, causing pulmonary hypertension and reversal of the shunt (pulmonary aortic or bidirectional), which results in differential cyanosis (caudal mucosal cyanosis). This pathophysiological situation is called Eisenmenger syndrome. Once diagnosed, the persistent ductus should be closed as soon as possible in order to avoid the development of heart failure or reversal of the shunt.

Several dog breeds are overrepresented among the population with patent ductus arteriosus, such as the Poodle, German Shepherd Dog, Border Collie, Pomeranian, Shetland Sheepdog, Maltese, English Springer Spaniel, Keeshond and Yorkshire Terrier. Females are more predisposed than males (3:1 ratio) (Buchanan, 2001; Oliveira et al., 2011).

2D and M Mode

- **Direct signs**: it is possible to visualise the ductus arteriosus using 2D echocardiography, using a right cranial short-axis view at the level of the aorta and pulmonary artery and a left cranial long-axis parasternal view (Fig. 7); these views allow its size and shape to be evaluated.
- **Indirect signs**: when blood diversion is moderate or severe, varying degrees of left-sided chamber overload (Fig. 7) and dilation of the aorta and main pulmonary artery are observed (Piantedosi et al., 2019).

Colour and Spectral Doppler

Turbulent flow (visualised as a mosaic image) from the descending aorta into the pulmonary artery through the ductus can be visualised using **colour Doppler** (Fig. 7). A high-speed (systolic–diastolic) spectrum (>4.5 m/s) is obtained using **continuous Doppler** due to the pressure gradient between the two arteries (Fig. 7) (Piantedosi et al., 2019). In cases where there is myocardial failure or when pulmonary hypertension begins to develop, the pressure gradient between the two arteries is reduced.

Ventricular Septal Defects

Ventricular septal defects (VSDs) consist of a communication between the two ventricles at different points in the ventricular septum. These are classified as:

- **membranous/paramembranous**: located in the upper part of the ventricular septum (the most common type in the dog)
- **infundibular, supracristal or subarterial**: located in the RVOT
- **muscular** (trabecular): located in the muscular septum.

Depending on their size, VSDs are **referred to as**:

- **restrictive**: when they are small in size and there is a large pressure difference between the two ventricles
- **nonrestrictive**: when they are large and the pressure gradient between the two ventricles is low.

As the systolic pressure in the left ventricle (120 mmHg) is higher than that in the right ventricle (20 mmHg), the shunt occurs from left to right. When the volume of blood flow through the VSD and into the pulmonary arteries is large, pulmonary hypertension and Eisenmenger syndrome can occur.

2D and M Mode

- **Direct signs**: from a right long-axis parasternal projection where the LVOT and the ascending aorta are seen, a VSD below the aortic valve leaflets can be directly visualised as a lack of echo in the ventricular septum with hyperechoic edges (Fig. 8). When the defect is located very close to the aortic valve, one of the leaflets may prolapse through the defect, partially closing it. In these cases, or when defects are small in size, they may be difficult to visualise using 2D mode. They may be suspected when an irregular area is observed between the highest part of the ventricular septum and the anterior wall of the aortic root. Likewise, colour flow Doppler (see below) can facilitate the detection and location of these small defects (Bomassi et al., 2015). A VSD is considered large when its diameter is >40% of the diameter of the aortic root.
- **Indirect signs**: if the defect is restrictive, it will have no haemodynamic significance and, therefore, the left-sided chambers may appear normal. In patients with nonrestrictive defects, varying degrees of left ventricular eccentric hypertrophy and left atrial overload are observed.

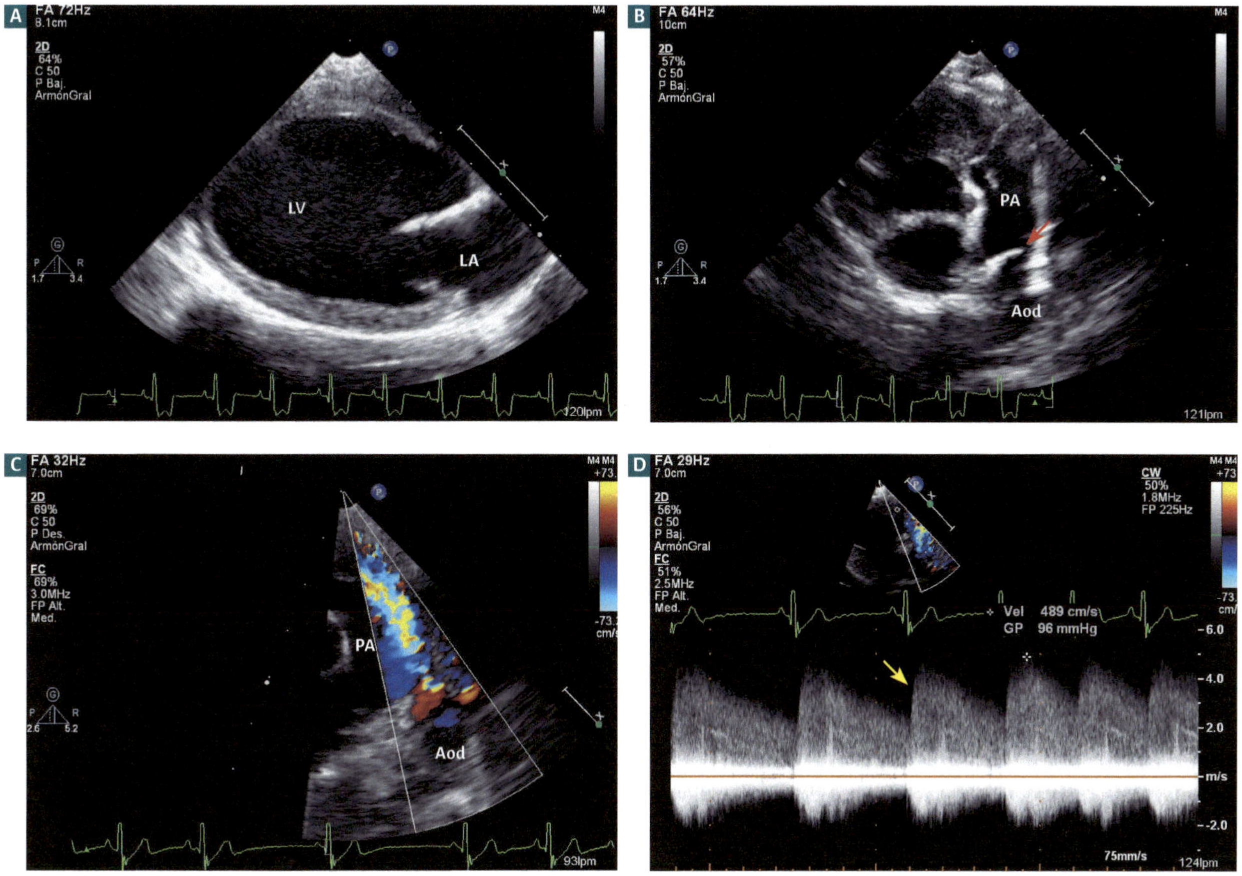

Figure 7. Echocardiograms of a dog with patent ductus arteriosus. **A**. 2D right long-axis parasternal access, four-chamber view, showing volume overload of the left-sided chambers. **B**. 2D left cranial long-axis parasternal access showing communication (arrow) between the descending aorta (Aod) and pulmonary artery (PA). **C**. Colour Doppler, left cranial long-axis parasternal access, showing turbulent flow (arrow) through the duct from the Aod to the PA. **D**. Continuous Doppler, left cranial long-axis parasternal access, in which a continuous flow is observed with DGP = 96 mmHg (arrow). LA: left atrium; LV: left ventricle.

Colour and Spectral Flow Doppler

Colour Doppler facilitates the detection of very small VSDs and allows the direction of blood flow between the ventricles to be determined (Fig. 8). Defects with restrictive left-to-right shunts cause a large pressure gradient, with a V_{max} through them, measured using continuous Doppler, of ≥5 m/s (Fig. 8). If the defect is large, the flow velocity is lower (<3 m/s) because the ventricular pressures are similar and the pulmonary flow velocity appears to be increased due to left-to-right blood diversion (relative pulmonary stenosis).

Calculation of the pulmonary flow/aortic flow ratio (Qp/Qs) allows VSDs to be classified as:

- restrictive: Qp/Qs <1.5:1.0
- moderately restrictive: Qp/Qs = 1.5–2.5:1.0
- nonrestrictive: Qp/Qs >2.5:1.0.

Atrial Septal Defects

An atrial septal defect (ASD) is a communication between the two atria. Depending on their location, these defects can be classified into several types, as follows.

- **Ostium secundum**, located in the middle part of the interatrial septum (in the fossa ovalis region).
- **Ostium primum** (or **incomplete common atrioventricular canal**), located in the lowest part of the interatrial septum and associated with endocardial cushion abnormality.
- **Sinus venosus**, located in the upper part of the interatrial septum and sometimes associated with abnormal venous return.
- **Coronary sinus**, located in the posteroinferior angle of the interatrial septum.

2D and M mode

- **Direct signs**: the presence of a defect between the two atria is observed as a result of signs such as a lack of echo in different parts of the atrial septum (Fig. 11). This should not be confused with the area of weaker echo corresponding to the fossa ovalis in the middle of the septum, which is present in normal animals. In ostium primum-type ASD the defect can be very large and the interatrial septum that persists is small, simulating a single chamber.

Colour and Spectral Flow Doppler

If pulmonary pressures are normal, a low-velocity shunt from the left to the right atrium is visualised through the defect because the pressure difference between the atria is small (Fig. 9). Sometimes, it is difficult to identify the flow through the defect due to drainage of the venae cavae and the coronary sinus into the right atrium. When ASDs are large, blood flow in the right-sided chambers and pulmonary artery is greater, causing an increase in pulmonary flow velocity.

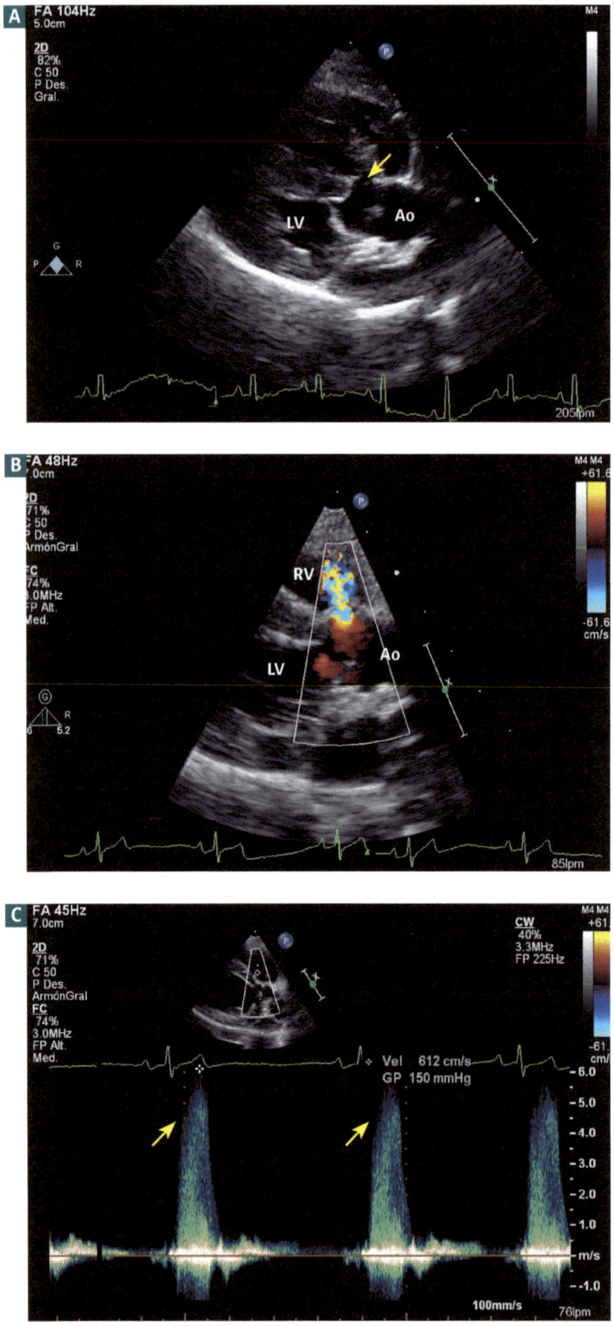

Figure 8. Echocardiograms of a dog with a perimembranous ventricular septal defect (VSD). **A**. 2D right long-axis parasternal access showing a subaortic VSD (arrow). **B**. Colour Doppler, right long-axis parasternal access, showing turbulent flow from the left ventricle (LV) to the right ventricle (RV) through the VSD. **C**. Continuous Doppler, showing high-velocity flow through the VSD (arrows) corresponding to a left-to-right shunt. Ao, aorta.

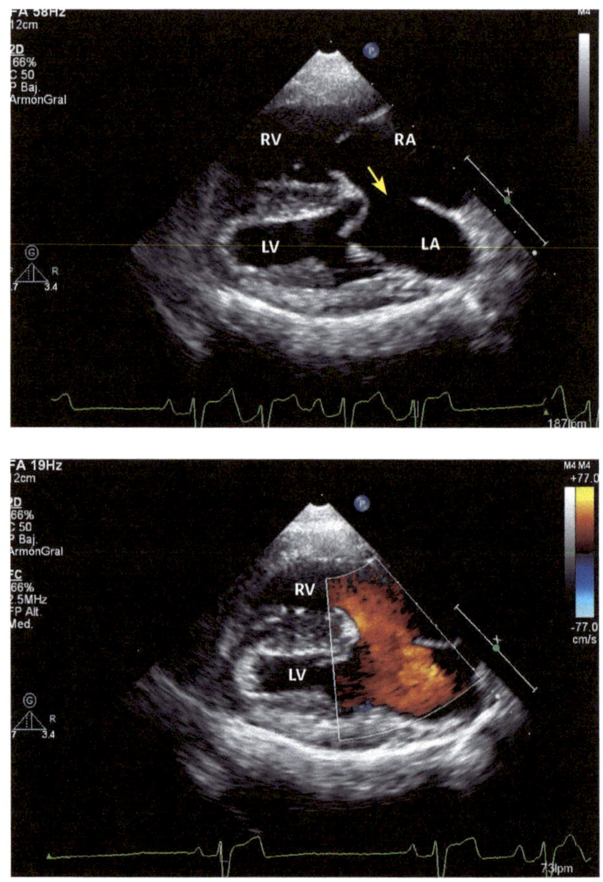

Figure 9. 2D and colour Doppler echocardiograms of a dog with ostium primum-type atrial septal defect (or incomplete endocardial cushion defect) obtained using a right long-axis parasternal access, four-chamber view, showing a large septal defect (arrow) and a septal leaflet of the tricuspid valve and anterior leaflet of the mitral valve with a common origin. LA: left atrium; LV: left ventricle; RA: right atrium; RV: right ventricle.

Atrioventricular Canal Defects or Endocardial Cushion Defects

These defects are a malformation of the central part of the heart, affecting the atrial and ventricular septa and the atrioventricular valves. They can be either complete or incomplete. The **complete form** includes an ostium primum defect of the atrial septum and a defect in the upper part of the interventricular septum, with a cleft of the anterior leaflet of the mitral valve and sometimes also of the septal leaflet of the tricuspid valve. In the **incomplete form**, or partial defect of the atrioventricular canal, in addition to the ostium primum-type atrial septum one or both of the atrioventricular valves is abnormal (Schrope, 2013).

2D Mode

In right long-axis parasternal and left apical four-chamber sections, a defect is observed in the upper part of the interventricular septum and another is observed in the lower part of the interatrial septum (in the complete form), together with malformation of the mitral valve (cleft in the anterior leaflet) and sometimes also of the tricuspid valve (Schrope, 2013). In the incomplete form, a defect in the lower part of the interatrial septum and malformation of the atrioventricular valves are visualised.

Colour and Spectral Doppler

Blood bypass through defects, usually bidirectional, and regurgitation of one or both atrioventricular valves is observed.

Eisenmenger Syndrome

This syndrome occurs when large volumes of blood shunt through atrial or ventricular septal defects and patent ductus arteriosus, initially from left to right, and cause severe pulmonary vascular damage, pulmonary hypertension and reversal of the direction of blood flow (from right to left) (Boon, 2011).

2D Mode

- **Direct signs**: visualisation of septal defects or patent ductus arteriosus along with secondary hypertrophy of the right ventricular free wall and dilation of the main pulmonary artery (Boon, 2011).

Contrast Echocardiography and Colour Doppler

These techniques can be used to visualise the right-to-left blood shunt. In patients with Eisenmenger syndrome secondary to patent ductus arteriosus, the diagnosis can be made using contrast echoaortography (injection of an echocardiographic contrast agent into the cephalic vein), which reveals opacification of the abdominal aorta (bypassing the left ventricle).

Spectral Doppler

Spectral Doppler allows pulmonary hypertension to be identified, that is, maximum rates of tricuspid regurgitation >3 m/s and pulmonary regurgitation >2.2 m/s (Johnson et al., 1999).

Vascular Anomalies

Persistent Left Cranial Vena Cava

Persistence of the left cranial vena cava is the result of abnormalities in the development of the cranial venous system; it can appear in isolation or coexist with the right cranial vena cava and sometimes other congenital heart defects. The persistent left cranial vena cava runs along the left side of the thorax, connects with the coronary sinus (causing it to dilate) and empties into the right atrium (Fernández del Palacio et al., 1997).

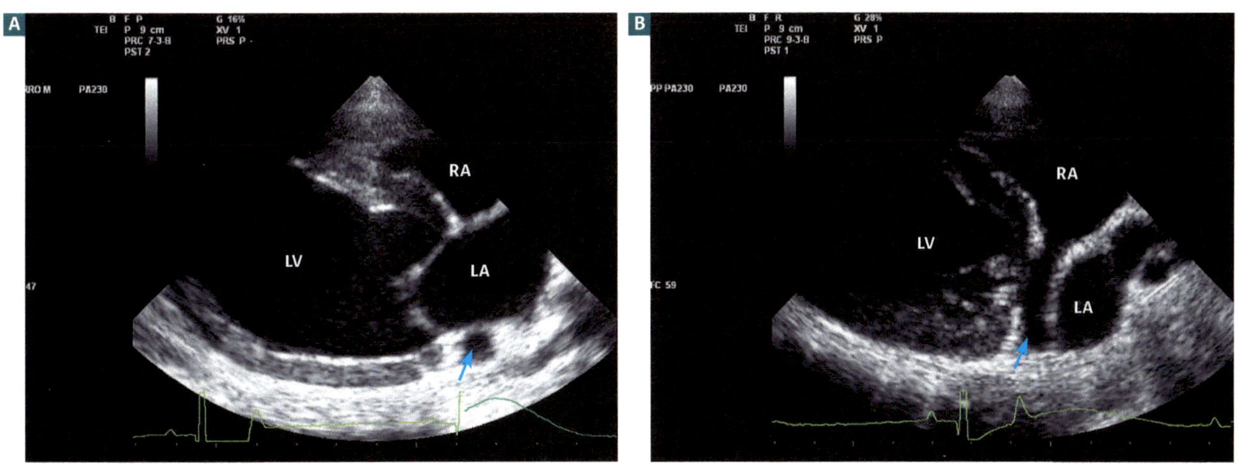

Figure 10. 2D echocardiogram of a dog with persistent left cranial vena cava, obtained through a right, long-axis parasternal access, four-chamber (**A**) and oblique (**B**) views, showing dilation of the coronary sinus (arrow) due to the drainage of the persistent vein. LA: left atrium; LV: left ventricle; RA: right atrium.

2D and M Modes

Dilation of the coronary sinus due to drainage of the left cranial vena cava is visualised in a right long-axis parasternal, four-chamber view at the atrioventricular junction, in a cross section of the aorta and the left atrium through the "floor" of the left atrium; it can also be observed in a left apical parasternal four-chamber view in the atrioventricular area (Fernández del Palacio et al., 1997). It is observed as a more or less circular, hypoechoic structure (Fig. 12).

Coronary sinus dilation may be due to the drainage of other veins (azygos veins) or to the intense increase in right atrial

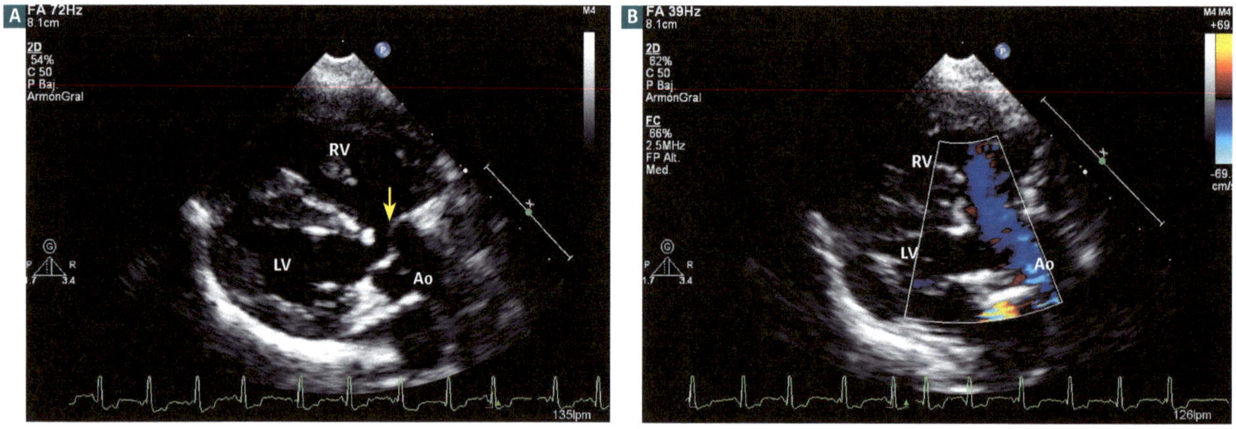

Figure 11. 2D (**A**) and colour Doppler (**B**) echocardiograms of a dog with tetralogy of Fallot, using a right long-axis parasternal access, at the level of the left ventricular outflow tract. Hypertrophy of the right ventricular (RV) free wall, a very large defect of the ventricular septum (arrow), dextroposition of the aorta (Ao) and a shunt from the RV to the ascending Ao can be seen. LV: left ventricle.

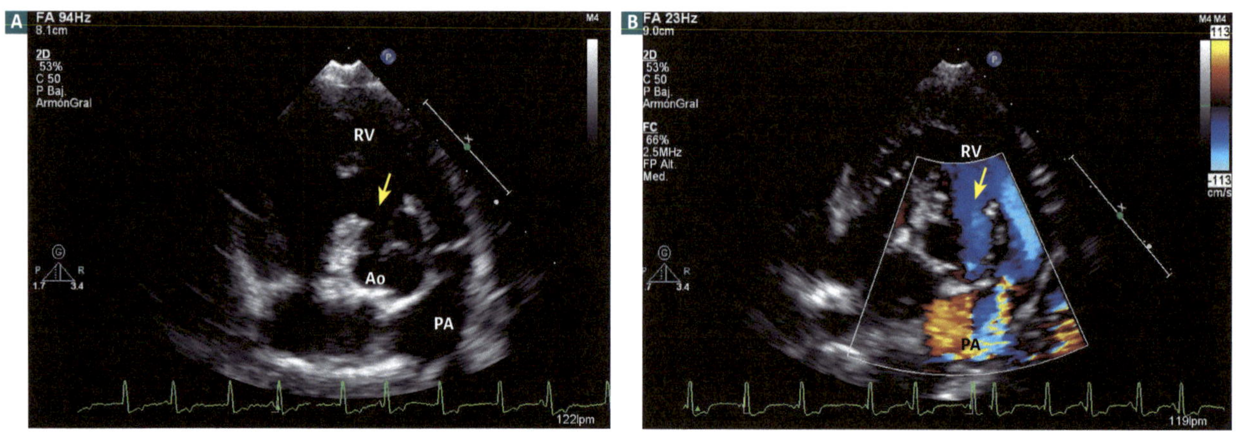

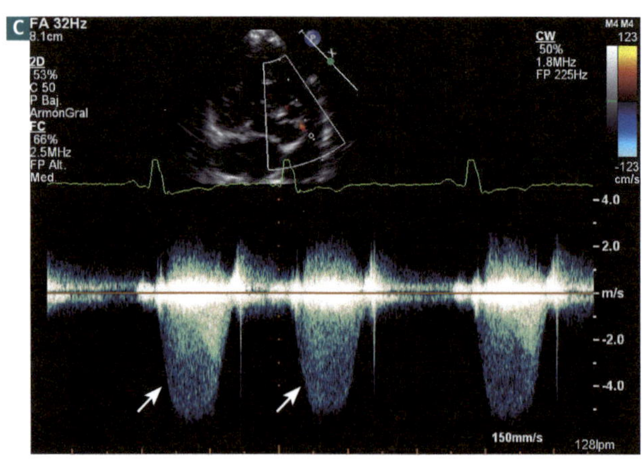

Figure 12. Echocardiograms of a dog with tetralogy of Fallot, right short-axis parasternal access. **A**. 2D ultrasound showing the communication between the right ventricle (RV) and the aorta (Ao) through a large septal defect (arrow), hypoplasia of the pulmonary artery (PA) and a stenotic valve. **B**. Colour Doppler showing the diversion of blood flow from the RV to the Ao (arrow) and turbulent flow in the pulmonary artery due to stenosis. **C**. Continuous Doppler showing high-velocity flow (V_{max} = 5 m/s and DPG = 100 mmHg) through the stenotic pulmonary valve.

pressure in cases of tricuspid dysplasia or severe obstruction of the RVOT. Confirmation of the diagnosis can be made by injecting agitated saline into both cephalic veins and checking that it drains into the right atrium through the coronary sinus. In oblique longitudinal sections, the path from the dilated coronary sinus to the right atrium can be visualised (Fig. 10).

Colour Flow Doppler

Colour flow Doppler allows visualisation of the blood flow from the coronary sinus towards the right atrium.

Complex Anomalies

Tetralogy of Fallot

Tetralogy of Fallot is considered a developmental anomaly of the conotruncal septum. It consists of the combination of a large VSD, pulmonary stenosis with hypoplasia, dextroposition of the aorta and hypertrophy of the right ventricular free wall. The result is the diversion of blood from the right ventricle to the aorta and consequent cyanosis.

2D and M Mode

In a right parasternal long-axis view at the level of the LVOT, a large subaortic VSD, dextroposition of the aorta and hypertrophy of the right ventricular free wall can be visualised (Fig. 11). Right parasternal short-axis access at the level of the aorta and left cranial parasternal long-axis access make evaluation of the RVOT and the pulmonary artery possible and reveal pulmonary stenosis (Chetboul et al., 2016).

Contrast Echocardiography

Injection of an echocardiographic contrast agent (agitated saline solution) allows identification of the right-to-left shunt.

Colour and Spectral Doppler

Colour Doppler can be used to visualise the passage of blood flow simultaneously from both ventricles to the ascending aorta (Fig. 11). Continuous Doppler allows the severity of pulmonary stenosis to be determined by measuring the flow velocity and the DPG (Fig. 12).

Acquired Cardiopathies

Chronic Degenerative Disease of the Atrioventricular Valves

Chronic degenerative disease of the atrioventricular valves, also called **endocardiosis**, is a chronic degenerative process affecting the atrioventricular valves due to glycosaminoglycan deposition, which causes deficient closure of the valves and valvular regurgitation (Menciotti et al., 2017; Wesselowski et al., 2015). Although the most commonly affected valve is the mitral valve, in many cases the tricuspid valve is also affected (Chetboul and Tissier, 2012; Keene et al., 2019).

It is a chronic process, and affected animals may remain free of clinical signs for months or even years until regurgitation is significant and causes cardiovascular remodelling with dilation of the left atrium, eccentric hypertrophy of the left ventricle, activation of neurohormonal mechanisms, increased pressure in the pulmonary veins and pulmonary oedema. Chronic increased pressure in the left atrium and pulmonary veins, hypoxia due to oedema, and other poorly defined mechanisms result in the development of postcapillary pulmonary hypertension, increased pressure in the right ventricle, tricuspid regurgitation and right-sided congestive heart failure.

This acquired heart disease is most common in small-breed and old dogs. It is also diagnosed in some large breed dogs such as the Boxer and German Shepherd. In the Cavalier King Charles Spaniel, the disease can occur in young animals from 1 year of age (Bagardi et al., 2020).

2D and M Modes

- **Direct signs**: in 2D and M modes, varying degrees of valve thickening can be visualised in both right long-axis parasternal (four chambers) and short-axis projections at the transmitral level (Fig. 13), as well as in left apical projections showing two, four and five chambers (Boon, 2011). Valve prolapse is characteristic of the initial stages of the disease, and is visualised as a valve protrusion towards the left atrium during systole (Olsen et al., 2003, Larouche-Lebel et al., 2019) (Fig. 13). In the case of rupture of the chordae tendineae, part of the valve cusp and the chordae are observed within the left atrium (Chetboul and Tissier, 2012).
- **Indirect signs**: these include varying degrees of left atrial and ventricular dilation depending on the clinical stage (Fig. 13). In the initial stages of the disease in asymptomatic dogs (**stage B**; ACVIM Consensus, Keene et al., 2019) there may not be any haemodynamic consequences (**stage B1**) or only slight dilation of the left atrium and ventricle (**stage B2**). In the symptomatic stage (**stage C**), severe dilation

of the left atrium and ventricle, and even dilation of the right atrium and ventricle, is observed when pulmonary hypertension develops. A left atrium/aorta ratio of ≥1.6, measured using 2D mode, in cross section (Swedish method), is indicative of left atrial dilation (Hansson et al., 2002) (Fig. 13). In advanced stages of the disease (**stage D**), pericardial effusion may be visualised, and even signs of tamponade in cases where the left atrium ruptures (Boon, 2011). In M mode, in the initial stages of the disease, thickening of the valve cusps is seen (Fig. 13). As the disease progresses, septal and parietal hyperkinesia and increased FS are observed; when this is normal or reduced, and coexists with severe mitral regurgitation, it suggests myocardial dysfunction.

Colour and Spectral Doppler Echocardiography

Doppler echocardiography makes evaluation of the haemodynamic consequences of valvular regurgitation possible. Valvular regurgitation can be detected early by **colour Doppler**, even before it is auscultable. Regurgitant flow appears as a turbulent flow that is directed from the ventricle into the atrium through the mitral valve (Figs. 13 and 14). It can be single or multiple and is usually eccentric. Calculation of the area of this type of flow has been used to semiquantitatively classify the severity of mitral regurgitation: if the flow is narrow and does not exceed more than half the length within the LA, it is considered mild; when the flow is broad and extends to the pulmonary veins it is considered moderate to severe (Fig. 13). In general, these same considerations can be applied to tricuspid regurgitation. There are other methods of assessing the severity of mitral regurgitation, such as the proximal isovelocity surface area (PISA) method or calculations using **spectral Doppler**.

When using continuous Doppler, high-speed mitral regurgitation flows (5–6 m/s) are obtained, according to the pressure gradient between the left-sided chambers (Fig. 14). When the rate of mitral regurgitation is >6.5 m/s it suggests the presence of systemic arterial hypertension. Tricuspid regurgitation rates >3 m/s (in the absence of RVOT obstruction) suggest pulmonary hypertension (Fig. 14).

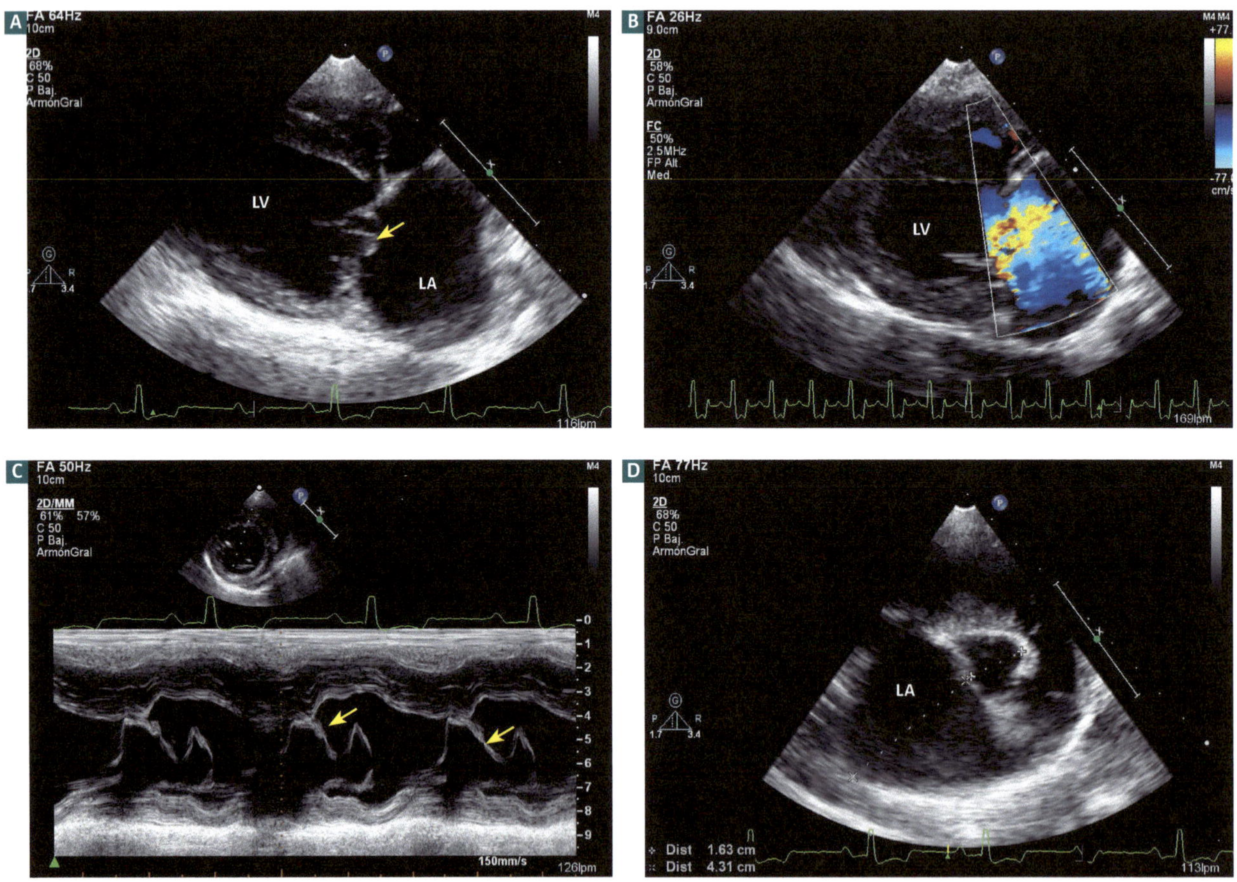

Figure 13. Echocardiograms of dogs with chronic degenerative mitral disease, obtained using a right parasternal access. **A**. 2D long-axis, four-chamber view showing dilation of the left atrium (LA) and left ventricle (LV), thickening of mitral valve leaflets and valve prolapse (arrow). **B**. Colour Doppler long-axis four-chamber view in which the turbulent flow due to mitral regurgitation is seen filling the entire LA. **C**. M mode, transmitral view showing thickening of the cusps of the mitral leaflets (arrows). **D**. 2D transaortic short-axis view showing severe dilation of the LA relative to the aorta (Ao), as well as measurements of both (LA/Ao ratio = 2.6; reference range <1.6).

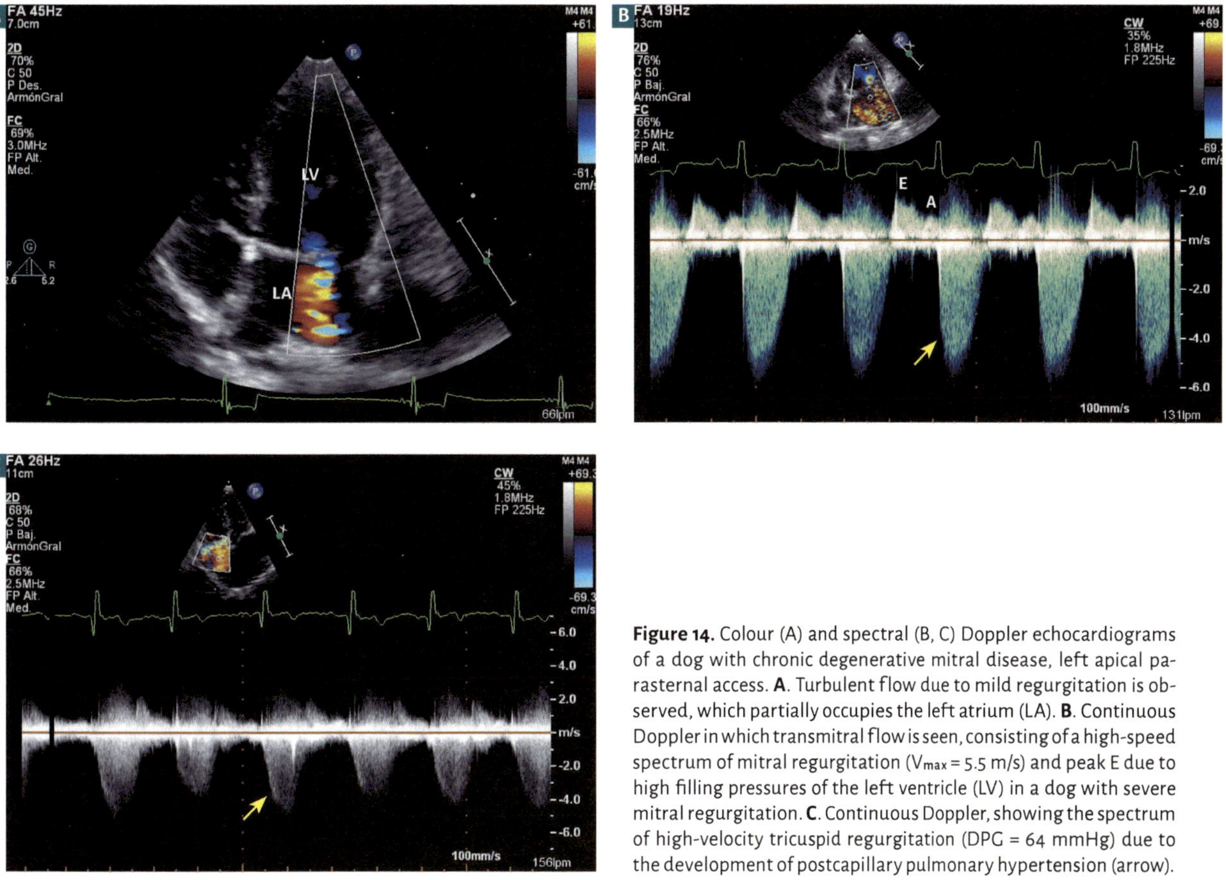

Figure 14. Colour (A) and spectral (B, C) Doppler echocardiograms of a dog with chronic degenerative mitral disease, left apical parasternal access. **A**. Turbulent flow due to mild regurgitation is observed, which partially occupies the left atrium (LA). **B**. Continuous Doppler in which transmitral flow is seen, consisting of a high-speed spectrum of mitral regurgitation (V_{max} = 5.5 m/s) and peak E due to high filling pressures of the left ventricle (LV) in a dog with severe mitral regurgitation. **C**. Continuous Doppler, showing the spectrum of high-velocity tricuspid regurgitation (DPG = 64 mmHg) due to the development of postcapillary pulmonary hypertension (arrow).

Bacterial Endocarditis

Bacterial endocarditis is uncommon in small animals. The aortic and mitral valves are most frequently affected, presenting proliferative vegetation-like or infiltrative lesions, which can even cause rupture of the valve leaflets (Sykes et al., 2006). Echocardiography is essential for the diagnosis and monitoring of endocarditis, especially when blood culture is not available or no murmur is detected.

2D and M Mode

- **Direct signs**: an increase in echogenicity and thickening of the affected valve leaflets is usually observed (Fig. 15), often with pedicles and mobile masses. Vegetative lesions can calcify, causing acoustic shadowing. Aortic vegetations are located on the ventricular aspect and those affecting the mitral valve are on the atrial aspect of the valve (Boon, 2011).
- **Indirect signs**: these are secondary to regurgitation of the affected valves, such as dilation of the left atrium and ventricle (Fig. 15) and septal and parietal hyperkinesia. When vegetations are located on the aortic valve, they cause insufficiency and diastolic vibration of the anterior leaflet of the mitral valve (Sykes et al., 2006).

It can be difficult to differentiate between chronic degenerative disease lesions of the mitral valve and endocarditis using echocardiography. The different clinical signs, as well as the location of the lesions, can help with diagnosis.

Colour and spectral Doppler echocardiography

Colour Doppler allows the regurgitation flow of the affected valve to be detected. The severity of aortic regurgitation can be determined by colour and **spectral Doppler**, evaluating the pressure half-time (Boon, 2011).

Canine Dilated Cardiomyopathy

Canine dilated cardiomyopathy (DCM) is a primary myocardial condition characterised by ventricular systolic dysfunction, varying degrees of left atrial and ventricular dilation, left-sided congestive heart failure and, in advanced stages, overall heart failure, with ascites and arrhythmias (Lee et al., 2002; Wess et al., 2017). DCM occurs mainly in large-breed dogs such as the Dobermann, German Shepherd Dog, Great Dane and Mastiff, and also in Cocker Spaniels; a juvenile form occurs in the Portuguese Water Dog.

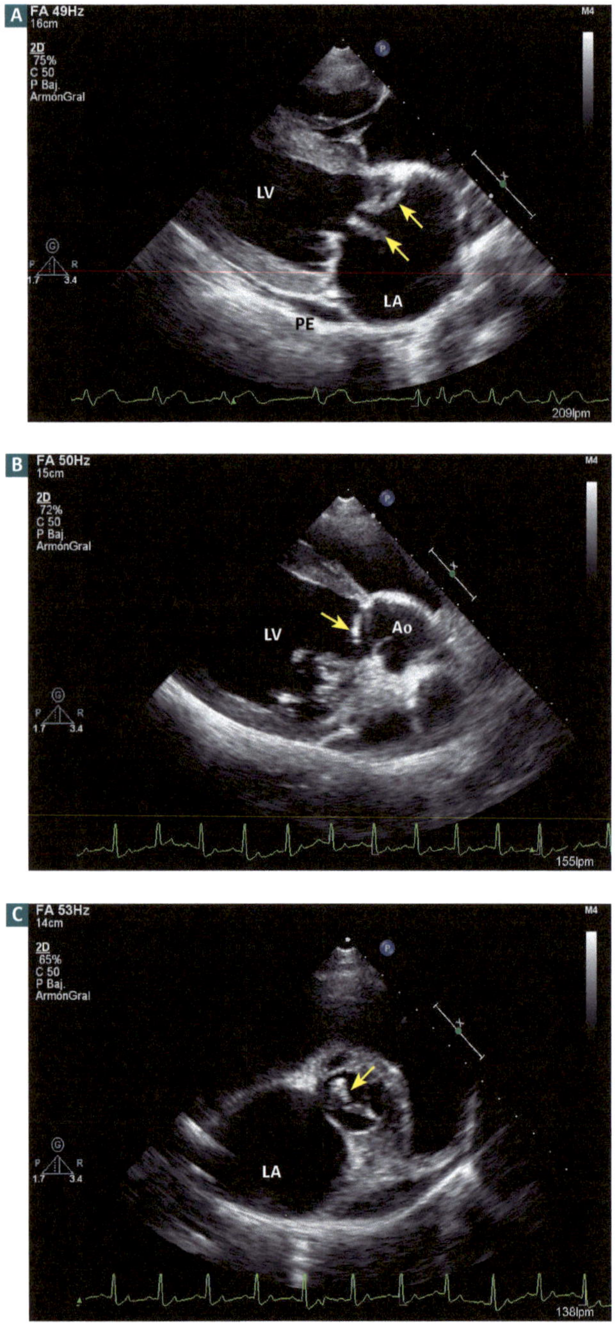

Figure 15. 2D echocardiograms, right long-axis parasternal access, showing bacterial endocarditis. Four-chamber (**A**) and five-chamber (**B**) views and transaortic short-axis view (**C**), showing vegetations on the mitral valve (A) and aortic valve (B, C) (arrows). (A) also shows dilation of the left-sided chambers and mild pericardial effusion (PE) due to congestive heart failure. Ao: aorta; LA: left atrium; LV: left ventricle.

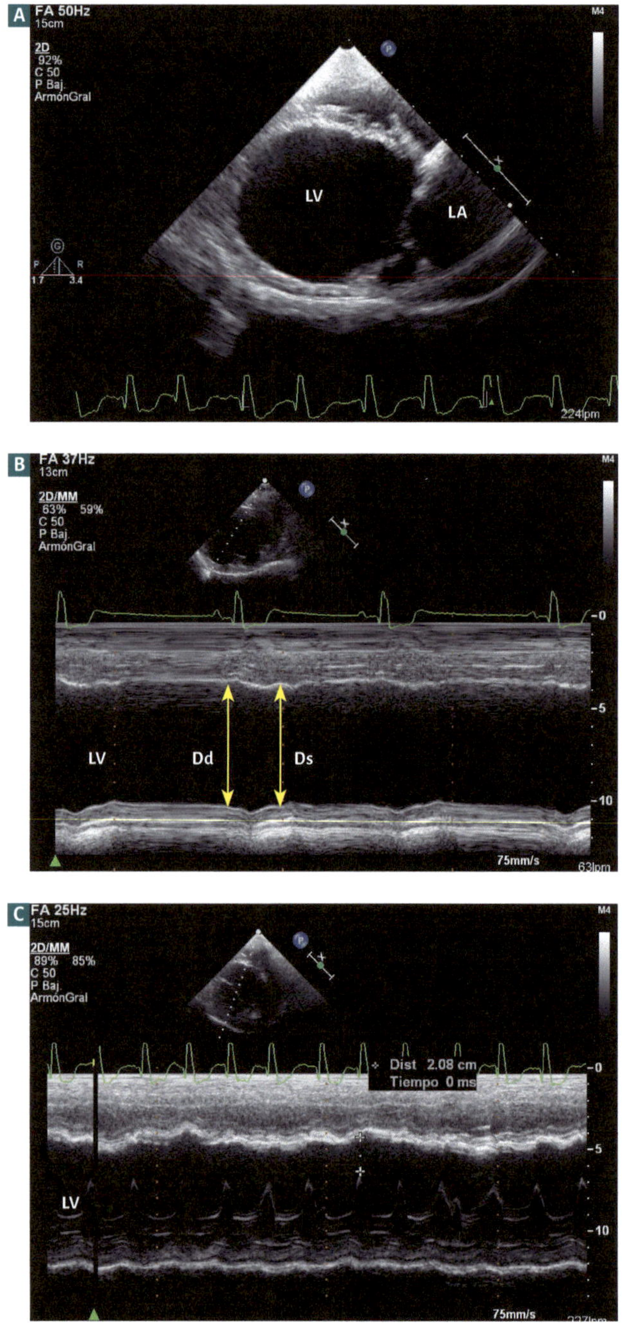

Figure 16. 2D and M mode echocardiograms of two dogs with dilated cardiomyopathy, obtained using a right parasternal access. **A.** 2D long-axis, four-chamber view showing severe dilation of the left-sided chambers, thinning of the septum and free wall of the left ventricle (LV), and atrial fibrillation. **B.** M mode, short transventricular axis view in which marked LV dilation is observed in both systole (Ds) and diastole (Dd), as well as greatly reduced fractional shortening (FS = 8%; reference range = 24–44%). **C.** M mode, short transmitral axis view showing an increased distance between the point of maximum opening for peak E of the mitral valve and the interventricular septum, compatible with severe LV dilation. Transmitral peak A is not observed due to atrial fibrillation.

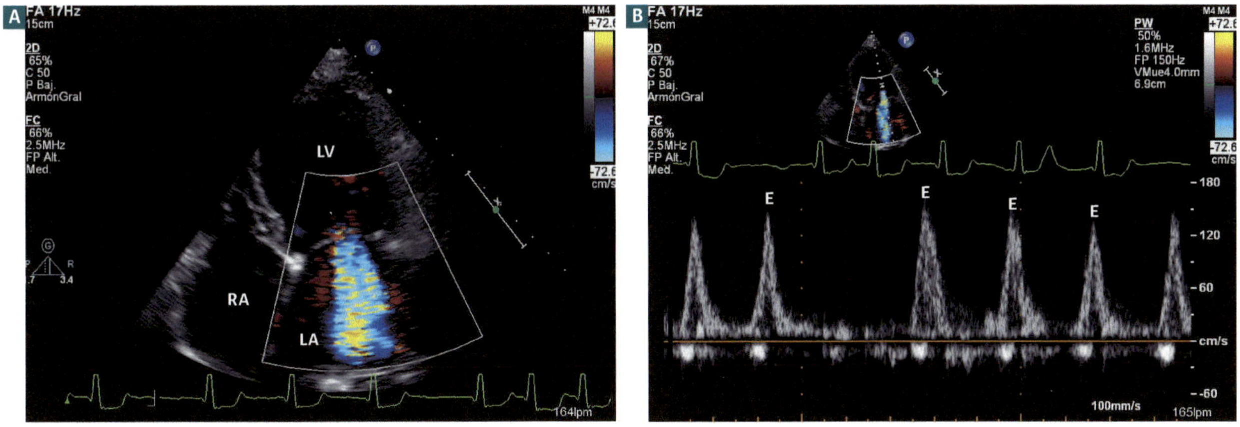

Figure 17. Doppler echocardiograms of a dog with dilated cardiomyopathy and atrial fibrillation, obtained using a left apical parasternal access. **A**. Colour Doppler showing dilation of the left-sided chambers and a high-velocity turbulent flow corresponding to mitral regurgitation (due to dilation of the mitral valve annulus). **B**. Pulsed Doppler showing peak E of high-velocity transmitral flow towards the left ventricle due to high ventricular filling pressures. LA: left atrium; LV: left ventricle; RA: right atrium.

2D and M Mode

Echocardiography is the most appropriate technique to identify signs of systolic dysfunction. Variable degrees of dilation of the left-sided chambers are mainly observed and, to a lesser extent, the right-sided ones, along with a decrease in myocardial contractility (Fig. 16). The thickness of the left ventricular free wall and the interventricular septum appears normal or decreased. Indices of systolic function such as FS, ejection fraction and circumferential shortening area decrease in proportion to the disease progression (Lee et al., 2002); the distance between the point of maximum opening of the mitral valve and the interventricular septum, evaluated in M mode, appears greatly increased in advanced cases (Fig. 16). Cutoff values for the sphericity index of <1.65 are used to identify DCM in the Dobermann (Wess et al., 2017).

Colour and Spectral Doppler

Colour Doppler reveals regurgitation of the atrioventricular valves secondary to dilation of the valve annuli (Fig. 17). The measurements obtained from the **Doppler spectra** of the aortic flow show systolic dysfunction, with increased pre-ejection time and decreased ejection time (ET), aortic flow velocity, mean acceleration and acceleration time.

Diastolic dysfunction present in dogs with DCM is assessed by evaluating transmitral flow (transmitral E/A peak ratio, mitral E peak deceleration time) and the flow in the pulmonary veins (S, D and R peaks). In dogs with atrial fibrillation, only peak E is observed because the atrial contraction disappears and therefore peak A is absent (Fig. 17). Increased mitral relaxation time and E/A ratio are associated with decreased exercise tolerance and decreased survival times. The restrictive pattern is indicative of a poor prognosis. The myocardial function index (MFI) allows a joint assessment of systolic and diastolic function, which may be useful for the early diagnosis of DCM. It is calculated using the formula: MFI = EA-ET / ET (Lee et al., 2022) where EA is the time between the E and A mitral flow waves and ET is the ejection time of the aortic flow.

Feline Hypertrophic Cardiomyopathy

Feline hypertrophic cardiomyopathy is characterised by the presence of left ventricular hypertrophy in the absence of hyperthyroidism, systemic arterial hypertension or LVOT stenosis (Fox et al., 1995; Häggström et al., 2015). Echocardiography makes it possible to assess the cardiac anatomy and functionality.

2D and M Mode

- **Direct signs**: using 2D, different degrees and patterns of left ventricular hypertrophy are observed (Ferasin, 2009; Luis Fuentes et al., 2020). Myocardial hypertrophy is considered when the diastolic thickness of the interventricular septum and/or left ventricular free wall measured on 2D is ≥6 mm. Values between 5.5 mm and 6 mm should be interpreted in the context of the cat's body weight, family history, morphology and ventricular function. Hypertrophy may be diffuse, primarily affecting the interventricular septum or left ventricular free wall, or located in the basal part of the septum (Fig. 18). The papillary muscles appear enlarged even in the initial stages of the disease.
- **Indirect signs**: the left atrium may be of normal size or enlarged. In cats with significant dilation of the left atrium (normal <1.5 cm), thrombi and/or signs of spontaneous contrast can be visualised as the "smoke sign" (Häggström et al., 2015).

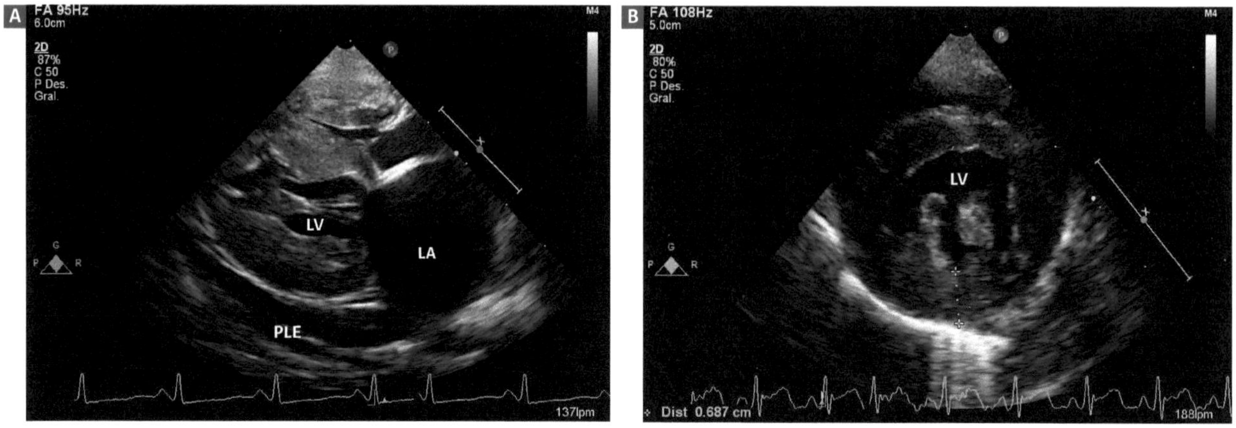

Figure 18. 2D echocardiograms of two cats with hypertrophic cardiomyopathy obtained using a right parasternal access. **A**. Long-axis four-chamber view in which concentric hypertrophy of the septum and the left ventricular (LV) free wall, dilation of the left atrium (LA), reduced LV chamber size and pleural effusion (PLE) are visualised. **B**. Short transventricular axis showing hypertrophy of the LV free wall and papillary muscles.

The diastolic dimensions of the left ventricle are usually normal, and the systolic dimensions are decreased; the FS usually appears normal or increased (Schober and Chetboul, 2015). In cats with congestive heart failure, mild pericardial effusion and/or pleural effusion may be observed.

In cases of dynamic obstruction of the LVOT (obstructive hypertrophic cardiomyopathy), systolic anterior motion of the mitral valve is observed in both M and 2D modes (Fig. 19); in some cats it is observed only in excited states (Ferasin, 2009).

Colour and Spectral Doppler

Colour Doppler may show a turbulent flow of mitral regurgitation, mainly in cases of dynamic obstruction; in this type of cardiomyopathy, turbulent flow in the LVOT and ascending aorta is characteristic. Transmitral flow may show varying degrees of diastolic dysfunction, ranging from an abnormal relaxation pattern (E/A ratio <1 and longer deceleration time and increased peak A amplitude with increased isovolumic relaxation time) to a restrictive pattern (E/A ratio >2 and greatly reduced peak E deceleration time and shortened isovolumic relaxation time).

The presence of turbulent flow in the left atrium and LVOT is indicative of obstructive hypertrophic cardiomyopathy (Fig. 19). The aortic flow spectrum is dagger shaped, characteristic of a dynamic obstruction (Fig. 19), with variable systolic velocities, which become higher with increasing heart rate or excitation (Ferasin, 2009).

Feline Restrictive Cardiomyopathy

Restrictive cardiomyopathy is defined as a myocardial condition resulting from an increase in myocardial rigidity, resulting in impaired ventricular filling and severe left atrial or biatrial dilation. Systolic function may be normal or near normal until advanced stages of the disease. Histologically, endocardial or endomyocardial fibrosis is observed.

2D and M Mode

The most characteristic abnormal findings include dilation of the left atrium (sometimes also the right atrium) and areas of endomyocardial hyperechogenicity, including hyperechoic bands in the lumen of the left ventricle. In some cats, thrombi and spontaneous contrast may develop in the left atrium.

Colour and Spectral Doppler

Most notable is the presence of varying degrees of mitral regurgitation and a restrictive pattern of transmitral flow, consisting of decreased isovolumic relaxation time, increased peak velocity E and reduced deceleration time E, decreased peak velocity A, and a greatly increased E/A ratio.

Pericardial Effusion and Cardiac Neoplasms

Echocardiography is the most sensitive and specific method for detection of the presence of pericardial effusion. The aetiology of pericardial effusion is very varied, including both congenital conditions (e.g. diaphragmatic pericardial peritoneal hernia, pericardial cysts) and acquired conditions (e.g. idiopathic pericarditis, neoplasms, valvular diseases, cardiomyopathies). When the volume of the effusion within the pericardial sac is greater than the pressure in the right-sided chambers, cardiac tamponade occurs.

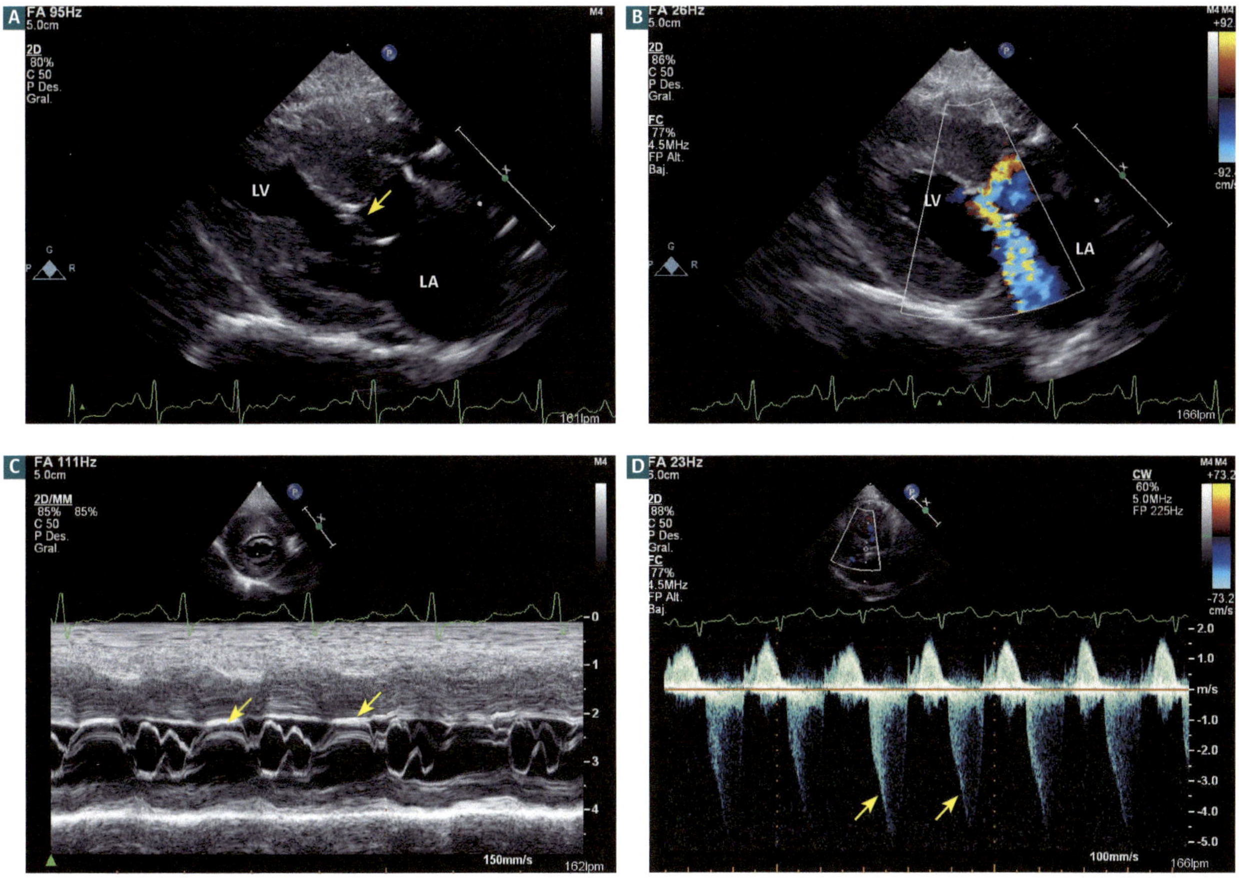

Figure 19. Echocardiograms of a cat with obstructive hypertrophic cardiomyopathy. **A.** 2D right oblique long-axis parasternal view showing systolic anterior motion (SAM) of the mitral valve towards the left ventricular (LV) outflow tract (arrow). **B.** Colour Doppler showing turbulent flow in the LV outflow tract due to SAM and mitral regurgitation. **C.** M mode transmitral view showing SAM (arrows). **D.** Continuous Doppler in which the spectrum of the transaortic flow is observed in systole as a dagger shape (arrows) at high speed (V_{max} = 4.5 m/s).

2D and M Mode

The fluid within the pericardial space is visualised as an anechoic or hypoechoic space between the pericardial layers in both long- and short-axis sections, as well as with both right and left parasternal accesses (Boon, 2011). The size of this space varies according to the volume of accumulated fluid, from an anechoic line that separates the two layers to a large separation that affects the entire cardiac contour from the apex to the base (Fig. 20). The most severe cases can cause cardiac tamponade, in which the heart appears to float within the fluid and is held at its base The right atrium and ventricle appear to collapse due to increased pressure within the pericardial sac (Fig. 20); the left-sided chambers show a reduced size due to low cardiac output (MacDonald et al., 2009).

Likewise, the causes of the effusion can be identified. In the case of the most common cardiac neoplasms, the areas that should be examined are the right atrium and the right atrioventricular junction in cases of haemangiosarcoma (Fig. 21), and the ascending aorta and the cardiac base to locate chemodectomas or ectopic thyroid carcinomas (Fig. 21). Diffuse pericardial tumours such as mesothelioma are difficult to visualise by ultrasonography (Rajagopalan et al., 2013).

In patients with constrictive pericarditis, the pericardium is rigid, and the volume of the pericardial effusion is generally reduced, in relation to the severity of the clinical signs. The morphology of the pericardium is difficult to examine echocardiographically due to the posterior enhancement of the echoes by the pericardial fluid (Boon, 2011).

Spectral Doppler

During cardiac tamponade and constrictive pericarditis, transmitral flow rates decrease during inspiration and increase on expiration; transtricuspid flow presents the opposite changes. This pattern is due to the respiratory variations in ventricular filling and the interdependence between the two ventricles.

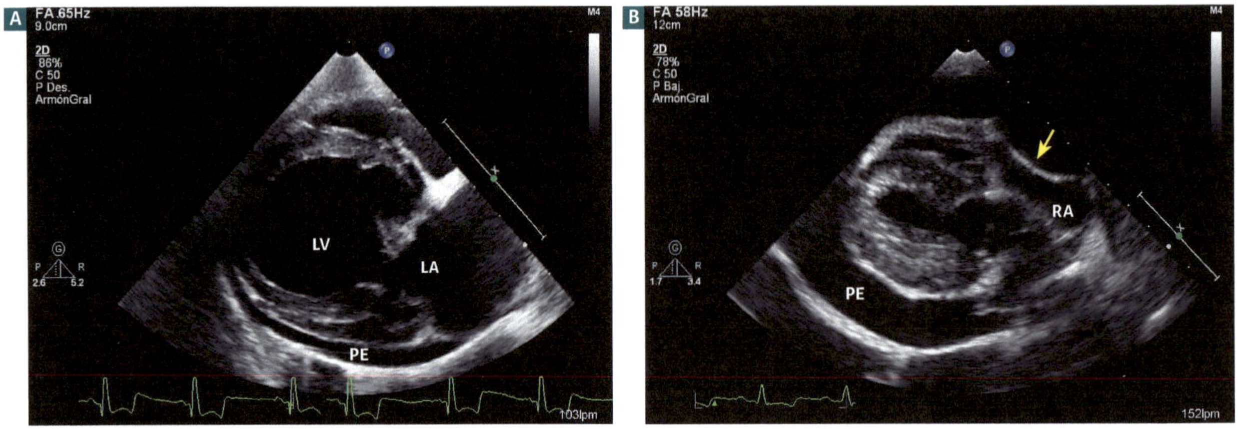

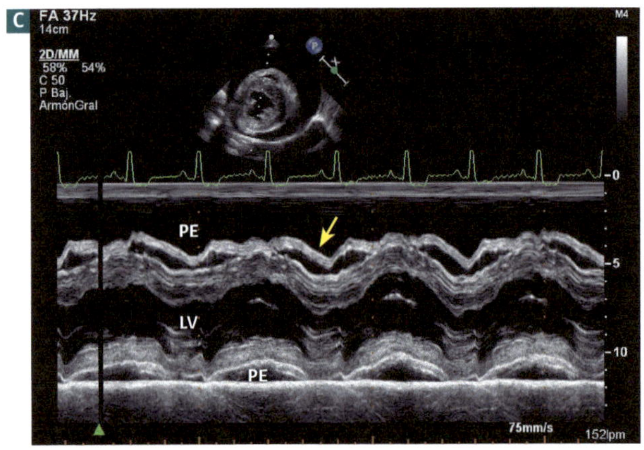

Figure 20. Echocardiograms of two dogs with pericardial effusion (PE) obtained using a right parasternal access. **A**. 2D long-axis four-chamber view showing mild effusion, dilation of the left-sided chambers and thickening of the mitral leaflets in a dog with chronic degenerative mitral disease and congestive heart failure. **B**. 2D long-axis four-chamber view showing severe PE and right atrial (RA) wall collapse (arrow) due to increased pressure within the pericardial sac (cardiac tamponade). **C**. M mode, short transventricular axis, in which PE is observed and there is variable collapse of the free wall of the right ventricle (arrow) depending on the phase of respiration. LA: left atrium; LV: left ventricle.

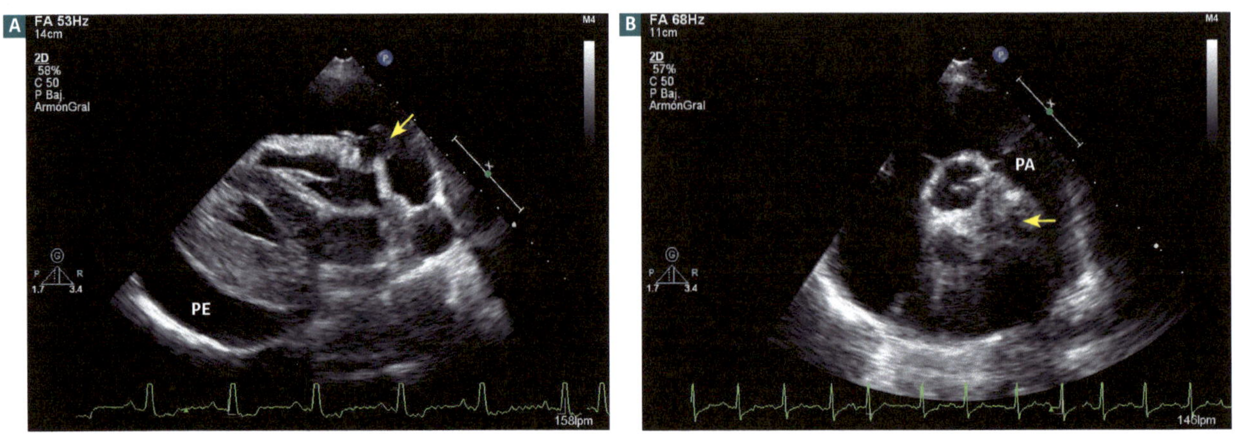

Figure 21. 2D echocardiograms of two dogs with cardiac neoplasms, obtained using a right parasternal access. **A**. Long-axis four-chamber view showing pericardial effusion (PE) and a mass in the wall of the right atrium compatible with a haemangiosarcoma (arrow). **B**. Transaortic short-axis view in which a large mass is observed in the cardiac base, compatible with a chemodectoma.

Pulmonary Hypertension

In pulmonary hypertension there is a sustained elevation of pressure in the pulmonary arteries, of very varied aetiology. Echocardiographic findings vary depending on the cause of pulmonary hypertension. A general diagnostic condition is the existence of a tricuspid regurgitation flow with velocity ≥2.8–3 m/s (Fig. 14) and/or pulmonary flow velocity ≥2.2 m/s, in the absence of pulmonary stenosis (Johnson et al., 1999; Reinero et al., 2020).

In 2D and M mode, varying degrees of right ventricular hypertrophy with variable right ventricular dilation (Vezzosi et al., 2018), paradoxical septal movement, and systolic septal flattening can be observed. It is sometimes possible to identify the causes of hypertension, as occurs in Eisenmenger syndrome (the presence of blood diversion), postcapillary hypertension (diseases of the left side of the heart) (Borgarelli et al., 2015) or dirofilariasis (parallel lines are seen due to the presence of adult heartworms) (Fig. 22) (Boon, 2011).

Systemic Hypertension

Systemic hypertension is a sustained elevation of systemic systolic or diastolic, or both, blood pressures. The consequence of increased afterload is an increase in left intraventricular pressure, resulting in concentric hypertrophy of the left ventricle. The most frequent echocardiographic findings include varying degrees of left ventricular hypertrophy with maintained systolic function. Colour and spectral Doppler can be used to detect aortic (Fig. 23) and mitral regurgitation, as well as a pattern of abnormal relaxation (Cortadellas et al., 2006) (Fig. 23).

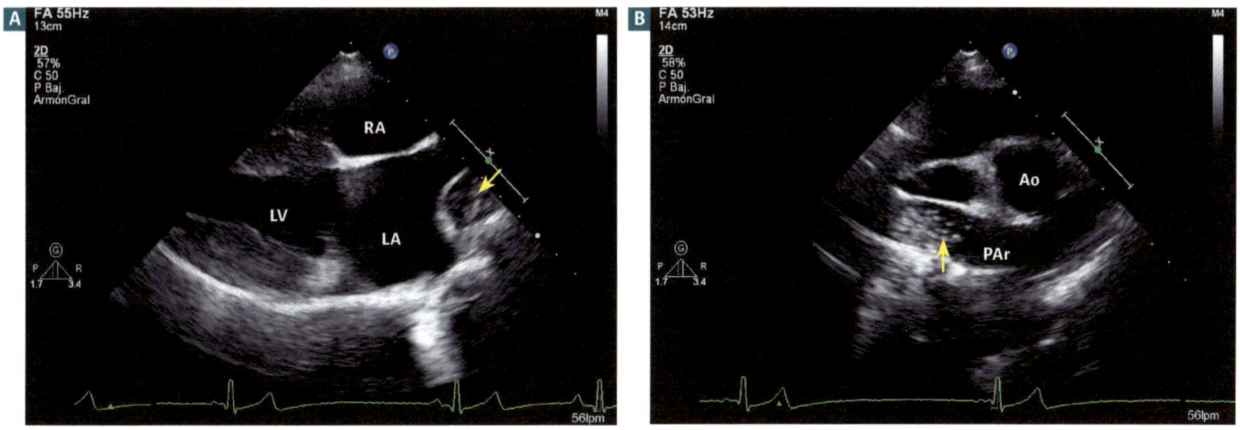

Figure 22. 2D echocardiograms of a dog with dirofilariasis, obtained using a right lateral access. **A**. Long-axis four-chamber view, in which dilation of the right atrium (RA) and occupation of the lumen of the right pulmonary artery (PAr) by parallel linear structures compatible with adult *Dirofilaria* worms (arrow) are observed. **B**. Transaortic short-axis view, in which dilation of the PAr is observed and its lumen is occupied by the same parallel structures (arrow) as seen in A, due to adult *Dirofilaria*. LA: left atrium; LV: left ventricle.

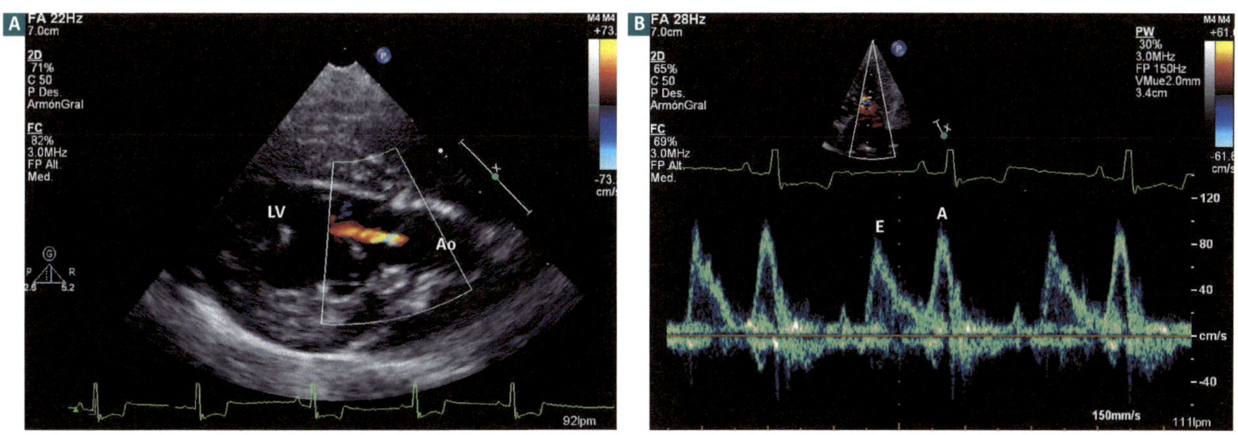

Figure 23. Doppler echocardiograms of a dog with systemic arterial hypertension. **A**. Colour Doppler, right long-axis parasternal access, in which flow indicating aortic insufficiency is observed. **B**. Pulsed Doppler, left parasternal apical access, showing transmitral flow from anomalous relaxation. LV: left ventricle; Ao: aorta.

Bibliography

- Bagardi, M., Bionda, A., Locatelli, C., et al. (2020) Echocardiographic evaluation of the mitral valve in Cavalier King Charles Spaniels. *Animals (Basel)*, 10(9):1454.
- Bonagura, J.D., Miller, M.W., Darke, P.G.G. (1998) Doppler echocardiography I. Pulsed-wave and continuous-wave examinations. *Vet Clin North Am Small Anim Pract*, 28(6):1325–1359.
- Bomassi, E., Misbach, C., Tissier, R., et al. (2015) Signalment, clinical features, echocardiographic findings, and outcome of dogs and cats with ventricular septal defects: 109 cases (1992–2013). *J Am Vet Med Assoc*, 247(2):166–175.
- Boon, J.A. (2011) *Veterinary Echocardiography*. 2nd ed. Wiley-Blackwell.
- Borgarelli, M., Abbott, J., Braz-Ruivo, L., et al. (2015) Prevalence and prognostic importance of pulmonary hypertension in dogs with myxomatous mitral valve disease. *J Vet Intern Med*, 29(2):569–574.
- Buchanan, J.W. (2001) Patent ductus arteriosus. Morphology, pathogenesis, types and treatment. *J Vet Cardiol*, 3(1):7–16.
- Bussadori, C., Amberger, C., Le Bobinec, G., et al. (2000) Guidelines for the echocardiographic studies of suspected subaortic and pulmonic stenosis. *J Vet Cardiol*, 2(2):17–24.
- Chetboul, V., Pitsch, I., Tissier, R., et al. (2016) Epidemiological, clinical, and echocardiographic features and survival times of dogs and cats with tetralogy of Fallot: 31 cases (2003–2014). *J Am Vet Med Assoc*, 249(8):909–917.
- Chetboul, V., Tissier, R. (2012) Echocardiographic assessment of canine degenerative mitral valve disease. *J Vet Cardiol*, 14(1):127–148.
- Cortadellas, O., Fernandez-del Palacio, M.J., Bayón, A., et al. (2006) Systemic hypertension in dogs with leishmaniasis: prevalence and clinical consequences. *J Vet Intern Med*, 20(4):941–947.
- Ferasin, L. (2009) Feline myocardial disease 2: diagnosis, prognosis and clinical management. *J Feline Med Surg*, 11(3):183–194.
- Fernández del Palacio, M.J., Bayón, A., Agut, A. (1997) Dilated coronary sinus in a dog with persistent left cranial vena cava. *Vet Radiol Ultrasound*, 38(5):376–379.
- Fernández del Palacio, M.J., Bayón, A., Bernal, L.J., et al. (1998) Clinical and pathological findings of severe subvalvular aortic stenosis and mitral dysplasia in a rottweiler puppy. *J Small Anim Pract*, 39(10):481–485.
- Fox, P.R., Liu, S.K., Maron, B.J. (1995) Echocardiographic assessment of spontaneously occurring feline hypertrophic cardiomyopathy. An animal model of human disease. *Circulation*, 92(9):2645–2651.
- Häggström, J., Luis Fuentes, V., Wess, G. (2015) Screening for hypertrophic cardiomyopathy in cats. *J Vet Cardiol*, 17 (Suppl 1):S134–S149.
- Hansson, K., Häggström, J., Kvart, C., Lord, P. (2002) Left atrial to aortic root indices using two-dimensional and M-mode echocardiography in cavalier King Charles spaniels with and without left atrial enlargement. *Vet Radiol Ultrasound*, 43(6):568–575.
- Johnson, L.R., Boon, J., Orton, E.C. (1999) Clinical characteristics of 53 dogs with Doppler-derived evidence of pulmonary hypertension: 1992–1996. *J Vet Intern Med*, 13(5):440–447.
- Keene, B.W., Atkins, C.E., Bonagura, J.D., et al. (2019) ACVIM consensus guidelines for the diagnosis and treatment of myxomatous mitral valve disease in dogs. *J Vet Intern Med*, 33(3):1127–1140.
- Lee, B.H., Dukes-McEwan, J., French, A.T., et al. (2002) Evaluation of a novel Doppler index of combined systolic and diastolic myocardial performance in Newfoundland dogs with familial prevalence of dilated cardiomyopathy. *Vet Radiol Ultrasound*, 43(2):154–165.
- Luis Fuentes, V., Abbott, J., Chetboul, V., et al. (2020) ACVIM consensus statement guidelines for the classification, diagnosis, and management of cardiomyopathies in cats. *J Vet Intern Med*, 34(3):1062–1077.
- Larouche-Lebel, É., Loughran, K.A., Oyama, M.A. (2019) Echocardiographic indices and severity of mitral regurgitation in dogs with preclinical degenerative mitral valve disease. *J Vet Intern Med*, 33(2):489–498.
- MacDonald, K.A., Cagney, O., Magne, M.L. (2009) Echocardiographic and clinicopathologic characterization of pericardial effusion in dogs: 107 cases (1985–2006). *J Am Vet Med Assoc*, 235(12):1456–1461.
- Menciotti, G., Borgarelli, M., Aherne, M., et al. (2017) Mitral valve morphology assessed by three-dimensional transthoracic echocardiography in healthy dogs and dogs with myxomatous mitral valve disease. *J Vet Cardiol*, 19(2):113–123.
- Menegazzo, L., Bussadori, C., Chiavegato, D., et al. (2012) The relevance of echocardiography heart measures for breeding against the risk of subaortic and pulmonic stenosis in Boxer dogs. *J Anim Sci*, 90(2):419–428.
- Navarro-Cubas, X., Palermo, V., French, A., et al. (2017) Tricuspid valve dysplasia: a retrospective study of clinical features and outcome in dogs in the UK. *Open Vet J*, 7(4):349–359.
- Nishimura, S., Visser, L.C., Bélanger, C., et al. (2018) Echocardiographic evaluation of velocity ratio, velocity time integral ratio, and pulmonary valve area in dogs with pulmonary valve stenosis. *J Vet Intern Med*, 32(5):1570–1578.
- Oliveira, P., Domenech, O., Silva, J., et al. (2011) Retrospective review of congenital heart disease in 976 dogs. *J Vet Intern Med*, 25(3):477–483.
- Olsen, L.H., Martinussen, T., Pedersen, H.D. (2003) Early echocardiographic predictors of myxomatous mitral valve disease in dachshunds. *Vet Rec*, 152(10):283–287.
- Oyama, M.A., Sisson, D. (2001) Evaluation of canine congenital heart disease using an echocardiographic algorithm. *J Am Anim Hosp Assoc*, 37(6):519–535.
- Piantedosi, D., Piscitelli, A., De Rosa, A., et al. (2019) Evaluation of left ventricular dimension and systolic function by standard transthoracic echocardiography before and 24-hours after percutaneous closure of patent ductus arteriosus in 120 dogs. *PLoS One*, 14(10):e0223676.

■ Pyle, R.L., Patterson, D.F., Chacko, S. (1976) The genetics and pathology of discrete subaortic stenosis in the Newfoundland dog. *Am Heart J*, 92(3):324–334.
■ Rajagopalan, V., Jesty, S.A., Craig, L.E., et al. (2013) Comparison of presumptive echocardiographic and definitive diagnoses of cardiac tumors in dogs. *J Vet Intern Med*, 27(5):1092–1096.
■ Reinero, C., Visser, L.C., Kellihan, H.B., et al. (2020) ACVIM consensus statement guidelines for the diagnosis, classification, treatment, and monitoring of pulmonary hypertension in dogs. *J Vet Intern Med*, 34(2):549–573.
■ Schober, K.E., Chetboul, V. (2015) Echocardiographic evaluation of left ventricular diastolic function in cats: hemodynamic determinants and pattern recognition. *J Vet Cardiol*, 17(Suppl 1):S102–S133.
■ Schrope, D.P. (2013) Atrioventricular septal defects: natural history, echocardiographic, electrocardiographic, and radiographic findings in 26 cats. *J Vet Cardiol*, 15(4):233–242.
■ Sykes, J.E., Kittleson, M.D., Pesavento, P.A., et al. (2006) Evaluation of the relationship between causative organisms and clinical characteristics of infective endocarditis in dogs: 71 cases (1992–2005). *J Am Vet Med Assoc*, 228(11):1723–1734.
■ Vezzosi, T., Domenech, O., Costa, G., et al. (2018) Echocardiographic evaluation of the right ventricular dimension and systolic function in dogs with pulmonary hypertension. *J Vet Intern Med*, 32(5):1541–1548.
■ Visser, L.C., Nishimura, S., Oldach, M.S., et al. (2019) Echocardiographic assessment of right heart size and function in dogs with pulmonary valve stenosis. *Vet Cardiol*, 26:19–28.
■ Wess, G., Domenech, O., Dukes-McEwan, J., et al. (2017) European Society of Veterinary Cardiology screening guidelines for dilated cardiomyopathy in Doberman Pinschers. *Vet Cardiol*, 19(6):405–415.
■ Wesselowski, S., Borgarelli, M., Menciotti, G., et al. (2015) Echocardiographic anatomy of the mitral valve in healthy dogs and dogs with myxomatous mitral valve disease. *J Vet Cardiol*, 17(2):97–106.

Noncardiac Thoracic Ultrasonography

Vicente Esteve Bernet and Patricia Laborda Vidal

INTRODUCTION

Ultrasonographic assessment of the thorax is a technique increasingly being used by veterinarians, mainly in cases of polytraumatised patients, in order to quickly identify the possible complications that the patient presents. It should be kept in mind that this technique offers less complete visualisation of the pulmonary field than other imaging techniques such as radiography or computed tomography (CT), and should not replace these modalities for assessment of the pathologies of the thoracic cavity.

Under normal conditions, ultrasonography provides little information due to the reverberation artefact caused by the air in the lungs. This artefact does not allow ultrasound waves to advance through the lung field, which prevents the use of ultrasonography for examination. The presence of an abnormality that replaces the gas that would normally be present in the lungs with other content is necessary so that the ultrasound waves can advance and be used to assess what is happening.

In some cases it is possible to assess the mediastinum using a subcostal window or through the thoracic inlet.

The main indications for noncardiac thoracic ultrasonography are:

- **free fluid/gas in the pleural cavity**
- **free fluid in the pericardial sac**
- **pulmonary pathologies (must be in contact with the costal wall)**
- **for ultrasound-guided sampling**
- **mediastinal pathologies (mainly in the cranial mediastinum).**

Technique and Patient Preparation

The patient is sedated and usually placed in sternal or lateral recumbency. It is important to clip the area to be scanned in order to achieve a good contact between the patient's skin and the transducer. In critically ill patients, a preliminary examination can be performed with the patient awake and without clipping so as not to waste time, wetting the hair coat and applying a large amount of gel. Once the patient is stable, performing a thorough examination with the hair coat clipped is recommended. It is also necessary to take into account the acoustic shadow that the ribs can cause. To avoid this, the transducer can be placed between two ribs at an intercostal space; this is easier to achieve with a microconvex probe than with a linear probe. Both hemithoraces must be scanned for a complete examination.

There are six regions where the transducer is placed that mark the **points of interest when searching for pathologies** (Fig. 1). The transducer should be positioned on the ventral part of the chest on both sides of the thorax, in the area where the heart can be felt beating against the costal wall. In the dorsal area, the examination should be carried out in the area where a thoracic drainage tube would be placed. Besides these four examination points, there is another access point to the thorax, through the abdomen, called the subcostal window. The transducer is placed just caudal to the xiphoid appendage and directed towards the patient's head. To assess the cranial mediastinum, there is an extra access point to the chest through the thoracic inlet. This window avoids the overlap of the lungs with the mediastinum and makes it more accessible. Placing the transducer at these six points provides an overview of what is happening in the chest. They are mainly used to assess traumatised patients or when a rapid examination is needed to stabilise the patient before performing further imaging.

If the aim is to obtain a more detailed view of the pulmonary parenchyma using ultrasonography, another protocol can be used to examine the pulmonary field (Fig. 2). In this protocol, the transducer is placed at four specific points in both hemithoraces to assess the pulmonary parenchyma in detail. Depending on the size of the patient, the transducer is moved by one intercostal space cranially or caudally from the locations described next. The first point is in the ninth intercostal space, in the caudodorsal aspect of the lung. The second point aims to assess the perihilar region by placing the transducer at or about the sixth intercostal space in the middle third of the thorax. The third and fourth points of examination begin at the level of the sixth intercostal space, in the ventral third of the thorax, displacing the probe two intercostal spaces cranially or caudally, respectively.

For examination of the chest, a 4–13 MHz microconvex probe is usually used because, depending on the lesion, deep areas of the chest will need to be assessed and, as mentioned above, this type of probe allows better intercostal access.

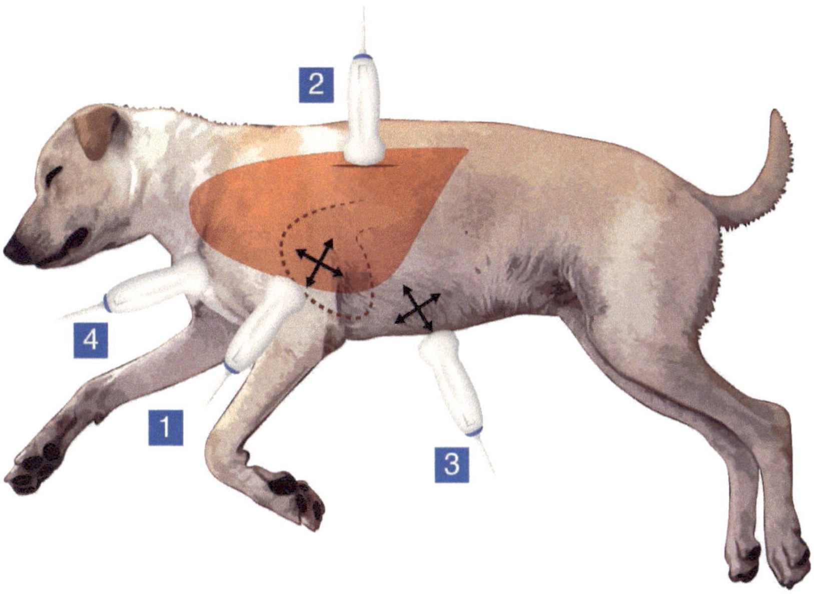

Figure 1. The points of interest used to assess thoracic pathologies by ultrasonography. Points 1 and 2 are assessed in both hemithoraces. Point 1 corresponds to the area where the transducer should be placed in the most sloping area of the chest, located where the tip of the heart can be felt beating. Point 2 corresponds to the area where the transducer is placed dorsally, at the same point as where a thoracic drain would be placed. Point 3 corresponds to the subcostal window, with the transducer placed caudal to the xiphoid process. Point 4 corresponds to the thoracic inlet, with the transducer placed pointing caudally.

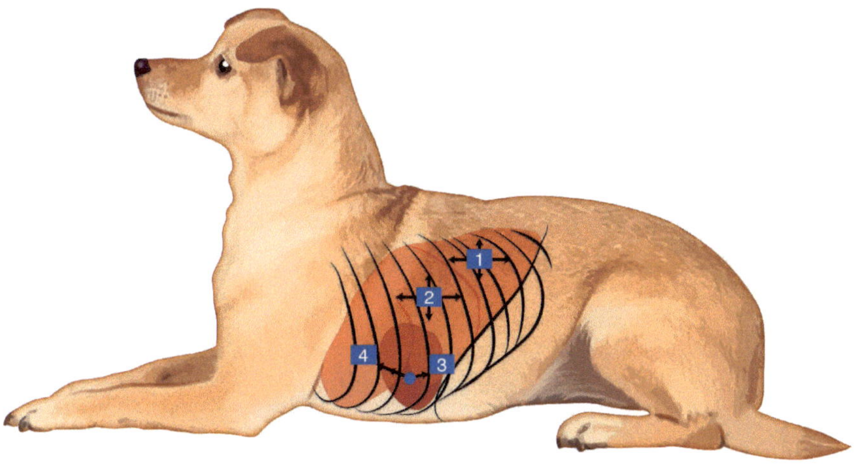

Figure 2. The points of interest used to examine the pulmonary parenchyma in more detail. Point 1 is located in the ninth intercostal space, in the caudodorsal aspect of the lung. Point 2 is around the sixth intercostal space in the middle third of the thorax, and aims to assess the perihilar region. Points 3 and 4 begin at the level of the sixth intercostal space, in the ventral third of the thorax, displacing the probe two intercostal spaces caudally and cranially, respectively.

Ultrasonographic Evaluation in Healthy Patients

Intercostal Access, Thoracic Inlet, Subcostal Access

As mentioned above, in healthy patients it is not possible to assess the lung field ultrasonographically because the air in the lungs creates a reverberation artefact that prevents the ultrasound wave from advancing into the parenchyma and also makes it difficult to visualise the mediastinal structures. In these patients, several layers of tissue with varying echogenicity corresponding to the skin, subcutaneous fat and muscle can be observed by **placing the transducer between the ribs** (Fig. 3). Deeper to these structures, the movement of the visceral pleura due to the patient's breathing can be visualised (this movement is known as the **sliding sign**); after the visceral pleura the reverberation artefact caused by the air in the lungs appears. If the transducer is positioned on a rib when it is placed on the chest, which usually occurs when obtaining a longitudinal section of the chest, an acoustic shadow produced by the ribs will appear on the screen. This is seen as a smooth, echogenic interface with a convex surface towards the transducer. When using this approach in young patients the thymus can be seen on the left side of the thorax. In obese patients, the accumulation of large quantities of fat can displace the lungs and allow a small access window through the ribs.

The presence of the thymus or large amounts of fat should not be confused with mediastinal masses. In case of doubt, performing advanced imaging studies such as CT is always recommended.

If the intention is to assess the cranial mediastinum, avoiding the overlap of the pulmonary parenchyma, the thorax can be accessed by **placing the transducer at the thoracic inlet** and directing it towards the diaphragm. From this position, in normal patients, mediastinal fat, the trachea and the oesophagus can be visualised. Sometimes blood vessels can also be seen.

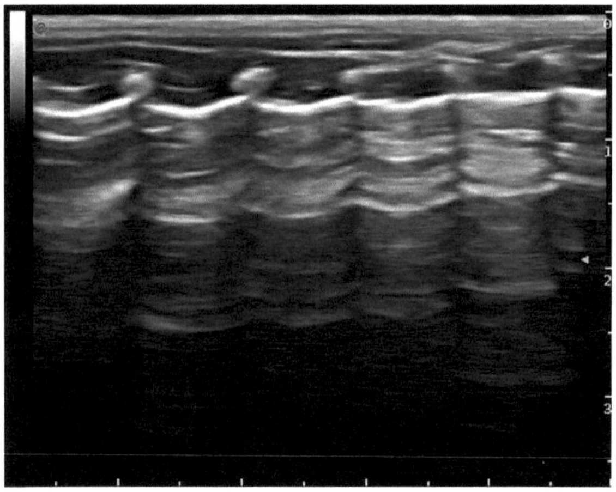

Figure 3. Ultrasound image, obtained using intercostal access, of a normal lung with the characteristic reverberation artefact (A lines). In the surface region of the image, the subcutaneous tissue is observed before reaching the lung. The visible acoustic shadows correspond to the ribs.

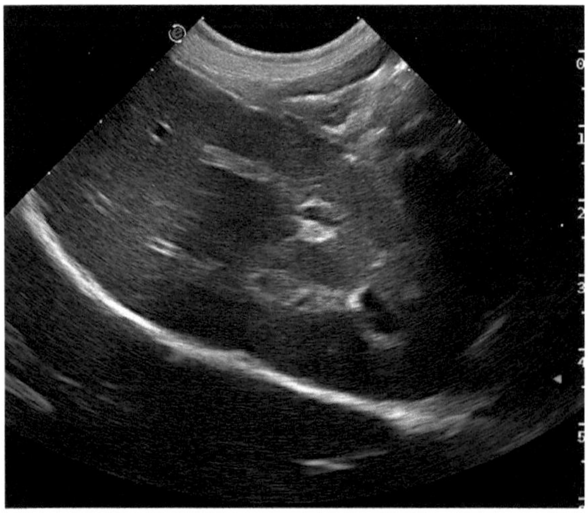

Figure 4. Ultrasound image obtained using subcostal access. In the field closest to the transducer, the liver is observed; the mirror image artefact appears deeper in the image.

Finally, if the **subcostal window** is used to access the thorax, the liver and diaphragm will appear next to the transducer. Under normal conditions in the deepest field, a mirror artefact generated by the change in acoustic impedance between the liver, the pulmonary parenchyma and the shape of the diaphragmatic dome will be present. In some patients the caudal oesophagus can be observed (Fig. 4).

Ultrasonographic Evaluation of Thoracic Pathologies

Pleural Cavity

The pleural cavity can present different pathologies, including inflammation, masses, and the accumulation of fluid or air. Ultrasonography is a useful technique for detecting these pathologies. In patients in which pleural effusion has been detected in a radiographic study, ultrasonography allows the underlying cause to be detected and samples to be taken under ultrasound guidance for further analysis. In cases of **pleuritis, neoplasms** (mesothelioma) or **metastases**, an increase in the thickness of the pleura or the presence of masses or nodules may be observed. Ultrasonography can reliably be used to identify whether masses are of pleural or lung origin: lung masses can be seen to move with the patient's breathing, whereas pleural masses are static and their position is not affected by breathing movements.

Pleural effusion is another pathology for which ultrasonography is useful. In this case there is a separation between the parietal and visceral pleurae where fluid accumulates that can be observed ultrasonographically; the fluid has different echogenicity depending on the cellular material it contains (Fig. 5). Fluids with low cellularity (pure transudate) are practically anechoic, whereas more cellular fluids (exudates, haemorrhage) are mainly hyperechoic. In cases where a mild pleural effusion is present, the fluid is located in the most dependent areas of the chest; as the volume of fluid increases, there is displacement and atelectasis of the pulmonary lobes, and the fluid starts to take up more space in the thoracic cavity. When there is a chronic pleural effusion, hyperechoic bands, which correspond to adhesions or fibrotic bands, can also be observed mixed with the fluid. In cases where there is pleural effusion, it is important not to drain the fluid until ultrasonography has been performed because the fluid provides the acoustic window necessary to try to identify the underlying cause. Only in cases where the patient is showing respiratory compromise is drainage of the pleural effusion recommended.

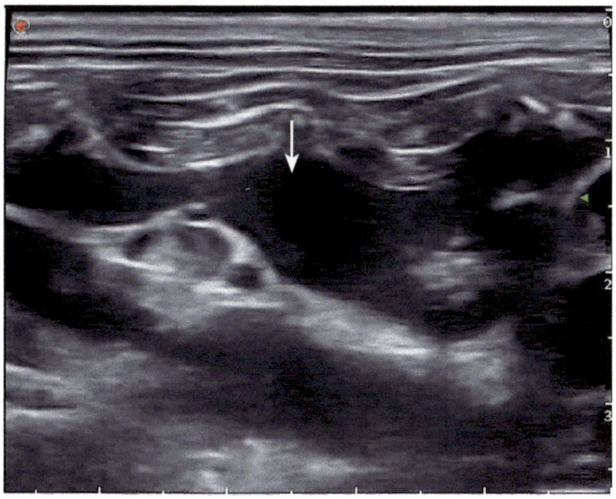

Figure 5. Ultrasound image of the thorax of a patient with pleural effusion. The left of the image is cranial. The presence of anechoic fluid is observed, located next to the left cranial lobe (arrow), which in this case was associated with pneumonia. The fluid was found to be a pyothorax.

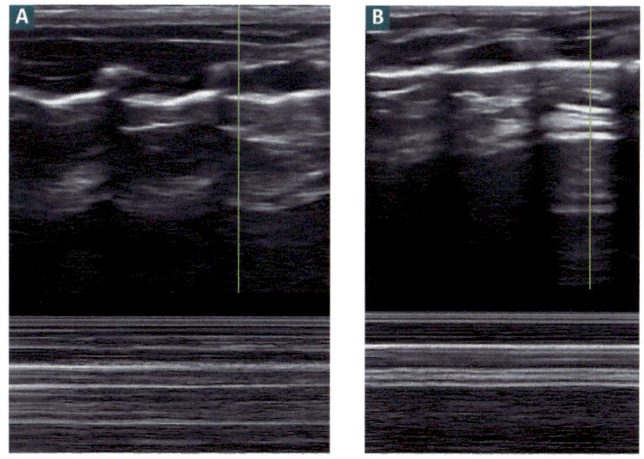

Figure 6. (**A**) M mode ultrasound image of a patient without pneumothorax in which the "seashore sign" is observed. (**B**) M mode ultrasound image of a patient with pneumothorax in which only the reverberation artefact caused by free gas in the pleura can be seen.

In cases of **pneumothorax**, ultrasonography can be used to detect it by assessing the sliding sign. In patients without pneumothorax, this sign is also observed, representing simply the sliding of the pleura over the chest wall during breathing. When patients have respiratory compromise and tachypnoea, assessment of whether or not there is movement of the pleura can be complicated, especially for less experienced operators. To improve the detection of pneumothorax, M mode can be used. In patients that do not have pneumothorax, the "seashore sign" is observed, which is the movement that occurs with breathing. In the case of pneumothorax, this sign is not present; instead, what is seen is an image with hyperechoic parallel lines that correspond to the reverberation artefact when it is still (Fig. 6). When the presence of pneumothorax is detected in a hemithorax, it is possible to use ultrasound to assess whether it is a partial pneumothorax or one that is occupying a large part of the pleural space. To do this, with the animal in sternal recumbency, the transducer is moved following the costal wall ventrally, while looking for the "sliding sign". If no pleural movement is observed from the least dependent area of the thorax to more sloping areas, it can be predicted that the pneumothorax occupies much or all of the affected hemithorax (Fig. 7).

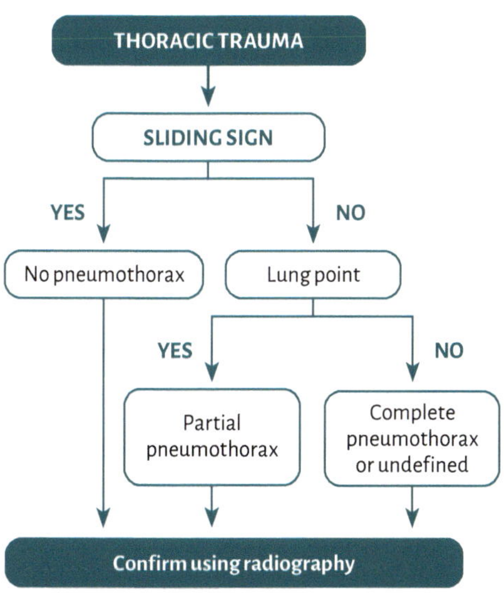

Figure 7. Flow chart outlining the technique for the detection of pneumothorax and whether pneumothorax is partial or total in a hemithorax.

It should be remembered that this technique can help when assessing the chest, mainly in polytraumatised or critically ill patients, but in no circumstances does it replace the need for radiography/CT to assess the presence and extent of pneumothorax (Fig. 8).

Mediastinum

Pathologies that affect the mediastinum will mainly cause an increase in mediastinal size. Mediastinal masses and accumulations of fat, gas or fluid can be found. **Masses** are the main pathology affecting the mediastinum. Solid masses, cysts or abscesses can be found, usually located in the cranial and ventral mediastinum. In the case of solid masses, they can be primary neoplasms such as lymphoma or thymoma. Inflammatory lesions such as granulomas can also be found. **Mediastinal cysts** are usually found mainly in brachycephalic breeds of dog and in cats. They appear as well-defined masses, with a thin wall and anechoic liquid content (Fig. 9).

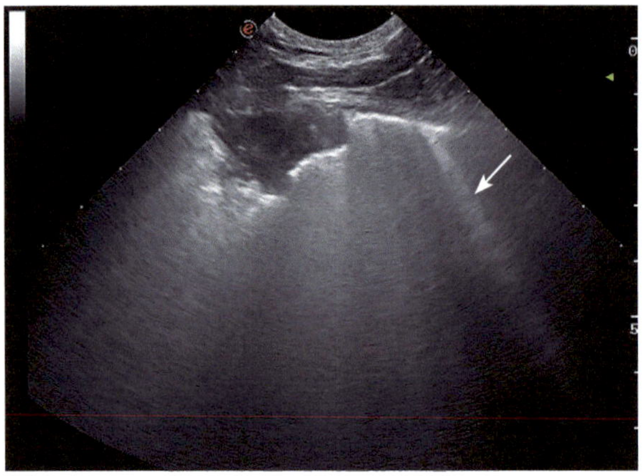

Figure 8. Ultrasound image of the thorax of a patient with pneumothorax, where the reverberation artefact caused by free gas in the pleural space can be seen.

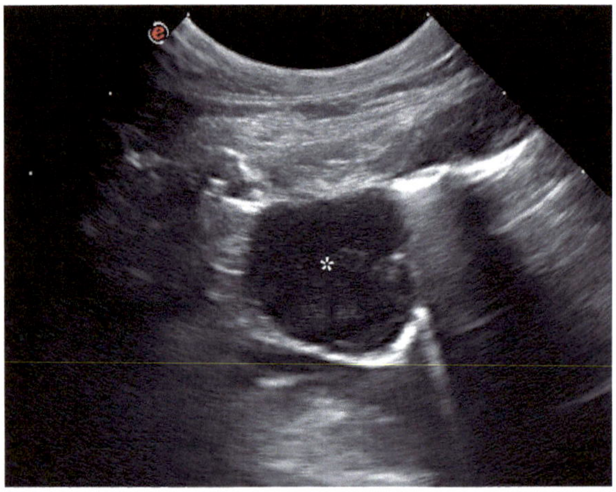

Figure 9. Ultrasound image of the thorax of a cat in which a thin-walled, well-defined mass with anechoic content, corresponding to a mediastinal cyst, is observed (*).

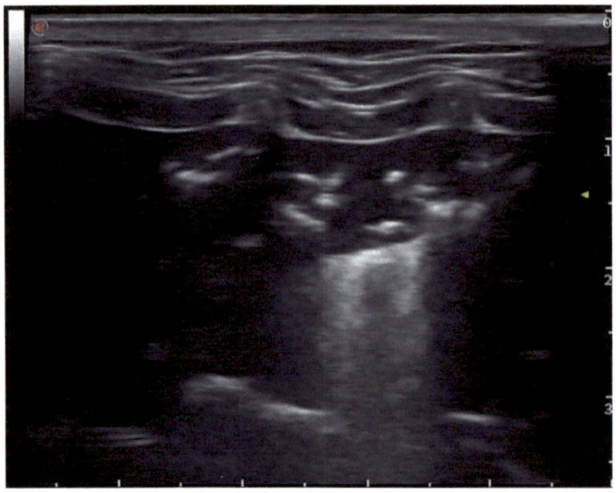

Figure 10. Ultrasound image of a patient in which hyperechoic lines perpendicular to the pleural surface are observed. These lines are known as B lines. The pulmonary lobe also presents with a hypoechoic nodular lesion.

Abscesses or **granulomas** have a more heterogeneous appearance than cysts, with hyperechoic content and a thicker, less well-defined wall. Lymph nodes can be visualised if they present either mild increases in size or cause mediastinal masses.

Differentiation between an increase in lymph node size due to primary neoplastic disease (lymphoma) or metastasis, or due to an inflammatory reaction is not possible ultrasonographically. In some cases it is also impossible to differentiate the presence of an abscess, a mass or an accumulation of fat. In these cases, ultrasonography allows the operator to search for an adequate acoustic window for fine-needle aspirate sampling or ultrasound-guided biopsy. For the detection of pathologies in the middle or caudal mediastinum, ultrasonography can be useful to detect masses affecting the cardiac base, taking advantage of the acoustic window provided by the heart. The main **neoplasms** that are located in this region are chemodectomas and haemangiosarcomas. Pathologies affecting the caudal mediastinum are more difficult to assess by ultrasonography. Lesions in this region (megaoesophagus, oesophageal neoplasm, mediastinal mass) may be assessed ultrasonographically depending on whether they are large enough to generate an adequate acoustic window.

Pulmonary Parenchyma

Assessment of the lung parenchyma using ultrasonography will depend on the location and extent of the lesion. Pathologies that are surrounded by healthy aerated lung will not have the necessary acoustic window to assess them. On the other hand, lesions that are on the surface of the pulmonary parenchyma in contact with the pleura, or when the pulmonary lobe is affected in its entirety, may be assessed ultrasonographically. It is also possible to observe hyperechoic lines perpendicular to the pleural surface. Fewer of these lines, called B lines, can be identified in healthy patients. An increase in the number of these lines can be linked to pathological processes such as pulmonary oedema, pulmonary contusion or acute respiratory distress syndrome (Fig. 10).

The main lesions that can be differentiated ultrasonographically are **pulmonary consolidations** (hepatisation of lobes), **nodules**, **masses** and **atelectasis**. When there is content that uniformly occupies the alveoli, whether it is blood, mucus, pus or cellular content, the pulmonary parenchyma becomes hypoechoic, with an echogenicity similar to that of the liver; this is termed pulmonary hepatisation. The bronchus may remain filled with gas; this will cause it to be observed as a hyperechoic structure within the pulmonary parenchyma. This image of the hepatised lung lobe with the hyperechoic bronchus is the ultrasonographic equivalent of a radiograph with an aerial bronchogram in an alveolar pattern. If the content that occupies the pulmonary lobe does not uniformly affect all the alveoli and there are groupings of alveoli filled with gas surrounded by other alveoli with other content, the ultrasound image will be heterogeneous, with areas of hepatised lung and areas with hyperechoic stippling that correspond to the trapped gas. These pulmonary consolidations are mainly caused by pneumonias, but they can also be caused by pulmonary contusions, haemorrhages, infiltrative neoplasms and lung lobe torsions.

Cases of pulmonary torsion or neoplasia are likely to be associated with pleural effusion, which is less common in cases of pneumonia. Pulmonary torsions also present a lack of blood flow that can be assessed with colour Doppler. In the case of infiltrative **neoplasms**, the lung lobe can be expected to be larger than normal, with changes in its shape (it can appear to have rougher and more rounded edges). In cases of **atelectasis** secondary to either pleural effusion, pneumothorax, bronchial obstruction or prolonged recumbency, a reduction in lung size will occur due to the lack of air inside, and the borders will continue to be thin and pointed. Atelectasis is easier to recognise in cases of pleural effusion because of the acoustic window it provides. In cases where there is a complete lack of gas, the ultrasound image will be the same as that of a hepatised lung.

Pulmonary Nodules and Masses

In cases of lung nodules or masses, it is important to remember that in order to visualise them, they must be in contact with the lung surface so as not to be surrounded by gas. It is possible to identify them as being of pulmonary origin due to the displacement they undergo during the patient's breathing, although this movement may be reduced or absent in the case of costal wall adhesions. These masses, unlike consolidations or atelectasis, can cause disruption of the lung surface. The main lesions that can be found are **neoplasms** or **metastases**, although infectious or inflammatory lesions such as abscesses and granulomas, as well as haematomas or cysts, can also be observed (Fig. 10).

Neoplasms are usually solid masses with hypoechoic or heterogeneous parenchyma. They generally form an acute angle with the costal wall and are surrounded by healthy lung, which generates a hyperechoic surface surrounding the mass (Fig. 11).

Rapidly growing pulmonary masses can generate central areas of necrosis or air entrapment, which can make them difficult to diagnose as they can be mistaken for abscesses or haematomas. Lung **abscesses** due to foreign bodies, for example, usually have a wall with variable thickness, without a defined shape, and a fluid content of variable echogenicity. **Cysts** contain anechoic content and have a thin wall and a well-defined rounded shape. As lung masses, metastases, abscesses. and so on may have similar characteristics on ultrasound examination, sampling is necessary for a definitive diagnosis.

Costal Wall and Diaphragm

It is also possible to assess the limits of the thoracic cavity, such as the costal wall and the diaphragm, ultrasonographically. Trauma, neoplasms and inflammatory processes in the costal wall can be assessed. **Neoplastic processes** are likely to originate from both bony structures (ribs, sternum, vertebrae) and soft tissue (fat, muscle). Depending on the origin, chondrosarcomas, osteosarcomas, fibrosarcomas, lipomas, among other types, can be found. These masses cause an irregular bone surface. When they grow into the thoracic cavity, they are characterised by presenting a convex surface towards the thorax, forming an obtuse angle with the healthy region of the costal wall. These masses can also be differentiated from lesions of pulmonary origin because they do not move with the patient's breathing. **Inflammatory lesions** of the costal wall include abscesses, granulomas and cellulitis. Ultrasonographically, it is possible to differentiate between these localised processes and infiltrative processes or accumulations of fluid.

The main pathology affecting the diaphragm are **diaphragmatic hernias**, whether congenital or traumatic. In these cases, ultrasonography can be very useful in reaching a diagnosis. Using ultrasonography, it is possible to locate the defect in the diaphragm and identify which abdominal organs are located in the thoracic cavity.

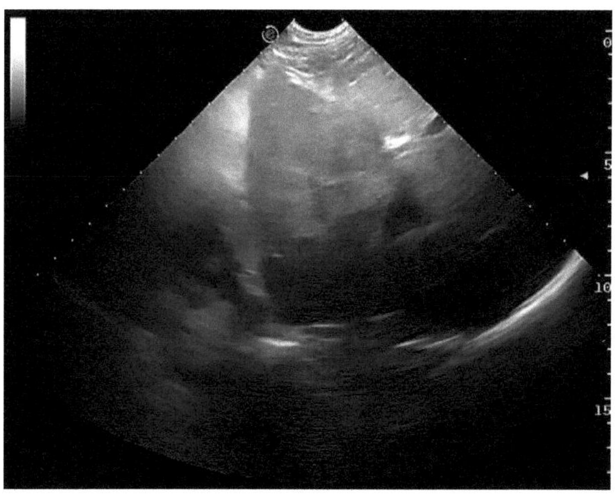

Figure 11. Ultrasound image of a patient with a primary pulmonary neoplasm occupying the right caudal lobe.

Bibliography

- Barr, F., Gaschen, L. (2011) *BSAVA Manual of Canine and Feline Ultrasonography.* 1st ed. BSAVA.
- Boysen, SR., Lisciandro, GR. (2013) The use of ultrasound for dogs and cats in the emergency room: AFAST and TFAST. *Vet Clin North Am Small Anim Pract*, 43(4):773–797.
- Cole. L., Pivetta, M., Humm, K. (2021) Diagnostic accuracy of a lung ultrasound protocol (Vet BLUE) for detection of pleural fluid, pneumothorax and lung pathology in dogs and cats. *J Small Anim Pract*, 62(3):178–186.
- Doyle, A.J., Miller, M.V., French, J.G. (2000) Ultrasound of soft-tissue masses: pitfalls in interpretation. *Australas Radiol*, 44(3):275–280.
- Mattoon, J.S., Nyland, T.G. (2015) *Small Animal Diagnostic Ultrasound.* 3rd ed. Elsevier Saunders.
- Penninck, D., d'Anjou, M-A. (2015) *Atlas of Small Animal Ultrasonography.* 2nd ed. Blackwell.
- Vezzosi, T., Mannucci, T., Pistoresi, A., et al. (2017) Assessment of lung ultrasound B-lines in dogs with different stages of chronic valvular heart disease. *J Vet Intern Med*, 31(3):700–704.
- Rademacher, N., Pariaut, R., Pate, J., et al. (2014) Transthoracic lung ultrasound in normal dogs and dogs with cardiogenic pulmonary edema: a pilot study. *Vet Radiol Ultrasound*, 55(4):447–452.

Notes

Musculoskeletal Imaging

Radiographic Diagnosis of the Musculoskeletal System

Marta Soler Laguía

Introduction

Radiography is a very useful technique in the study of the musculoskeletal system. Generally, radiographs of good technical quality can be obtained when working with dogs and cats, even with less powerful equipment, because the osseous tissue attenuates a large portion of the X-ray beam.

Certain processes or pathologies require the use of advanced techniques, such as computed tomography (CT) and magnetic resonance imaging (MRI), which avoid the overlapping of structures. This is necessary for the correct detection and visualisation of these lesions.

Bone tissue is a living tissue that undergoes rapid development during the first year of the animal's life, determined by a series of genetic, hormonal and nutritional factors. During this period there are variations in the size of the bones and the progressive calcification of the bones can be observed radiographically. There are two main types of ossification (Barreiro and Vila, 2014).

- **Intramembranous ossification**, by which flat bones, such as those of the skull, are formed from fibrous tissue.
- **Endochondral ossification**, by which most of the bones of the skeleton are formed from preformed cartilaginous models. A normal long bone develops from three primary centres of ossification: a diaphysis and two epiphyses.

Several characteristic anatomical parts of long bones can be differentiated on radiographs (Fig. 1).

1. **Epiphysis**: located at the ends of the bone and usually formed from a secondary ossification centre. At birth the epiphyses consist of cartilaginous tissue and are therefore less radiopaque, but with the progressive calcification that occurs in the first months of life, their radiodensity increases at the same time as their degree of calcification.
2. **Epiphyseal line**: also known as epiphyseal cartilage, growth plate or physis. This is a radiotransparent line located between the epiphysis and the metaphysis that should not be confused with a fracture line. It is seen only in young animals before the end of their growth period. From this line, which is a very active layer of cartilage, growth in bone length is promoted. This line is very sensitive to local trauma, which can cause premature fusion between the epiphysis and metaphysis, preventing the longitudinal growth of the bone. When the animal completes its growth stage, the cartilaginous tissue is replaced by bone tissue and, in some bones, it is visualised as a radiodense line that is known as an "epiphyseal scar". The epiphyseal line disappears at different times in each bone.
3. **Metaphysis**: an area of intermediate/high radiopacity that corresponds to porous bone that is forming from the epiphyseal line. During the growth period, it is highly vascularised and very active because it contributes to the growth in bone length, and as the animal develops it undergoes a process of involution and remodelling.
4. **Diaphysis**: contains a radiodense external area of compact bone called cortical bone. The cortex or cortical bone has an external surface called periosteum and an internal surface called endosteum. The internal area of cancellous bone is known as the medullary cavity, which is seen on radiographs as an area of less opacity.

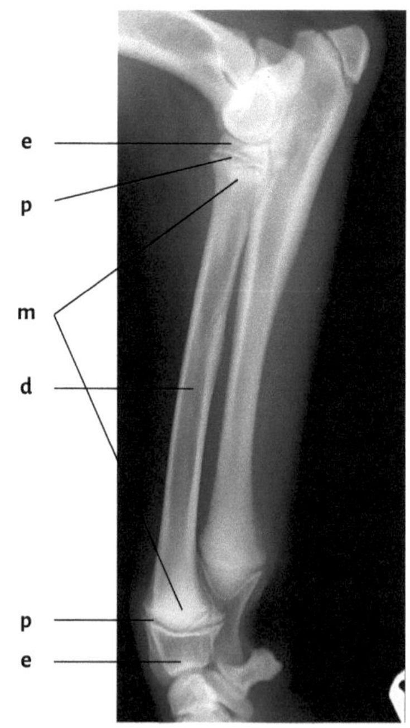

Figure 1. Mediolateral radiograph of the ulna and radius of an immature animal in which the different parts of a long bone are visualised: epiphysis (e), metaphysis (m), diaphysis (d), epiphyseal line (physis, growth plate) (p).

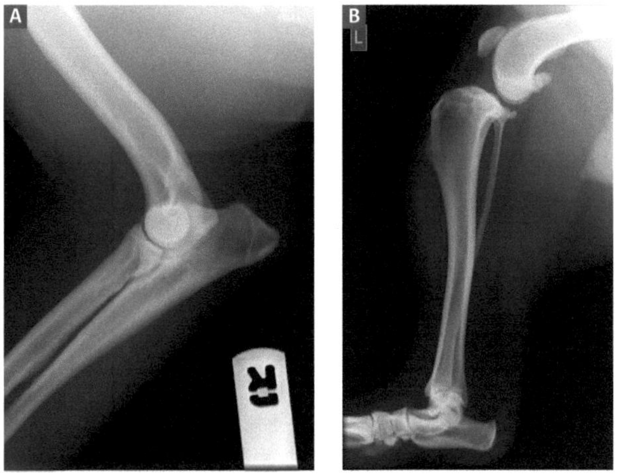

Figure 2. Mediolateral radiograph of the elbow (**A**) and tibia (**B**) of a radiologically adult dog, showing how the X-ray beam should be focused on the area of interest depending on the region to be radiographed, either in the centre of the joint or on the long bone and encompassing the proximal and distal joints.

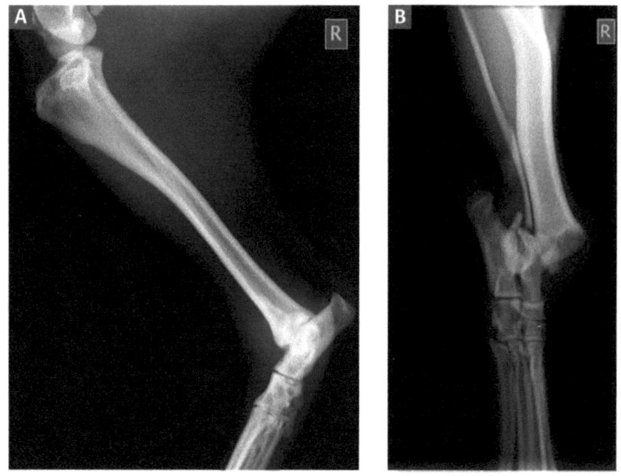

Figure 3. Mediolateral (**A**) and dorsoplantar (**B**) radiographs of the tarsal joint of a radiologically mature dog. These images demonstrate the importance of obtaining at least two orthogonal projections to obtain all the information in the three dimensions of the study area, because the distal fracture of the tibia and fibula is obscured in the mediolateral view.

Radiographic Technique

To optimise radiographic technique and achieve radiographs of optimal quality, the following aspects must be taken into account (Morgan, 1993).

1. Beam Centring

- **Joint**: the X-ray beam should be centred on the joint being studied (Fig. 2).
- **Long bone**: the proximal and distal joints related to the bone should always be included; this allows the angles between the different parts of a limb to be studied (Fig. 2).

2. Radiographic Projections

- At a minimum, **two orthogonal views** of the area being studied should always be obtained in order to assess its three dimensions; with only a single projection, essential information might not be obtained (Fig. 3). On certain occasions oblique views are also useful.
- Flexion/extension and traction/rotation manoeuvres are useful for the study of possible ankylosis of a joint or in cases of sprains or the presence of small bone fragments around a joint. These manoeuvres are called "stressed" projections.
- Sometimes it is necessary to perform radiographs of the contralateral limb, especially in young (radiologically immature) animals to compare the growth lines at the level of the epiphyses and the closures of the apophysis (secondary ossification centres).

3. Exposure Parameters: Kilovoltage/Milliampere Time (kV, mAs)

- When possible, a high milliamperage and a low kilovoltage should be used to decrease the production of scattered radiation and thus obtain greater radiographic contrast.
- It is advisable not to use a grid (as long as the area to be radiographed is less than 10 cm thick) because its use increases the exposure dose and does not contribute to better image definition.

4. Scattered Radiation

- The production and effect of scattered radiation can be reduced by collimating the primary X-ray beam as much as possible.
- When radiographing areas that are more than 10 cm thick, the grid should be used to avoid scattered radiation.

Radiographic Interpretation

When interpreting a radiograph, whether of the osseous system or of any other part of the body, a systematic approach should be used to ensure that nothing is overlooked (Barreiro and Vila, 2014). An example of how to do this is as follows.

1. Assessment of the Soft Tissues Adjacent to the Bone, Looking for the Presence of

- **inflammation**, which is sometimes visible as a deviation of the fasciae between muscle planes (Fig. 4);
- **gas**, which indicates the existence of an open wound or the presence of infection with gas-producing organisms. The presence of gas is normal after surgery;
- **fatty opacity**, which is normally related to the existence of a lipoma but may sometimes indicate the presence of a liposarcoma (Fig. 5);
- **mineral opacity**, which may indicate the presence of a foreign body or dystrophic or metastatic soft tissue mineralisation; or
- **metal opacity**, due to either implants or foreign bodies.

2. Evaluation of Bone

- **Diaphysis**: the cortices should be evaluated (external surface: periosteum; internal surface: endosteum); they should be smooth and continuous. The medullary cavity is less radiopaque than cortical bone due to its spongy component; it should have a homogeneous opacity with a trabeculated pattern and, sometimes, the nutrient canal can be seen. Trabeculation is best observed in the metaphyseal areas and in the epiphyses, whereas it is less visible towards the centre of the diaphysis.
- In young animals, the **physis (epiphyseal line, growth plate)** is visualised as radiolucent lines separating the epiphysis from the metaphysis. When the animal ceases growing, the epiphysis merges with the metaphysis and the physis is no longer observed. Sometimes, lines with greater opacity are visualised in this area; these are called "epiphyseal scars" and consist of closed physes. In the dog, growth is completed between 10 months and 14 months of age, but there may be variations in the closure time of the physis, even in animals of the same breed. The proximal epiphysis of the humerus is the last to fuse in the dog.

3. Evaluation of Joints

- The articular surface should be smooth, without irregularities. The subchondral bone should be of a homogeneous opacity (when it is increased in opacity, this is called subchondral bone **sclerosis**).
- The periphery of the articular surface is examined for the presence of **osteophytes** or **enthesophytes**.
- The joint space or synovial area should be examined for the presence of **synovial effusion**, a **mass** or **mineralisation**.

4. Assessment of Angles

- **In long bones**: there may be alterations due to previous fractures that have resolved abnormally or malformations.
- **In joints:** valgus or varus joints may be seen. Comparison with the contralateral limb should always be made, and comparing the length of the same bones in both limbs is very useful.

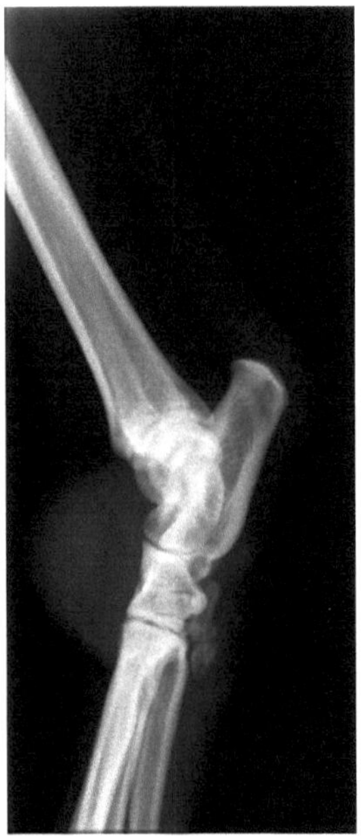

Figure 4. Mediolateral radiograph of the tarsal joint of an adult dog showing an increase in the thickness and local opacity of the soft tissues dorsal to the joint. This increase in thickness has well-defined edges and a homogeneous soft tissue opacity; possible differential diagnoses include a haematoma, abscess, cyst, granuloma or neoplasm. Further investigations such as ultrasonography and fine-needle aspiration are necessary to reach a definitive diagnosis.

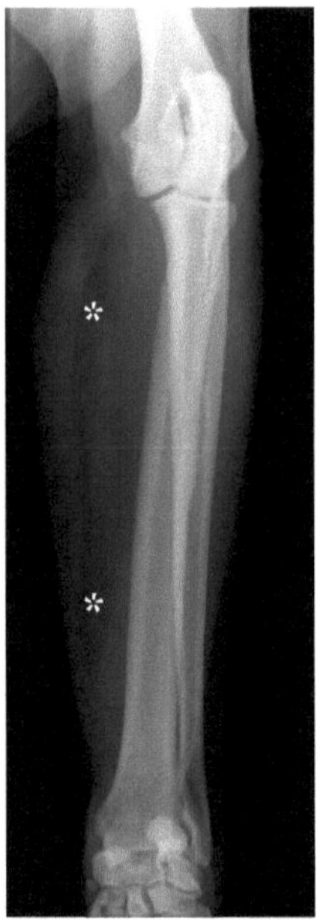

Figure 5. Craniocaudal radiograph of the ulna and radius of an adult dog in which an increase in the thickness of the soft tissues medial to the radius, with heterogeneous opacity due to the presence of an area of less opacity than that of the soft tissues (asterisks), is seen. This area of reduced opacity corresponds to fatty opacity, so the most likely diagnosis is an intermuscular lipoma. To reach a definitive diagnosis, histopathology is necessary.

Aggressive Versus Nonaggressive Lesions

Many bone pathologies can present similar bone lesions. Often, the specific diagnosis cannot be made from radiographs alone, meaning that fine-needle aspiration (FNA) or biopsy of the lesion is needed for a definitive diagnosis. However, if certain criteria are applied when evaluating radiographs, lesions can be classified as aggressive or nonaggressive, and a basic list of differential diagnoses can be used, according to which aggressive lesions are usually mainly due to infection or neoplasms, whereas nonaggressive lesions can correspond to traumatic lesions or benign neoplasms (Thrall, 2018).

Osseous System Response to All Lesions

The bone is constantly remodelled throughout the animal's life and responds in the same way to various aetiologies, stimuli or agents, even if they are different. It may show osteolysis (which causes a decrease in radiopacity due to the destruction of bone tissue), osteogenesis (which causes an increase in radiopacity due to a process of bone neoformation) or a combination of both.

Osteolytic changes can be detected radiographically at 7–10 days after the start of the aetiological agent/stimulus, whereas productive changes due to **osteogenesis** cannot be radiographically evidenced for at least 10–14 days.

As the same type of bone response occurs regardless of the aetiological agent that caused it, it is difficult and complicated to reach a definitive diagnosis of a lesion based solely on its radiographic appearance. Therefore, it is useful to define a bone injury as aggressive or nonaggressive, thus reducing the number of possible differential diagnoses. Even so, it is very important to note that, on many occasions, **FNA or biopsy** is needed to reach a definitive diagnosis and that the evaluation of other organs, such as the lungs and lymph nodes, can be useful to locate the presence of disease in other areas of the body. Thus, whenever there is a suspicion that a bone lesion might be neoplastic, a **thoracic radiograph** should be performed to detect the presence of pulmonary metastases as soon as possible, which will affect the prognosis and/or treatment (Barreiro and Vila, 2014; Thrall, 2018).

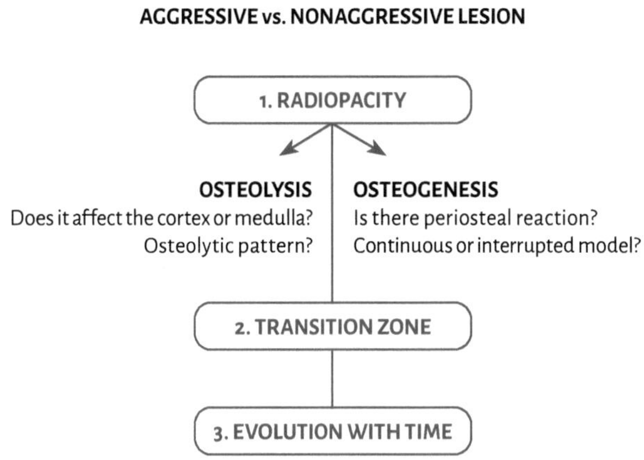

Figure 6. Representative diagram of the elements of a bone lesion to be evaluated to determine its degree of aggressiveness.

Radiographic Criteria for Differentiating Aggressive and Nonaggressive Bone Diseases

There are several factors that must be evaluated on a radiograph to classify a bone lesion according to its aggressiveness (Thrall, 2018) (Fig. 6).

- First, the radiopacity of the lesion should be noted: if osteolysis is present, the integrity of the cortical bone and the appearance or involvement of the medullary cavity should be studied. If osteogenesis is present, the appearance or type of the periosteal reaction should be examined.
- Next, the characteristics of the transition zone and the margins of the lesion should be examined.
- Finally, the evolution of the lesion over time should be assessed.

Osteolytic Patterns

The presence of lysis in the cortical bone and medullary cavity is a sign of aggressiveness of the bone lesion. Such aggressiveness varies depending on the model or pattern of osteolysis present. Three patterns of osteolysis have been described, from least to greatest severity (Thrall, 2018).

- **Geographic**: characterised by a large area of lysis, usually more than 1 cm in diameter, located in the medullary cavity of the bone. This pattern usually presents sharp and sclerotic margins and intact cortical bone, corresponding to nonaggressive processes, with a narrow transition zone. This type of pattern is usually seen with benign lesions such as bone cysts. However, if there is destruction of the cortex, the lesion should be considered aggressive.

- "**Moth-eaten**": there are multiple osteolytic foci of between 3 mm and 10 mm, which are not well defined and can merge together, forming a focus of "geographic" appearance at the centre of the lesion. The cortex may or may not be affected. This pattern can be observed in cases of infections as well as malignant neoplasms, and has a wide transition zone to healthy bone. It is therefore considered an aggressive pattern (Fig. 7).
- **Permeative**: there are small osteolytic foci 1–2 mm in diameter. These foci can converge, forming larger radiotransparent osteolytic foci, so this pattern is sometimes difficult to differentiate from the "moth-eaten" pattern. The cortical bone is affected (small osteolytic foci are better visualised in the cortex than in the medulla due to its trabecular pattern). This pattern is observed in very aggressive processes such as very active malignant neoplasms and in cases of severe fungal osteomyelitis (Fig. 8).

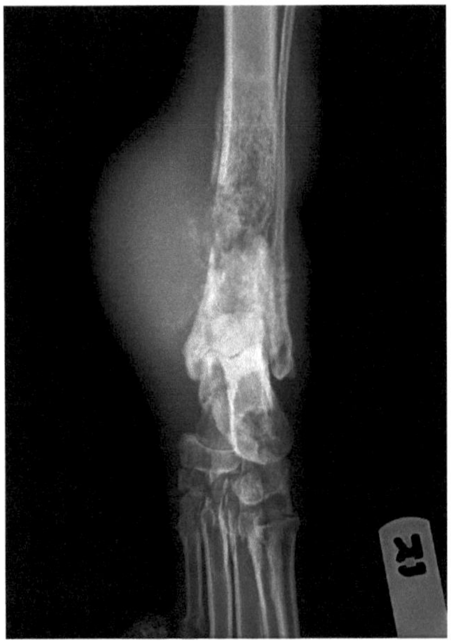

Figure 7. Craniocaudal radiograph of the distal portion of the tibia and fibula. A marked "moth-eaten" pattern of osteolysis is observed that affects both the medullary cavity and the cortex.

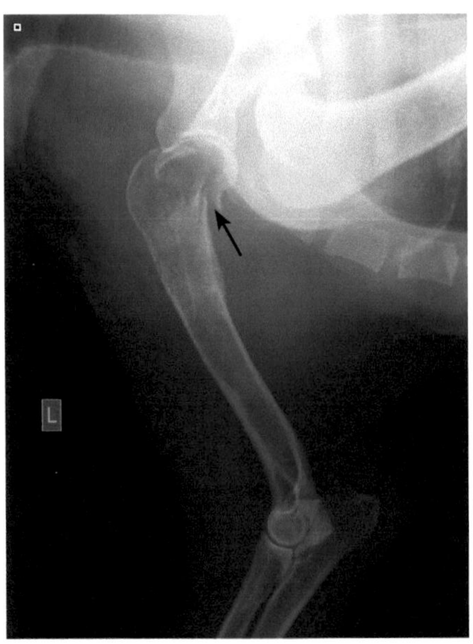

Figure 8. Mediolateral radiograph of the humerus of an adult dog. Small osteolytic foci of the same size are observed. These foci converge, affecting the medullary cavity and the cortices at the level of the proximal metaphysis of the humerus, causing a pathological fracture (arrow).

Periosteal Reaction

Periosteal reactions can occur due to multiple causes, including trauma, infection, and invasion of the periosteum by neoplastic bone cells or those from adjacent soft tissues. Periosteal reactions are grouped into **continuous** and **interrupted** models, although, depending on the literature consulted, there are small differences in classification (Barreiro and Vila, 2014). Within the continuous model there are the following models: solid (smooth or irregular), lamellar, "palisade" and "brush border". Interrupted models include: spiculated, "radial" spiculated (sunburst) and amorphous (Fig. 9). Continuous models are considered to originate from processes that evolve slowly over time or sometimes to be early stages of aggressive injury, whereas interrupted models are caused by aggressive pathologies that evolve rapidly over time.

- **Unilamellar, smooth solid and irregular solid** model: these are usually inactive periosteal reactions, with homogeneous, well-defined margins, appearing in nonaggressive lesions such as subperiosteal haematomas or periostitis. In these types of models there is variable thickening of the cortex, and the margins can be smooth or wavy/irregular. The changes in shape and opacity depend on the time at which the lesion occurred (Fig. 10).

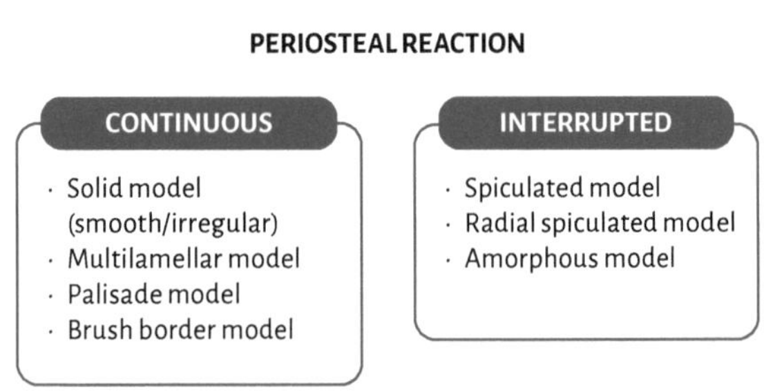

Figure 9. Periosteal reaction models grouped by whether they are continuous or interrupted.

- **Multilamellar** model: caused by intermittent elevations of the periosteum, which indicate that the lesion is semi-aggressive and cyclical; they are very rare.
- "**Palisade**" reaction: the bone neoformation extends outwards as columns forming a right angle with the cortex. This type of periosteal reaction is seen in cases of hypertrophic osteopathy (and, over time, can remodel and transform into a continuous solid model) (Fig. 11).

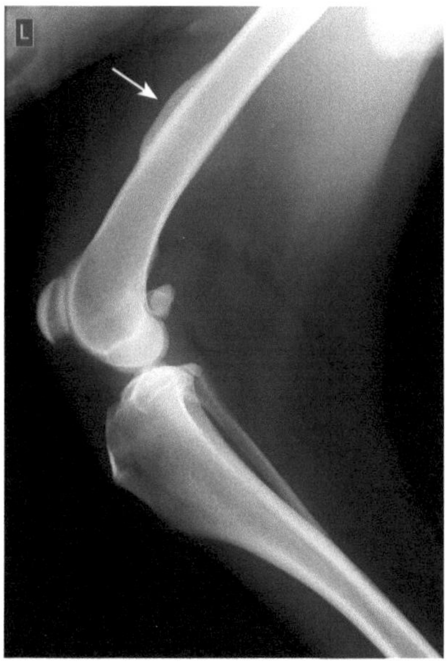

Figure 10. Mediolateral radiograph of the stifle and distal femur in which a solid and smooth continuous periosteal reaction model is visualised in the cranial cortex of the medial diaphysis of the femur (arrow). The integrity of the cortex can be seen and there is no involvement of the medullary cavity.

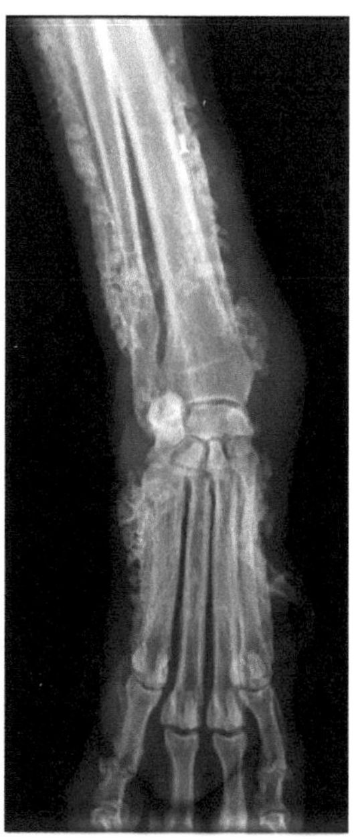

Figure 11. Dorsopalmar radiograph of the carpus, metacarpus and distal diaphysis of the ulna and radius in which a palisade periosteal reaction is observed in the cortices of the second and fifth metacarpals, as well as in those of the ulna and radius. At the level of the medial cortex of the second metacarpal, the reaction has been remodelled into a solid model. There is inflammation of the soft tissues adjacent to the medial area of the carpal joint.

- "**Brush border**" reaction: the speed of growth determines the thickness of the spicules of new bone, which are thicker in slow processes and thinner in fast, more aggressive ones. This model is seen in osteomyelitis and leishmaniasis. In these cases, despite being in the group of continuous models, they are considered semi-aggressive. There may be destruction/discontinuity of the cortex.
- **Spiculated** model: this consists of active periosteal reactions characterised by irregular margins, which occur in cases of aggressive lesions. Thin spicules of bone tissue are visualised extending outwards from the bone lesion. This type of reaction is indicative of an aggressive process, usually present in malignant bone neoplasms, so there is clear destruction of the cortex. The term "sunburst" applies to an exuberant spiculated model (Fig. 12).
- **Amorphous** model: this last model indicates that the lesion is expanding very rapidly; it is the least organised and corresponds to very aggressive lesions, mostly bone tumours. There are often areas of osteolysis associated with injury and invasion of adjacent soft tissues that show infiltration with bone tissue (Fig. 13).

In active periosteal reactions, an elevation of the periosteum is visualised at the edge of the lesion (between the fibrous layer of the periosteum and the cortical layer) that adopts a triangular shape known as "Codman's triangle". Although it is often seen at the margins of primary bone tumours, it is not pathognomonic of tumours (or in particular of osteosarcomas, as described previously) since it occurs in cases of both aggressive and nonaggressive active lesions, where the periosteum has elevated rapidly from the cortex (Fig. 14).

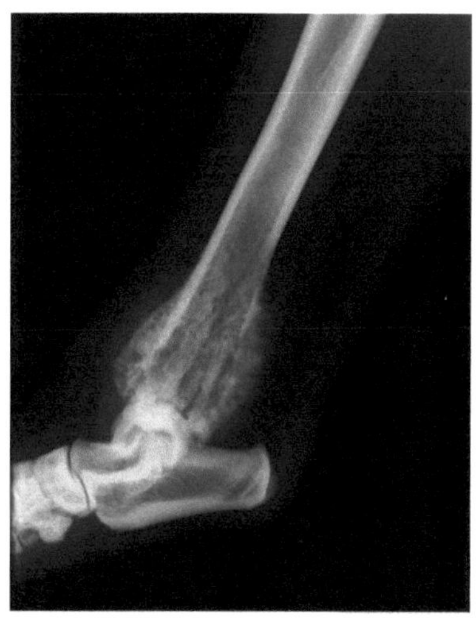

Figure 12. Lateral radiograph of the distal portion of the tibia in which an aggressive bone lesion is visualised affecting the distal metaphysis of the tibia, with an interrupted spiculated periosteal reaction, especially in the caudal cortex, which is thinned and shows some discontinuity. There is also involvement of the medullary cavity, with the presence of osteolytic foci.

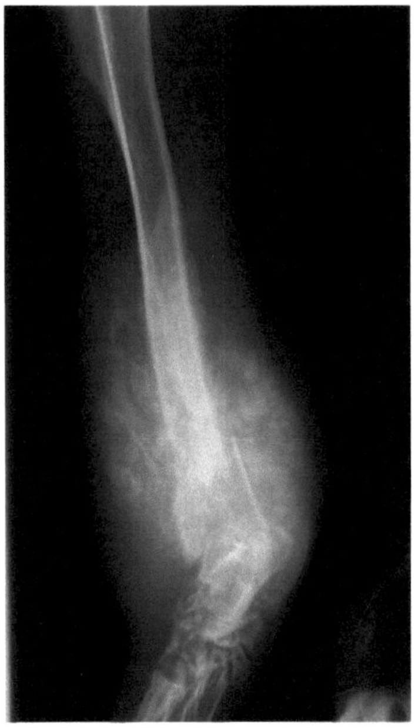

Figure 13. Oblique lateral radiograph of the distal diaphysis of the tibia in which an aggressive bone lesion with an interrupted amorphous periosteal reaction is visualised. This lesion has caused a pathological fracture of the bone. There is severe inflammation of the adjacent soft tissues, which have been infiltrated by neoplastic bone tissue.

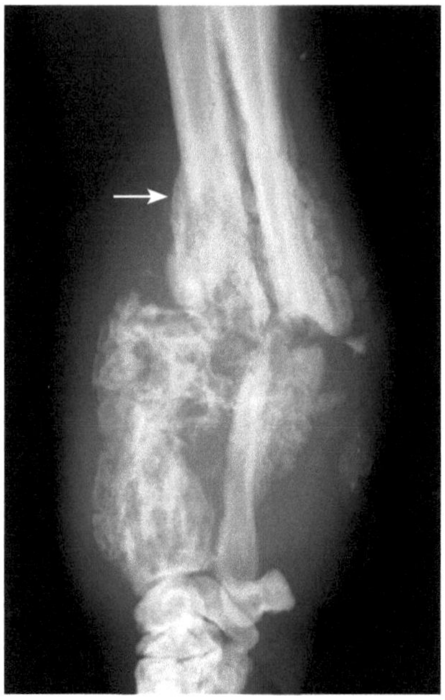

Figure 14. Lateral radiograph of the distal diaphysis of the ulna and radius showing an aggressive bone lesion with an interrupted amorphous-type periosteal reaction, in addition to pathological fracture of both bones. At the level of the cranial cortex of the proximal fragment of the radius, "Codman's triangle" (arrow) can be seen.

Transition Zone, Lesion Margins and Soft Tissues

Once the lesion has been evaluated, the area around it should be examined, observing whether the limits of the lesion are well defined, which is more typical of nonaggressive lesions, or whether they are very irregular and unclear, which suggests an aggressive lesion.

At the same time, the transition zone (the area between the affected bone and healthy bone) should be assessed, and it should be noted whether it is narrow or wide, and well defined or poorly defined. If the transition zone is narrow and well defined (where the healthy bone ends and where the affected bone begins can be clearly differentiated), it indicates a nonaggressive lesion, whereas aggressive lesions have a broad, poorly defined transition zone (it is difficult to see where the healthy bone ends and the affected bone begins). However, the two characteristics are not always linked; for example, a lesion may have a clear transition zone, in which the periosteal reaction can be seen decreasing in depth and the bone gradually becomes totally normal in appearance, but affects a significant length of the bone, which means that it is more aggressive due to its extension.

The soft tissue adjacent to the bone does not usually show any changes in the case of nonaggressive lesions, whereas with aggressive lesions there tend to be soft tissue changes, especially in cases of tumours and osteomyelitis, resulting in inflammation and/or infection (Barreiro and Vila, 2014).

Evolution of Lesions Over Time

Performing serial radiographic examinations over time is useful to assess the extent of change between one examination and another, and to evaluate the response to treatment. When evaluating the evolution of a lesion over time, nonaggressive lesions can be seen to change slowly, whereas aggressive lesions can show dramatic changes that occur over a very short period of time.

After evaluating the radiographs using these criteria, an idea of the degree of aggressiveness of the lesion (Table 1) can be gained and a list of differential diagnoses established, according to which aggressive lesions are usually due to infections or neoplasms, whereas nonaggressive lesions are usually chronic traumatic lesions undergoing recovery, bone cysts, developmental pathologies or nonaggressive neoplasms (Thrall, 2018).

From this point on in this chapter, other factors such as the location (Table 2), number and distribution (Table 3) of the lesion(s) will be considered to define which of these lesions is the most likely, because certain bone diseases have a tendency to be located in a particular area of the bone, and may affect either a single bone or more than one bone; in these cases knowledge of the distribution of the lesion(s) in the skeleton is also very important to reach a definitive diagnosis.

Table 1. Characteristics of aggressive and nonaggressive lesions.

	Nonaggressive	Aggressive
Type of osteolysis	Geographic	Moth-eaten/ permeative
Periosteal reaction	Continuous	Interrupted
Margins	Well defined, sclerosis present	Poorly defined, infiltrating, without sclerosis
Transition zone	Small, well defined	Extensive, poorly defined
Cortex	Intact	Irregular, shows destruction
Change over time	Slow	Fast
Inflammation of soft tissue	No	Yes

Table 2. Location of bone pathologies.

Epiphysis	Physis	Metaphysis	Diaphysis
Osteochondrosis	Physitis Rickets	Primary tumour	Metastatic tumour
Chondrodysplasias	Premature closure	Haematogenous osteomyelitis	Panosteitis Hypertrophic osteopathy
Arthritis, synovial neoplasms	Fractures	Metaphyseal osteopathy	Fractures

Table 3. Monostotic (single bone) versus polyostotic (several bones) distribution of certain bone pathologies.

Monostotic	Polyostotic
Trauma	Trauma
Primary bone tumour	Metastatic tumour
Local osteomyelitis	Bone marrow tumour
Congenital/ developmental disorder	Haematogenous osteomyelitis
	Metabolic/nutritional disease

Nonneoplastic Pathologies of the Musculoskeletal System

In this section anomalies that generally affect the skeleton will be discussed.

Congenital Diseases

Osteochondrodysplasia

Osteochondrodysplasia is the term used to describe a group of skeletal developmental pathologies in various canine and feline breeds, which have a genetic basis and often cause disproportionate dwarfism (Martínez et al., 2006). Although radiographically they may present a similar appearance, histologically and biochemically they are a rather heterogeneous group of diseases. They are characterised by abnormalities in growth and development at the level of the growth plate (physis), the bone or both. Some of these disorders mainly affect the epiphyses, others the physes and others the metaphyses (Pollard and Phillips, 2018). The most representative are described here.

- **Chondrodystrophy**: considered as a set of anatomical variations in certain breeds (which are described as chondrodystrophic), such as the Dachshund, Basset Hound and Corgi. There is an alteration in endochondral ossification that causes the long bones to be short (in proportion to the length of the skull and spine), to have thickened cortices and to be slightly curved (Fig. 15). These animals have lateral deviation of the limbs (valgus deformity) at the level of the carpus (Brown et al., 2017) (Fig. 16).
- **Chondrodysplasia**: causes autosomal and recessive hereditary dwarfism. Numerous types of chondrodysplasia have been described depending on the breed of dog that is affected, for example, that affecting the Labrador Retriever (associated with ocular dysplasia and hip dysplasia), Alaskan Malamute, Beagle or Norwegian Elkhound. It has also been identified in breeds of cat such as the Scottish Fold. In all cases, there is marked shortening of the long bones, which are curved. These abnormalities may be associated with a delay in the development of secondary ossification centres at the level of the elbow joint (anconeal process, medial coronoid), as occurs in chondrodysplasia of Labradors, or asynchronous growth of the ulna and radius together with involvement of the cuboid bones of the carpus, which has been observed in both Labradors and Alaskan Malamutes, resulting in angular deformations of the forelimbs (radius curvus) (Pollard and Phillips, 2018).
- **Multiple epiphyseal dysplasia** (**MED**): mainly described in Beagle puppies and Miniature Poodles. This is a rare type of chondrodysplasia caused by an alteration of endochondral ossification, associated with hypoplasia of the growth plates of the long bones, which results in a failure in the ossification of the epiphyses. Affected animals exhibit disproportionate dwarfism with short limbs, kyphosis of the spine and thickened joints (Rubenstein and Christakis, 2006). The epiphyses of the femur and humerus are the most affected, but lesions can

be seen in the carpus, tarsus, metacarpals, metatarsals and vertebral bodies. The radiographic pattern of MED is characterised by the presence of stippling on the epiphyses, which also have irregular margins and, according to the literature, present an appearance reminiscent of a blackberry (Agut et al., 2008) (Fig. 17).

Metabolic and Nutritional Diseases

Congenital Hypothyroidism

This is a very rare pathology, which is caused by **aplasia or hypoplasia of the thyroid** that results in an absence or delay in the development of the epiphyses. Affected dogs and cats

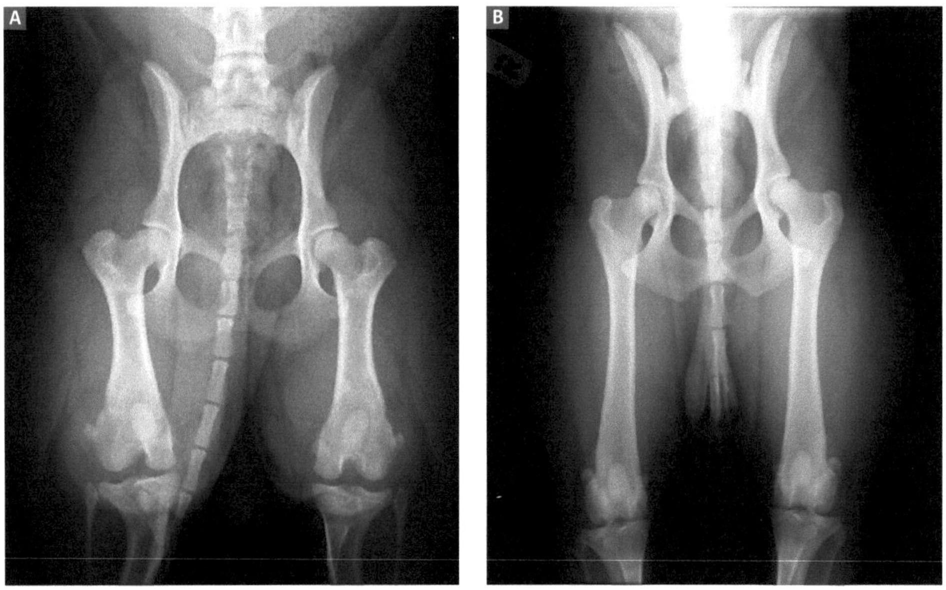

Figure 15. Ventrodorsal radiographs of the hip of (**A**) a chondrodystrophic and (**B**) a nonchondrodystrophic dog. Note that the femurs of the chondrodystrophic dog are shorter (relative to hip size) than those of the nonchondrodystrophic dog.

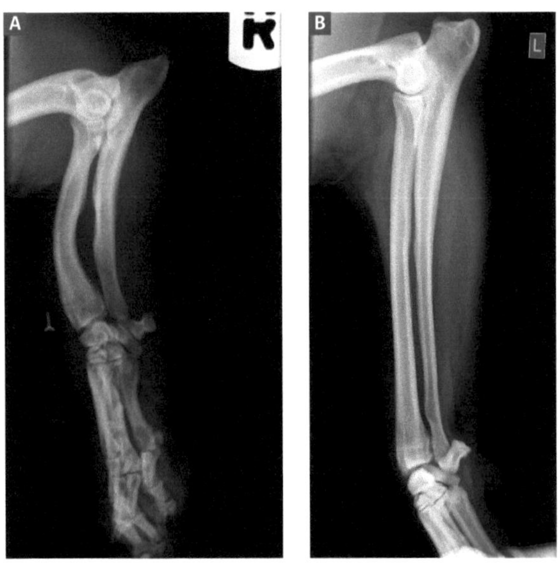

Figure 16. Mediolateral radiographs of the ulna and radius of (**A**) a chondrodystrophic and (**B**) a nonchondrodystrophic dog. Note the shortening of the ulna and radius in the chondrodystrophic dog, as well as the slight cranial curvature of the radius (in this image a cranial artefact is observed at the distal epiphysis of the radius that corresponds with a catheter).

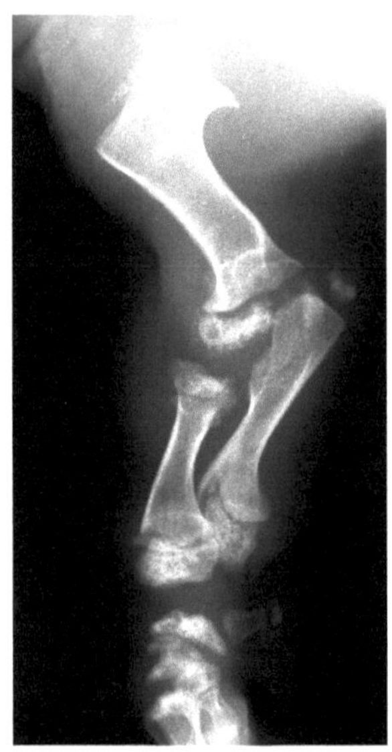

Figure 17. Mediolateral radiograph of the ulna and radius of a 10-week-old mixed-breed dog, which was smaller than the rest of the litter and had difficulty walking and standing. The epiphyses of the long bones have a heterogeneous, dotted opacity and irregular margins. A diagnosis of multiple epiphyseal dysplasia was obtained by histopathological study.

have smaller skulls than normal due to delayed closure of the fontanelles, thickening of the cortices of the radius and ulna, bowing of the forelimbs and shorter spines (sometimes with kyphosis due to dysplasia of the articular surfaces of the vertebral bodies), causing disproportionate dwarfism.

Among the most characteristic radiographic findings of this disorder are delay in the ossification of cuboid bones (smaller carpal and tarsal bones) and delay in the closure of the enlarged growth plates (Pollard and Phillips, 2018). If the disorder is diagnosed early, the abnormalities may regress with treatment.

Secondary Nutritional Hyperparathyroidism

This pathology affects young dogs and cats whose diet have very little calcium intake or with a serious imbalance in calcium and phosphorus content (very low in calcium and very rich in phosphorus), causing secondary hyperparathyroidism (Langley-Hobbs, 2012). When there is hyperphosphataemia, there is a drop in blood calcium levels, and this hypocalcaemia stimulates increased production of parathyroid hormone. This causes a decrease in the renal reabsorption of phosphates and an increase in the reabsorption of calcium from the bones. In addition, there is an increase in the activity of osteoclasts in the bones, causing an increase in bone resorption that results in a greater amount of calcium in the blood.

Radiographically, generalised demineralisation (osteoporosis, osteopaenia) of the entire skeleton can be observed, so that there is little contrast between the opacity of the bone and that of the soft tissue. The cortices of the bones appear very thin and pathological "greenstick" or folding fractures can occur, and the spine can present an abnormal shape with lordosis in the lumbar area, especially in cats. All of these radiographic changes can be resolved with dietary modification, although some deformities of the spine or those that are the result of pathological fractures can persist (Stander and Cassel, 2016) (Fig. 18).

Secondary Renal Hyperparathyroidism

This pathology can occur in animals of any age as a result of **chronic renal failure**. The changes are more evident in the skull, producing what is known as "rubber jaw" as it starts to become softer and more flexible. Radiographically, there is demineralisation of the mandible and maxilla, especially around the roots of the teeth, with loss of definition of the lamina dura, giving the impression that the teeth are "floating". There may be soft tissue calcifications, for example, at the level of the gastric mucosa or in the walls of some vessels (Stander and Cassel, 2016).

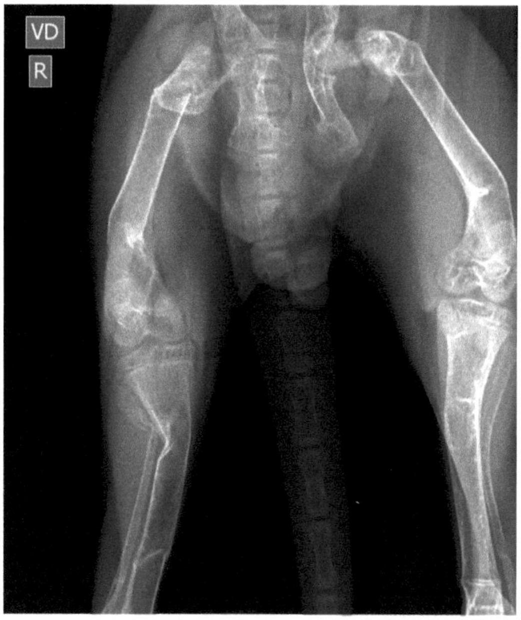

Figure 18. Craniocaudal radiograph of the hindlimbs of a 4-month-old cat with weakness in all four limbs. The cat was fed only tuna and ham. Generalised osteopaenia is seen, and is especially marked at the level of the right femoral head. Both femurs and tibias have changes in their morphology that could lead to pathological fractures. The diagnosis was secondary nutritional hyperparathyroidism.

Rickets

Nowadays, it is rare for animals to present with rickets, also known as juvenile osteomalacia. This pathology may be due to the inability of the animal to synthesise vitamin D or to a deficiency of vitamin D in the diet (Carrera, 2014). On radiographs, the physes of the long bones can be seen wider than normal and somewhat irregular, the metaphyses show a flared shape (especially in the distal radius, ulna and tibia), and the cortices are thinned; however, the epiphyses are normal in appearance (Fig. 19).

Hypervitaminosis A

Hypervitaminosis A is mainly seen in adult cats that are fed predominantly on raw beef liver, which contains excessive vitamin A. The pathophysiology of hypervitaminosis A involves suppression of osteoclast and chondrocyte activity at the level of the physis (Hough et al., 1988).

Radiographic changes in affected young animals include shortening of the long bones with premature closure of the growth plates (physes). In chronic processes in adult animals, bone proliferation predominates, with bone neoformations at the origin and insertion of tendons and ligaments and at the level of the joint capsule in joints with more activity, such as the cervical and thoracic vertebrae and elbows; these changes result in ankylosing spondylopathy of the cervical and thoracic spine (Fig. 20), and ankylosing enthesopathy or arthropathy and degenerative joint disease (DJD) at the level of the shoulders and elbows (Allan and Davies, 2018).

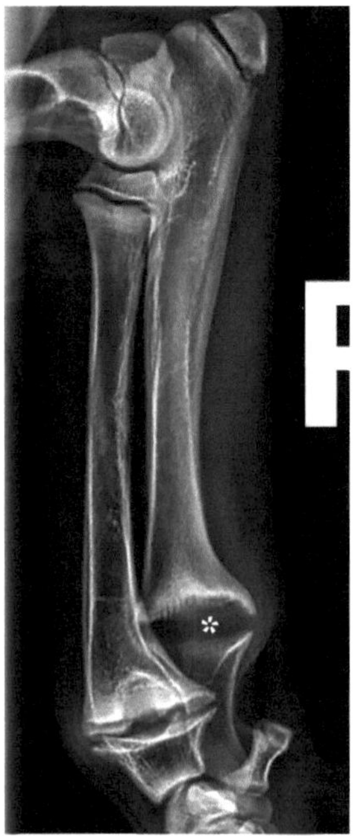

Figure 19. Mediolateral radiograph of the ulna and radius of a 5-month-old Newfoundland with generalised enlargement of the physes in all long bones, which is very marked in the distal physis of both the ulna and radius (asterisk) and the distal physis of both tibias. These findings are compatible with rickets. (Image courtesy of A. Navarro, Nexo Menescal Novelda.)

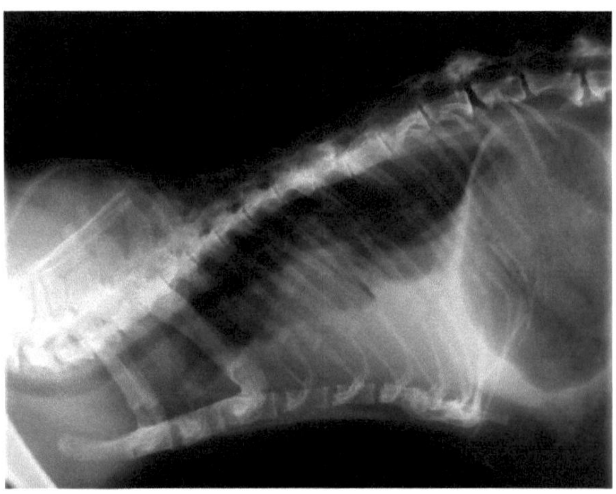

Figure 20. Lateral radiograph of the thoracic spine of an adult cat with changes in the spinous processes, which have remodelled and fused, resulting in ankylosing spondylopathy, compatible with hypervitaminosis A.

Mucopolysaccharidosis

The mucopolysaccharidoses are a rare group of autosomal recessive diseases. They are caused by a deficiency of different enzymes that cause a decrease or absence of the catabolism of glycosaminoglycans. This causes abnormal lysosomal storage of mucopolysaccharides that are not degraded, resulting in a multisystemic chronic progressive disease (Carrera, 2014).

Depending on the enzyme involved, several types of mucopolysaccharidosis are described (classed as I to VII). They usually give rise to epiphyseal dysplasia of the articular surfaces of the vertebral bodies and fusion of the vertebrae, dwarfism, facial deformities (by affecting the frontal sinuses and other bony structures of the skull), pectus excavatum, hip dysplasia and epiphyseal dysplasia in the long bones, which, over time, gives rise to osteoarthritis (degenerative joint disease).

Mucopolysaccharidoses are rare in the dog and more common in the cat, especially in the Siamese breed. In cats, it is necessary to differentiate the disease from hypervitaminosis A (Allan and Davies, 2018).

Fractures

A fracture is defined as a disruption of continuity in a bone that occurs intensely and rapidly. There are **predisposing factors** for a fracture to occur, such as the shape and position of the bone (the ulna and radius are more liable to fractures than bones such as those of the carpus), as well as factors extrinsic to the bone that have previously weakened or altered it, such as neoplasms or infections, which result in so-called pathological fractures. There are also the **determining factors** that cause the fracture itself, such as external trauma or excessive contraction of the muscles or tendons (Soler and Agut, 2014).

When naming a fracture, several aspects must be referred to in order to define it with accuracy (Henry and Cole, 2018). To do this, the following classification can be followed.

1. According to the Extension of the Fracture Line

Complete or incomplete. If the fracture is complete, there is a discontinuity along the entire thickness of the bone, affecting the two visible cortices in each projection, whereas in an incomplete fracture there is still continuity in some of the cortices, as occurs in the case of fissures (Fig. 21) or in so-called "greenstick" fractures that occur in young animals.

2. According to Whether there is External Communication

Open or closed. In an open fracture, there is a wound that communicates the focus of the fracture with the outside of

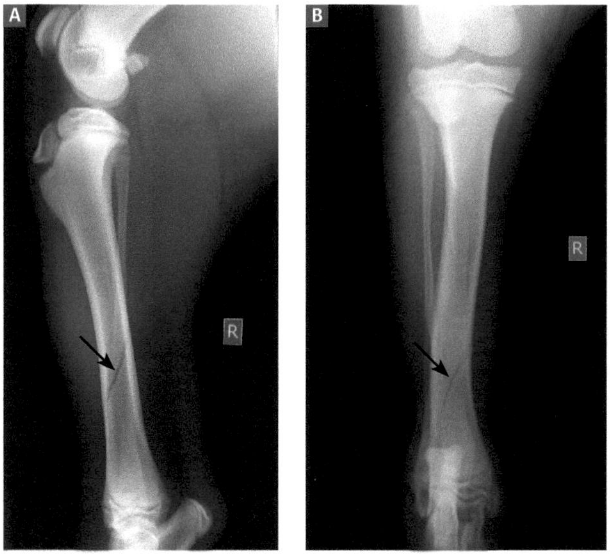

Figure 21. Mediolateral (**A**) and craniocaudal (**B**) radiographs of the tibia of a 6-month-old Rottweiler showing an oblique radiotransparent line in the distal third of the diaphysis (arrows) in a craniodistomedial–caudoproximolateral direction, which affects the medullary cavity but not the cortex, so it is considered an incomplete fracture or fissure.

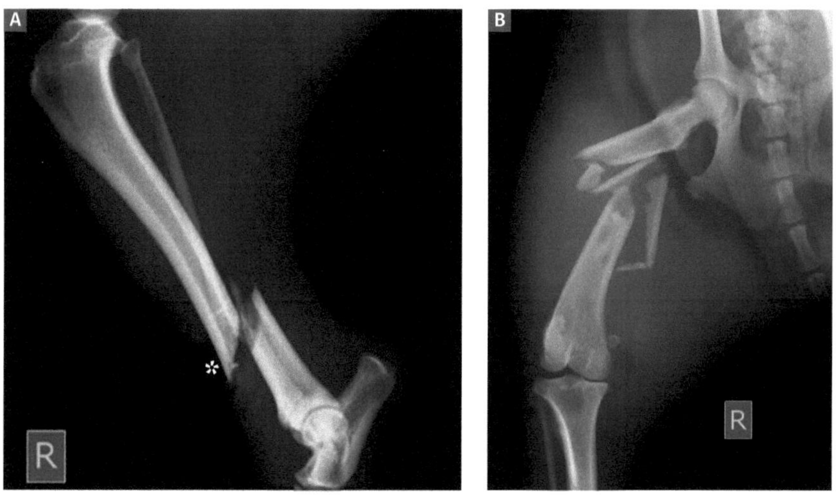

Figure 22. A. Mediolateral radiograph of the tibia of an adult dog in which a fracture is observed in the distal third of the diaphysis. The fracture is complete, simple and oblique and there is loss of continuity of the cranial soft tissues external to the focus of the fracture (asterisk), therefore it is an open fracture. **B**. Craniocaudal radiograph of the femur of an adult dog that has a multiple comminuted fracture in the mid-diaphysis. Several fragments can be seen that converge at the focus of the fracture.

the body; there may be loss of material from the soft tissues and adjacent skin (Fig. 22 A). **Open fractures can be subclassified** (**type I to type IV**) depending on the major or minor defect/involvement in the skin and soft tissues.

3. According to the Number of Fragments

Single or multiple. A single fracture has only one fracture line and two fragments; a multiple fracture has two or more fracture lines. Multiple fractures can be subclassified into **segmental**, where several fracture lines usually appear that do not communicate with each other and usually give rise to large fragments, and **comminuted**, in which the different fracture lines communicate at a point (Fig. 22 B).

4. According to the Direction of the Fracture Line

Transverse, oblique or spiroidal. This refers to the direction of the fracture line in a single fracture. If the fracture forms a 90° angle with the longitudinal axis of the bone, it is transverse; if it forms another type of angle, it is oblique; and if it forms a spiral along the long axis of the bone, it is spiroidal (Fig. 23).

5. According to the Location in the Bone

- **Articular**: the fracture line extends to an articular surface (Fig. 24). One type of joint fracture is a slab fracture, which occurs when the fracture line extends from one articular surface to another; this type is rare and could be found, for example, in the intermediate carporadial bone.
- **Diaphyseal**: a diaphyseal fracture is located in the diaphysis of a long bone; its location in the proximal, middle or distal third of the diaphysis should be described.
- **Metaphyseal**: a metaphyseal fracture affects the proximal or distal metaphysis of a long bone (Fig. 25).

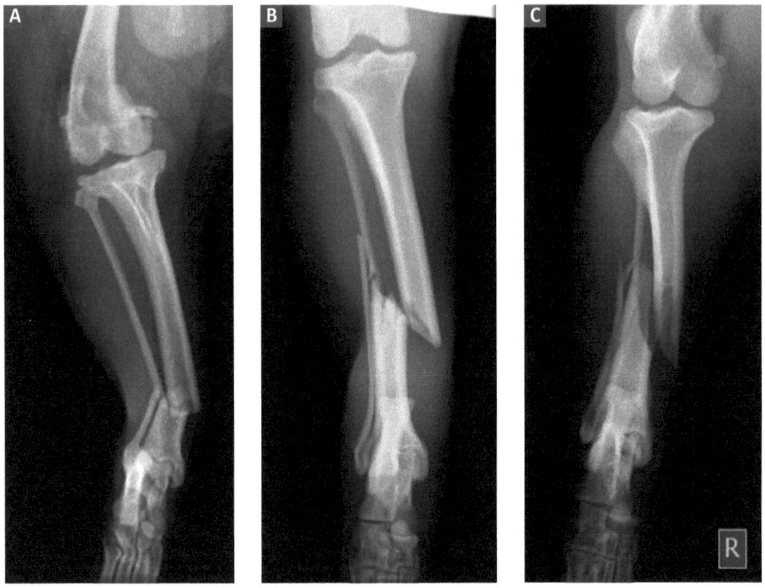

Figure 23. Craniocaudal radiographs of the tibia of three adult dogs with complete, simple, and transverse (**A**), oblique (**B**) and spiroidal (**C**) fractures.

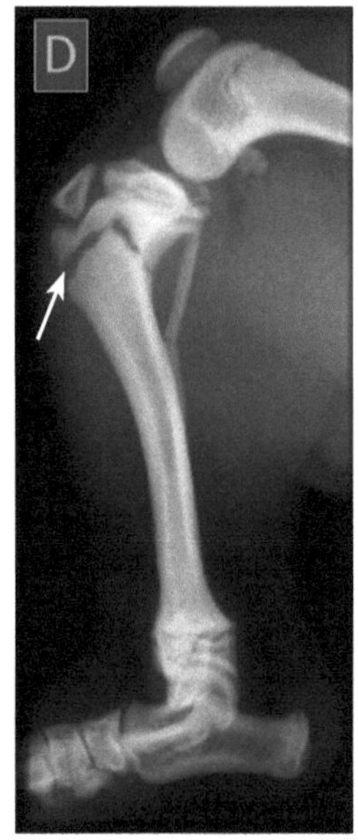

Figure 25. Mediolateral radiograph of the tibia of a 7-month-old dog with a complete fracture of the proximal metaphysis of the tibia (arrow).

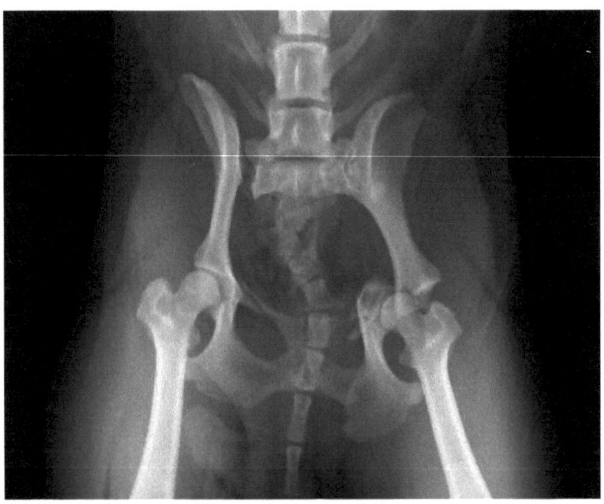

Figure 24. Ventrodorsal radiograph of the pelvis of an adult dog with a left acetabular joint fracture, also considered an impaction fracture. In addition, fractures are seen in the left ischium and in the cranial branches of the left and the right pubis, as well as a right sacroiliac luxation.

– **Epiphyseal**: may involve only the epiphysis, but it usually affects the physeal area. If it occurs in a young animal where the physis is still open, the fracture should be named using the **Salter–Harris** classification system, in which five or six types of fracture are differentiated depending on the structures that are involved (Burk and Feeney, 2003).
  - **Type I**: the fracture line is visualised at the level of the physis, so a separation between the epiphysis and the metaphysis is observed (Fig. 26).
  - **Type II**: the fracture affects the physis and also a portion of the metaphysis (Fig. 27).
  - **Type III**: the fracture extends through part of the epiphysis and along part of the physis, so it involves the physis and the epiphysis.
  - **Type IV**: the fracture line crosses the epiphysis and physis and affects a portion of the metaphysis, thus involving all three structures (Fig. 28).
  - **Type V**: affects the physis; there is no fracture line, but crushing or compression of the physis causes premature closure of the growth plate. Some authors differentiate a **type VI** fracture when the entire physis is not affected and only a portion of the physis undergoes premature closure. These types of fractures cause angular deformations in the long bones.

Other Types of Fractures

– **Avulsion fracture**: when an avulsion fracture occurs, a fragment of bone into which a tendon or ligament is inserted is separated from the bone of origin due to excessive traction by the muscle or tendon. This type of fracture is more common in young animals because these bone fragments coincide with secondary ossification centres that have not yet fused with the main bone, for example, the tibial tuberosity, the olecranon or the calcaneus (Fig. 29). In cases where there is doubt whether the separation between the bones is physiological or due to avulsion, a radiograph of the contralateral limb is indicated.

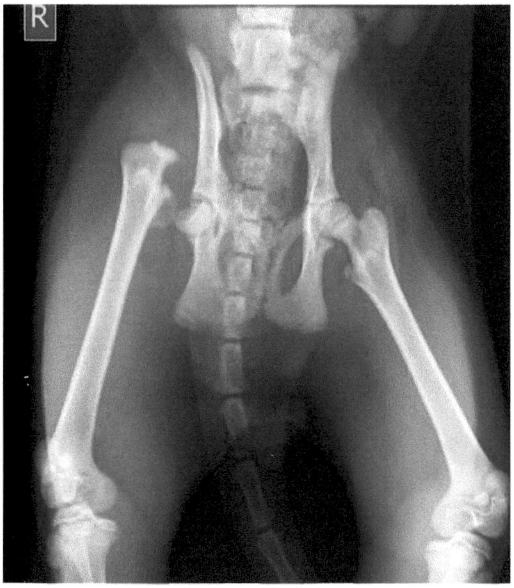

Figure 26. Ventrodorsal radiograph of the hip of an immature cat with a Salter–Harris type I fracture of the right femoral head. The fracture line crosses the physis (growth plate).

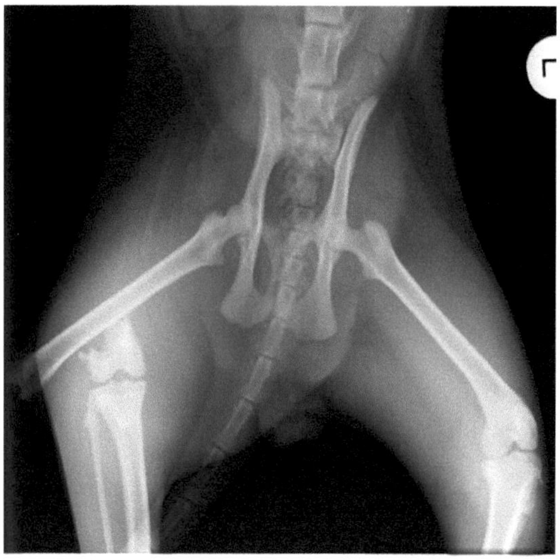

Figure 27. Ventrodorsal radiograph of the hip of an immature cat with a Salter–Harris type II fracture of the distal epiphysis of the right femur. The fracture line affects the physis and also a portion of the metaphysis.

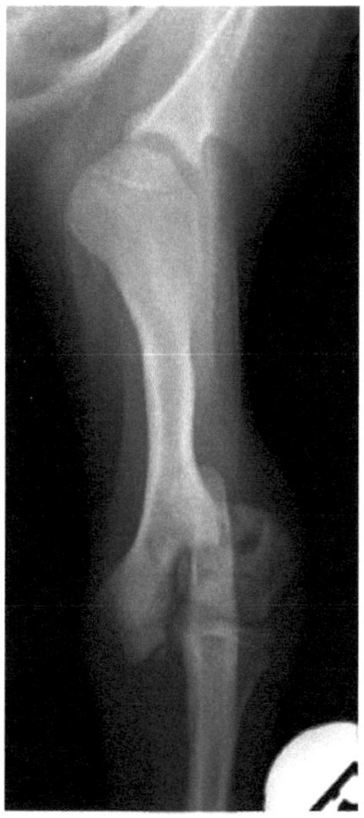

Figure 28. Craniocaudal radiograph of the elbow of a 3-month-old dog. A Salter–Harris type IV fracture is visualised affecting the distal epiphysis of the humerus and involving the epiphysis, the physis and a portion of the metaphysis.

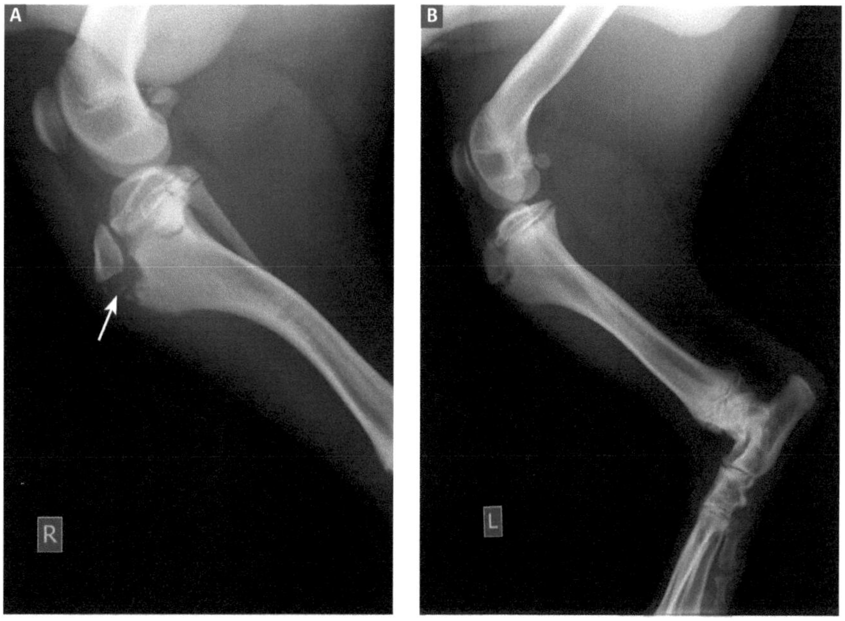

Figure 29. Mediolateral radiographs of both stifles of a 6-month-old dog that was run over. In the right stifle (**A**), the tibial tuberosity is visualised with an abnormal separation of the plateau and metaphysis of the tibia (arrow), while in the left stifle (**B**), the tibial tuberosity remains in a normal position, and there is a separation from the rest of the tibia appropriate for the age of the animal. The diagnosis was an avulsion fracture of the right tibial tuberosity.

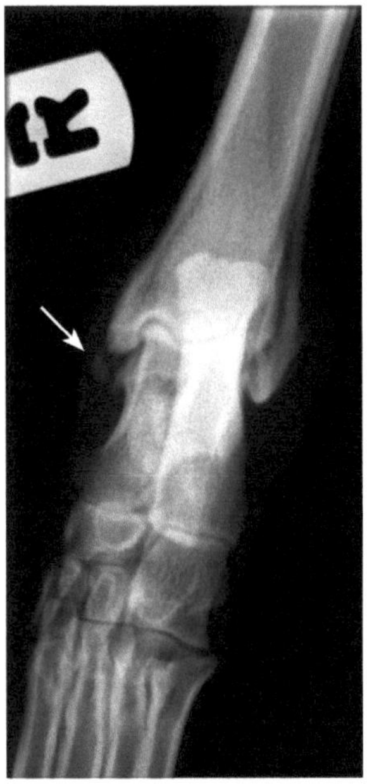

Figure 30. Dorsoplantar radiograph of the tarsus of an adult dog. A "chip-like" fracture is visualised, with a small fragment coming from the medial surface of the talus (arrow), probably due to avulsion produced by the medial collateral ligament of the tarsus.

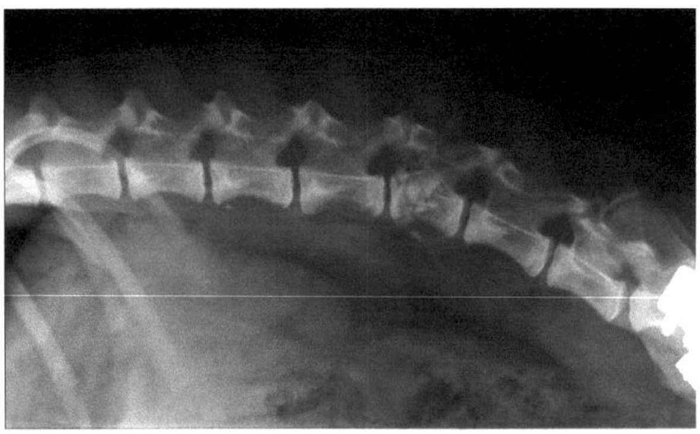

Figure 31. Lateral radiograph of the lumbar spine of an adult dog in which a compression/impact fracture is seen in the vertebral body of L5. The length of the vertebral body of L5 can be seen to be shorter in length than the adjacent vertebral bodies.

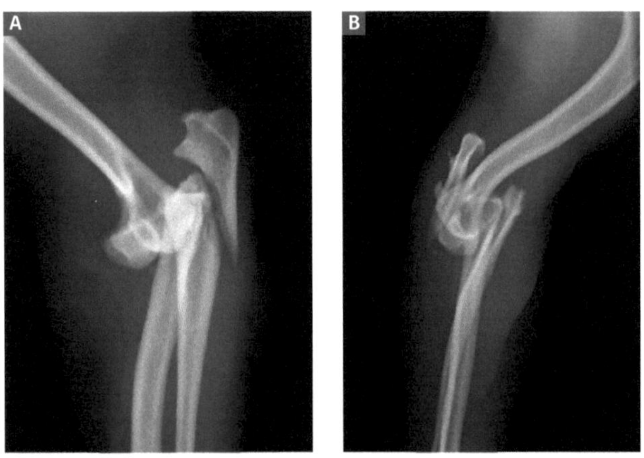

Figure 32. Mediolateral (**A**) and craniocaudal (**B**) radiographs of the elbow of an adult dog in which a Monteggia fracture has occurred: a proximal ulnar fracture and a humeroradial luxation are both visualised. In this case it is a Monteggia type II, as the radius has luxated caudally.

- "**Chip-like" fracture**: this is usually a type of avulsion fracture, in which the resulting fragment is small in size and the gap left where the fragment originated is visible (Fig. 30).
- **Impact or compression fracture**: these fractures occur when trauma causes compression or crushing of the bone, which results in a reduction in the size of the bone; it usually happens in the vertebral bodies (Fig. 31).
- **Monteggia fracture**: this is a special type of fracture in which the fracture line is located in the proximal third of the ulna and, in addition, a humeroradial luxation occurs. There are several subtypes depending on the direction of the radial luxation:
  - cranial luxation: type I
  - caudal luxation: type II
  - lateral luxation: type III
  - cranial luxation together with radial fracture: type IV (Fig. 32).

Fracture Repair

After repairing a fracture, orthogonal radiographs should be performed after surgery and then, ideally, check-ups should be done every 4–6 weeks or so, if there are no complications.

To help carry out a review of the fracture and not overlook the assessment of any element involved, a system that can be easily followed by means of a mnemonic should be used (**ABCDS**, where the letters refer to **A**: **alignment**, evaluation of alignment of fragments; **B**: **bones**, assessment of the evolution of bone callus; **C**: **cartilage**, referring to the surface of the articular cartilage; **D**: **devices**, assess the appearance of the fixation systems (devices) in case there is any movement of these or if there is a reaction of the bone due to their presence; **S**: **soft tissues**, look for changes in them, such as inflammation or the presence of gas).

Bone repair can occur by two mechanisms (Henry and Cole, 2018).

- **Direct repair or primary healing**, by intramembranous ossification. This occurs when rigid fixation systems are used to ensure the fragments are perfectly aligned, achieving an excellent anatomical reduction of the fracture. In these conditions there is growth of the periosteum and endosteum by intramembranous ossification, and there is no formation of bone callus. The space between the fragments is minimal and the continuity between the cortices is restored in a short period of time (Fig. 33).
- **Indirect repair or secondary healing**. This is caused by intramembranous and endochondral ossification, in which the formation of a callus occurs from undifferentiated mesenchymal tissue that matures over time, going from granulation tissue to cartilage, which subsequently mineralises and finally transforms into bone.

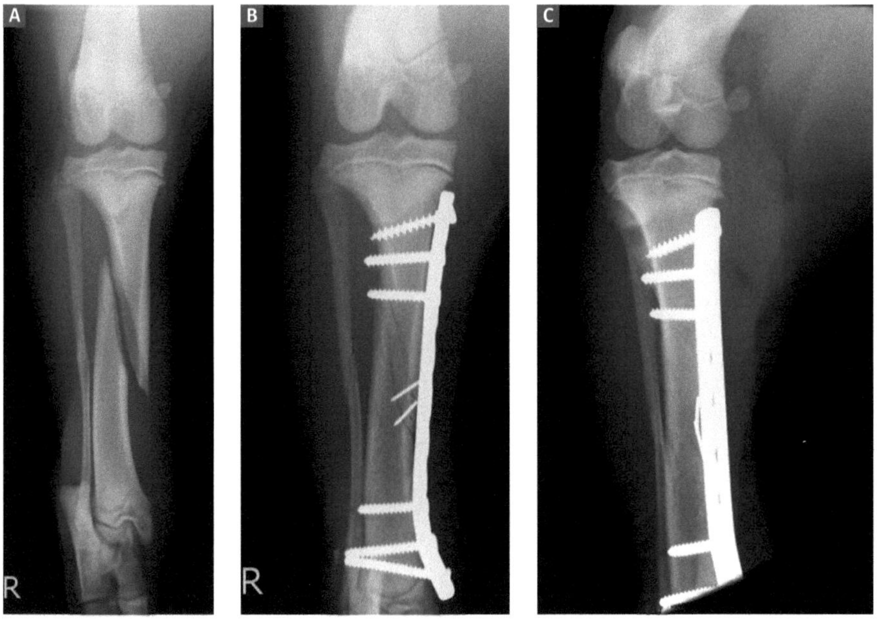

Figure 33. Craniocaudal radiographs of the tibia of a 5-month-old dog with a simple, closed, complete, oblique, mid-diaphyseal fracture of the tibia and fibula. **A**. Before surgical resolution. **B**. After surgical resolution. **C**. One week after surgical resolution. Primary repair of the fracture is evident, without the presence of bone callus and with a rapid restoration of cortical continuity.

This type of repair occurs in cases where the fixation system does not achieve exact apposition of the fragments, or with external fixators, which are not as rigid as osteosynthesis plates and other internal fixation systems; in these cases, there is some movement between the fragments, which favours the formation of bone callus at the fracture.

The process of bone callus formation and remodelling is variable over time because it depends on many factors. Among them, the following should be taken into account (Soler and Agut, 2014).

- **Blood supply**. Cell differentiation and the evolution of bone callus depend on the oxygen supply the callus receives. In cases where the blood supply is poorer, fracture repair is slower. This can happen when there is serious damage to the soft tissues adjacent to the fracture site or if there is excessive pressure from internal fixators on the cortices of the bone fragments.
- **The type of bone and the area of the fractured bone**. Different locations have different resolution times: fractures affecting the metaphysis heal more quickly than those located in the diaphysis of a long bone. In addition, in small-breed dogs, diaphyseal fractures of the ulna and radius heal more slowly.
- **Immobilisation system**. Internal fixation systems lead to better anatomical reduction of the fracture and less space between the fragments, which favours faster fracture repair than with external fixation systems.
- **Fracture type**. A simple fracture will repair more quickly than a comminuted fracture.
- **Fragment alignment**. When the fracture reduction is near the ends of the fragments with good apposition and little space between them, the repair process is faster.
- **Age and any systemic diseases affecting the animal**. In a young, healthy animal, a fracture will resolve more quickly than in a mature or geriatric animal. On the other hand, in animals with systemic pathologies such as hyperparathyroidism, diabetes or hypothyroidism, or in those that are receiving treatment with certain drugs, such as corticosteroids, the process may be slower.

In a simple fracture with no initial complications that is repaired by endochondral ossification, it can be expected that **radiographic changes** in the weeks following fracture resolution will usually follow the following sequence (Sande, 1999).

- **Phase 1** (initial occurrence): the surfaces of the fragments are sharp and well defined, and the soft tissues are inflamed.
- **Phase 2** (during the 1st week): the fracture line widens, and the margins of the fragments are blurred. There is minimal early periosteal reaction, and the soft tissues are no longer as inflamed.
- **Phase 3** (during the 2nd and 3rd weeks): the fracture focus narrows, an unstructured bone callus can be visualised and the ends of the fragments are less opaque because there is bone resorption.
- **Phase 4** (from the 4th week until the 8th–10th weeks): the fracture line gradually disappears, and the callus increases in opacity and remodels, making its surface appear smoother.
- **Phase 5** (from 3 months onwards): the callus reduces in volume, and there is total repair (continuity) of the cortices and the trabeculation pattern of the medulla.

Fracture Complications

Complications can arise after the resolution of a fracture. The most common complications are malunion, delay in union or nonunion between fragments, and osteomyelitis (Henry and Cole, 2018).

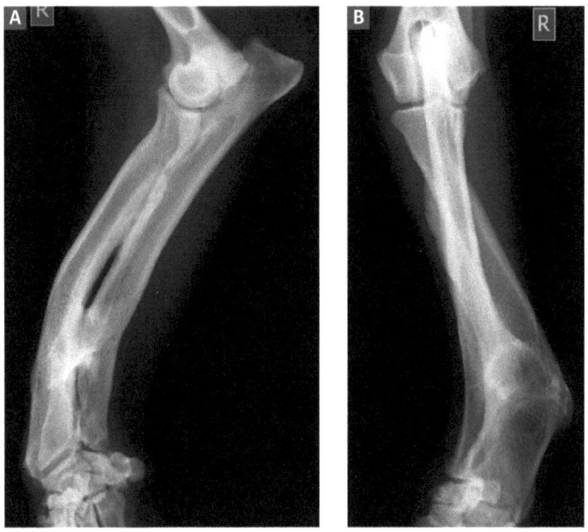

Figure 34. Mediolateral (**A**) and craniocaudal (**B**) radiographs of the ulna and radius of an adult dog presenting with a malunion of an old fracture in the distal part of the middle third of the diaphysis. As a consequence of the malunion, there has been an antecurvatum (A) and valgus (B) deviation.

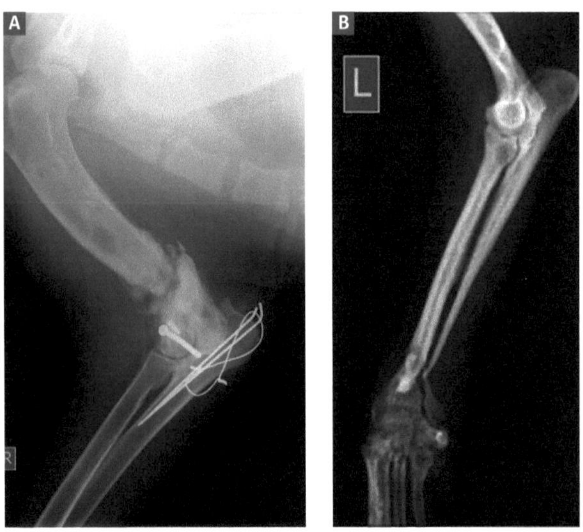

Figure 35. A. Mediolateral radiograph of the humerus of an adult dog in which a biologically active, hypertrophic nonunion in the distal third of the diaphysis of the humerus can be seen; there is evidence of bone callus formation. **B**. Mediolateral radiograph of the ulna and radius of an adult dog in which a biologically inactive, atrophic nonunion is visualised, with pointed and sclerotic fragments at the ends. Note the generalised osteopaenia of the distal fragments and the rest of the bones due to disuse of the limb.

Malunion

When the fragments are not well aligned, the formation of a callus causes abnormal consolidation between the fragments, producing angulation or rotation between them. As a consequence of poor attachment, the proximal or/and distal joint of the fractured bone may undergo angulations, which can be classified depending on their alignment and angulation into valgus, varus, antecurvatum, recurvatum, torsional or translational (Fig. 34).

Delay in Union and Nonunion

In these cases, the fracture line persists and there is an absence of bone callus. This may be mainly due to an inadequate fixation system, a decrease or absence of blood supply to the site or the presence of an infection. In delayed union there is some evidence of bone activity present but union between the fragments takes longer than expected, although with enough time the fracture consolidates. However, if fracture consolidation does not happen, the process evolves to a nonunion, in which the repair of the fracture ceases (from 12 weeks after the fracture occurs) and the fragments do not come together.

Nonunion used to be classified into two possible types, hypertrophic nonunion and atrophic nonunion; however, there is now a **new classification** depending on whether or not the fragments are viable or biologically active (Butterworth, 2016).

Nonunion with Viable or Biologically Active Fragments

- **Hypertrophic nonunion**: the formation of bone callus is visualised at the end of each fragment, which stopped and did not join the fragments. Therefore, the edges of the fragments are smooth, rounded, sclerotic and well defined. The medullary cavity appears closed, showing a radiotransparent line at the fracture site. In the literature, this type of nonunion has been called "elephant foot" or "horse foot", and a pseudojoint with fibrous tissue can form between the fragments (Fig. 35 A).
- **Nonoligotrophic union**: described as a nonunion in which there was no formation of bone callus or the callus is small in size and there is fibrous tissue between the fragments. This type of nonunion is difficult to differentiate from a nonviable nonunion.

Nonunion with Nonviable or Biologically Inactive Fragments

This type is uncommon. Several subtypes have been described: **dystrophic, necrotic** and **atrophic**. In all of them, there is a decrease or total loss of blood supply to one or both fragments, with the ends of the resorbed fragments appearing pointed and the medullary cavity "closed". There may be generalised osteopaenia of the fragments and even of the rest of the bones in the limb due to disuse (Fig. 35 B).

Osseous Infections

Osteomyelitis or bone infection can occur by different mechanisms and, depending on these, is classified as **localised** or **generalised** osteomyelitis (McAllister and Tobin, 2016).

Localised Osteomyelitis

Localised osteomyelitis is associated with penetrating wounds (bites, open fractures), the spread of infections affecting adjacent soft tissues or an iatrogenic cause after surgical procedures with inadequate asepsis.

Radiographic findings in cases of localised osteomyelitis are usually the appearance of "brush border" or "palisade" periosteal reactions, which, with treatment and time, are remodelled into a smooth, continuous periosteal reaction. Osteolytic lesions may also appear and are accompanied by inflammation of the soft tissues adjacent to the bone lesion, in which gas or fistulous tracts may be present (Fig. 36).

Sometimes, although infrequently, **bone sequestrum** can occur. A bone sequestrum is a fragment of dead bone that exhibits increased opacity because its trabeculae have collapsed. Surrounding this fragment there is a radiotransparent area called the involucrum, which consists of granulation tissue. Sequestration is a chronic process that develops over time and usually triggers the formation of an external fistula (Henry and Cole, 2018) (Fig. 37).

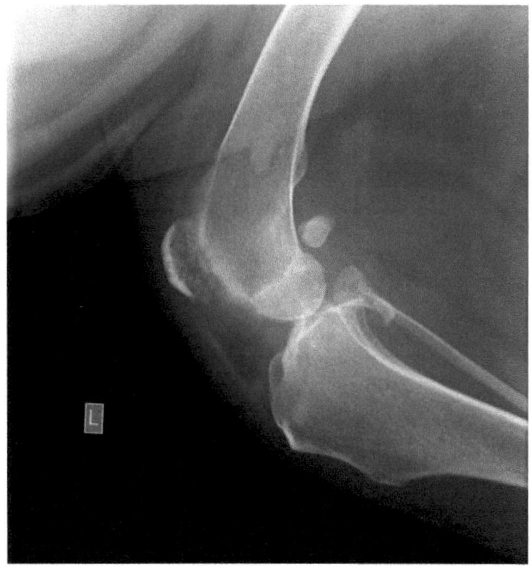

Figure 36. Mediolateral radiograph of the stifle of an adult dog with soft tissue inflammation and infection in the medial aspect of the thigh and stifle, with the presence of fistulas. The image shows an aggressive osteolytic bone lesion affecting the patella, and a periosteal reaction in the cranial cortex of the distal metaphysis of the femur. The diagnosis was osteomyelitis due to the spread of the infection present in the adjacent soft tissues.

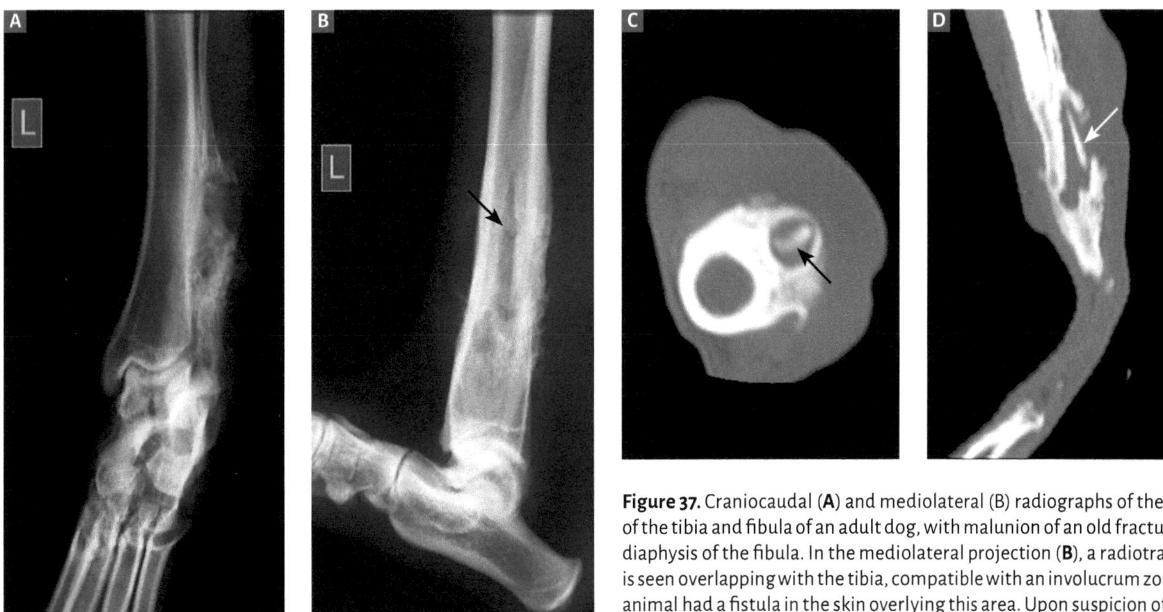

Figure 37. Craniocaudal (**A**) and mediolateral (B) radiographs of the distal portion of the tibia and fibula of an adult dog, with malunion of an old fracture in the distal diaphysis of the fibula. In the mediolateral projection (**B**), a radiotransparent area is seen overlapping with the tibia, compatible with an involucrum zone (arrow); the animal had a fistula in the skin overlying this area. Upon suspicion of bone sequestrum, a CT scan was performed, based on which the presumptive diagnosis of sequestration was confirmed. **C.** CT image in the transverse plane and bone window in which the bone fragment (sequestrum) surrounded by hypoattenuated tissue (involucrum) is observed (arrow). **D.** CT reconstruction in the dorsal plane, in which the length of the sequestrum is visualised (arrow).

Generalised Osteomyelitis

This pathology is caused by pathogens that are transported in the blood, and is therefore also called haematogenous or disseminated osteomyelitis. The causative agents can be, from highest to lowest frequency, bacteria, fungi and protozoa (the latter transmitted by ticks). Animals with weakened immune systems and puppies are more likely to have haematogenous osteomyelitis than healthy adult animals. Radiographically, lesions are observed in the metaphysis of the long bones and appear as poorly defined foci of less opacity than the surrounding bone, accompanied by inflammation of the adjacent soft tissues (Stander and Cassel, 2016) (Fig. 38).

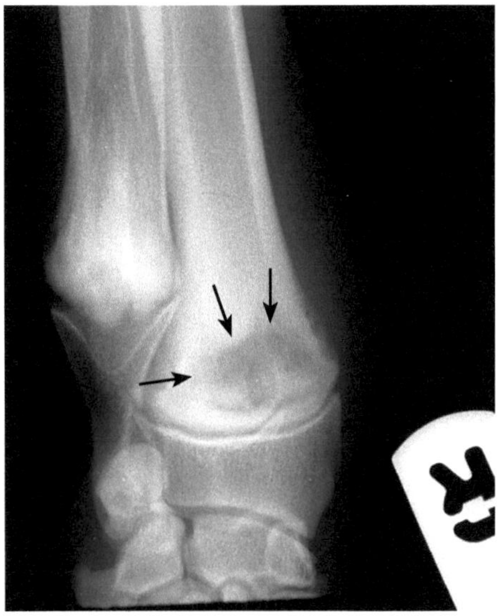

Figure 38. Craniocaudal radiograph of the distal portion of the radius and ulna of a 4-month-old dog with pain and swelling at the ends of the long bones. Two weeks earlier, the animal had suffered a urinary tract infection. The image shows an ill-defined osteolytic lesion in the distal metaphysis of the radius (arrows) with minimal periosteal reaction in the medial cortex. Similar lesions were observed in the metaphysis of other long bones. Bacterial haematogenous osteomyelitis was confirmed by blood culture.

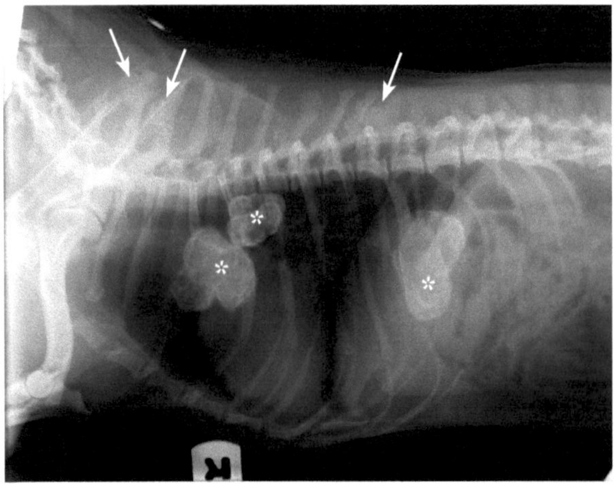

Figure 39. Lateral thoracic radiograph of an adult dog with multiple cartilaginous exostoses (osteochondromatosis). Several bone neoformations are visualised in the ribs (asterisks) and in some of the spinous processes (arrows).

Sometimes it is not possible to distinguish between neoplastic and infectious lesions of the bone on the basis of radiographic images alone. Other factors, such as the age of the animal, clinical history, physical examination and laboratory data should be taken into account, although histopathology will specify the origin of the lesion and is necessary to reach a definitive diagnosis and a prognosis, as well as for the implementation of treatment.

Neoplasia

Benign Bone Neoplasms

- **Osteochondroma** (single location)/**osteochondromatosis** or multiple cartilaginous exostoses (multiple locations): these are uncommon and considered a type of dysplasia rather than a neoplastic process. In the dog, this lesion is located in the metaphysis of the long bones, ribs and costochondral junctions, pelvis and vertebrae (any bone with endochondral ossification) and is hereditary. It is characterised as an expansive lesion, with well-defined margins and a trabeculated interior, which is often disorganised (McAllister and Tobin, 2016) (Fig. 39).
- **Enchondroma**: this is an intramedullary cartilaginous tumour of short tubular bones, usually found in the metacarpals and metatarsal bones of dogs. These tumours expand the bone by thinning the cortices and can cause pathological fractures. They are very rare.

Malignant Bone Neoplasms

Primary Bone Tumour

There are several types of primary bone neoplasms, among which **osteosarcoma** is the most common, while others such as fibrosarcoma, chondrosarcoma, haemangiosarcoma, lymphoma or mastocytoma account for only 5–10% of cases. Adult large- and giant-breed dogs are most predisposed to osteosarcomas, although some studies have confirmed a peak in the appearance of these neoplasms between 18 months and 24 months of age. Pulmonary metastases are common, which worsens the prognosis, so in the presence of a possible osteosarcoma, performing radiographs or CT of the thoracic cavity is indicated to rule out the presence of metastasis. Osteosarcomas are less frequent in the cat than in the dog, and metastases appear more slowly. These tumours are mostly located in the metaphysis of long bones, and they do not usually affect the joint or more than one bone, but there may be exceptions. The radiographic appearance is very variable: periosteal reactions in a spiculated or amorphous model, which have a predominantly osteoproductive nature, may be seen, or lesions may be predominantly osteolytic; however, most commonly, mixed lesions are observed (Fig. 40). As in osteomyelitis, osteosarcoma can cause pathological fractures (Keally et al., 2011).

Bone Metastases

Bone metastases have a low incidence. They have a variable radiographic appearance, although most often they present as solitary osteolytic lesions that can appear in locations where it is unusual for primary bone tumours to appear, such as in the diaphysis of a long bone. In addition, it should be taken into account whether the animal has a clinical history of current or previous neoplasia. Differentiating bone metastasis from a primary bone tumour is not possible by radiographic imaging.

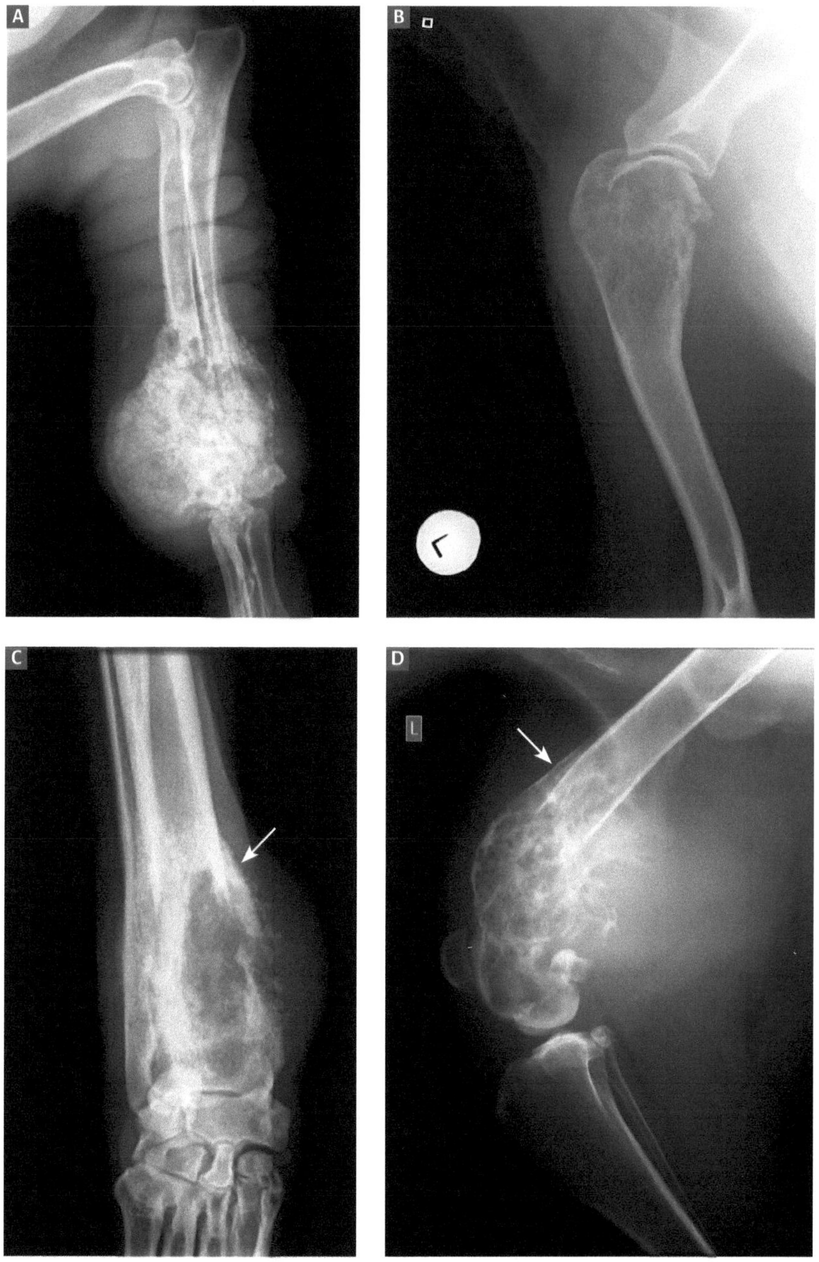

Figure 40. Radiographs corresponding to four primary bone neoplasms with variable appearance, predominantly osteogenic (**A**), osteolytic (**B**) and mixed (**C**, **D**). Note the presence of "Codman's triangle" in images C and D (arrows).

Joint Neoplasms

Synovial Cell Sarcoma

This is a rare periarticular tumour that originates in the synoviocytes of the joint capsule or the sheath of a tendon. It usually affects adult medium- or large-breed dogs and is more common in large joints such as the stifle, shoulder or elbow, although it can occur in any joint (Keally et al., 2011).

Radiographically, marked to severe inflammation of the periarticular soft tissues and osteolytic lesions in the bones that make up the joint are seen, with minimal or no periosteal reaction (Fig. 41). These tumours have a medium potential to metastasise to regional lymph nodes and the lungs. Biopsy is necessary to make a definitive diagnosis and rule out other tumour types such as periarticular histiocytic sarcoma or anaplastic carcinoma, or other types of pathological process such as septic arthritis (Davies et al., 2016).

JOINT PATHOLOGIES

Degenerative Joint Disease

Degenerative joint disease (**DJD**), also referred to as **osteoarthrosis**, is defined as a noninflammatory joint pathology that involves a loss of joint cartilage and can affect one or multiple joints.

It can be **primary**, which is uncommon and has been seen in animals in which there is no apparent reason for them to have joint degeneration, or **secondary**, which is the more common form and develops as a result of a joint being subjected to abnormal stress. Any pathology that interferes with the normal function of a joint can trigger secondary degenerative changes. The first change that occurs is fissuring and fragmentation of the articular cartilage, so it stops protecting the subchondral bone correctly. This causes remodelling changes in the articular surfaces and bone neoformations around the edges of the joint (Keally et al., 2011).

Considering the appearance of a normal joint, it should not be too difficult to find the alterations typical of degenerative joint disease. Thus, a series of **radiographic signs** are established for these pathologies (Fig. 42).

- Changes in the articular surfaces, which are irregular and do not have a uniform and smooth appearance.
- Presence of periarticular neoformations, known as osteophytes.
- Increased intra-articular opacity and synovial volume due to increased production of synovial fluid.
- Changes in the opacity of the subchondral bone; the most common is an increase in opacity, that is, sclerosis of the subchondral bone, although sometimes foci of decreased opacity due to the presence of small subchondral cysts can be seen.
- Changes in the joint space, which may be increased in size

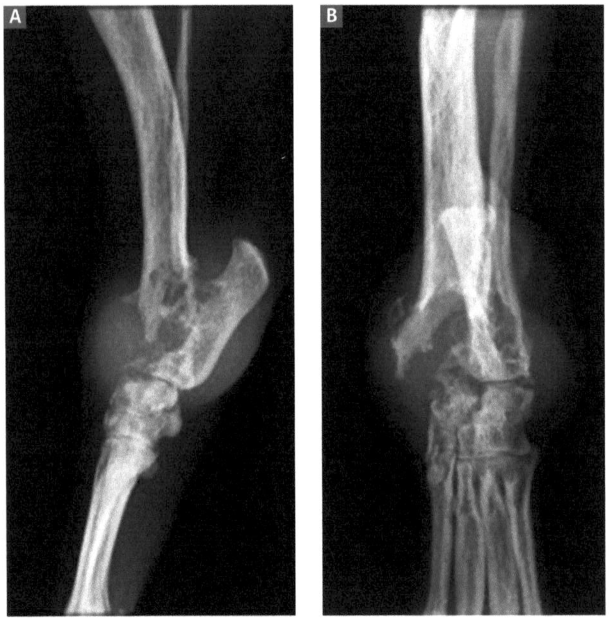

Figure 41. Mediolateral (**A**) and dorsoplantar (**B**) radiographs of the tarsus of an adult dog in which osteolysis of all the bones that make up the tibiotarsal joint is observed, as well as marked inflammation of the periarticular soft tissues. Results of fine-needle aspiration were consistent with synovial cell sarcoma despite this joint not being the most frequent location for this tumour type.

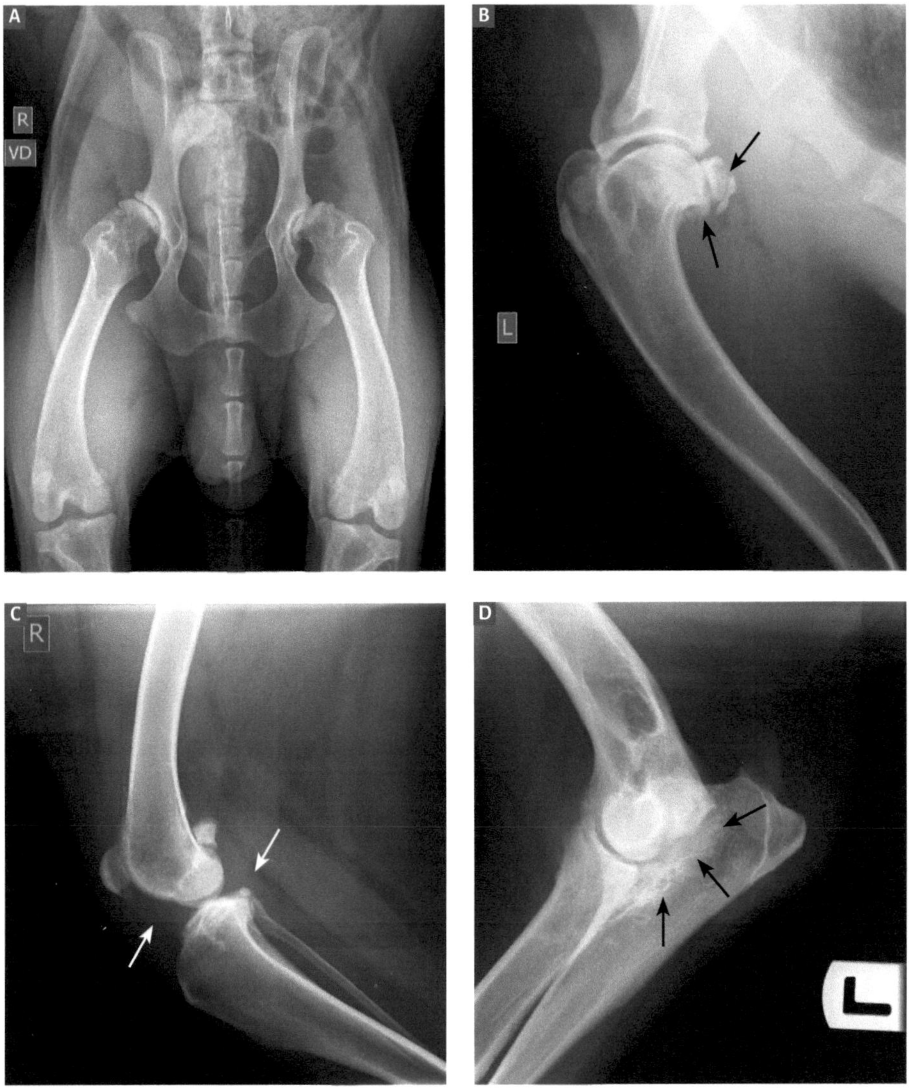

Figure 42. Radiographs of different joints of adult dogs showing radiographic signs of degenerative joint disease. **A**. Ventrodorsal projection of hip joints with irregular articular surfaces. **B**. Mediolateral projection of a shoulder with periarticular bone neoformations (arrows). **C**. Mediolateral projection of a stifle with increased intra-articular opacity (arrows). **D**. Mediolateral projection of an elbow with subchondral sclerosis of the semilunar trochlea of the ulna (arrows).

in cases in which there is abundant synovial effusion, or decreased in chronic cases in which the reduction or even disappearance of the thickness of the articular cartilage causes a smaller joint space to be observed.
- Intra-articular calcifications, which usually correspond to fragments of detached articular cartilage that become mineralised.
- Incongruity of the articular surfaces, which can become subluxations or luxations.

Not all of these signs appear at the same time or in all the joints that are affected; the radiographic appearance always depends on the evolution of the disease and the point in time at which the animal presents for examination.

There are many pathologies found in different joints that can cause degenerative joint disease; those that occur most frequently in cats and dogs will be covered hereunder.

Immune-Mediated Arthritis

The different types of immune-mediated arthritis are rare pathologies. They are classified as erosive or nonerosive depending on whether or not there is involvement of the bones of the joint, or only an inflammatory component in the soft tissue (Davies et al., 2016).

Erosive

The most common type is **rheumatoid arthritis**. It occurs in small breeds of dog (such as the Poodle and the Shetland Sheepdog), with an average age of onset of 4 years (range 1–9 years) and without a sex predisposition.

The joints that are most commonly affected are the carpus and tarsus. The radiographic changes are bilateral, with the presence of osteolytic foci (Fig. 43), loss of bone density, progressive destruction of the bone at the joint margins and an irregular joint space, which can cause subluxations.

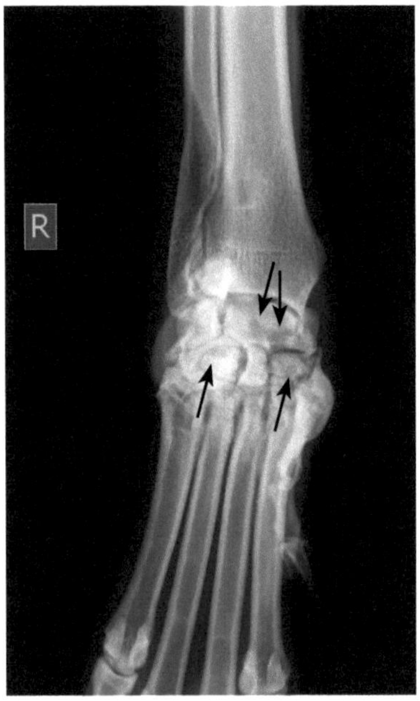

Figure 43. Dorsopalmar radiograph of the carpus of an adult dog with rheumatoid arthritis. Multiple small osteolytic foci are visualised in the carpal bones, especially in the intermedioradial, II and IV (arrows).

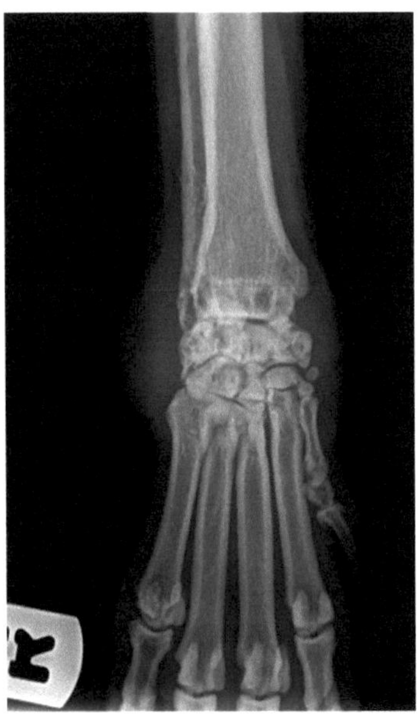

Figure 44. Dorsopalmar radiograph of an adult dog with inflammation and fistulous tracts of the soft tissues of the carpus. Marked inflammation of the soft tissues adjacent to the carpus is seen, especially laterally, and there are osteolytic foci in the carpal bones and in the distal epiphysis of the radius. After sampling by fine-needle aspiration and biopsy, the diagnosis was septic arthritis.

Inflammation of the soft tissues adjacent to the affected joints is also seen (Keally et al., 2011). To reach a definitive diagnosis, differentiation from other types of nonimmune-mediated erosive polyarthritis such as that caused by leishmaniasis, especially in endemic areas, is necessary. To do this, arthrocentesis and analysis of the synovial fluid should be performed, as well as an analysis/test for the rheumatoid factor.

Nonerosive

The changes are not as obvious as in the erosive form, and sometimes the only radiographic alteration that is visualised is inflammation of the periarticular soft tissues. There are no erosive changes in the bones. The animal may present with fever and signs of pain.

The most representative example of this type of pathology is **lupus erythematosus** (Allan and Davies, 2018).

Septic Arthritis

Septic arthritis can be classified as localised or generalised (the latter being less common). **Localised septic arthritis**, as in osteomyelitis, is usually caused by open wounds (bites, trauma), migration of foreign bodies from the skin or surgical procedures (iatrogenic).

Radiographically, moderate to marked inflammation of the periarticular soft tissues is seen, and the presence of osteolytic foci that affect the bones that make up the joint usually stands out (Keally et al., 2011) (Fig. 44). A differential diagnosis must be made with an articular neoplasm (synovial cell sarcoma) and the radiographic image must be interpreted in the context of the physical examination and patient's clinical history, although the definitive diagnosis should be reached by sampling (FNA, analysis of synovial fluid, biopsy).

Other Bone Pathologies

Panosteitis

Canine panosteitis is a condition of unknown aetiology that affects the long bones of large-breed dogs that have rapid bone growth. It usually arises between 5 months and 18 months of age, although it has been described in dogs over 2 years old. The most commonly affected breed is the German Shepherd Dog, and there is a sex predisposition for males.

Insufficient blood supply to the medullary cavity due to inadequate opening of the nutrient foramina, some viral infections or nutritional disorders (diets very high in calories and calcium) have been proposed as possible causes, but none has been proven.

Panosteitis produces pain on deep palpation in the diaphysis of the affected bone, which manifests as intermittent lameness of one or more limbs; it can disappear in one bone only to reappear in another.

Radiographically, panosteitis is characterised by a focal increase in bone opacity (sclerosis) in the medullary cavity of the long bones. The humerus is the most common site of occurrence, followed by the femur, ulna, radius and, finally, the tibia. Radiographic changes are usually seen initially in the vicinity of the nutrient canal and then spread to other areas of the bone.

These focal lesions continue to develop with progressive speckling and thickening of the cortices, and sometimes there is also a focal periosteal reaction (Carrera, 2014). Panosteitis is considered a self-limiting process, and radiographs taken sequentially, over a period of 2–3 months, show a gradual remodelling of the lesions with disappearance of the radiopaque foci (Fig. 45).

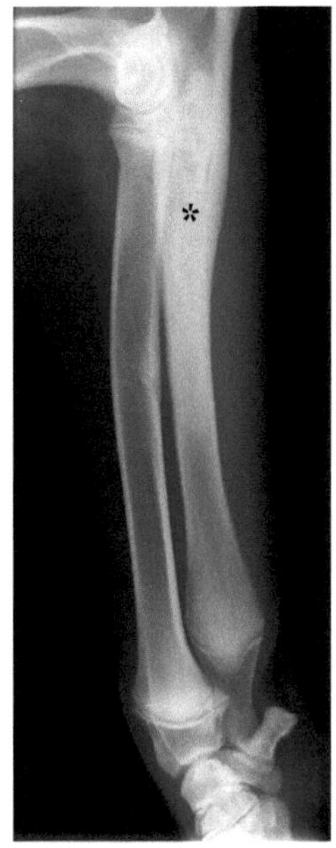

Figure 45. Mediolateral radiograph of the ulna and radius of an 8-month-old Spanish Mastiff with left forelimb lameness. The image shows a marked increase in intramedullary opacity in the middle and proximal third of the diaphysis of the ulna (asterisk) compatible with panosteitis.

Metaphyseal Osteopathy

This is also known as **hypertrophic osteodystrophy**. It affects large-breed dogs with rapid growth between 3 months and 6 months of age. The aetiology is unknown; previously it has been associated with inadequate nutritional supplementation, dietary calcium/phosphorus imbalance and vitamin C deficiency, although the latter has not been proven, and in more recent years an association with canine distemper virus has been proposed.

Lesions are usually located in the distal metaphysis of the ulna and radius, although they can occur in all long bones, in the jaw and even in flat bones such as the scapula and ribs.

Animals show lameness of the affected limbs, sometimes refuse to stand up or move, and show signs of pain when walking and/or on palpation of the metaphyseal areas, which appear inflamed and warm; fever is present in most cases (Pollard and Phillips, 2018). Valgus deviation of the carpus can be a sequel.

Radiographic signs are usually bilateral and symmetrical. The **initial changes** consist of the appearance of a thin radiotransparent band in the metaphyseal area immediately proximal to the physis (growth plate), which is referred to as the "double physis sign" (Fig. 46). Next, there is an increase in the opacity (sclerosis) of the metaphysis. In **more advanced stages**, there is marked development of the metaphysis, with widening, and deposits of periosteal neoformations may appear adjacent to the metaphyseal cortex (Fig. 47).

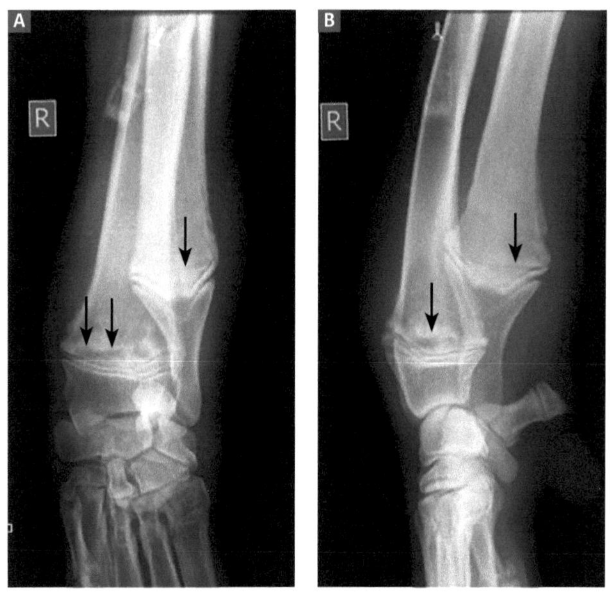

Figure 46. Dorsopalmar (**A**) and mediolateral (**B**) radiographs of the carpus of a 5-month-old Great Dane. The images show a poorly defined radiotransparent band in the distal metaphysis of the radius, immediately proximal to the physis (arrows), corresponding to an initial stage metaphyseal osteopathy lesion ("double physis sign"). A similar band is less evident in the ulna.

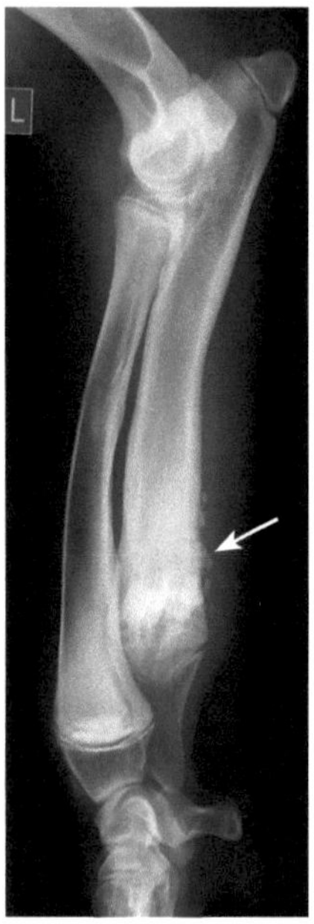

Figure 47. Mediolateral radiograph of the ulna and radius of the same dog shown in Fig. 46, obtained 1 month later. Marked sclerosis is visualised in the distal metaphysis of the ulna that extends proximally, as well as multiple periosteal neoformations in the caudal cortex of the ulna (arrow), resulting from the evolution of metaphyseal osteopathy.

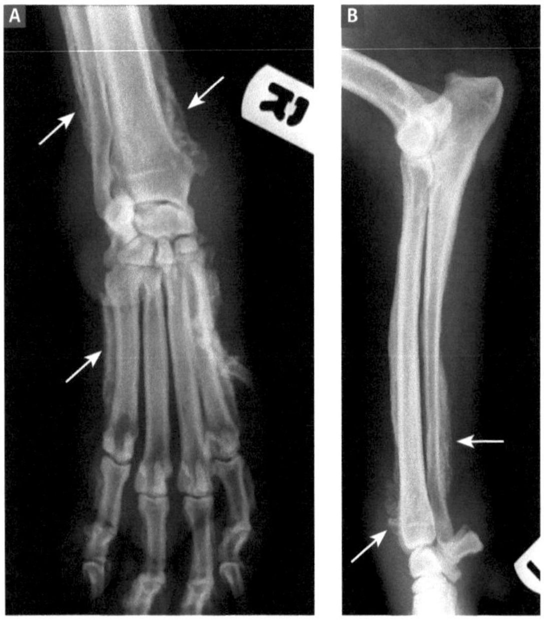

Figure 48. Dorsopalmar radiograph of the right carpus and metacarpus (**A**) and mediolateral radiograph of the ulna and left radius (**B**) of a 10-year-old German Shepherd Dog with hypertrophic osteopathy. Multiple periosteal reactions are visualised in a solid model, with an irregular and smooth surface in the cortices of the ulna, radius and metacarpals (arrows), as well as marked inflammation of the adjacent soft tissues. The lesions were bilateral and symmetrical. Lung masses were observed on thoracic radiographs.

Subsequently, the bone neoformation may converge with the cortex, producing a marked radiopaque widening of the metaphyseal area, which may progress and envelop the diaphysis (Stander and Cassel, 2016).

Hypertrophic Osteopathy

Hypertrophic osteopathy is a syndrome characterised by periosteal proliferation along the long bones that begins in the distal part of the limbs (metacarpals, metatarsals and phalanges). It is an acquired bone disorder that appears secondary to other processes, mainly as a paraneoplastic syndrome associated with primary lung tumours. It has also been described to be associated with metastatic lung tumours and oesophageal tumours, as well as other primary extrathoracic tumours (usually in the abdomen) and even nontumourous masses, such as lung abscesses and granulomas of fungal or parasitic origin (Allan and Davies, 2018). The clinical history of affected dogs typically includes alternating lameness or resistance to movement. All four limbs are usually affected, with swollen, warm and painful both carpi and tarsus.

The presumptive diagnosis of hypertrophic osteopathy is made by observation of radiographs of the affected bones, which show periosteal reactions in a continuous model, either a palisade (Fig. 11) or a solid model with an irregular or smooth surface (since, depending on the time that has elapsed since the reaction began to be evident, remodelling occurs) (Fig. 48). Lesions begin distally and extend proximally, are bilateral and symmetrical, and are accompanied by inflammation of the adjacent soft tissues. In cases where these signs are observed, a radiographic study of the thoracic cavity is indicated to search for the underlying cause and, if thoracic radiographs appear normal, radiography and ultrasonography of the abdomen should be performed (McAllister and Tobin, 2016).

Leishmaniasis

Leishmaniasis, apart from producing cutaneous, renal and ocular changes, can also cause orthopaedic problems, which manifest as lameness due to polyarthritis, polymyositis and/or bone injuries.

In the joints, these are usually bilateral injuries, which mainly affect the carpi and the stifles. The lesions that can be observed are small osteolytic foci in the subchondral bone with a "moth-eaten" pattern and inflammation of the periarticular soft tissues, creating an image of an erosive polyarthritis (Fig. 49). In the long bones, a small periosteal reaction has been observed in an irregular solid model, as well as increased intramedullary opacity (Agut et al., 2003).

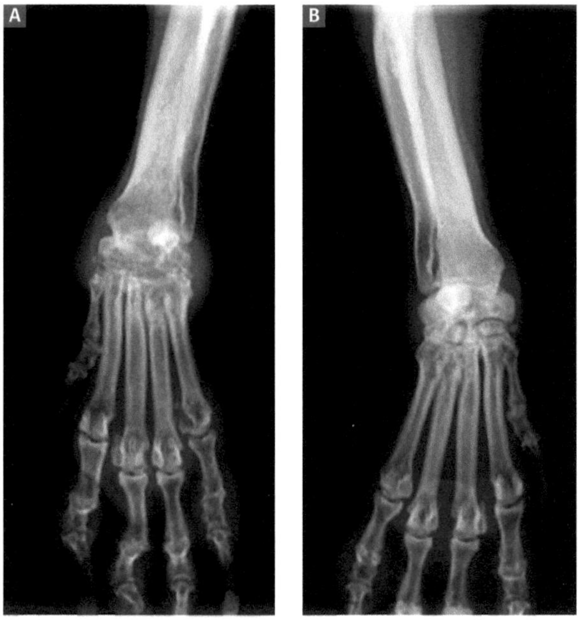

Figure 49. Dorsopalmar radiographs of the right (**A**) and left (**B**) carpus of an 11-year-old, 4 kg mixed-breed dog. Osteolytic foci are seen in the carpal bones, which are mild in the left carpus and very severe in the right, with loss of bone morphology and marked periarticular inflammation. Lesions are also observed in the proximal area of the metacarpals and the distal area of metacarpal V. After performing arthrocentesis for analysis of synovial fluid, Leishmania amastigotes were detected inside macrophages, confirming the cause of the polyarthritis.

Bone Cyst

Bone cysts are very rare and usually benign. They mostly affect young dogs. A cyst appears as a well-defined area of reduced opacity. They originate in the metaphysis, causing an expansive lesion of the bone. There is loss of the normal bony trabeculae, and there may be septa inside and thinning of the cortices, but no associated inflammatory reaction. Because the cyst weakens the bone, pathological fractures may occur near the cyst (McAllister and Tobin, 2016).

Bibliography

- Agut, A., Corzo, N., Murciano, J., et al. (2003) Clinical and radiographic study of bone and joint lesions in 26 dogs with leishmaniasis. *Vet Rec*, 153(21):648–652.
- Agut, A., Haro, P., Soler, M., et al. (2008) What is your diagnosis? Multiple epiphyseal dysplasia. *J Am Vet Med Assoc*, 233(8):1235–1236.
- Allan, G., Davies, S. (2018) Radiographic signs of joint disease in dogs and cats. In: Thrall, D.E. (ed). *Textbook of Veterinary Diagnostic Radiology*. 7th ed, pp. 403–433. Elsevier Saunders.
- Barreiro, A., Vila, M. (2014) Interpretación radiológica del sistema óseo. In: Agut, A. (ed). *Diagnóstico por Imagen en Pequeños Animales*, pp. 109–122. Multimédica Ediciones Veterinarias.
- Brown, E.A., Dickinson, P.J., Mansour, T., et al. (2017) *FGF4* retrogene on CFA12 is responsible for chondrodystrophy and intervertebral disc disease in dogs. *Proc Natl Acad Sci U S A*, 114(43):11476–11481.
- Burk, R., Feeney. D. (2003) The appendicular skeleton. In: *Small Animal Radiology and Ultrasound. A Diagnostic Atlas and Text*. 3rd ed, pp. 477–606. Saunders.
- Butterworth, S.J. (2016) Long bones – fractures. In: Kirberger, R.M., McEvoy, F.J. (eds), *BSAVA Manual of Canine and Feline Musculoskeletal Imaging*. 2nd ed, pp. 133–155. BSAVA.
- Carrera, I. (2014) Enfermedades del desarrollo. In: Agut, A. (ed). *Diagnóstico por Imagen en Pequeños Animales.*, pp. 163–173. Multimédica Ediciones Veterinarias.
- Davies, S., Allan, G., Nicoll, R. (2016) Joints – general. In Kirberger, R.M., McEvoy, F.J. *BSAVA Manual of Canine and Feline Musculoskeletal Imaging*. 2nd ed, pp. 156–170. BSAVA.
- Henry, G.A., Cole, R. (2018) Fracture healing and complications in dogs. In: Thrall, D.E. (ed). *Textbook of Veterinary Diagnostic Radiology*. 7th ed, pp. 366–389. Elsevier Saunders.
- Hough, S., Avioli, L.V., Muir, H., et al. (1988) Effect of hypervitaminosis A on the bone and mineral metabolism of the rat. *Endocrinology*, 122(6):2933–2939.
- Keally, J.K., McAllister, H., Graham, J.P. (2011) Bones and joints. In: *Diagnostic Radiology and Ultrasonography of the Dog and Cat*. 5th ed, pp.351–446. Elsevier Saunders.
- Langley-Hobbs, S. (2012) Musculoskeletal oddities in the cat: an overview of some curious causes of lameness. *J Feline Med Surg*, 14(1): 31–42.
- Martínez, S., Fajardo, R., Valdés, J., et al. (2006) Histopathologic study of long-bone growth plates confirms the basset hound as an osteochondrodysplastic breed. *Can J Vet Res*, 71(1):66–69.
- McAllister, H., Tobin, E. (2016) Long bones – mature. In: Kirberger, R.M., McEvoy, F.J. (eds). *BSAVA Manual of Canine and Feline Musculoskeletal Imaging*. 2nd ed, pp. 108–132. BSAVA.
- Morgan, J.P. (1993) *Techniques of Veterinary Radiography*. 5th ed, pp. 3–272. Iowa State University Press.
- Pollard, R.E., Phillips, K.L. (2018) Orthopedic diseases of young and growing dogs and cats. In: Thrall, D.E. (ed). *Textbook of Veterinary Diagnostic Radiology*. 7th ed, pp. 348–365. Elsevier Saunders.
- Rubenstein, J.D., Christakis, M.S. (2006) Case 95: Fracture of double-layered patella in multiple epiphyseal dysplasia. *Radiology*, 239(3):911–913.
- Sande, R. (1999) Radiography of orthopedic trauma and fracture repair. *Vet Clin North Am Small Anim Pract*, 29(5):1247–1260.
- Soler, M., Agut, A. (2014) Traumatismos. Fracturas. In: Agut, A. (ed). *Diagnóstico por Imagen en Pequeños Animales*, pp. 175–186. Multimédica Ediciones Veterinarias.
- Stander, N., Cassel, N. (2016) Long bones – juvenile. In: Kirberger, R.M., McEvoy, F.J. (eds). *BSAVA Manual of Canine and Feline Musculoskeletal Imaging*. 2nd ed, pp. 87–107. BSAVA.
- Thrall, D.E. (2018) Principles of radiographic interpretation of the appendicular skeleton. In: Thrall, D.E. (ed). *Textbook of Veterinary Diagnostic Radiology*. 7th ed. pp. 334–347. Elsevier Saunders.

Notes

327

Radiographic Diagnosis, Computed Tomography and Magnetic Resonance Imaging of the Limbs

Marta Soler Laguía

Forelimb

Scapula

Projections

- **Mediolateral** (ML): the animal is positioned in lateral recumbency with the side under study on the table; generally, it is necessary to use a grid, although this will depend on the size of the animal. The head and cervical spine should be moved cranially and dorsally, the limb being studied should be pulled cranially and the unaffected contralateral limb should be positioned with the elbow in slight flexion. This position allows the neck of the scapula and the shoulder joint to be assessed; however, study of the rest of the scapula is difficult due to the overlap of part of the thorax and the spine (Barreiro and Vila, 2014) (Fig. 1).
- **Mediolateral "swimmer's" view**: this is a variation of the ML projection, which aims to avoid overlap with the vertebrae in order to better visualise the body and the spine of the scapula. For this projection, the affected limb is pulled cranially and dorsally, and the head and neck of the animal are placed over the limb in a ventral direction (Fig. 2).
- **Caudocranial** (CdCr): the animal is positioned in dorsal recumbency, the affected limb is stretched cranially by pulling it, trying to position the scapula as parallel to the table as possible, and the unaffected limb is held cranially or caudally, slightly rotating the patient's body to the unaffected side (Morgan, 1993) (Fig. 3).

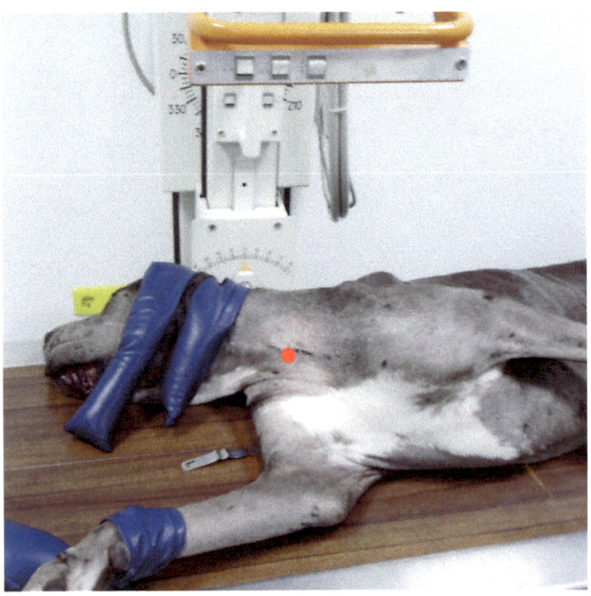

Figure 1. Positioning for performing a ML projection of the scapula. The X-ray beam should be focused on the scapula at the point indicated by the red dot.

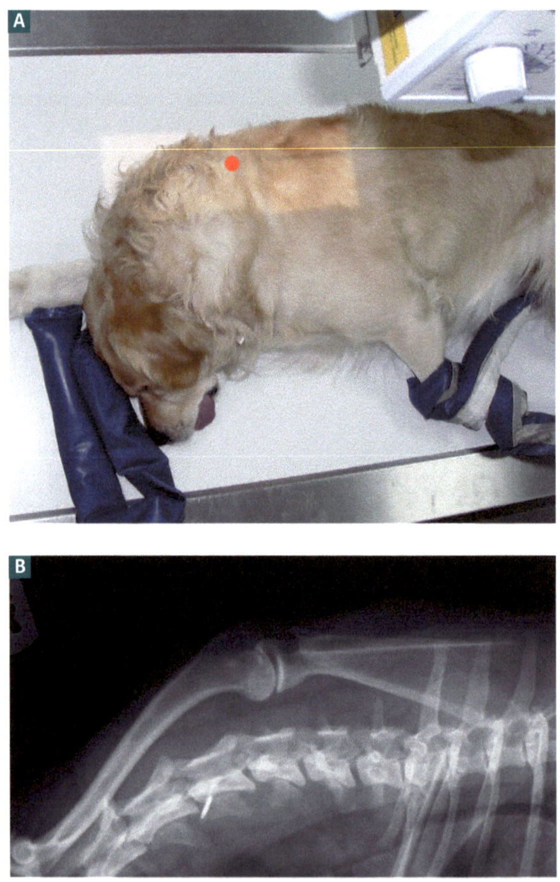

Figure 2. Positioning for performing a ML "swimmer's" projection of the scapula (**A**) and the resulting radiographic image (**B**). The red dot in (A) indicates the point at which the X-ray beam should be focused .

Trauma: Fractures and Avulsions

Fractures and avulsions of the scapula are not usually very common, but they often occur due to road traffic accidents. Fractures can affect any part of the scapula, although they are more likely to occur in the neck and body than in the spine of the scapula. In young animals in which the acromion has not yet fused to the rest of the scapula, avulsions of the acromion tuberosity may be seen (Fig. 4). Nowadays, computed tomography (CT) is also usually performed to obtain further detail of the fracture, avoiding overlaps with other anatomical structures and at the same time exploring neighbouring areas, such as the vertebrae, ribs and lungs, that may have suffered traumatic damage (Fig. 5).

Tumours

Neoplasms in the scapula are rare in both dogs and cats. Animals show lameness, although the first sign of the presence of a neoplasm is a mass or bulge in the adjacent soft tissues. As in any other bone, the most common type of neoplasm is **osteosarcoma**, although others, such as chondrosarcoma, haemangiosarcoma, soft tissue sarcoma and histiocytic sarcoma, can occur. Thoracic radiographs should be performed to check for pulmonary metastases, as osteosarcoma in particular is very aggressive and highly metastatic (Montinaro et al., 2013) (Fig. 6).

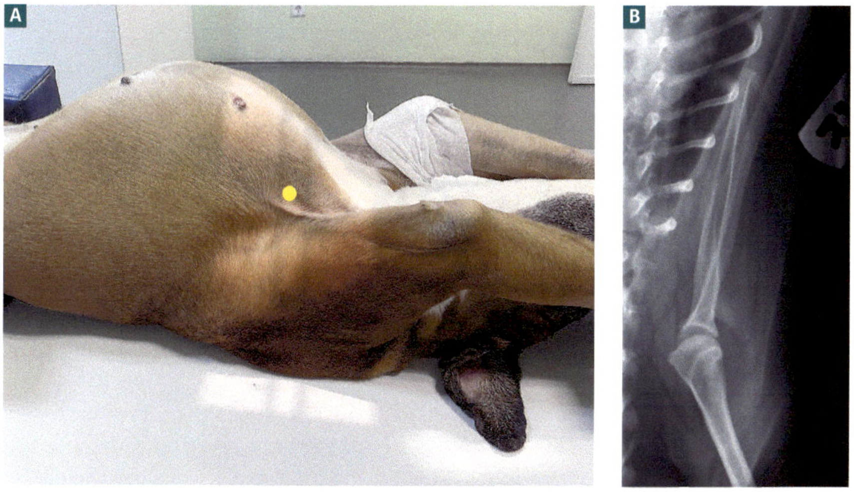

Figure 3. Positioning for a CdCr projection of the scapula (**A**) and the resulting radiographic image (**B**). The yellow dot in (A) indicates the point at which the X-ray beam should be focused.

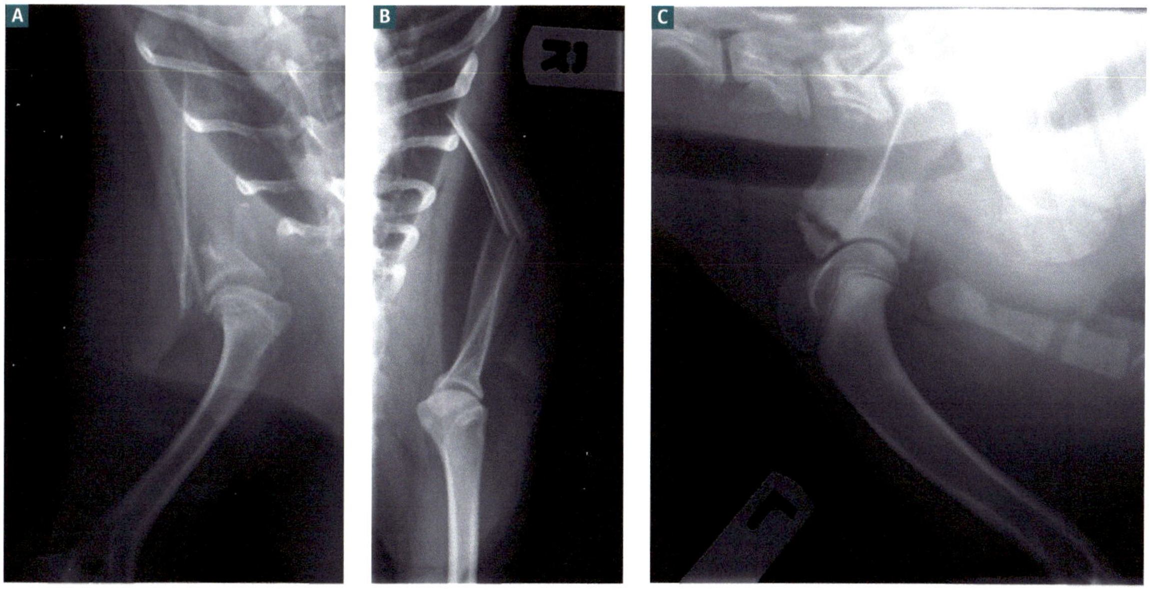

Figure 4. Radiographs of scapular fractures. **A**. Neck of scapula. **B**. Scapular body. **C**. Avulsion of the acromion tuberosity in a young animal.

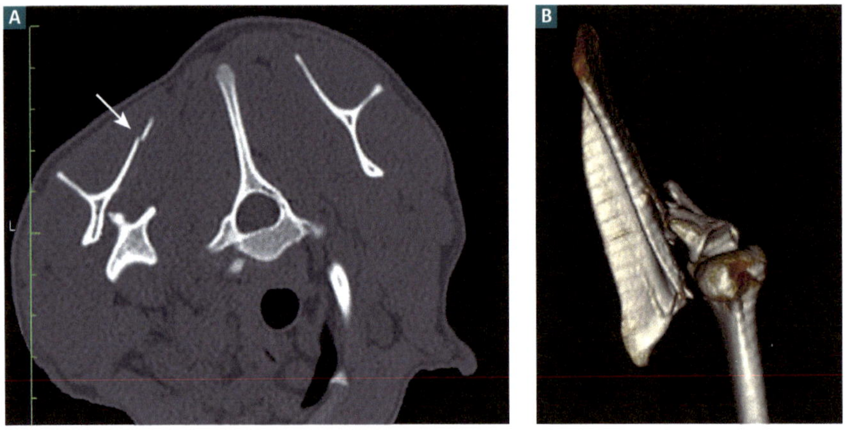

Figure 5. CT image in a transverse plane and bone window (**A**) and three-dimensional reconstruction using volume rendering (**B**) of a dog with a fracture of the scapular neck. A fracture can also be seen in the cranial border of the scapula (arrow).

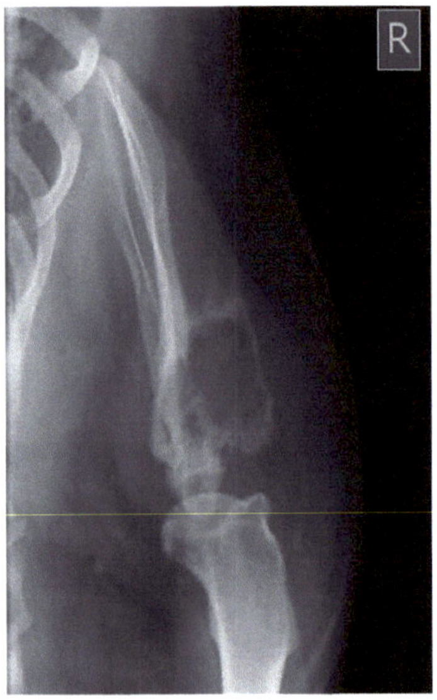

Figure 6. CdCr radiograph of the scapula of an adult dog with an osteolytic lesion showing a geographic model with irregular edges, compatible with an aggressive bone lesion of a neoplastic nature.

Shoulder Joint

Projections

- **Mediolateral** (ML): similar to that described for a ML scapula projection, but the X-ray beam is focused on the joint at the level of the acromion with collimation of the joint region (Fig. 7).
- **Caudocranial** (CdCr): similar to that described for a CdCr scapula projection, but the X-ray beam is focused on the joint and with collimation of the joint region (Barreiro and Vila, 2014) (Fig. 7).
- **Tangential/"skyline"**: the animal is positioned in sternal recumbency with the head elevated, ideally above the shoulders. The unaffected limb is flexed at the elbow and raised to head height. The limb being studied must be flexed at the shoulder and elbow at the same time, displacing the carpus outwards. The X-ray beam is focused on the intertubercular groove of the humerus (Barreiro and Vila, 2014) (Fig. 8).

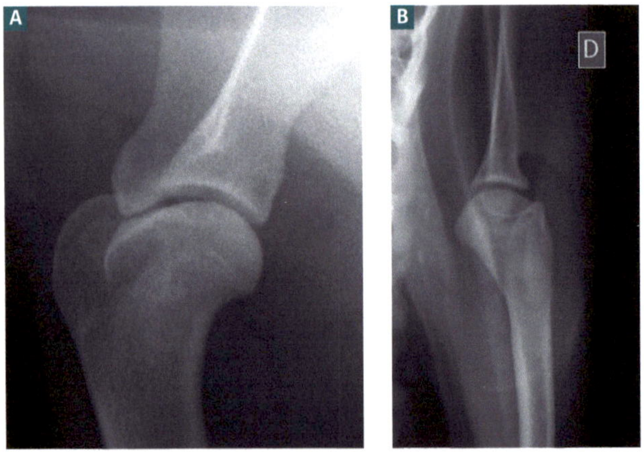

Figure 7. ML (**A**) and CdCr (**B**) radiographs of the shoulder of an adult dog without abnormalities.

Osteochondrosis/ Osteochondritis Dissecans

Osteochondrosis (OC) is a developmental disease that causes alterations in the joint surfaces of weight-bearing joints. It is most common in large and giant breeds of dog with rapid growth rates, which usually develop the pathology and clinical signs between 5 months and 10 months of age. At a pathophysiological level, there is a failure in endochondral ossification of the articular surface. Some authors consider that local ischaemia triggers the entire process as it causes necrosis of the articular cartilage, producing an intracartilaginous separation between mineralised and nonmineralised layers of articular cartilage, which leads to abnormal thickening of the cartilage that can become necrotic (Pollard and Phillips, 2018). Cracks may develop in the cartilage, resulting in flaps or

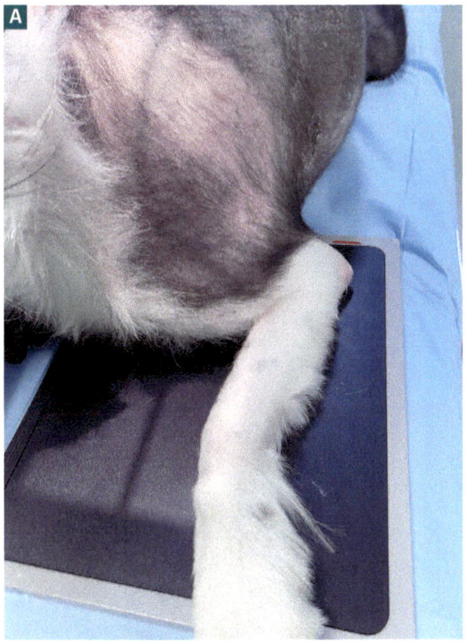

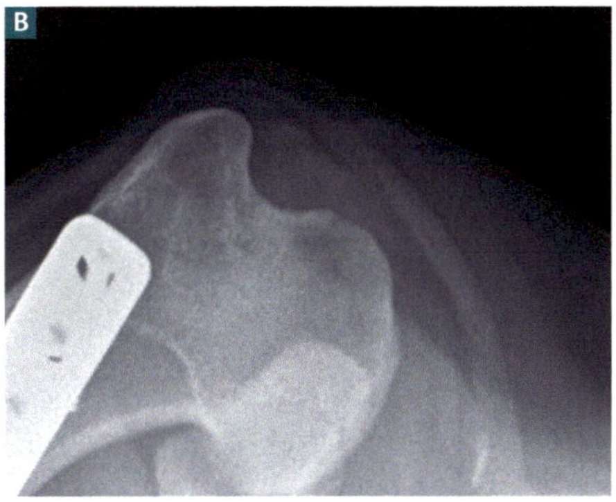

Figure 8. A. Image showing the correct positioning to perform a skyline projection of the shoulder. **B**. The resulting radiograph.

fragments of cartilage, which are radiologically visible if they are mineralised. When a cartilaginous fragment separates from the adjacent subchondral bone and mineralises, the disease is called **osteochondritis dissecans** (OCD). If left untreated, it usually progresses to degenerative joint disease (DJD). It is common for it to occur bilaterally, although the animal is lame on only one limb (Pollard and Phillips, 2018).

In addition to the shoulder, in which the caudal portion of the head of the humerus is mainly affected, other joints can be affected by this pathology.

- **Elbow**: the lesion is visualised at the medial level of the trochlea of the humerus.
- **Stifle**: the pathology can be seen in both the lateral and medial condyles, but the lateral condyle is affected more often.
- **Tarsus**: the medial border and, to a lesser extent, the side of the trochlea of the talus are affected.

The radiographic signs that are observed are (Pollard and Phillips, 2018) (Fig. 9):

- **radiotransparent defects** of the subchondral bone with flattening of the articular surface, surrounded by a halo of sclerosis of the subchondral bone
- the presence of a **mineralised joint flap/fragment**, also referred to as a "joint mouse"
- **degenerative joint changes**, which are often the only radiological sign when the affected joint is the elbow or tarsus.

In the case of the shoulder, arthrography was commonly used in the past as a diagnostic tool as it was an especially useful technique to highlight this type of injury when flaps of cartilage are not evident due to the lack of calcification, or to identify cartilaginous fragments in the caudal sac or around the bicipital tendon. Nowadays, when this pathology is suspected but is not completely evident in the radiographic image, **CT** is normally used; this latter technique is much more sensitive to early bone changes (Fig. 10).

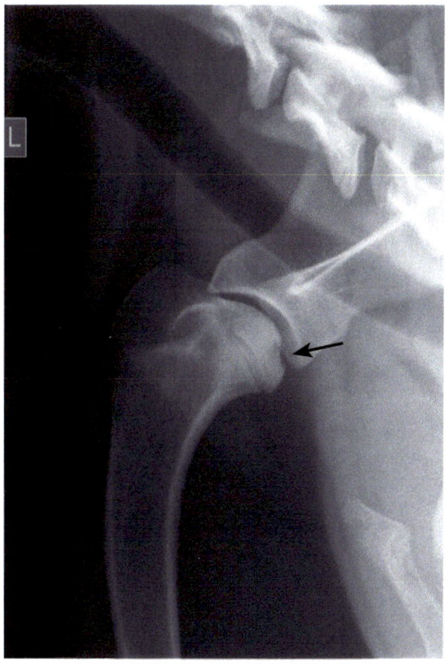

Figure 9. ML radiograph of the shoulder of an immature dog with osteochondrosis. There is a loss of the rounded morphology of the caudal surface of the head of the humerus, which presents a slight depression and hypodense area, with adjacent sclerosis (arrow).

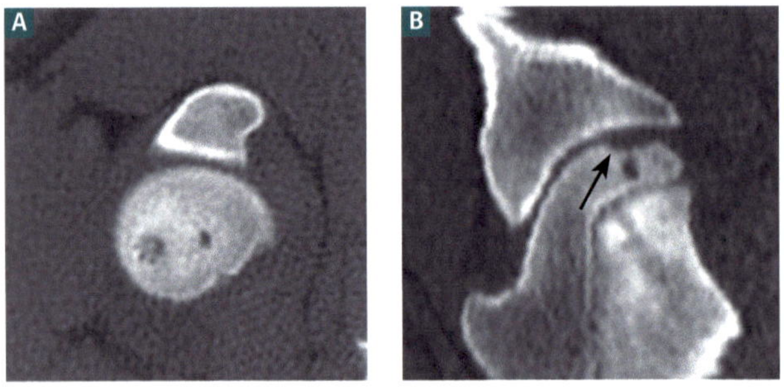

Figure 10. Transverse plane CT image (**A**) and sagittal plane reconstruction (**B**) of the shoulder of a 6-month-old Boxer with osteochondrosis. Small hypoattenuated foci are visualised in the head of the humerus, in addition to a loss of its rounded morphology, with a depression caudally (arrow).

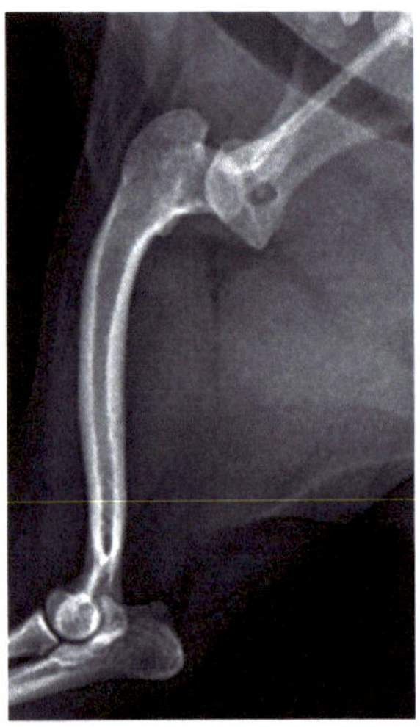

Figure 11. ML radiograph of the shoulder of a dog with a congenital luxation. Incongruence of the articular surfaces is visualised, with the head of the humerus displaced medially and craniodorsally, overlapping with the scapula, which presents an anomalous flattened conformation of the glenoid cavity. (Image courtesy of Dr. A. Navarro, Nexo Menescal Novelda.)

Congenital Shoulder Luxation

Congenital shoulder luxation is a rare pathology that has generally been described in small-breed dogs (Miniature Poodle) (Barreiro and Vila, 2014). The clinical signs become especially evident when animals reach 3–4 months of age, and a nonpainful mechanical lameness becomes apparent. Radiographically, there is medial displacement of the head of the humerus, which may appear enlarged and flattened, as well as flattening or convexity of the glenoid cavity of the scapula (Fig. 11).

MRI in Shoulder Pathologies

Magnetic resonance imaging (MRI) of the shoulder is one of the most common uses of musculoskeletal MRI in dogs, because shoulder disorders are not always caused by bone lesions that can be easily diagnosed by radiography or CT. MRI provides superb soft tissue contrast and resolution. Ultrasonography may also be used to evaluate the soft tissues of the shoulder joint but is limited by its small field of vision and inability to evaluate the structures of the medial compartment of the shoulder joint.

MRI of the shoulder allows visualisation of all components of the joint: the joint capsule, articular cartilage, tendons (supraspinatus, infraspinatus, bicipitalis, teres minor, subscapularis and glenohumeral), muscles and bones. In addition, adjacent areas such as the caudal cervical spine and brachial plexus structures can be evaluated at the same time (Zalcman et al., 2018) (Figs. 12 and 13).

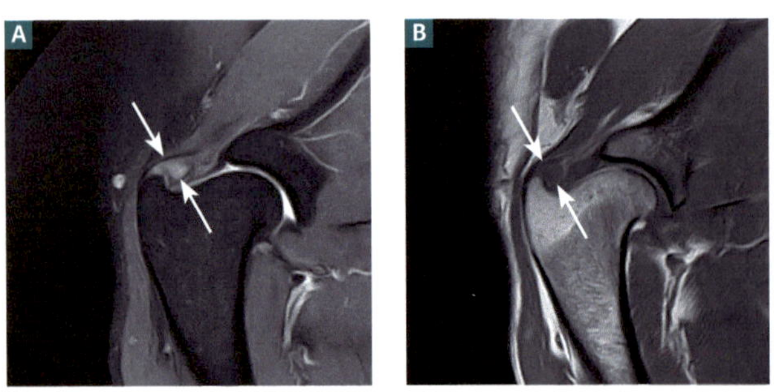

Figure 12. MRI images in a dorsal plane enhanced in T2 (**A**) and T1 (**B**), in which the insertion of the supraspinatus tendon is seen without abnormalities (arrows). (Images courtesy of Dr. A. Ansón, Tufts University.)

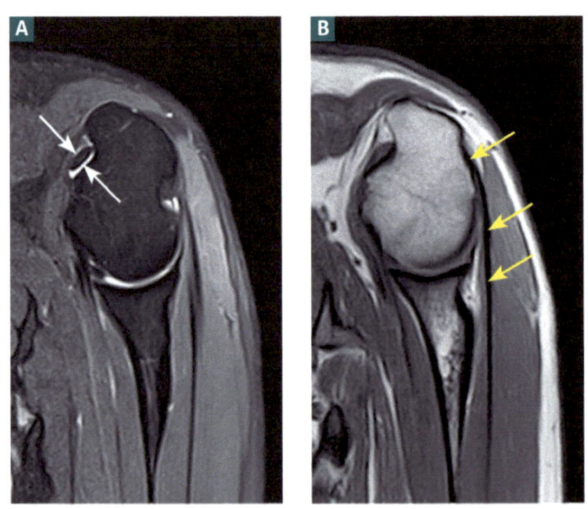

Figure 13. MRI images in a transverse plane enhanced in T2 (**A**) and T1 (**B**), in which the biceps tendon (white arrows) and the infraspinatus tendon (yellow arrows) are visualised without abnormalities. (Images courtesy of Dr. A. Ansón, Tufts University.)

Supraspinatus Tendinopathy

Supraspinatus tendinopathy is a condition that usually affects large-breed dogs. It can range from an incidental finding to the animal presenting pain on shoulder flexion, causing chronic intermittent lameness of the affected limb. The aetiology is unknown, although there are factors that contribute to the disease (e.g. age, trauma, excessive movement) that cause myxomatous degeneration, cartilaginous metaplasia and the formation of an area of disorganised collagen fibres in the tendon. It may present mineralisation; thus, it is also called **calcifying tendinopathy of the supraspinatus**. The increase in size of the supraspinatus tendon can cause medial displacement of the biceps tendon from the bicipital groove and result in pain (Spall et al., 2016) (Figs. 14 and 15).

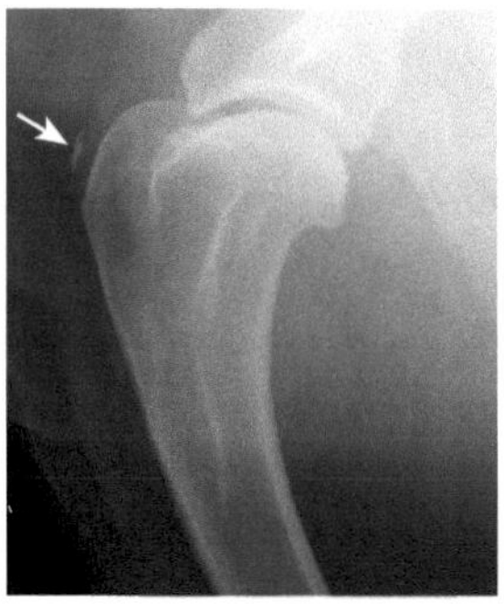

Figure 14. ML radiograph of the shoulder of an adult dog in which a mineralisation can be seen in the area of insertion of the tendon of the supraspinatus muscle (arrow). In this case it was an incidental finding.

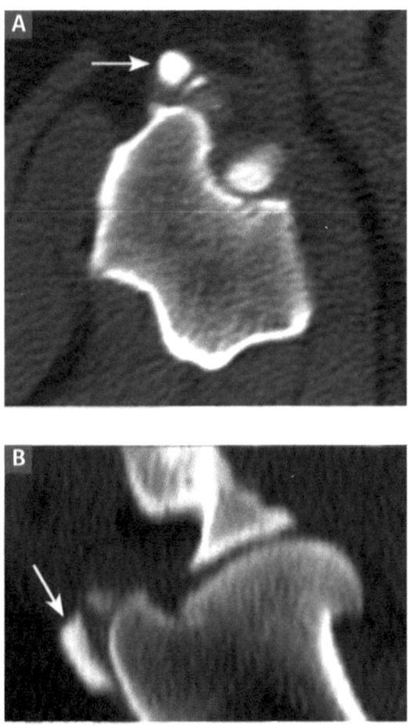

Figure 15. CT image in a transverse plane (**A**) and reconstruction in a sagittal plane (**B**) of the right shoulder of a 7-year-old, 40 kg mixed-breed dog with lameness in the right forelimb, which presented a calcifying tendinopathy of the supraspinatus. Hyperdense mineralised areas (arrows) are visualised cranially to the greater tubercle of the humerus where the supraspinatus tendon is located.

Brachial Biceps Tendon Tenosynovitis

Inflammation of the tendon and synovial sheaths is usually caused by direct irritative processes due to pre-existing pathologies (supraspinatus tendinopathy, OC, presence of joint mice, degenerative joint conditions, etc.) or as a result of traumatic rupture of the bicipital tendon. Radiographically, degenerative changes or the presence of joint mice can be detected in the bicipital groove, as well as calcification of the synovial membrane. Occasionally, osteolysis can be seen at the point of insertion of the tendon into the supraglenoid tubercle. Arthrography and ultrasonography can be of great help in identifying the presence of nonmineralised cartilage fragments, checking the condition of the tendon and showing the presence of adhesions within the tendon sheath, although MRI is becoming relevant for the diagnosis of this type of pathology (Pollard and Phillips, 2018) (Fig. 16).

Elbow Joint

Projections

See also Morgan (1993).

- **Mediolateral** (ML): the animal is positioned in lateral recumbency with the joint under study on the table; the contralateral limb is withdrawn caudally. This projection can be obtained in a neutral position by flexing the elbow between 45° and 90°, in forced flexion by flexing the joint to the maximum, and in extension by pulling the limb cranially (Fig. 17).

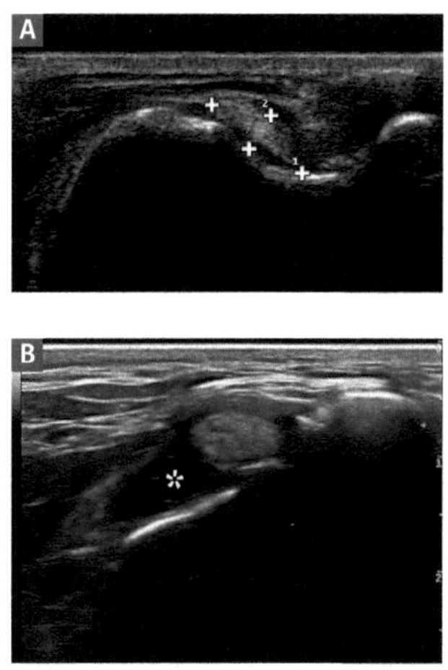

Figure 16. A. Ultrasound image of a normal bicipital tendon (between crosses) in the transverse plane. **B.** Ultrasound image of a patient with bicipital tendon tenosynovitis. An increase in the echogenicity of the tendon and marked presence of synovial fluid in the bursa (asterisk) are visualised in the transverse plane.

- **Craniocaudal** (CrCd): the animal is placed in sternal recumbency in the "sphinx position"; the head is raised and tilted to the opposite side to the affected limb. It is not normally necessary to use the grid, so the elbow to be radiographed is placed on the plate and, to avoid rotation, a piece of foam can be placed under the elbow (Fig. 18).
- **Caudocranial** (CdCr): a CdCr projection can be obtained by positioning the animal in the same way as for a CdCr shoulder projection, but centring the X-ray beam on the elbow.
- **Cranio 15° lateral–caudomedial oblique**: this projection is not usually performed on a regular basis. It is useful to better assess the medial aspect of the trochlea of the humerus and the area around the medial coronoid process. The animal is positioned as for a CrCd projection but the limb is turned inwards (medially) (Fig. 19).

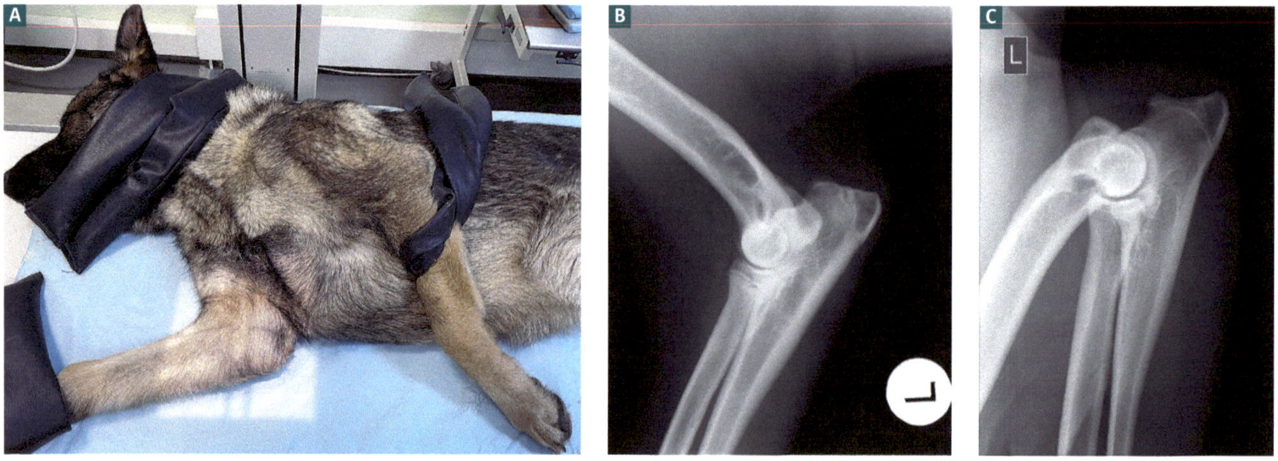

Figure 17. A. Positioning for performing neutral ML radiography of the elbow. **B**. The resulting radiographic image. **C**. Radiographic image obtained with forced flexion.

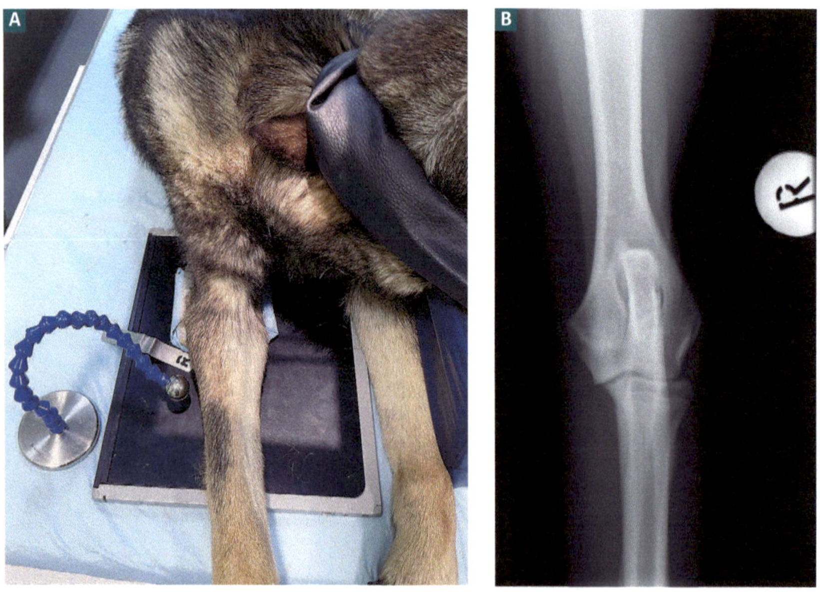

Figure 18. A. Positioning for a CrCd elbow projection. **B**. Corresponding radiographic image.

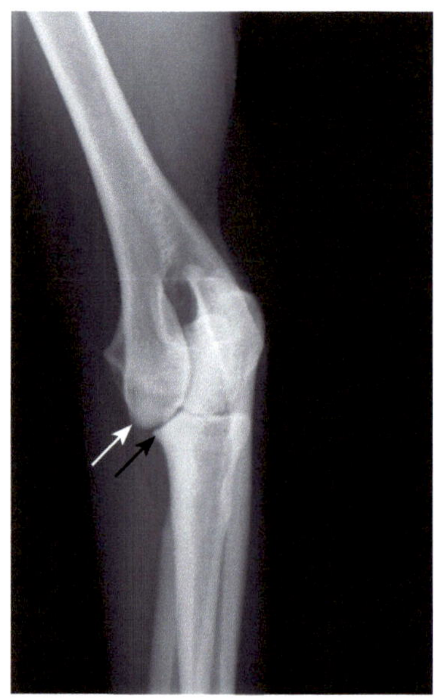

Figure 19. Cranio 15° lateral–caudomedial oblique radiograph of the elbow of an adult dog without abnormalities. This projection evaluates the articular surface of the medial aspect of the trochlea of the humerus (white arrow) and the region around the medial coronoid process (black arrow).

Elbow Dysplasia

Elbow dysplasia is the most common cause of lameness of the forelimb in the dog. It encompasses several developmental diseases that affect the elbow joint, including **nonunion of the anconeal process, fragmentation of the coronoid process, OC of the medial aspect of the trochlea of the humerus** and **joint incongruence** (Soler et al., 2015). These pathologies may or may not occur together, but the presence of only one is sufficient for the use of the term elbow dysplasia, which describes a misalignment of the articular surfaces of the elbow. There are authors who also include incomplete ossification of the humeral condyle as a cause of elbow dysplasia.

The International Elbow Working Group recommends performing several radiographic projections of the elbow to study its articular surfaces and make a diagnosis of elbow dysplasia. These projections include ML in flexion and extension, CrCd and cranio 15° lateral–caudomedial oblique. However, due to the overlap that exists between the radius and the ulna, it is sometimes difficult to visualise certain pathologies, especially those of the medial compartment, which is why CT is currently used to study the elbow joint when it is suspected that the animal may have elbow dysplasia.

Nonunion of the Anconeal Process

Nonunion of the anconeal process affects large-breed dogs and is very common in the German Shepherd. Other predisposed breeds are the Bernese Mountain, Mastiff, Rottweiler and Saint Bernard. In these cases, the anconeal process (which is an accessory ossification centre) does not fuse to the olecranon, as would be expected, at 5 months of age (in German Shepherd and other breeds somewhat later, at 5.5 months). In certain animals, excessive growth of the radius or a delay in the growth of the ulna causes the lateral portion of the humeral condyle to create a force in the proximal direction, causing excessive pressure on the anconeal process. This hinders the endochondral ossification of the cartilage, causing the nonunion of the anconeal process. Over time, this abnormality gives rise to DJD. Radiologically, if an ML projection is carried out in forced flexion to avoid the superimposition of the medial epicondyle of the humerus on the anconeal process region, a defect or radiotransparent line is observed that separates the anconeal process from the olecranon; usually, no other imaging technique is needed to reach a diagnosis (Michelsen, 2013) (Fig. 20).

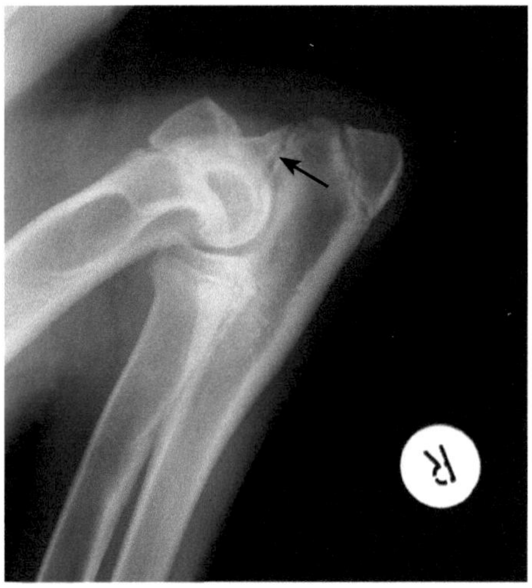

Figure 20. ML radiograph of the elbow of a 6-month-old German Shepherd Dog with nonunion of the anconeal process (arrow).

Fragmentation of the Medial Coronoid Process

Fragmentation of the medial coronoid process (FMCP) is the most common pathology affecting the elbow joint and therefore the most frequent cause of elbow dysplasia. Currently, many authors use the terminology **medial compartment disease**, which encompasses fragmentation or fissuring of the medial coronoid process and also abnormalities of the articular cartilage and subchondral bone of the medial coronoid process and the medial aspect of the humeral condyle. It is a very common pathology in young animals, seen at around 4–13 months of age (although clinical signs are frequently observed between 4 months and 6 months of age) in large breeds such as the Labrador, Rottweiler, Chow Chow, German Shepherd, Irish Wolfhound, Saint Bernard and Bullmastiff, and there seems to be a greater predisposition in males than in females (Cook and Cook, 2009). Fragmentation of the coronoid process is attributed to a delay in the growth of the radius relative to the ulna and is associated in many cases with OC of the medial humeral condyle, which causes a poor distribution of loads in the joint (Soler et al., 2015).

Radiographically, the free fragment of the coronoid process in the medial area (in a CrCd projection of the elbow) is not usually visualised due to the overlap of the radial head and its variable degree of mineralisation. Sometimes a step between the radial head and the coronoid process can be seen in the lateral projection, but in this view, it is very difficult to visualise fragments. Diagnosis is usually guided by the presence of radiographic signs associated with the joint instability caused by this pathology (osteophytic reaction at the proximal end of the anconeal process, in the medial aspect of the humeral condyle and in the cranial aspect of the radial head, sclerosis of the trochlear notch in the ulna, humeroradial incongruence, etc.) (Fig. 21). In theory, the radiographic projection that best shows FMCP is the cranio 15° lateral–caudomedial oblique view (Fig. 22); however, the best means of diagnostic imaging to visualise this pathology is CT.

Computed Tomography Findings

To be able to detect CT abnormalities related to FMCP, knowledge of the **normal tomographic anatomy** of the elbow joint is essential (Fig. 23).

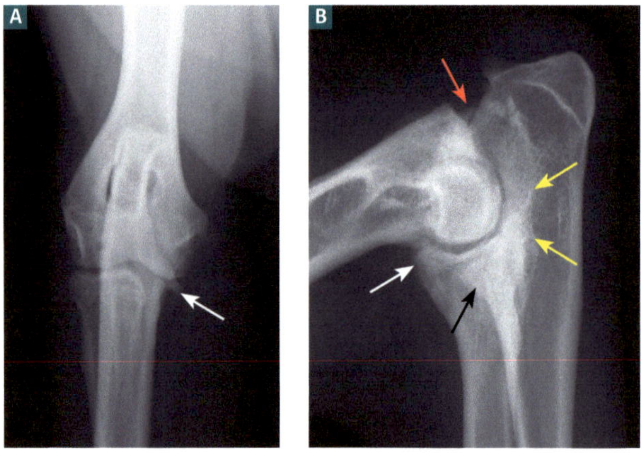

Figure 21. CrCd (**A**) and ML (**B**) radiographs of the elbow of a 7-month-old Labrador with fragmentation of the medial coronoid process confirmed after arthroscopy. In the CrCd projection, an osteophyte is visualised in the projection area of the medial coronoid process (MCP) (arrow), as well as an irregular surface of the medial aspect of the humeral condyle. The ML projection shows an irregular cranial surface of the head of the radius with abnormal morphology (white arrow), a bone neoformation dorsal to the anconeal process (red arrow) and sclerosis of the subtrochlear notch of the ulna (yellow arrows), as well as a hypodense line that could correspond to the fragmentation of the MCP (black arrow).

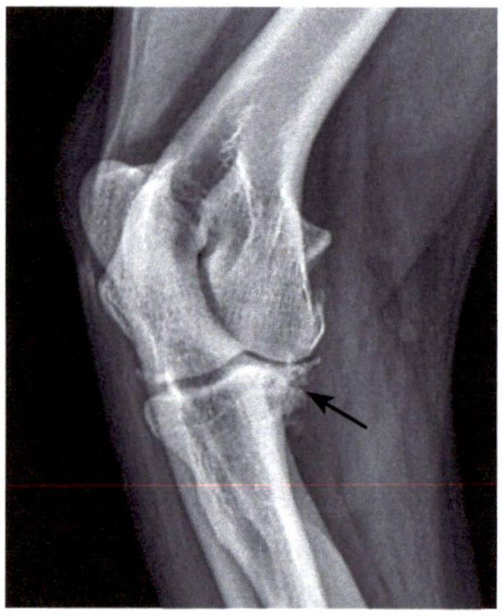

Figure 22. Cranio 15° lateral–caudomedial oblique radiograph of the elbow of a 6-month-old dog with fragmentation of the medial coronoid process that was confirmed by CT, in which an irregular surface with bone neoformation and the fragmented medial coronoid process itself can be observed (arrow). (Image courtesy of A. Navarro, Nexo Menescal Novelda.)

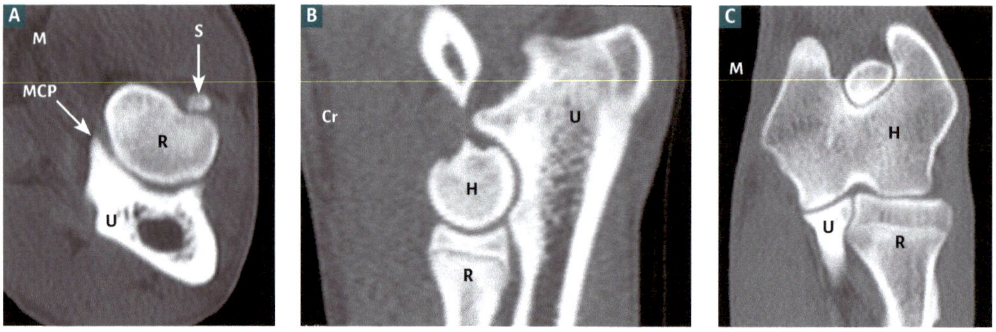

Figure 23. CT images in a bone window, in the transverse plane (**A**) at the level of the medial coronoid process (MCP), and reconstructions in the sagittal (**B**) and dorsal (**C**) planes to assess the joint congruence of a normal elbow of a 7-month-old dog. R: radius, U: ulna, H: humerus, S: sesamoid of supinator muscle (not always present), M: medial, Cr: cranial.

In the transverse plane, findings concerning the medial coronoid process are variable: they can range from changes in its shape and/or a decrease in attenuation to subtle lines due to fissures or fragmentation with or without displacement of the fragment. At the level of the radial notch of the ulna, an irregular surface and the presence of small subchondral cysts can be observed. In the sagittal and dorsal planes, a greater or lesser degree of articular incongruence can be seen, with a small step between the proximal articular surfaces of the radius and ulna. Finally, and depending on each case, there will be changes related to DJD, such as osteophytosis and subchondral bone sclerosis (Villamonte-Chevalier, et al., 2015) (Fig. 24).

Osteochondrosis/Osteochondritis Dissecans Affecting the Medial Aspect of the Humeral Trochlea

In the elbow joint, the medial area of the humeral trochlea is the usual site of presentation of OC/OCD. It most often affects large-breed dogs, especially Rottweilers and Golden Retrievers, with a bilateral presentation being common. The radiographic signs of OC are similar to those previously described for OC of the shoulder: visualisation of a radiotransparent defect in the subchondral bone of the medial surface of the humeral trochlea or the loss of its convex shape, so that it appears flatter or even concave, together with a more radiopaque

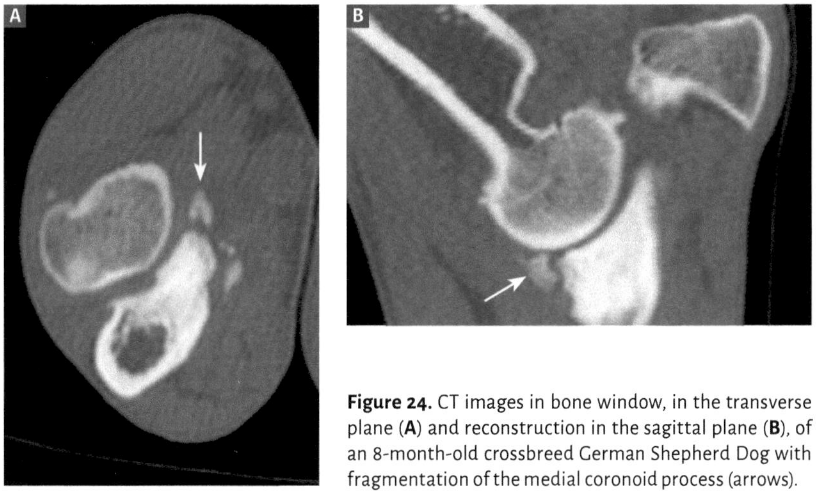

Figure 24. CT images in bone window, in the transverse plane (**A**) and reconstruction in the sagittal plane (**B**), of an 8-month-old crossbreed German Shepherd Dog with fragmentation of the medial coronoid process (arrows).

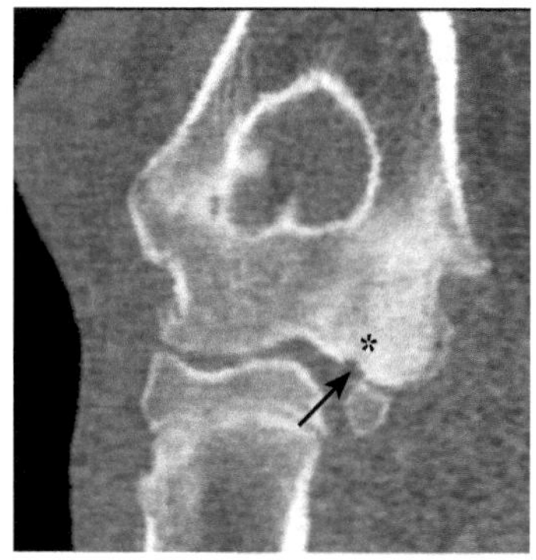

Figure 26. CT image, reconstructed in the dorsal plane, of the elbow of a 9-month-old Mastiff. There is marked sclerosis of the medial aspect of the humeral condyle (asterisk) as well as a small hypoattenuated focus in the subchondral bone and a defect in the articular surface (arrow). These findings are compatible with osteochondrosis.

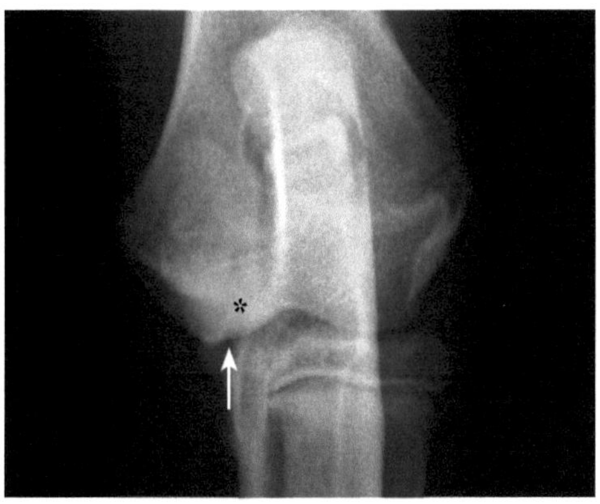

Figure 25. CrCd radiograph of the elbow of a 6-month-old Dogue de Bordeaux. The image shows sclerosis of the subchondral bone of the medial aspect of the humeral trochlea (asterisk) and a small radiotransparent focus in the articular surface (arrow) compatible with osteochondrosis.

area of subchondral sclerosis (Fig. 25). On rare occasions, a small mineralised joint mouse is visualised. Secondary signs of DJD as a result of OC/OCD are commonly found, with the presence of osteophytes on the margins of the articular surfaces. It is estimated that in 12% of cases, OC appears together with FMCP (Soler et al., 2015).

Sometimes it is difficult to show the radiographic changes when the disease is in its early stages and other techniques are necessary to reach a diagnosis. Changes similar to those described in conventional radiography can be observed by CT but are detectable in the initial stages of the disease due to the greater sensitivity and resolution of this modality. Hypoattenuated defects in the articular surface surrounded by subchondral sclerosis (hyperattenuated area) can be visualised (Samii et al., 2011) (Fig. 26).

Articular Incongruence

Articular incongruence is a pathology in which the articular surfaces of any of the components of the elbow joint (humeroradial, humeroulnar or both) have an altered alignment. It is observed in young animals from 4 months of age and in most cases it occurs together with other abnormalities such as nonunion of the anconeal process, disease of the medial compartment or OC. In the event of suspicion of an articular incongruence of the elbow joint, ML and CrCd projections should be obtained, but the X-ray beam should not be focused on the joint but should cover the entire length of the ulna and radius, and the carpal joint should also be evaluated. Thus, it can be observed whether, in addition to a step between the radius and the ulna at the proximal level, there is some alteration at the level of the distal growth plates of these bones and some deformity of these bones or of the carpus. A CT evaluation in multiplanar reconstructions, in both the sagittal and dorsal planes, can be used to more reliably examine whether there is a discrepancy between the proximal articular surface of the radius and that of the ulna (Soler et al., 2015) (Fig. 27).

Incomplete Ossification of the Humeral Condyle

Incomplete ossification of the humeral condyle (IOHC) is an inherited disorder affecting purebred and crossbred Springer Spaniels, resulting in a higher than normal incidence of condylar fractures associated with normal activity, and DJD of the elbow. The humeral condyle has two ossification centres (lateral portion: trochlea; medial portion: capitulum) that should fuse at 12 weeks of age.

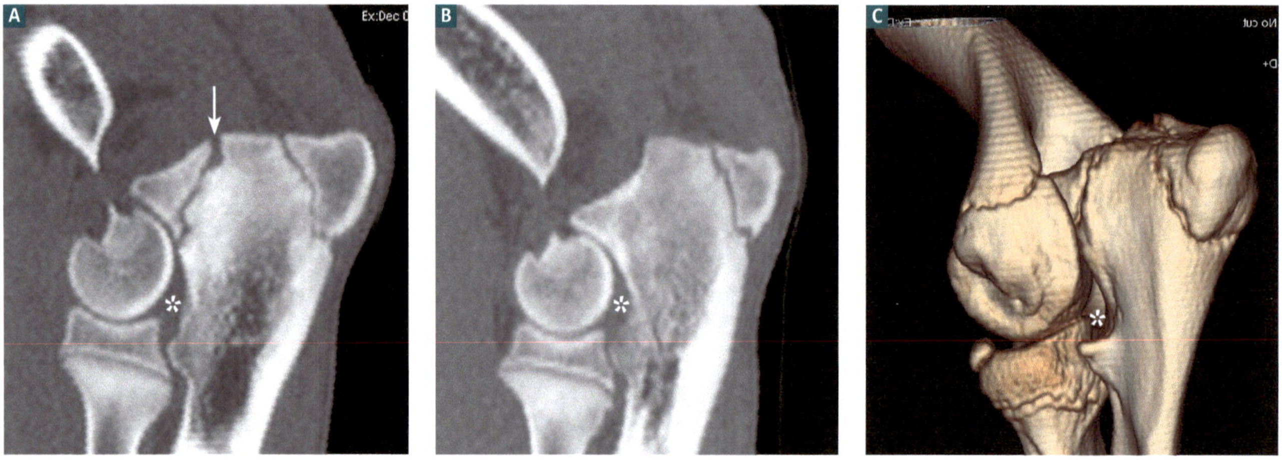

Figure 27. Reconstructed CT images in the sagittal plane (**A**, **B**) and a volume rendering reconstruction (**C**). In both elbows, a humeroulnar incongruence is visible, with loss of the normal curvature of the trochlear notch of the ulna (asterisk). In addition, in one of the elbows (A) a nonunion of the anconeal process is observed (arrow).

Radiographically, a vertical radiotransparent line can be observed in the intercondylar region, which can extend from the margin of the subchondral bone of the trochlea to the distal edge of the supratrochlear foramen. There seems to be a greater predisposition in males than females. Both elbows should be assessed because IOHC is usually bilateral. The best way to diagnose this pathology early is by CT, because it cannot always be clearly visualised on a CrCd radiograph, sometimes because it is not very pronounced or because the olecranon overlaps it (Carrera et al., 2008) (Fig. 28).

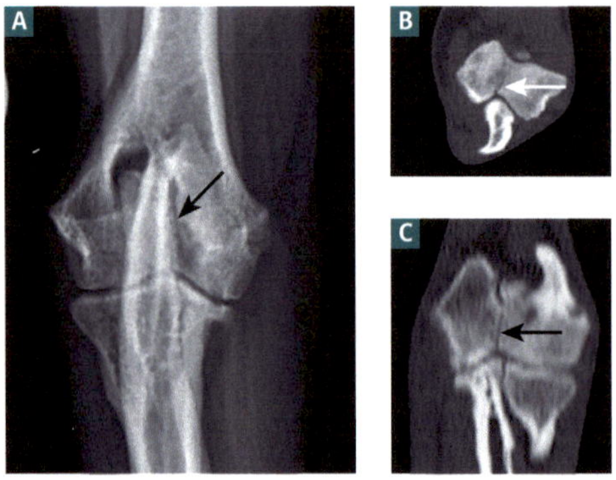

Figure 28. A. CrCd radiograph of the elbow in which a radiotransparent line can be seen in the middle of the humeral condyle. **B**. Transverse plane CT image in a bone window. **C**. CT reconstruction in the dorsal plane. In (B) and (C), a thin hypoattenuated line (arrow) is observed, indicating the incomplete ossification of the humeral condyle. (Images courtesy of A. Navarro, Nexo Menescal Novelda.)

As in the case of the hip, there is a scale for classifying elbow dysplasia:

- **Grade 1 dysplasia: medium osteoarthritis with the presence of osteophytes of <2 mm on any surface of the elbow.**
- **Grade 2 dysplasia (moderate osteoarthritis): with osteophytes of 2–5 mm in one or more of the locations described.**
- **Grade 3 dysplasia (severe osteoarthritis): with osteophytes of >5 mm in one or more of the locations described for the other two grades.**

Fractures

The articular fractures with the highest incidence in the elbow are condylar (intercondylar) and supracondylar fractures of the humerus (Fig. 29), and fractures of the olecranon (Fig. 30) (Barreiro and Vila, 2014). The lateral portion of the humeral condyle (capitulum) is fractured most frequently. In young animals it corresponds to a type III or IV Salter–Harris fracture, as described in Chapter 18.

Luxations

Elbow luxations are of congenital or traumatic origin, the latter being more frequent.

Two grades for **congenital luxations** have been established (Milton and Montgomery, 1987).

- **Grade I** (radial head luxation): affects a wide variety of small breeds (especially chondrodystrophic breeds); seen sporadically in large breeds. Luxation of the head of the radius occurs in a caudolateral direction, leaving the humeroulnar joint relatively normal. Sometimes it results in a clinically silent subluxation. It can result from damage to the growth plate of the ulna or an alteration of the intra-articular ligaments, among other causes. The head of the radius may appear to have a flattened or convex articular surface (Fig. 31).
- **Grade II**: occurs in miniature breeds. Clinical signs may start from birth or go unnoticed until 2–3 months of age. It occurs as a result of aplasia of the medial collateral ligament, causing hypoplasia of the anconeal and coronoid processes. The ulna is rotated 45–90° laterally.

Ulna and Radius

Agenesis of the Ulna/Radius

In puppies, it is possible to observe complete or partial agenesis or hypoplasia of a long bone. The most frequently involved bones are the radius, ulna, tibia and fibula, although the metacarpals and metatarsals may also be affected. If the ulna or radius is affected, the longitudinal growth of the forelimb is severely restricted. Agenesis of the ulna leads to deformation of the radius, and vice versa, causing serious malformations in the elbow and carpal joints.

Premature Closure of the Physis of the Ulna or Radius

Correct growth of the forelimb is dependent on synchrony in the development of the ulna and radius. Any disorder that alters the growth rate of one of the bones will have serious consequences in the proximal and distal joints. Premature closure of the distal physis (growth plate) of the ulna causes shortening of the ulna with arching of the radius (radius curvus) and incongruence in the elbow and carpal joints (carpal valgus) (Fig. 32). Early closure of the distal and/or proximal physis of the radius causes shortening, with incongruence in the elbow joint and deformity in the carpus (carpal varus).

Cartilage Retention (Endochondral)/ Cartilaginous Nucleus

Cartilage retention primarily affects the distal epiphyseal cartilage of the ulna in large and giant breeds of dog between 6 months and 12 months of age, and usually occurs along with

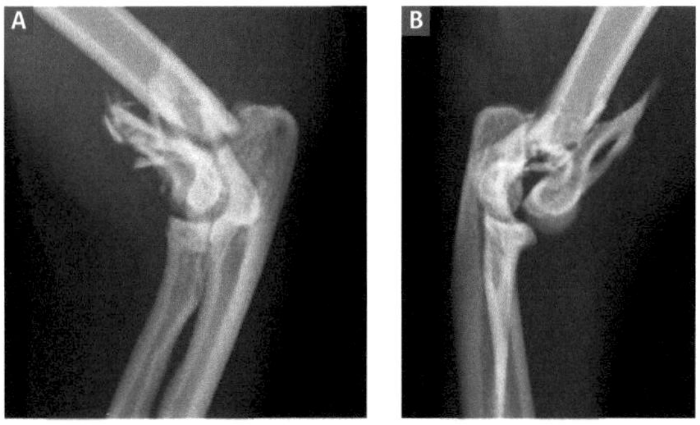

Figure 29. ML (**A**) and CrCd (**B**) radiographs of a cat with supracondylar and intercondylar fractures of the elbow.

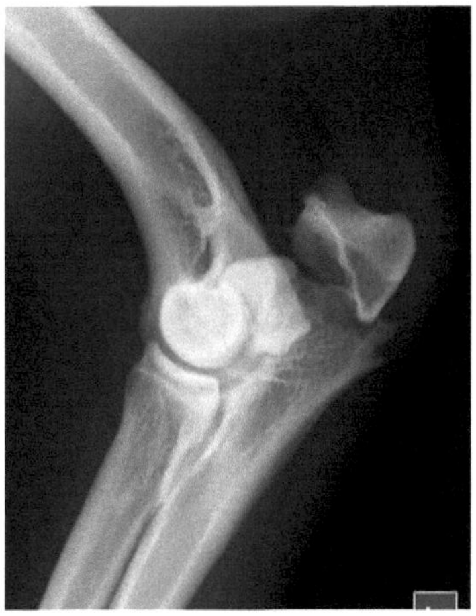

Figure 30. ML radiograph of the elbow of a 3-year-old dog with an olecranon fracture.

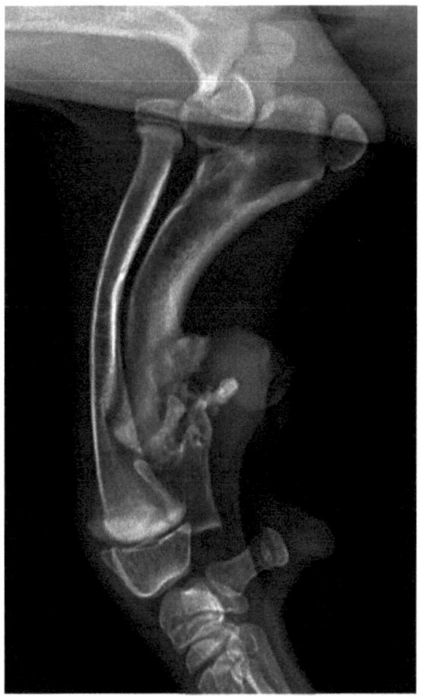

Figure 31. ML radiograph of the antebrachium of a 3-month-old dog with a congenital grade I elbow luxation. (Image courtesy of A. Navarro, Nexo Menescal Novelda.)

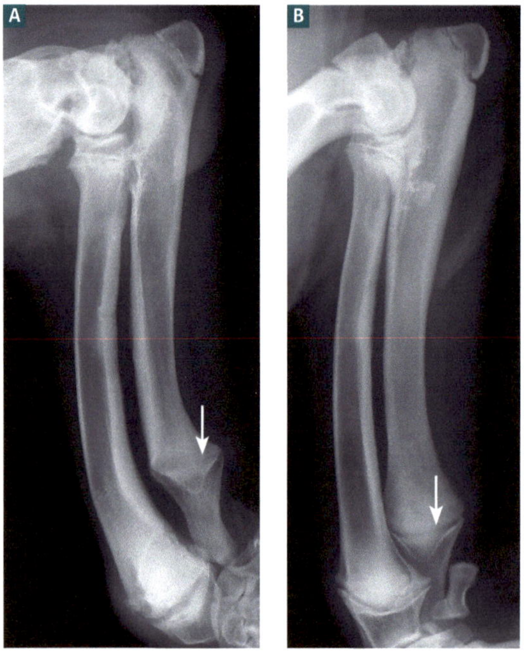

Figure 32. ML radiographs of the antebrachium of a 6-month-old dog. In (**A**), the distal physis of the ulna appears closed (arrow), causing shortening of the ulnar length and abnormal curvature of the radius (radius curvus), in addition to an articular incongruence at the humeroulnar level. Image (**B**) corresponds to the contralateral limb, in which the distal physis of the ulna is still open (arrow) and there is normal growth of the ulna. Both elbows presented nonunion of the anconeal process.

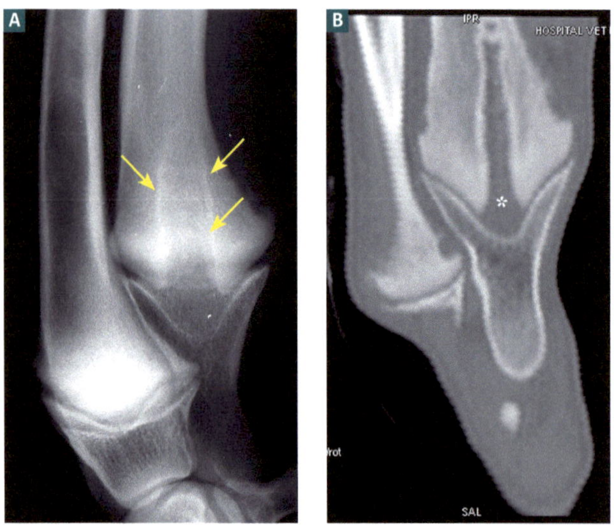

Figure 33. A. ML radiograph of the distal ulna and radius in which the retention of the distal endochondral cartilage of the ulna is visualised in the shape of a "flame" or cone (arrows). **B**. Sagittal section reconstructed CT image of the distal portion of the ulna and radius of a 6-month-old Great Dane with retention of the distal endochondral cartilage of the ulna visualised as a hypoattenuated area (asterisk).

other developmental disorders. It may be an incidental finding with no clinical significance.

It is usually a self-limiting condition but can occasionally cause a delay in growth of the ulna and result in deformation of the limb (radius curvus) and valgus deformation of the carpus. The cause is unknown; there are authors who consider it to be a form of OC of the distal growth cartilage of the ulna, because the cartilaginous tissue of the growth line does not transform into bone, producing a cartilaginous centre retained in the metaphyseal area, that is, retention of the endochondral cartilage in the distal metaphysis of the ulna. This can be temporary or permanent (Pollard and Phillips, 2018).

Radiographically, the lesion appears as a cone-shaped radiotransparent area with smooth margins extending from the epiphyseal line into the metaphysis of the ulna in the medullary cavity, which does not affect the cortices (Fig. 33 A). In CT images, it is visualised as a hypoattenuated area that is directed from the epiphyseal line proximally, extending through the metaphysis towards the diaphysis (Fig. 33 B).

When it affects the growth of the ulna and radius, the lesion can be seen to have irregular edges and extends into the cortices of the bone.

Carpal Joint

Projections

The animal is positioned in the same way as for radiography of the elbow joint, with the X-ray beam focused on the carpal joint.

- **Dorsopalmar** (DP): the animal is placed in sternal recumbency in the "sphinx position"; the head is raised and tilted to the opposite side from the affected limb. Using the grid is not necessary, so the carpus to be radiographed is placed on the plate. In the carpal area, a good evaluation of the adjacent soft tissues is particularly important, so an attempt should be made to reduce the kilovoltage (kV) to avoid excessive penetration of the X-ray beam (Fig. 34).
- **Mediolateral** (ML): the animal is positioned in lateral recumbency with the joint under study on the table; the contralateral limb is withdrawn caudally (Barreiro and Vila, 2014). It is important to obtain a true lateral position because rotation can make interpretation difficult (Fig. 35).
- **Stress projections**: in certain circumstances, pathologies such as small fractures and subluxations may not be visualised in neutral DP and ML images. In order to perform these projections, it may be necessary to sedate or anaesthetise the animal, depending on the suspected pathology and the degree of pain.

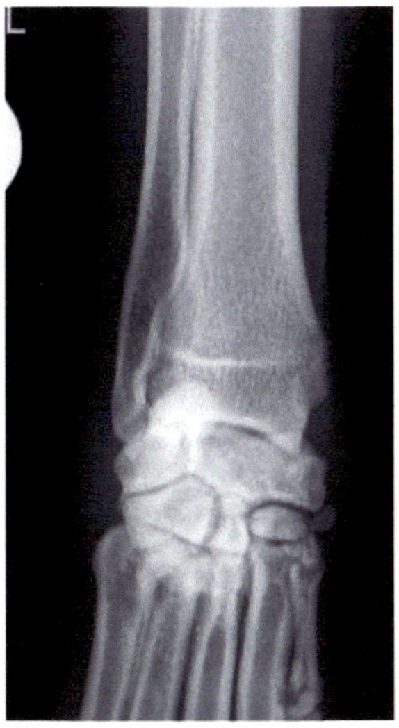

Figure 34. DP radiograph of the carpus of a radiologically mature dog without abnormalities.

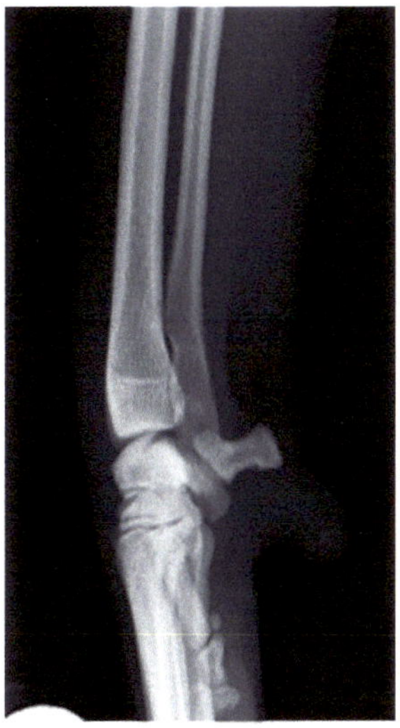

Figure 35. ML radiograph of the carpus of a radiologically mature dog without abnormalities.

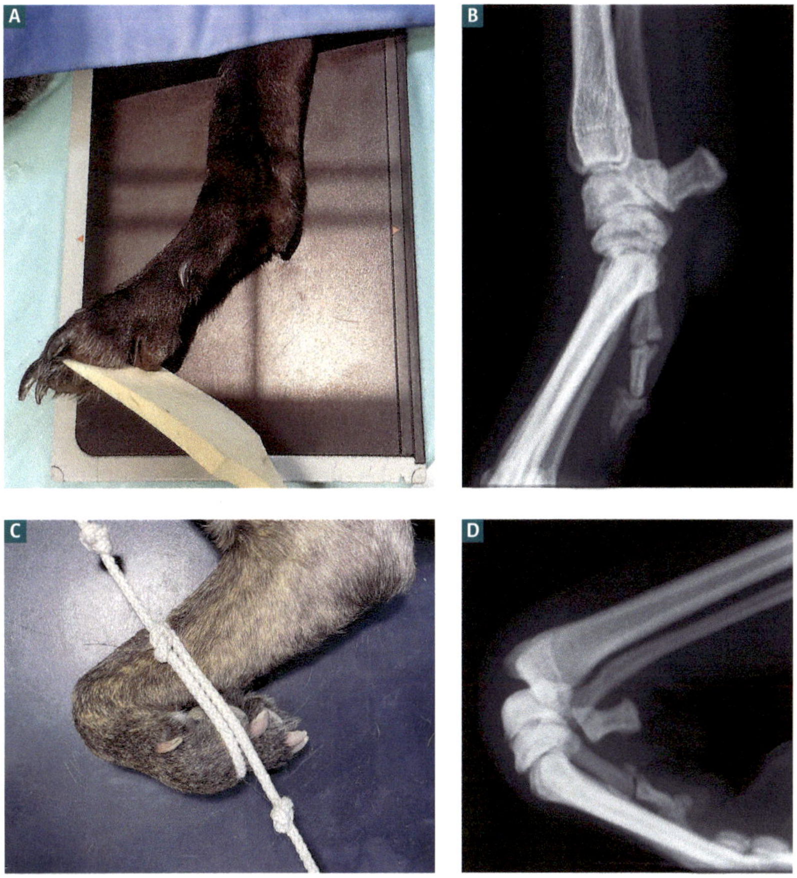

Figure 36. A. Positioning for a stress ML projection of the carpus with dorsal extension. **B**. The resulting radiograph. **C**. Positioning for performing the ML projection of the carpus in flexion. **D**. The resulting radiograph.

- **Stress mediolateral projection**: the animal is placed in the same position as described above for the ML projection but the limb under study is forced into flexion or dorsal hyperextension with the help of ropes, gauze bandages or other aids (Fig. 36).
- **Stress dorsopalmar projection**: the animal is placed in the same position as described above for the DP projection but the limb under study is forced laterally or medially by means of ropes or gauze bandages (Fig. 37).

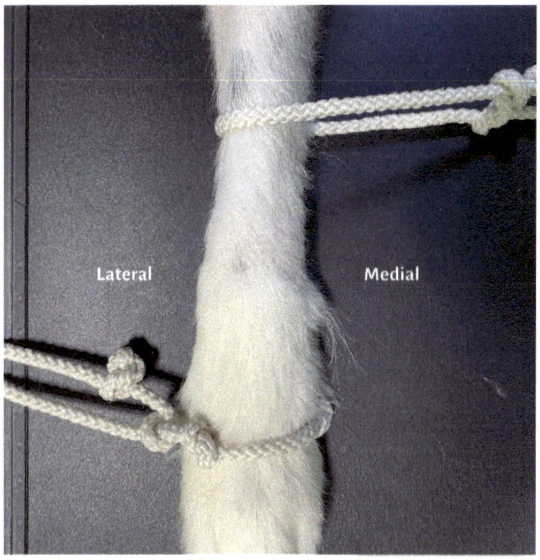

Figure 37. Positioning to perform a forced/stressed DP radiograph of the carpus. In this case, the metacarpals are forced laterally and the forearm medially, which reveals abnormalities in joint spaces/surfaces medially. Performing another radiograph applying opposing forces is recommended.

Luxations/Subluxations

Luxations/subluxations can occur in any joint, with carporadial and carpometacarpal luxations being most common (Barreiro and Vila, 2014). When collateral ligament tears occur, forced/stressed projections of the joint in both DP and ML views should be performed in order to evidence the subluxations radiographically (Fig. 38).

Fractures

Fractures of the carpal joint are not very common. After trauma or falling from a height, luxations and subluxations usually occur due to ligament rupture; however, when fractures do occur, they usually involve the styloid process of the ulna (Fig. 38 A), the intermediate radial bone and the accessory bone (Fig. 39). Fractures of the accessory bone in particular are more frequent in Greyhounds and are classified into five types (Johnson, 1987).

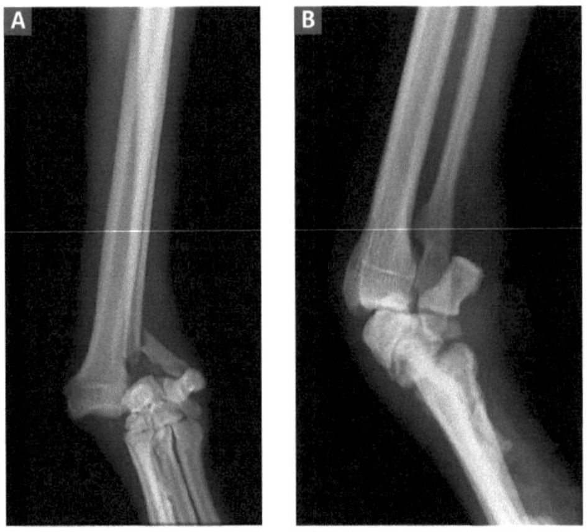

Figure 38. A. DP radiograph of an adult dog with complete carporadial luxation and fracture of the distal epiphysis of the ulna. **B**. Stress ML radiograph in which a carporadial subluxation is evident.

- **Type I**: fractures affecting the distal articular surface of the accessory bone.
- **Type II**: fractures of the proximal articular surface.
- **Type III**: fractures at the origin of the accessory metacarpal ligaments.
- **Type IV**: avulsion fractures of the insertion of the flexor carpi ulnaris tendon.
- **Type V**: comminuted fractures.

On some occasions a CT study is necessary when a fracture of the carpal bones is suspected but is not clearly identifiable by radiography (Fig. 40).

Arthritis

Arthritis usually causes joint strain and pain, although the radiographic signs vary depending on the origin and severity of the injury. In types of arthritis considered erosive, which can be septic or immune mediated, there is initially a synovial effusion that causes distension of the joint capsule and widening of the joint spaces. Next, the destruction of the cartilage of the articular surfaces causes the joint spaces to decrease in size. Finally, there is destruction of the subchondral bone and osteolytic foci can be seen, which cause heterogeneous opacity of the carpal bones and an irregular appearance of the articular surfaces.

Tenosynovitis of the Abductor Muscle of the First Phalanx

Stenosing tenosynovitis of the abductor muscle of the first phalanx (pollicis longus) is a pathology that mainly affects medium/large-breed dogs that perform frequent exercise (e.g. military, hunting, agility demonstrations). It causes inflammation and pain on flexion of the carpus (Grundmann and Montavon, 2001). The radiographic changes that are sometimes seen can be subtle; among others, inflammation of

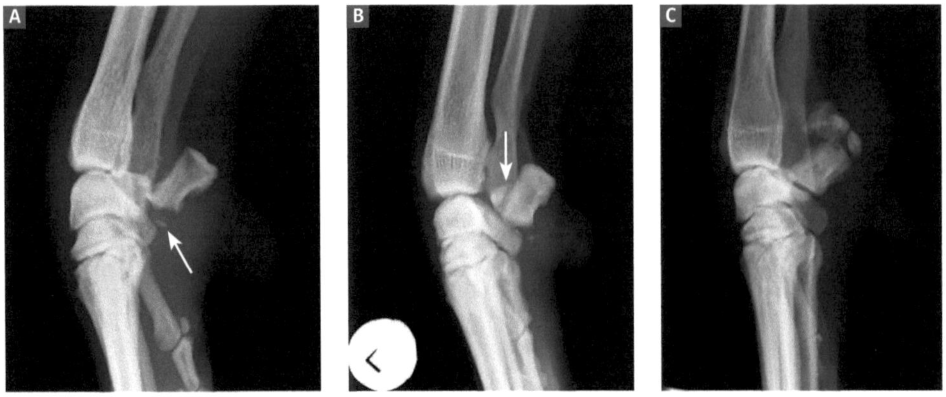

Figure 39. ML radiographs of different types of accesory carpal bone fractures. **A**. Type I; **B**. Type II; **C**. Type V.

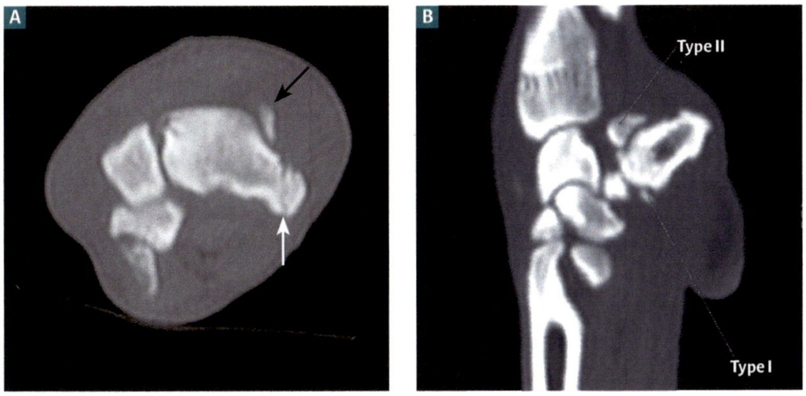

Figure 40. A. CT image in a transverse plane at the level of the proximal row of carpal bones, in which a fracture is visualised at the medial level of the intermediate radial bone (white arrow) in addition to a small bone fragment dorsal to this bone (black arrow). **B**. Reconstructed sagittal plane CT image of a dog with accessory carpal bone fractures (type I and type II).

the soft tissues of the medial aspect of the carpus and the presence of osteophytes affecting the distal radius in the dorsomedial area (area of the sulcus that runs through the tendon) may be visualised (Fig. 41). Ultrasonography seems to be much more accurate and better for diagnosis in these cases because, as well as inflammation and osteophytes, it is able to detect fluid in the tendon sheath and inflammation and small mineralisations of the tendon sheath (Hittmair et al., 2012).

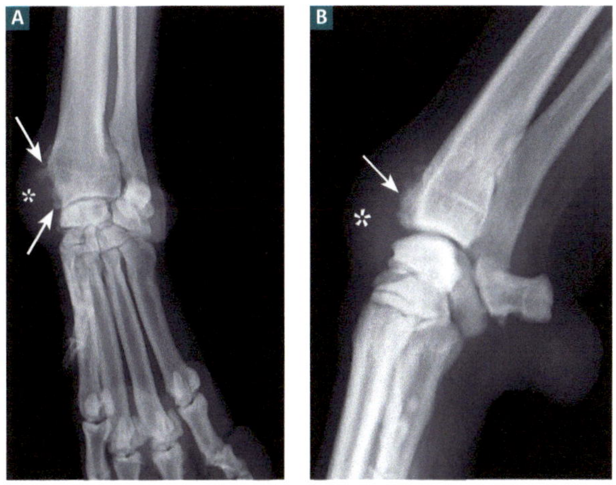

Figure 41. DP (**A**) and ML (**B**) radiographs of the carpus of a 6-year-old Boxer with chronic stenosing tenosynovitis of the abductor muscle of the first phalanx, in which there is inflammation of the soft tissues dorsomedial to the carpal joint (asterisk) and bone neoformations on the medial and dorsal surfaces of the distal portion of the radius (arrows), corresponding to the groove of the tendon of the abductor muscle of the first phalanx.

Metacarpals and Phalanges

Projections

The animal is positioned in the same way as for the radiographic projections of the carpal joint. Although when the carpus is radiographed it is not necessary to encompass all the phalanges distally, when an animal presents with suspected abnormalities of the metacarpals or phalanges, the carpal joint should be encompassed proximally (Morgan, 1993).

- **Dorsopalmar** (DP): the main X-ray beam is focused on the metacarpophalangeal joint. To facilitate radiographic interpretation, balls of clean, dry cotton wool can be placed between the toes to separate them (Fig. 42).
- **Mediolateral** (ML): due to the overlap of the different metacarpal bones and phalanges, it is difficult to visualise abnormalities other than metacarpophalangeal luxations. For this reason, ropes or gauze bandages can be used to separate the toes to try to identify fractures or dislocations of the phalanges, dorsally extending the phalanx in which the abnormality is suspected (Fig. 43).

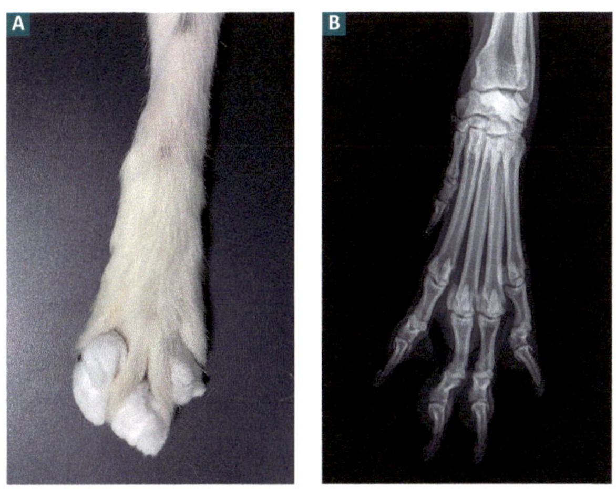

Figure 42. A. Positioning for radiography of the phalanges in the DP projection by placing cotton wool in the interdigital spaces. **B**. The resulting radiograph.

Fractures and Luxations

Fractures and luxations are the pathologies that are most often found in the metacarpal bones and phalanges of animals that have fallen from a certain height (Fig. 44).

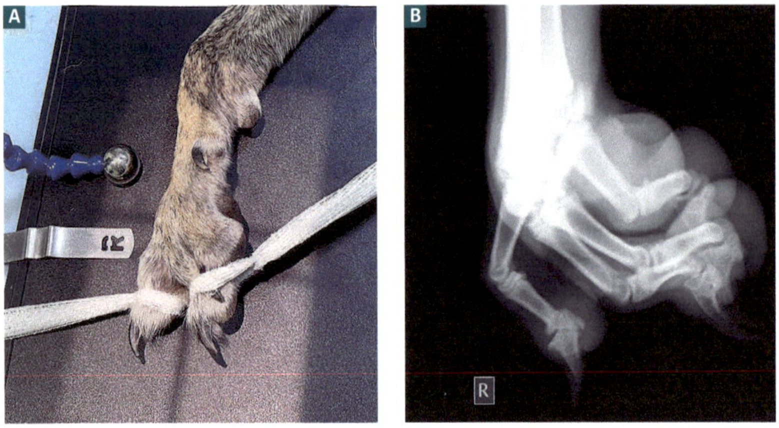

Figure 43. A. Positioning for radiography of the phalanges; in this case the third phalanx is being held dorsally with the help of gauze bandages. **B**. The resulting radiograph.

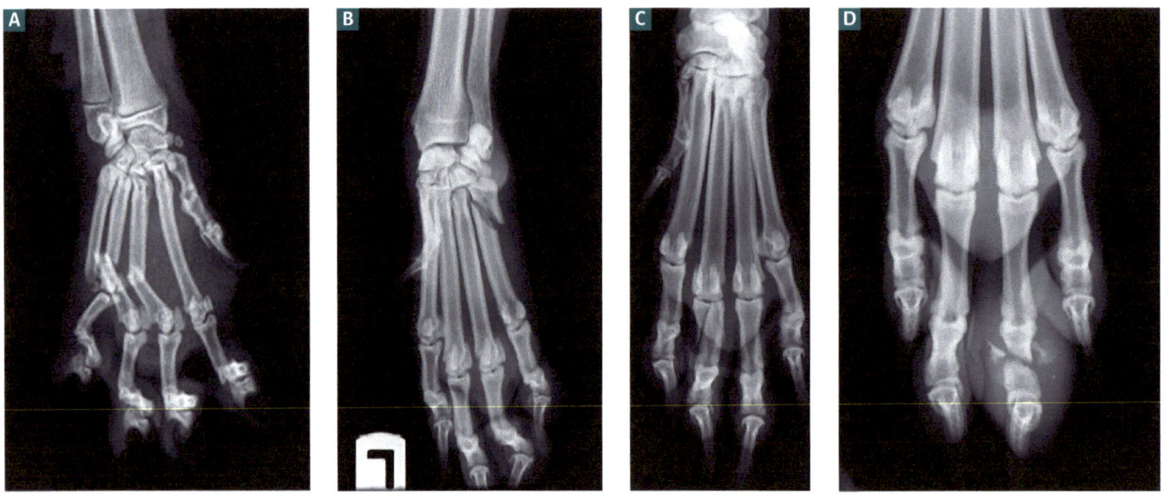

Figure 44. Dorsopalmar radiographs of different cases with fractures of the metacarpals and phalanges. **A**. Radiograph of an immature cat with fractures of the III, IV and V metacarpals. **B**. Radiograph of an adult dog with a proximal V metacarpal fracture. This type of fracture is relatively common in racing Greyhounds. **C**. Radiograph of an adult dog with an oblique fracture of the proximal phalanx of the third toe. **D**. Radiograph of an adult dog with a fracture of the middle phalanx of the third toe; note the marked inflammation of the adjacent soft tissues.

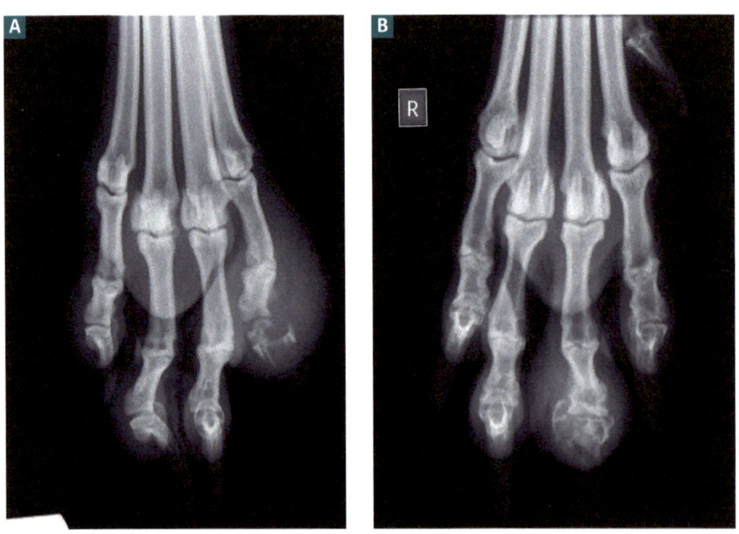

Figure 45. Dorsoplantar (**A**) and dorsopalmar (**B**) radiographs of the phalanges of two adult dogs with aggressive osteolytic bone lesions of the distal phalanx of the second and third toes, respectively, with marked inflammation of the adjacent soft tissues. In both cases, after amputation of the affected phalanges and histopathological study, the diagnosis was squamous cell carcinoma of the nail matrix.

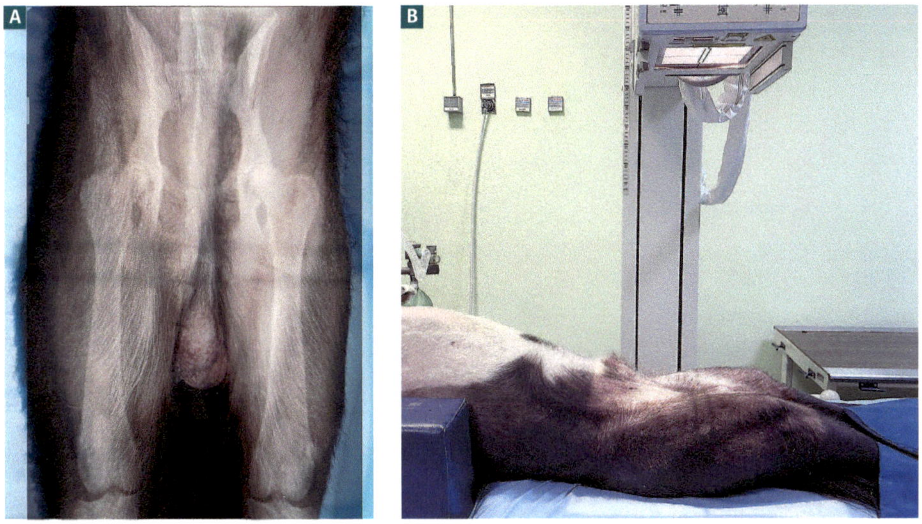

Figure 46. Ventrodorsal (**A**) and lateral (**B**) images of positioning for VD radiography of the hip in extension. The X-ray beam is centred at the base of the penis or at the level of the last pair of nipples and extends from the wings of the ilium to the tibial tuberosities. The limbs are rotated slightly medially, leaving the patellae centred on the femoral condyles.

Neoplasms and Osteomyelitis

Aggressive bone lesions of the phalanges (especially the distal phalanges) are more frequently caused by neoplasms (83%) than by osteomyelitis (17%).

Among the neoplasms, the most common are **subungual squamous cell carcinoma** and **melanoma** (Marino et al., 1995). All these pathologies usually cause marked osteolysis (bone destruction) of the distal phalanx, with considerable inflammation of the adjacent soft tissues, and can also affect the middle phalanx. In order to reach a definitive diagnosis, a histopathological study is necessary as these neoplasms cannot be differentiated radiographically from each other, nor from an infection (Fig. 45).

Hindlimb

Hip Joint

Hip Dysplasia

It is well known that hip dysplasia is an abnormal development of the joint, which has a hereditary, multifactorial aetiology. It is much more prevalent in large and giant breeds of dog that grow rapidly. It is believed that, although the hip may be normal at birth, an increase in joint laxity is the cause of subsequent radiographic findings such as coxofemoral luxation or subluxation and DJD.

As osteoarthritis progresses, the acetabulum begins to lose its depth and becomes flattened. The femoral head also loses its rounded shape and becomes flattened, and the femoral neck presents irregular edges and becomes thicker due to the formation of osteophytes. Hip dysplasia is generally bilateral, although in some cases only one joint is affected (Pollard and Phillips, 2018).

An extended ventrodorsal (VD) projection is the standard radiographic projection proposed by the Orthopaedic Foundation for Animals (OFA) and is the one established in most countries for making an official diagnosis and assessing the degree of dysplasia. Correct positioning is essential, and for this the animal must be under general anaesthesia or deeply sedated. The animal is positioned in dorsal recumbency, using holders or sandbags around the forelimbs and with the hindlimbs fully extended by manual traction by an assistant wearing protective clothing, or by means of ropes and sandbags (Barreiro and Vila, 2014) (Fig. 46).

The radiograph must meet a series of requirements (Fig. 47):

- it should cover the area from the pelvis to the tibial tuberosities
- it must be symmetrical in position:
  1. the wings of the ilium should have a similar contour
  2. the obturator foramina should be the same size on each side
  3. the femurs should be parallel to each other and parallel to the table, forcing a slight medial rotation so that the patellae are centred between the femoral condyles (in the midline above the femoral condyles)
  4. both femurs should overlap the ischial tuberosities in the same way.

Radiographic findings of hip dysplasia include the following (Pollard and Phillips, 2018) (Fig. 48).

- **Coxofemoral luxation or subluxation**: present when 50% or more of the femoral head is not encompassed by the dorsal acetabular border. The acetabulum is considered to be flat when its depth is less than half the width of the femoral head, it is normal for the dorsal acetabular border to encompass two-thirds of the head of the femur.

- **Signs of DJD**.
  - Remodelling of the femoral head and neck. Remodelling of the femoral head causes the loss of its rounded shape so that it appears flattened, and the area of attachment to the femoral neck becomes indistinct as it becomes wider.
  - Visualisation of osteophytes has been described as an early sign of future osteoarthritis and development of hip dysplasia. The osteophytes form a curved line in the caudolateral area of the femoral neck (area of insertion of the joint capsule) that is called a caudolateral curvilinear osteophyte; radiographically, a radiopaque curved line, also known as "Morgan's line", is visualised (Powers et al., 2004).
  - Remodelling of the acetabulum. When the acetabulum is remodelled, it adopts a semi-elliptical or egg shape, losing its semicircular shape, and the medial margin becomes thickened.
  - Periarticular osteophytes on the margin of the femoral head and acetabulum.
  - Osteophytes on the margin of the femoral head parallel to the epiphyseal scar.
  - Subchondral sclerosis of the acetabular border.

The degree of coxofemoral subluxation and involvement of hip dysplasia can be quantified by measuring the **Norberg angle**.

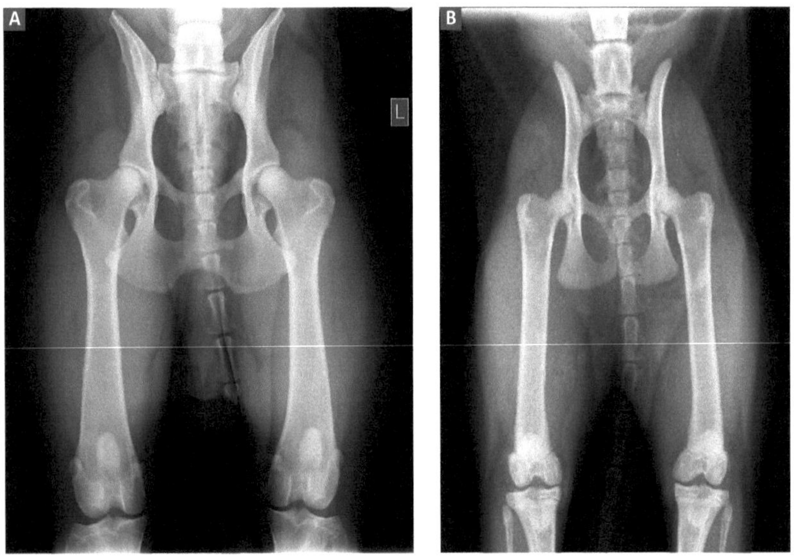

Figure 47. VD radiographs of the hip of an adult dog (**A**) and cat (**B**) correctly positioned for evaluation. The view extends from the wings of the ilium to the tibial tuberosities, the obturator foramina are symmetrical, the femurs are parallel to each other and the patellae are centred on the femoral condyles, overlapping equally with both ischial tuberosities.

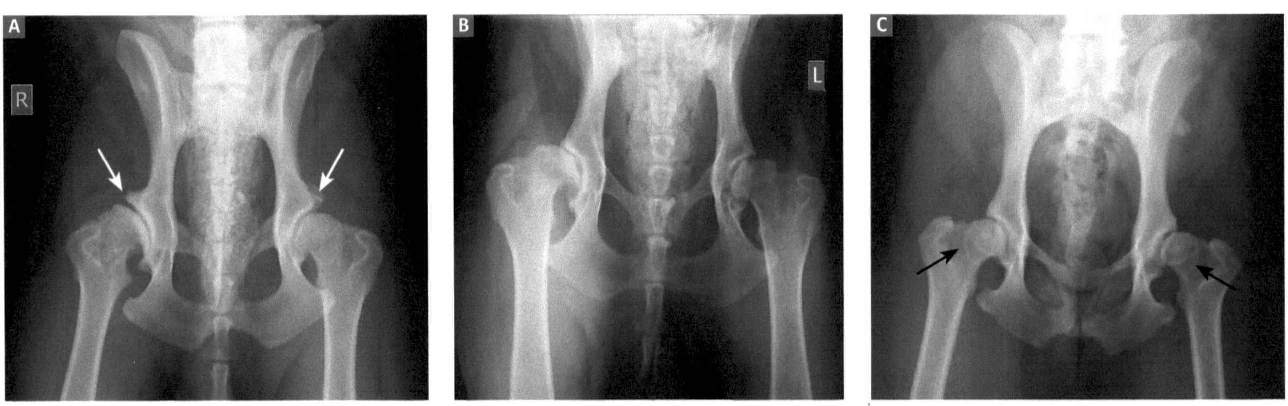

Figure 48. VD radiographs of the hip of adult dogs with different degrees of osteoarthritis due to dysplasia. **A**. Remodelling of the femoral heads and necks; the heads have lost their rounded morphology and the necks are thickened by the presence of bone neoformations. The acetabula are flattened, especially on the right side, the dorsal acetabular edges do not cover 50% of the femoral heads and osteophytes are present on the cranial acetabular edges (white arrows). **B**. Changes in the femoral heads and necks as well as flattening of the acetabula. **C**. Marked flattening of the acetabula; there is left coxofemoral subluxation and the presence of a caudolateral curvilinear line ("Morgan's line") at the level of the femoral necks (black arrows).

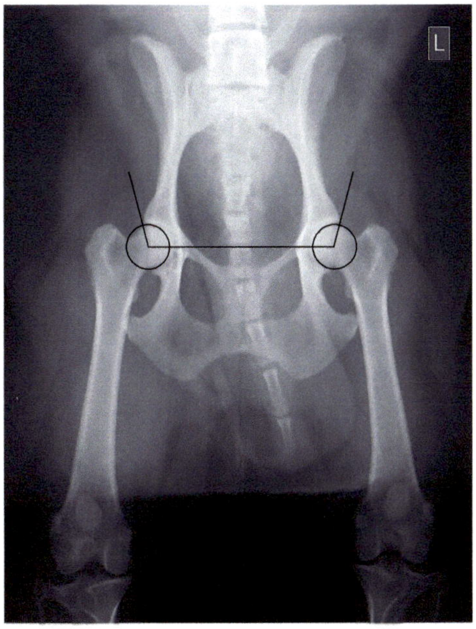

Figure 49. VD radiograph of the hip of an adult dog in which the Norberg angle has been calculated for both hip joints; the angle for each joint is 105°.

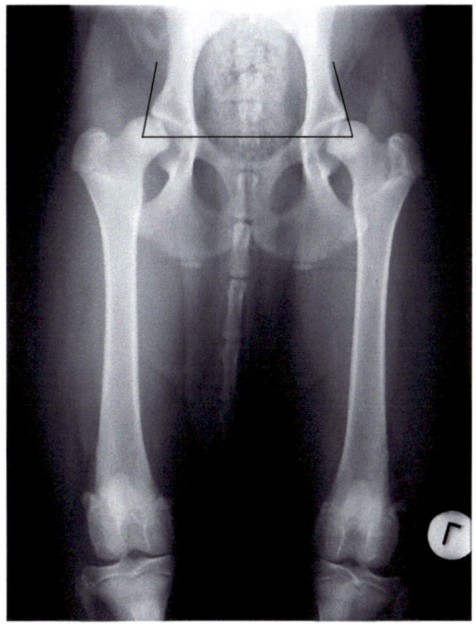

Figure 50. VD radiograph of the hip of an immature dog in which measurement of the Norberg angle reveals angles less than 90°, indicating severe hip dysplasia. There are no signs of DJD (osteoarthrosis).

To determine this angle, a line is drawn that crosses the pelvis and joins the centre of both femoral heads; then, from the centre of each femoral head another line is drawn that tangentially touches the craniolateral acetabular edge (Fig. 49). The resulting angle between the two lines is the Norberg angle; it should be 105° or greater in the dog and 95° or greater in the cat (Barreiro and Vila, 2014).

Thus, there are various degrees of involvement.

- **Mild dysplasia**: there is slight coxofemoral subluxation and the Norberg angle is between 100° and 105°.
- **Moderate dysplasia**: there is coxofemoral dislocation, the Norberg angle is between 90° and 100°, and flattening of the acetabular border and secondary degenerative changes are visualised.
- **Severe dysplasia**: there is coxofemoral dislocation, the Norberg angle is less than 90°, and severe degenerative changes and flattening of the femoral head are evident (Fig. 50).

In immature patients, an early diagnosis of hip dysplasia can be made by manipulating the hip joint of the anaesthetised animal to evidence passive laxity of the hip joint (Ortolani sign). This can be shown radiographically, using a VD projection in which the hindlimbs are raised and the stifles are brought closer towards each other, placing a rigid radiotransparent structure between them. In this way, the femurs are positioned at a 90° angle with respect to the spine and the tibias at a 90° angle with respect to the femurs (Fig. 51). If the animal has joint capsule laxity, coxofemoral subluxation (increase in the joint space) will be seen; the joint space should not

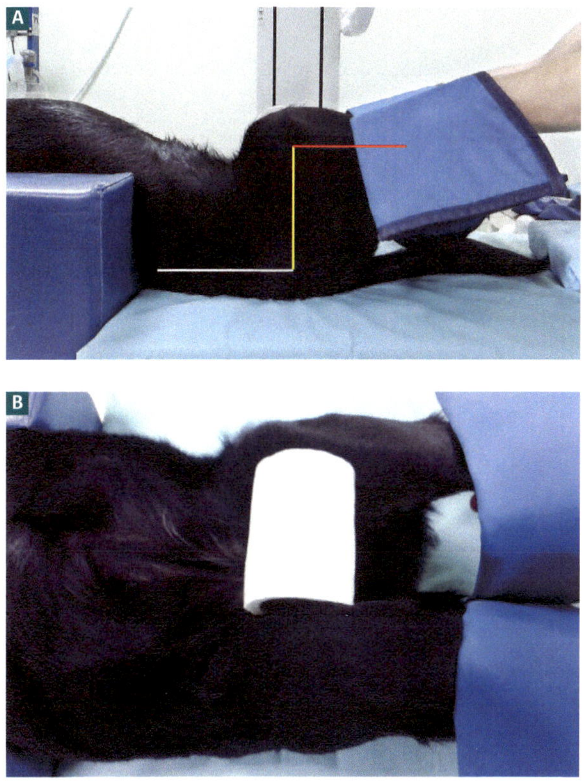

Figure 51. Positioning to perform a VD radiograph of the hip with distraction. The animal is in dorsal recumbency, the femurs are raised so that they form a 90° angle with the spine and the stifles are bent at 90° with respect to the femurs. In addition, a firm but radiotransparent object is placed between the stifles in order to create pressure from one stifle to the other, to force distraction of the coxofemoral joints.

vary if the animal does not have the pathology (Fig. 52). This method is a variation of the so-called "PennHIP method" developed at the University of Pennsylvania.

Another option to assess the laxity of the coxofemoral joints without the need to perform distraction radiography is to use **CT**. Several studies have been carried out using this modality in which, by assessing certain parameters, predictive indicators of dysplasia in the hip joints of immature animals could be obtained (Kishimoto et al., 2009). CT studies are also performed in radiographically mature animals to more accurately measure the different angles and distances for a possible surgical approach. For these studies, the animal is positioned in sternal recumbency, in the "prayer position", so that the tibias are parallel to the table and at a 90° angle with the femurs, which in turn form a 90° angle with the spine (Fujiki et al., 2004) (Fig. 53).

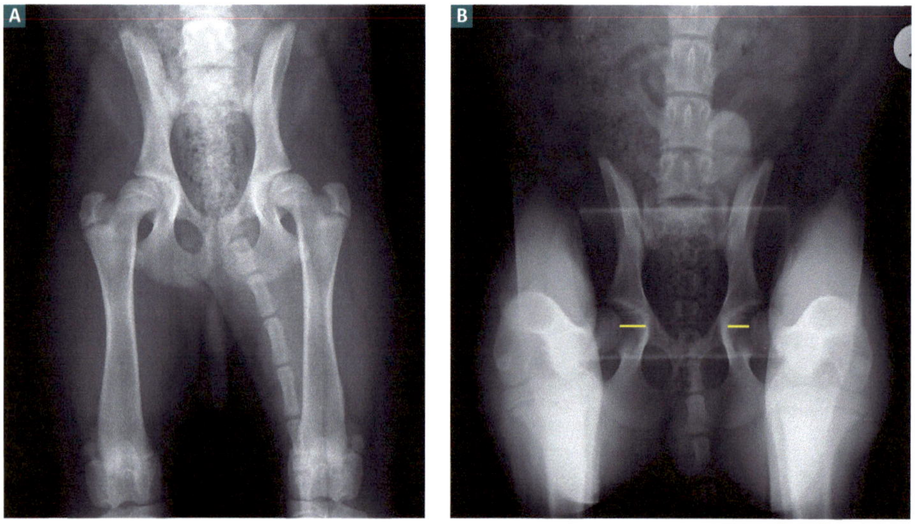

Figure 52. VD radiographs of hip extension (**A**) and distraction (**B**) of a 4-month-old Golden Retriever with altered gait and positive Ortolani sign. In the VD radiograph in extension (A) there are no evident abnormalities; however, in the distraction projection (B) a marked increase in the joint spaces (yellow lines) is observed, showing the presence of coxofemoral laxity. This projection allows an early identification of the pathology, providing the possibility of implementing preventive treatments such as pubic symphysiodesis.

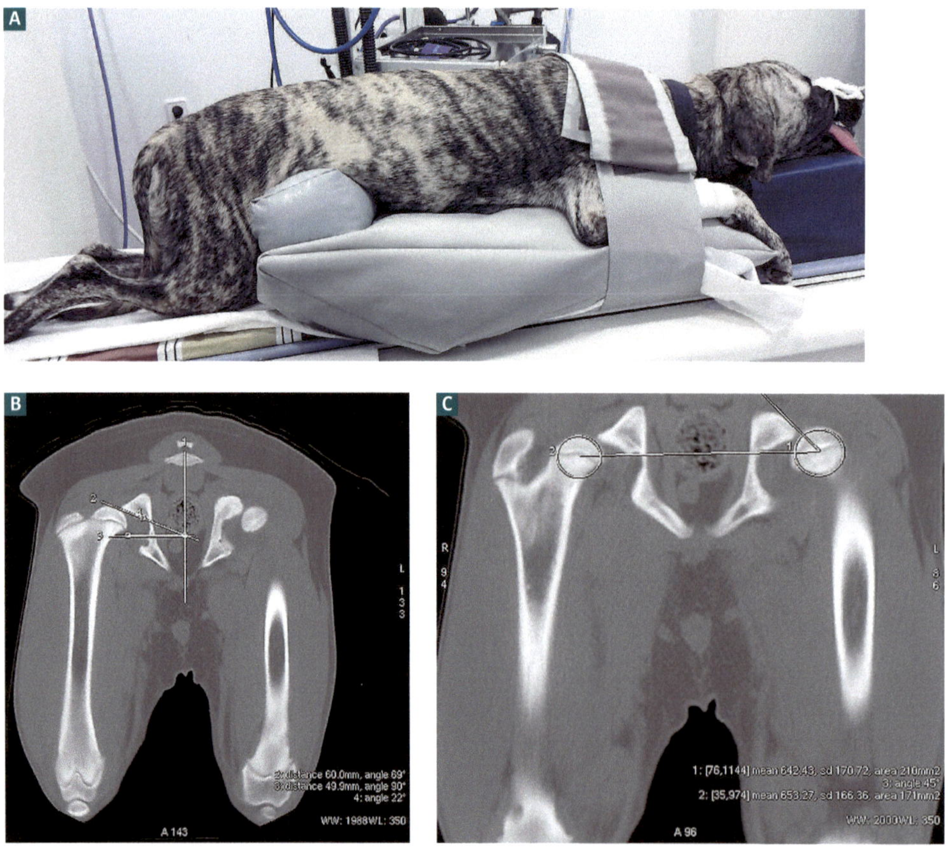

Figure 53. A. Positioning of a dog for a hip CT scan. **B**, **C**. The resulting CT images, in which a series of measurements are made to assess the best treatment to apply.

Aseptic/Avascular Femoral Head Necrosis

Avascular femoral head necrosis (AFHN), also known as Legg–Calvé–Perthes disease, has an unknown aetiology, although the pathological findings are typical of avascular bone necrosis. This condition is also known as aseptic femoral head necrosis.

This disease occurs more frequently in young animals of miniature breeds, weighing less than 12 kg, and has no sex predisposition. It is generally unilateral, although it occasionally occurs bilaterally (10–15% of cases). Avascular necrosis is a hereditary disorder caused by an autosomal recessive gene in breeds such as the Miniature Poodle, Yorkshire Terrier and West Highland White Terrier. Affected animals show lameness at an early age, between 4 months and 10 months of age (Barreiro and Vila, 2014).

Early **radiographic signs** include an increase in poorly defined opacity in the femoral head and neck. In later stages, the joint space increases (subluxation) and radiotransparent foci are visualised (osteolysis due to bone necrosis) in the subchondral bone of the femoral head, which loses its rounded shape. Pathological fractures of the femoral head occasionally occur and degenerative changes in the joint are usually observed, as well as muscular atrophy of the affected limb (Pollard and Phillips, 2018) (Fig. 54).

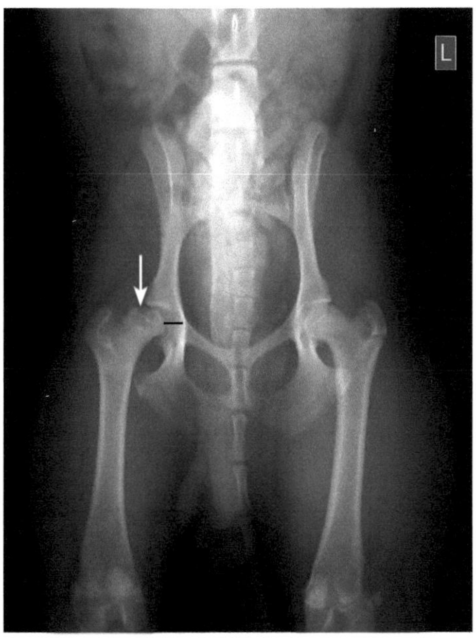

Figure 54. VD radiograph of the hip of a 7-month-old Poodle with right-sided avascular femoral head necrosis, in which the right femoral head is observed to have abnormal morphology and heterogeneous opacity with the presence of radiotransparent areas (arrow), and the joint space is increased (subluxation) (black line).

Feline Metaphyseal Osteopathy of the Femoral Neck

Feline metaphyseal osteopathy is of unknown aetiology, although histopathological findings are typical of necrosis and bone resorption in the proximal metaphysis of the femur, leading to a pathological fracture (Queen et al., 1998). There are other conditions that can cause this bone lesion, such as a Salter–Harris type I fracture of the femoral head with secondary resorption of the neck (spontaneous epiphyseal fracture of the femoral head), Legg–Calvé–Perthes disease with secondary fracture, and osteomyelitis with secondary bone resorption; a relationship with herpesvirus has also been described. It occurs more frequently in young cats and even more frequently in those that are overweight, especially in neutered males of any breed, and is very common in mixed breeds (Craig, 2001). It is generally a unilateral condition, although it can occur bilaterally. Affected animals show lameness at an early age, between 5 months and 24 months of age, with a lot of pain on extension of the hip joint, which does not subside with rest and administration of anti-inflammatory drugs. Closure of the epiphysis of the femoral head in the cat occurs at 10 months of age; in male animals castrated before this age, this closure is delayed by the persistence of the capital physis, and therefore immature vascular modelling in this area could be the aetiology of vascular disorders.

Radiographically, a loss of definition can be observed as well as areas of osteolysis in the femoral neck. A complete radiotransparent line or space is also observed in the epiphyseal area of the femoral neck, which shows a discontinuity in the femoral head, which may be in a normal position and/or of normal opacity (Schwartz, 2013). Extended VD radiograph should be performed, but there may be occasions on which the abnormality is not visible on this projection; in those cases, a flexed (frog-leg) radiograph of the pelvis should be performed or a CT study is recommended (Fig. 55).

Slipped Capital Femoral Epiphysis/ Spontaneous Femoral Capital Physeal Fracture

In this pathology, separation of the capital epiphysis (head of the femur) occurs in the absence of previous trauma. It usually happens in immature animals. An acute, unstable slippage of the femoral head occurs but, according to some authors, is not itself an epiphysiolysis (Salter–Harris type I) (Moores et al., 2004). In children, it may be associated with endocrine disorders such as hypothyroidism or hypogonadism, but in most cases it is idiopathic. In dogs, the aetiology is unknown and uncertain, although the most widely accepted hypothesis is that it is related to a delay in endochondral ossification of the proximal physis (i.e. a type of OC or dysplasia that precedes the slippage of the epiphysis). OC has a multifactorial origin, and both hereditary and nutritional factors, such as rapid growth, previous trauma, and a decrease in vascular supply at the junction of the physis and metaphysis, may be involved in the process.

The animal presents with lameness and/or limb stiffness. In many cases, remodelling of the femoral neck is seen due to chronicity of the process both before and after separation of the epiphysis (Fig. 56), although sometimes the radiographic changes are so subtle in the VD projection that more projections are required to visualise the abnormality. This pathology also occurs in cats and may be associated with feline metaphyseal osteopathy of the femoral neck, from which it can be differentiated only by histology (Gemmill et al., 2012).

Luxations

The coxofemoral joints luxate more frequently compared with the rest of the joints, and the vast majority of cases are caused by traffic accidents. Coxofemoral luxations are usually seen in mature animals; in young animals (less than 10 months of age) it is more common for trauma to cause a fracture in the proximal physis (Salter–Harris type I). Luxation occurs in the craniodorsal direction. Although two radiographic projections (VD and lateral) are required to confirm this displacement, usually only a VD projection is performed. Luxation is usually unilateral, but cases of bilateral luxation can occur (Harasen, 2005) (Fig. 57).

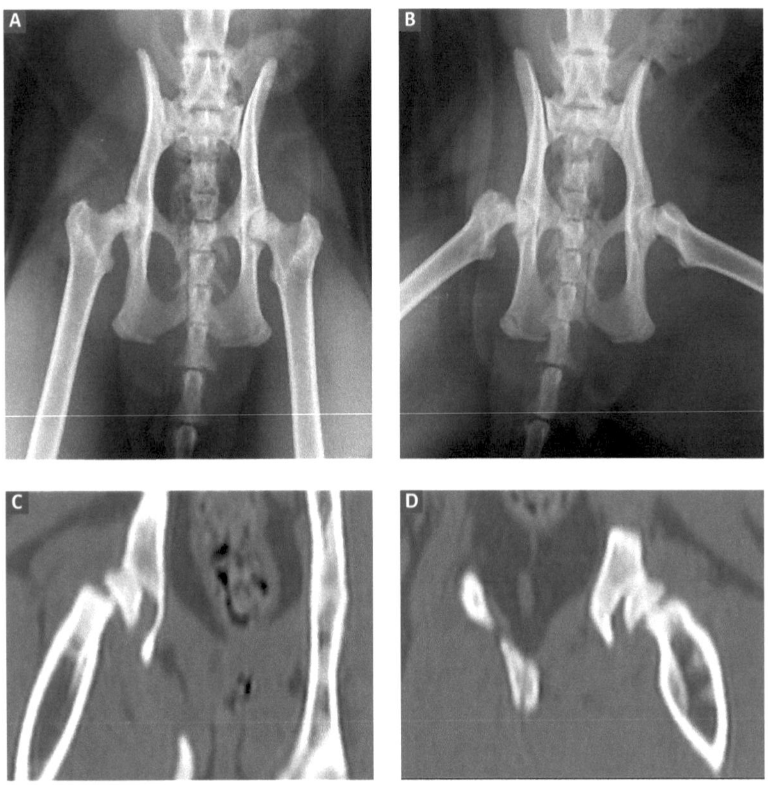

Figure 55. VD radiographs of the hip in extension (**A**) and in the "frog position" (**B**) of a 6-month-old castrated male Siamese cat with metaphyseal osteopathy of the femoral neck that has caused slippage of the capital epiphysis (femoral head), visible in the frog position projection (B) on the right side. **C**, **D**. Reconstructed CT images in the dorsal plane, in which the condition can be seen to be bilateral because the discontinuity (hypoattenuated line) is observed at the level of the right (C) and the left (D) femoral neck.

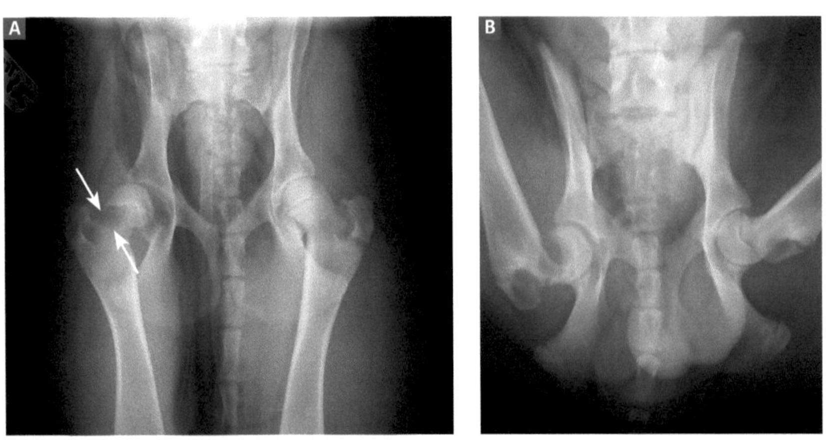

Figure 56. Hip radiographs of a 6-month-old Presa Canario dog in extension (**A**) and in the "frog position" (**B**), in which a decrease in opacity and remodelling of the proximal metaphysis of the right femur (femoral neck) (arrows) with sliding of the femoral head is observed.

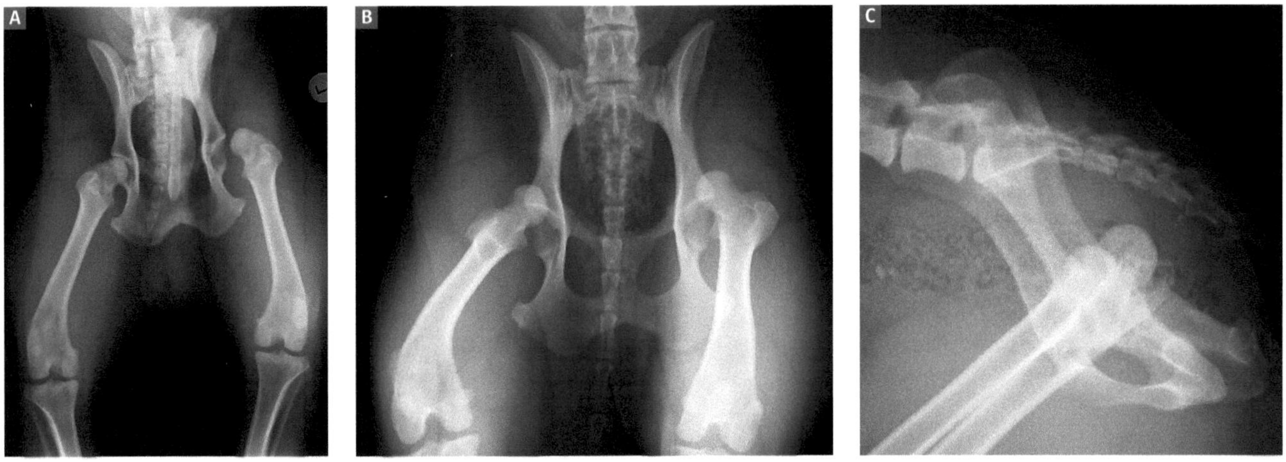

Figure 57. VD radiographs of the hip of two adult dogs with left coxofemoral luxation (**A**) and bilateral coxofemoral luxation (**B**). **C**. Lateral radiograph of the hip of the same animal as in image (B), in which dorsal displacement of the femoral heads with respect to the acetabulum can be seen.

Fractures

As with luxations, most hip fractures are caused by road traffic accidents. Due to the conformation of the hip, fractures may involve one or more bones (Fig. 58). Depending on whether the hip is stable or unstable, medical treatment with strict restriction of movement or surgical treatment will be recommended (Harasen, 2007).

Stifle Joint

Projections

Sedation is recommended, as a conscious animal will usually not allow correct positioning (Barreiro and Vila, 2014).

- **Mediolateral** (ML): with the animal conscious or sedated depending on the pathology and the degree of pain it presents, it should be placed in lateral recumbency with the affected stifle on the table, with a triangular foam wedge placed under the tarsus so that the tibia remains parallel to the table, thus preventing axial rotation. The X-ray beam should be centred on the cranial joint space, caudal to the patellar ligament at an average distance between the patella and tibial tuberosity (Fig. 59).
- **Caudocranial** (CdCr): the patient is placed in sternal recumbency; the unaffected limb is flexed, displaced cranially and elevated by using foam or sandbags. The affected limb is extended caudally by placing a small foam wedge or cotton wool under the patella so that it does not rotate and is centred between the femoral condyles (Fig. 60).
- **Craniocaudal** (CrCd): some clinicians prefer to position the patient in dorsal recumbency and perform this projection instead of the CdCr projection described above.

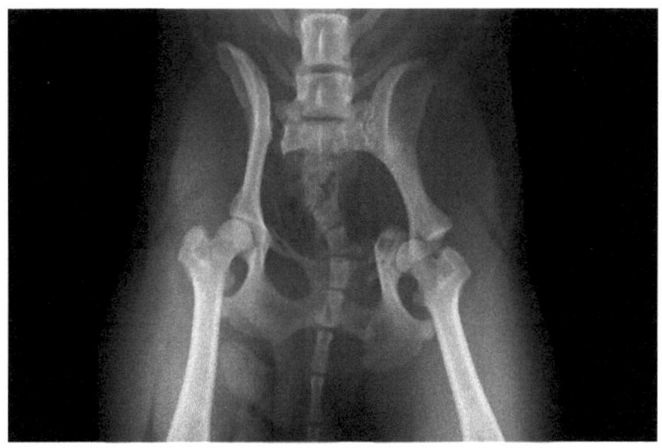

Figure 58. VD radiograph of the hip of an adult dog with right sacroiliac luxation and fractures of the left acetabulum (impact fracture), the cranial branches of the left and right pubis, and at the level of the left ischiatic table.

The hindlimbs are extended in the same way as for a VD hip radiograph, but the X-ray beam is focused on the stifle being studied.

- **Caudocranial with horizontal beam**: on occasion, although it is rare, it may not be possible to extend the hip joint; in these situations, in order to obtain an image of the stifle in extension, it is possible to resort to performing a radiograph of the stifle with the beam horizontal, if the X-ray machine allows this (Fig. 61).
- **Tangential "skyline" projection of the stifle** (craniodistal–cranioproximal) with horizontal beam: with the patient in dorsal recumbency, the limb to be studied is flexed and the cassette is placed vertically as close to the femur as possible. The X-ray beam is centred on the patella. This projection is performed to assess the trochlear groove of the stifle (Barreiro and Vila, 2014) (Fig. 62).

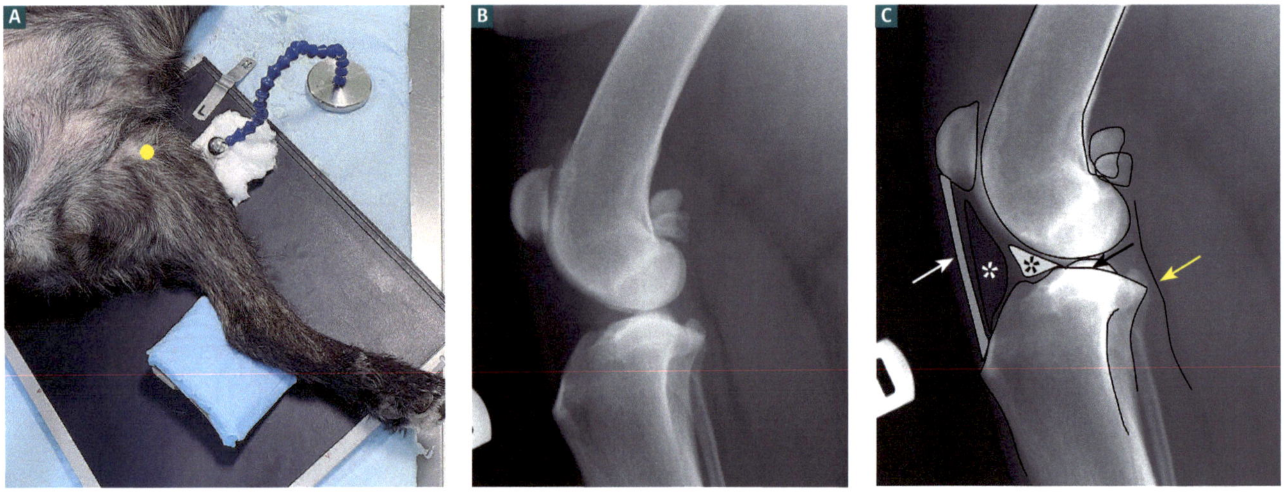

Figure 59. A. Positioning of the animal to perform a ML radiograph of the stifle, with the X-ray beam centred on the joint (yellow dot). **B**. The resulting radiograph. **C**. Diagram superimposed on a radiographic image in which various components of the joint are shown: patellar tendon (white arrow), infrapatellar adipose body (white asterisk), intercondylar area with soft tissue opacity (presence of menisci, portions of cruciate ligaments and a minimum amount of normal synovial fluid) (black asterisk), intercondylar eminences (black arrow), and fascial line caudal to the joint (yellow arrow).

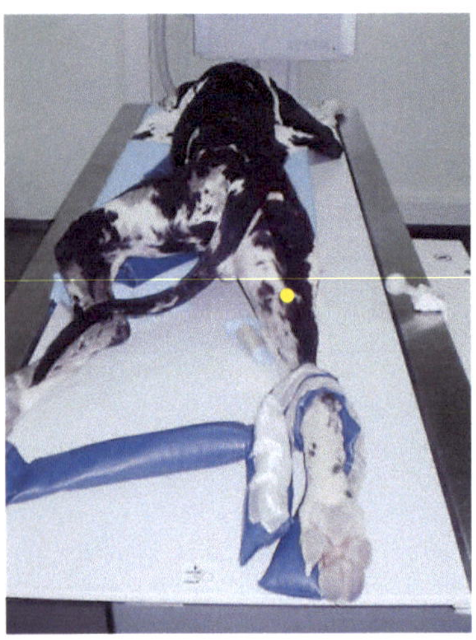

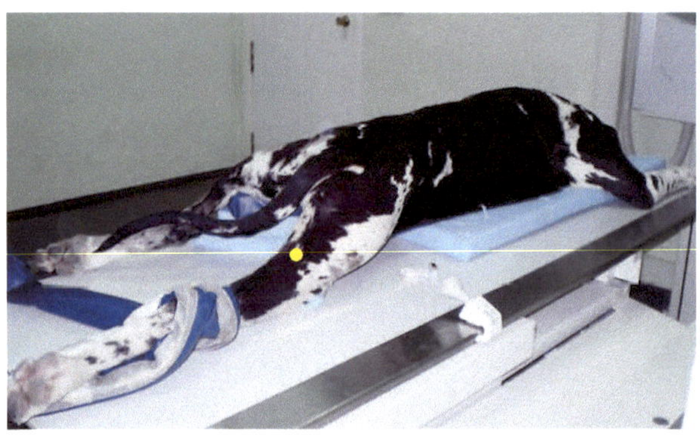

Figure 60. Positioning of the animal to perform a CdCr projection of the stifle, with the X-ray beam centred on the joint (yellow dot).

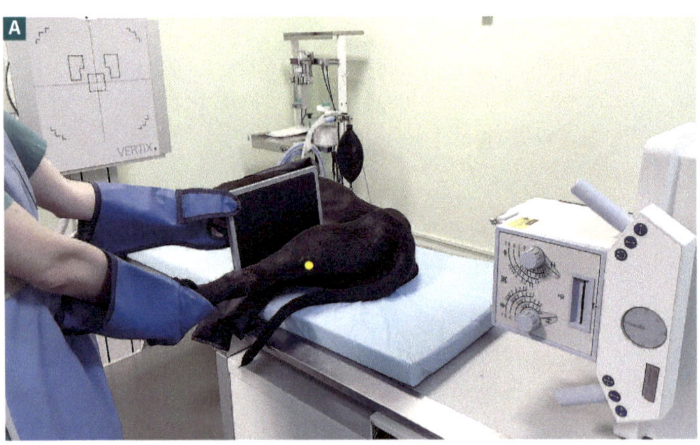

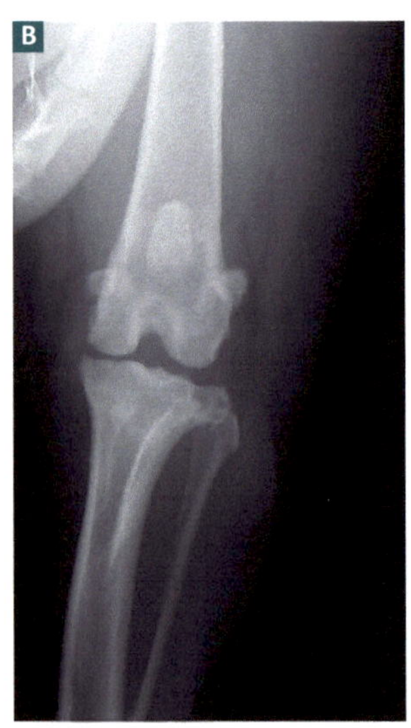

Figure 61. A. Positioning of the animal to perform a CdCr projection of the stifle, with the X-ray beam horizontal and centred on the joint (yellow dot). **B**. CdCr radiograph of the stifle.

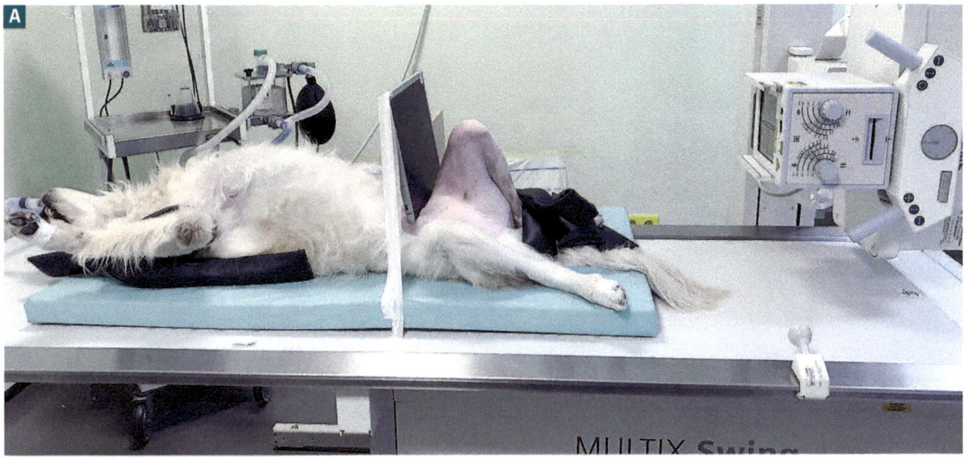

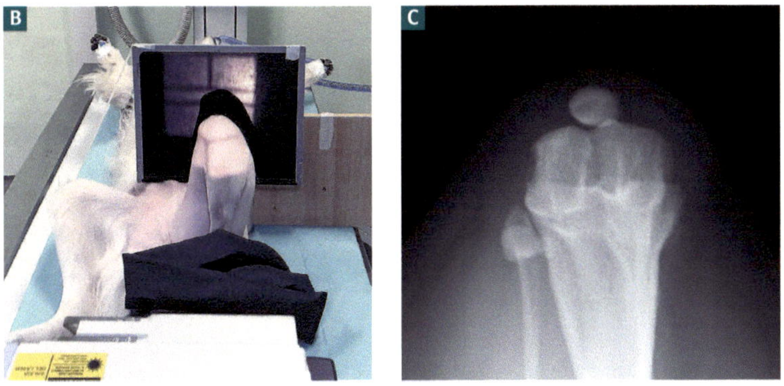

Figure 62. A, B. Positioning of the animal to perform a tangential (skyline) projection of the stifle. **C**. The resulting radiograph.

Cranial Cruciate Ligament Rupture

A presumptive radiographic diagnosis of cranial cruciate ligament rupture is obtained if cranial displacement of the tibia with respect to the femur is observed in a forced ML projection (with the stifle and tarsal joints flexed). In a stable stifle, the intercondylar eminences of the tibia are located at the midpoint of the articular surface of the femoral condyles (Barreiro and Vila, 2014) (Fig. 59).

Depending on the degree of rupture (partial or complete), the weight of the animal and how long it has had the injury, signs of DJD may be present. One of the first radiographic signs seen is increased opacity of the joint space due to an increase in the amount of synovial fluid. The presence of excess synovial fluid causes cranial displacement of the infrapatellar adipose body, which is normally visualised as a triangular shape of fatty opacity, occupying the cranial joint space (Fig. 59). Other common findings of joint degeneration are the presence of periarticular osteophytes, located in the supratrochlear area, laterally and medially to the trochlea of the femur, at the proximal and distal ends of the patella, on the tibial articular surface and in the tibial tuberosity. The sesamoid bones of the gastrocnemius muscles may also be affected (Fig. 63).

Ultrasonography or MRI can be used to investigate this pathology, especially when the rupture is not complete, as well as for the assessment of lesions of the caudal cruciate ligament, the patellar ligament or the menisci (Sage and Gavin, 2016) (Fig. 64).

Patellar Luxation

Patellar luxation can be congenital or acquired. **Acquired** luxation is of traumatic origin and can produce medial or lateral displacement of the patella. **Congenital** luxation is more common and occurs mainly in small breeds (Poodle, Yorkshire Terrier, etc.). In 90% of cases the luxation is medial. Congenital patellar luxation may be accompanied by a greater or lesser degree of rotation of the tibia, curvature of the diaphysis of the femur, or hypoplasia or aplasia of the trochlear groove of the femur.

Four degrees of severity can be established (Di Dona et al., 2018).

- **Grade I**: intermittent luxation that causes occasional lameness and may not be evident on radiography.
- **Grade II**: frequent luxation that in certain cases starts to be more or less permanent; the tibial tuberosity is usually observed as normal or slightly rotated (Fig. 65).

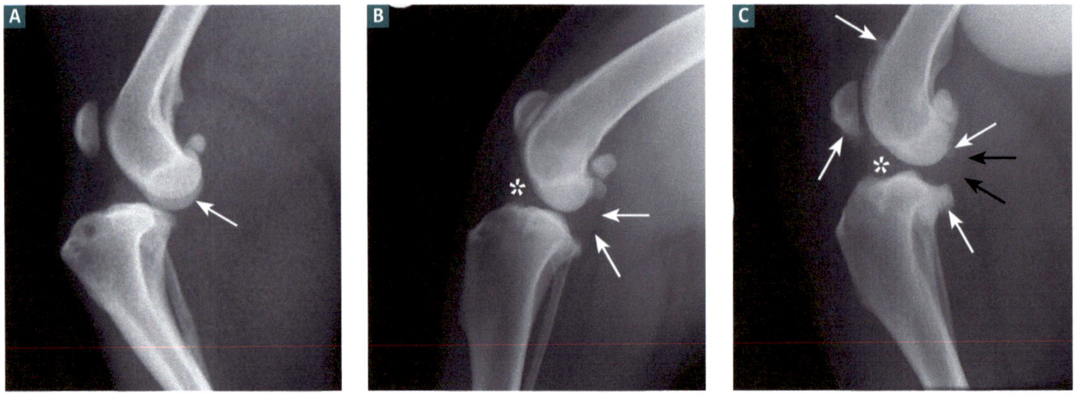

Figure 63. ML radiographs of the stifle of adult dogs with cranial cruciate ligament rupture. **A**. Caudal displacement of the femoral condyles with respect to the tibia (arrow) are visualised. **B**. An increase in opacity is observed intra-articularly (synovial effusion) that obliterates the fatty opacity of the infrapatellar adipose body (asterisk), as well as caudal displacement of the fascial line (arrows). **C**. Signs of DJD are visualised, with osteophytes on articular surfaces (white arrows) in addition to synovial effusion (asterisk, black arrows).

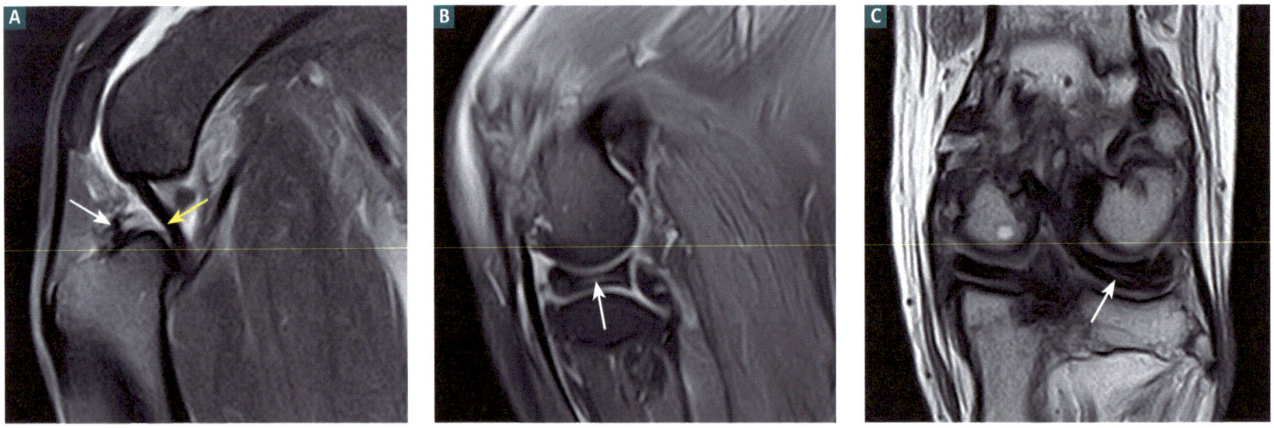

Figure 64. MRI study of the stifle joint. **A**. T2-weighted image in the sagittal plane, showing the ruptured cranial cruciate ligament (white arrow marks the distal end) and the caudal cruciate ligament without alterations (yellow arrow). **B**. T2-weighted image in the sagittal plane, in which a hyperintense line is visualised in the lateral meniscus, compatible with a fissure (arrow). **C**. PD-weighted image (proton density) (same animal as in image B), in which the fissure in the lateral meniscus (caudal horn) is visualised (arrow). (Images courtesy of Dr. A. Ansón, Tufts University.)

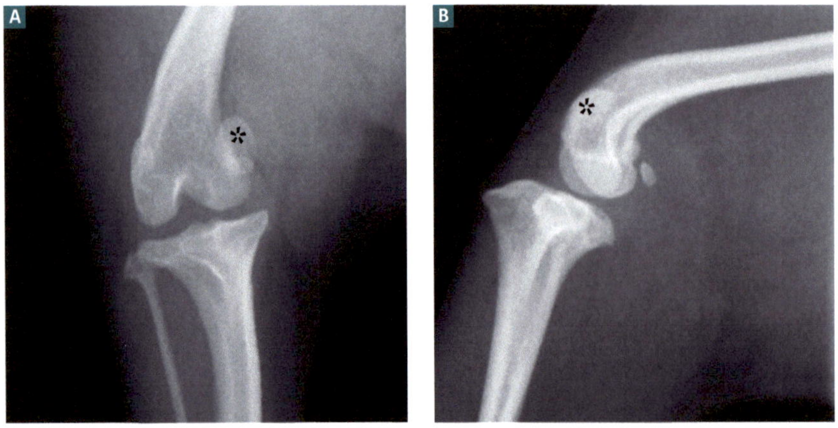

Figure 65. CdCr (**A**) and ML (**B**) radiographs of the stifle of a 14-month-old Yorkshire Terrier with grade II congenital medial patellar luxation. The patella is visualised medially overlapping with the supratrochlear area of the femur (asterisk).

- **Grade III**: the patella is permanently luxated, with rotation of the tibia and deviation of the tibial tuberosity between 30° and 50° from its CrCd plane.
- **Grade IV**: the tibia is tilted medially and can even be seen caudal to the femur in a lateral projection, the tibial tuberosity can show a greater medial deviation of between 50° and 90° in its CrCd plane, and there is curvature of the distal third of the femoral diaphysis (Fig. 66).

This pathology is easily recognised on radiographs; however, in advanced cases that require surgical treatment, CT studies are usually carried out, spanning the area from the coxofemoral joint to the tarsus of both limbs, to assess the degree of curvature of the bones (Dudley et al., 2006; Fox and Tomlinson, 2018) and the area of the trochlear groove of the femur in order to adequately plan corrective surgery (Petazzoni et al., 2018) (Fig. 67).

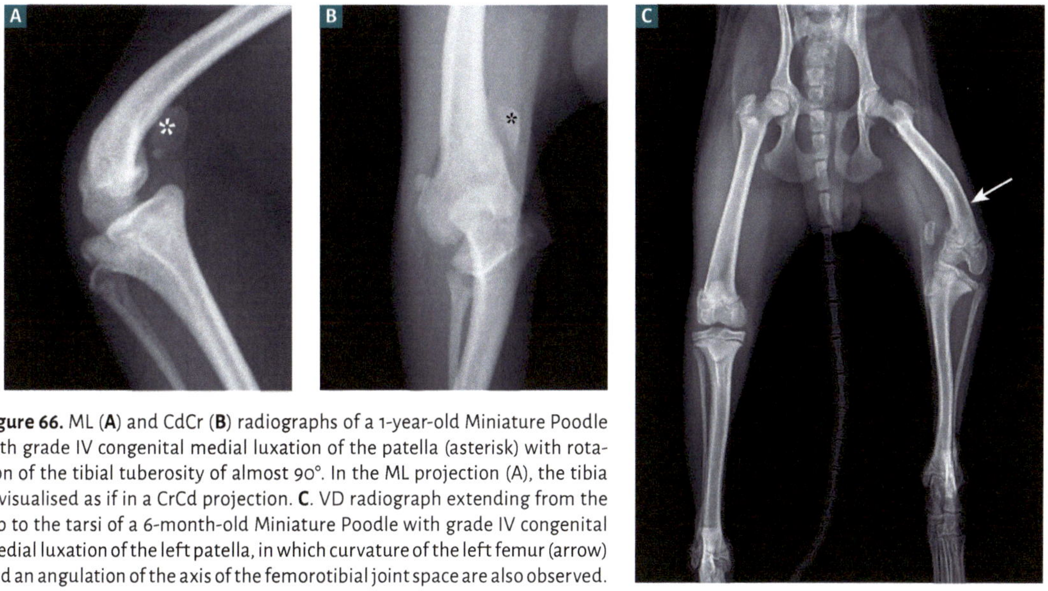

Figure 66. ML (**A**) and CdCr (**B**) radiographs of a 1-year-old Miniature Poodle with grade IV congenital medial luxation of the patella (asterisk) with rotation of the tibial tuberosity of almost 90°. In the ML projection (A), the tibia is visualised as if in a CrCd projection. **C**. VD radiograph extending from the hip to the tarsi of a 6-month-old Miniature Poodle with grade IV congenital medial luxation of the left patella, in which curvature of the left femur (arrow) and an angulation of the axis of the femorotibial joint space are also observed.

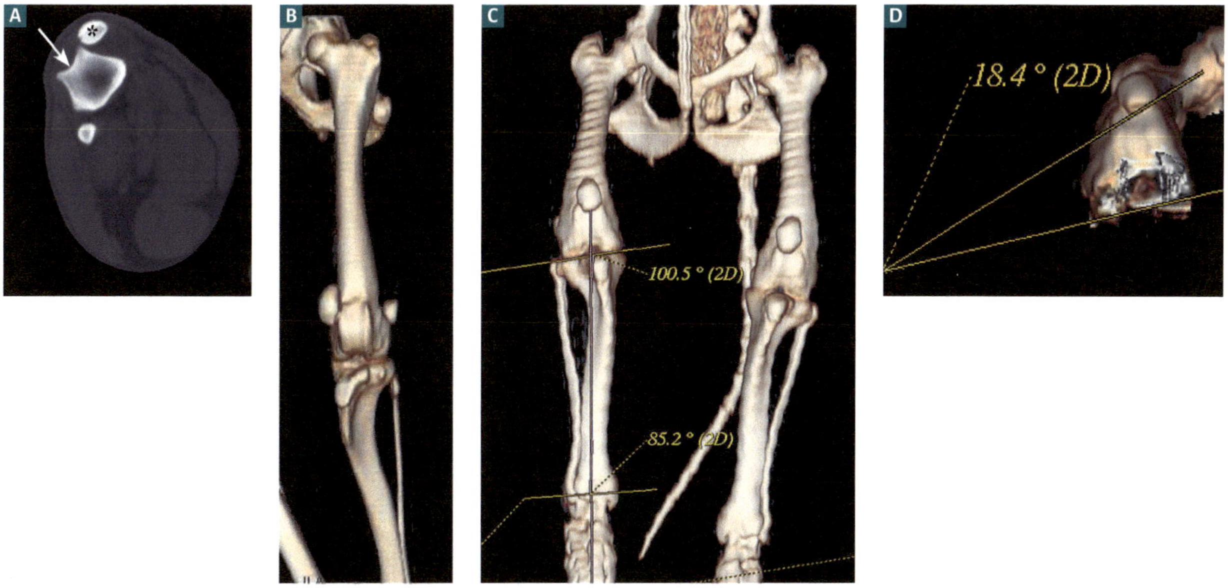

Figure 67. A. CT image in a transverse plane and a bone window of the right stifle of a 10-month-old Dogue de Bordeaux with bilateral medial patellar luxation. The patella is visualised in an abnormal medial position (asterisk). In addition, the trochlear groove of the femur (arrow) can be assessed in this image. **B**. Reconstructed image using volume rendering (VR) of the same animal as in image A. **C**, **D**. VR reconstructions of a CT study of the hindlimbs of a 9-month-old Maltese with patellar luxation. With these images, the necessary measurements can be made (proximal and distal medial tibial angle (C), anteversion angle (D)) to plan an adequate approach for corrective surgery.

Osteochondrosis/Osteochondritis Dissecans of the Femoral Condyles

In the stifle joint, this developmental disease mainly affects the lateral condyle and, less frequently, the medial condyle. Large-breed puppies (Saint Bernard, Rottweiler, Retrievers, etc.) aged between 5 months and 11 months are most frequently affected.

Radiographically, signs of joint inflammation, radiotransparent defects in the subchondral bone with adjacent sclerosis and flattening of the condylar surface, and the possible presence of joint mice can be observed. The differential diagnosis includes avulsion of the tendon of the long digital extensor muscle, which can create a radiotransparent defect in the lateral femoral condyle on radiographic imaging. Since tendon avulsion is an extra-articular pathology, changes associated with DJD are not present. It is important to remember to examine the contralateral stifle, because this pathology frequently has bilateral involvement (Pollard and Phillips, 2018) (Fig. 68).

Tibial Tuberosity Avulsion

This is a lesion of traumatic origin, typically seen in puppies. The tibial tuberosity detaches from the tibia, which leads to the dorsal displacement of the patella, as this is the point of insertion of the patellar tendon (Soler and Agut, 2014). If it is not very clearly visible, and in order not to confuse it with a physiological separation of the tibial tuberosity that is not yet fused with the tibia, performing a radiograph of the contralateral limb for comparison is recommended (Fig. 69).

Tarsal Joint

Projections

As for other areas of the hindlimb, sedation is recommended so that the animal can be properly positioned (Morgan, 1993).

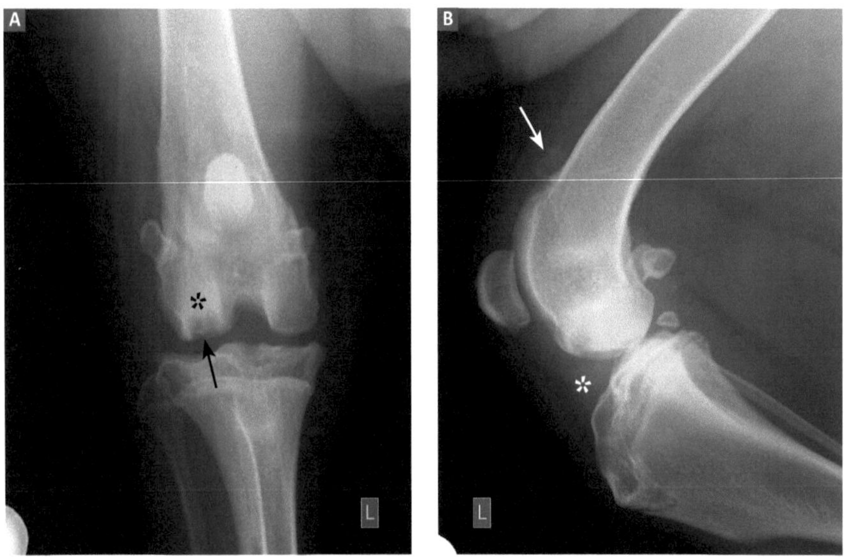

Figure 68. CrCd (**A**) and ML (**B**) radiographs of the left stifle of a 9-month-old German Shepherd Dog in which a radiotransparent focus (black arrow) with sclerosis of the adjacent subchondral bone (black asterisk), consistent with an osteochondrosis lesion, is visualised affecting the lateral femoral condyle. In addition, other signs of degenerative joint disease are observed, such as increased intra-articular opacity (synovial effusion) (white asterisk) and the presence of osteophytes in the supratrochlear region (white arrow).

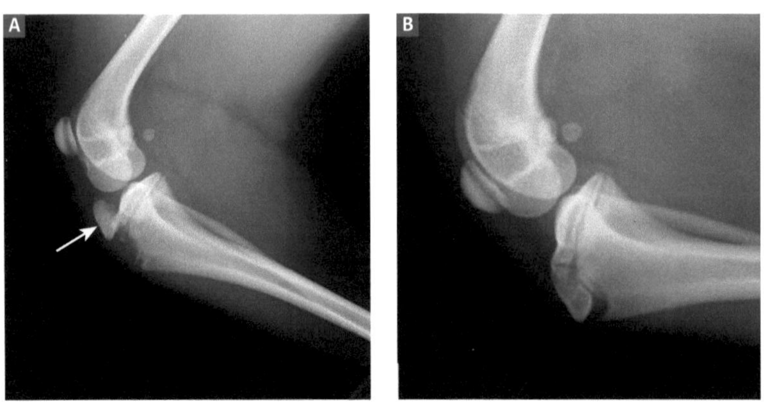

Figure 69. ML radiographs of both stifles (**A**: right, **B**: left) of a 5-month-old mixed-breed dog with lameness of the right hindlimb, which presented an avulsion fracture of the tibial tuberosity (arrow) and secondary proximal displacement of the patella. In the contralateral stifle, the tibial tuberosity has not yet fused to the tibia and presents a physiological separation.

- **Mediolateral** (ML): the position is the same as for the ML stifle projection but the X-ray beam is focused on the tarsal joint (Fig. 70 A).
- **Dorsoplantar** (DPt): the animal is positioned in dorsal or sternal recumbency (plantaro-dorsal projection, positioning the animal in the same way as for the CdCr projection of the stifle). The limb with the affected tarsus is extended and the X-ray beam is centred on the joint, avoiding rotation of the limb (Fig. 70 B).
- **Stress views**: as for the carpus, these types of projections are sometimes necessary. There are two stress ML views: flexed ML, that approximates the metatarsal bones toward the tibia and fibula using a tape, and the hyperextended ML: where a tape or rope is applied around the tibia and fibula and pulled cranially and at the same time another rope is placed around the metatarsal bones and pulled caudally. The DPt views of the tarsus with lateral or medial stress applied are obtained by placing two tapes: one around the proximal metatarsal bones and the second around the fibula and tibia. The tapes pull in opposite directions, one medially and the other laterally to obtain one of the stress DPt views and then it is repeated but pulling in a reverse way.
- **Flexed dorsoplantar/tangential "skyline" projection of the tarsus**: due to the overlap of the calcaneus in a DPt projection, the assessment of the trochlear groove of the talus and the lateral malleolus (distal end of the fibula) is complicated. To visualise these structures, the skyline projection can be performed. The patient is positioned in dorsal recumbency, using a holder or sandbags to ensure that its body does not rotate; the limb with the affected tarsus is flexed to place the tibia at a 90° angle with the femur, resting on a support; in turn, the foot is flexed and supported so that the metatarsals and phalanges are at a 90° angle with the tibia. The X-ray beam is centred on the tarsus (Fig. 71).

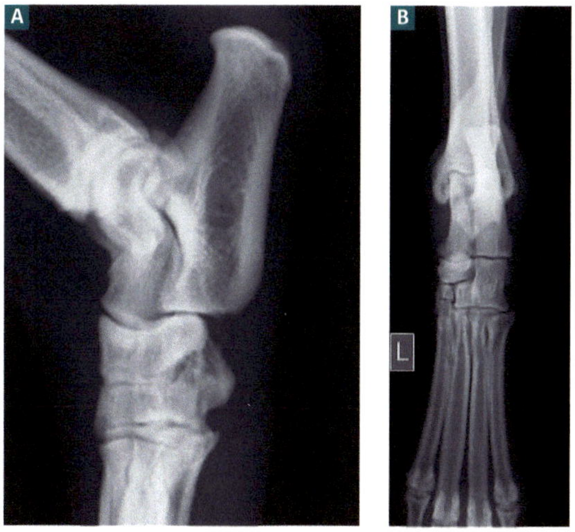

Figure 70. ML (**A**) and DPt (**B**) radiographs of the tarsus of an adult dog without abnormalities.

Fractures

Malleolar fractures are common joint fractures. Medial (tibial) malleolus fractures are more common than those of the lateral (fibular) malleolus (Fig. 72).

Fractures of the tarsal bones are not very common, with the order of incidence being fractures of the calcaneus, talus and central tarsal bone.

Luxation and Subluxation

These lesions lead to the rupture of joint ligaments. As with luxation of the carpus, they are revealed on forced/stressed projections of the joint, and in certain cases it is necessary to carry out a CT study to assess small fractures (Fig. 73).

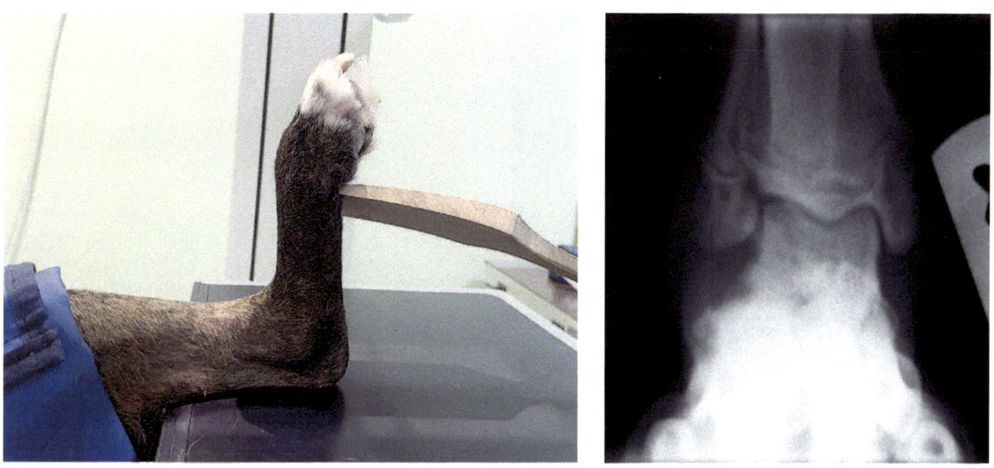

Figure 71. Positioning for performing the DPt projection in tarsal flexion (or tarsal skyline) and a resulting radiograph, in which the calcaneus is not superimposed on the trochlea of the talus or the lateral malleolus of the fibula.

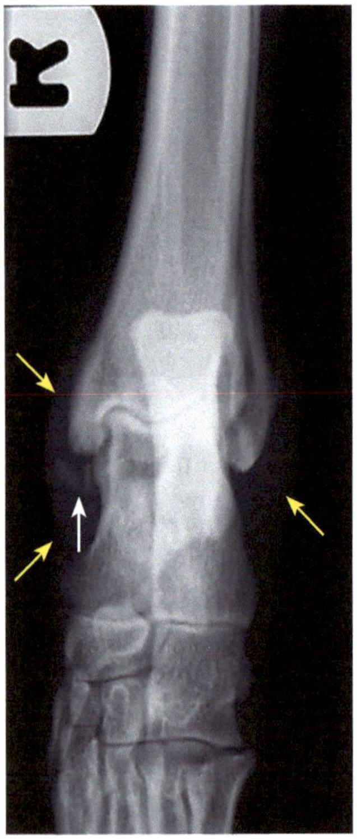

Figure 72. DPt radiograph of the tarsus of an adult dog presenting with a fracture of the medial malleolus of the tibia with two small "chip-like" fragments (white arrow). There is also an increase in the thickness of the periarticular soft tissues (yellow arrows).

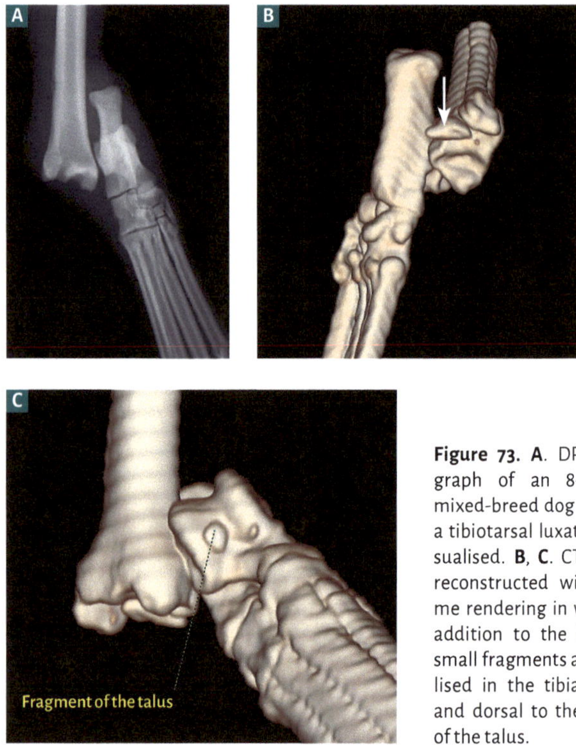

Figure 73. A. DPt radiograph of an 8-year-old mixed-breed dog in which a tibiotarsal luxation is visualised. **B**, **C**. CT images reconstructed with volume rendering in which, in addition to the luxation, small fragments are visualised in the tibia (arrow) and dorsal to the surface of the talus.

Tarsal Osteochondrosis/ Osteochondritis Dissecans

This pathology usually occurs more frequently in the medial trochlear border of the talus but can affect the lateral border. Although rare, lateral lesions have been reported to be larger than those seen medially (Samii et al., 2011). Radiographically, an increase in the joint space is observed and, sometimes, in the ML projection, the defect in the articular surface can be detected, although it is difficult to see it clearly. Degenerative changes (DJD) are observed in old lesions (Pollard and Phillips, 2018). In order to better observe the bone abnormality, performing a DPt projection is indicated with the tarsus flexed to form a 90° angle with the tibia and centring the X-ray beam on the distal tibia, so that the trochlea of the talus can be visualised without overlapping the calcaneus; alternatively, a CT study can be performed (Fig. 74).

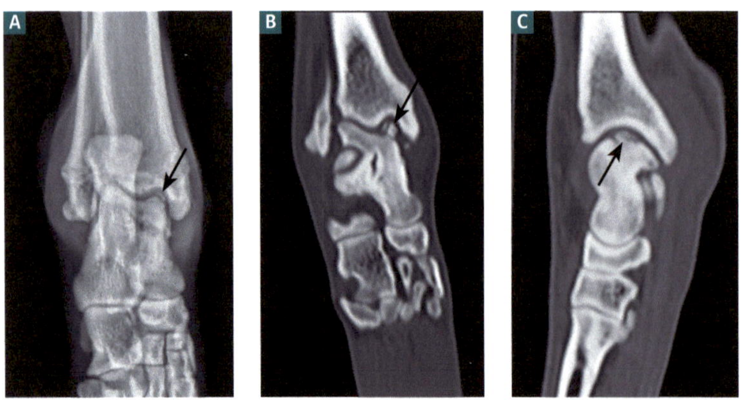

Figure 74. DPt radiograph (**A**) and reconstructed CT images in the dorsal (**B**) and sagittal (**C**) plane in a bone window of an adult dog with an osteochondritis dissecans lesion on the medial aspect of the trochlea of the talus. A mineralised fragment of articular cartilage is visualised (arrow). (Images courtesy of Dr. A. Ansón, Tufts University.)

Metatarsals and Phalanges

Projections

Mediolateral (ML) and **dorsoplantar** (DPt): positioning is the same as when these projections are performed on the tarsal joint. The X-ray beam is focused on the metatarsophalangeal joints and the tarsal joint should be included in the collimation. In the event that an abnormality in the phalanges is suspected, projections similar to those described for the phalanges of the forelimb (separating the toes with cotton wool balls) should be obtained (Morgan, 1993).

Fractures

As is the case for the metacarpals, fractures are the most common pathology that affect the metatarsal bones, especially when an animal falls from a height (more common in cats), and can be accompanied by luxation of the tarsus due to ligament rupture (Fig. 75).

Fragmentation of Metacarpal/ Metatarsophalangeal Sesamoid Bones

This syndrome has been described in large breeds of dog and occurs more frequently in Rottweilers. The aetiology is not fully known, but the most likely hypothesis is that of underlying osteonecrosis affecting the sesamoids. Although there are eight sesamoid bones in each limb, the sesamoid bones that are affected by this pathology are mainly the II and VII (numbered from medial to lateral) (Fig. 76). This pathology is evident in a DP/DPt projection, but if it cannot be clearly seen, oblique projections can be used while applying traction on the toes (Thrall and Robertson, 2011).

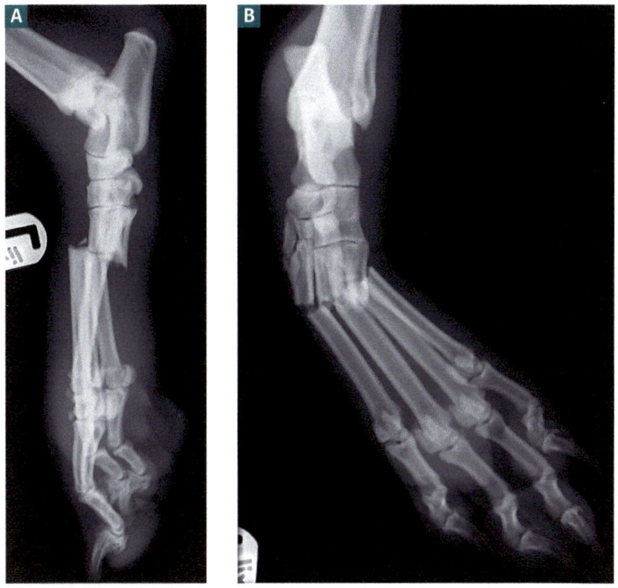

Figure 75. ML (**A**) and DPt (**B**) radiographs of a 9-year-old Labrador Retriever with fracture of the four metatarsal bones in the proximal third of the diaphysis, with dorsal and lateral displacement of the distal fragments.

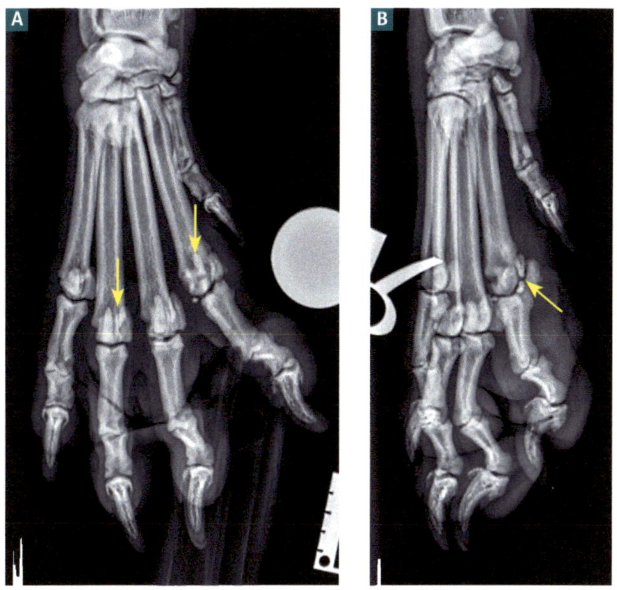

Figure 76. DP (**A**) and lateral oblique (**B**) radiographs of the forefoot of a 7-year-old Rottweiler with fragmentation of the II and V sesamoid bones (arrows). (Image courtesy Dr. A. Navarro, Nexo Menescal Novelda.)

Bibliography

■ Barreiro, A., Vila, M. (2014) Articulaciones y enfermedades articulares. In: Agut, A. (ed). *Diagnóstico por Imagen en Pequeños Animales*, pp. 123–161. Multimédica Ediciones Veterinarias.

■ Carrera, I., Hammond, G., Sullivan, M. (2008) Computed tomographic features of incomplete ossification of the canine humeral condyle. *Vet Surg*, 37(3):226–231.

■ Cook, C.R., Cook, J.L. (2009) Diagnostic imaging of canine elbow dysplasia: a review. *Vet Surg*, 38(2):144–153.

■ Craig, L.E. (2001) Physeal dysplasia with slipped capital femoral epiphysis in 13 cats. *Vet Pathol*, 38(1):92–97.

■ Di Dona, F., Della Valle, G., Fatone, G. (2018) Patellar luxation in dogs. *Vet Med (Auckl)*. 9:23–32.

■ Dudley, R.M., Kowaleski, M.P., Drost, W.T., Dyce, J. (2006) Radiographic and computed tomographic determination of femoral varus and torsion in the dog. *Vet Radiol Ultrasound*, 47(6):546–552.

■ Fox, D.B., Tomlinson, J.L. (2018) Principles of angular limb deformity correction. In: Johnston SA, Tobias KM (eds). *Veterinary Surgery. Small Animal*. 2nd ed, pp. 2152–2184. Elsevier.

■ Fujiki, M., Misumi, K., Sakamoto, H. (2004) Laxity of canine hip joint in two positions with computed tomography. *J Vet Med Sci*, 66(8):1003–1006.

■ Gemmill, T.J., Pink, J., Clarke, S.P., McKee, W.M. (2012) Total hip replacement for the treatment of atraumatic slipped femoral capital epiphysis in dogs. *J Small Anim Pract*, 53(8):453–458.

■ Grundmann, S., Montavon, P.M. (2001) Stenosing tenosynovitis of the abductor pollicis longus muscle in dogs. *Vet Comp Orthop Traumatol*, 14(2):95–100.

■ Harasen, G. (2005) Coxofemoral luxations part 1: diagnosis and closed reduction. *Can Vet J*, 46(4):368–370.

■ Harasen, G. (2007) Pelvic fractures. *Can Vet J*, 48(4):427–428.

■ Hittmair, K.M., Groessl, V., Mayrhofer, E. (2012) Radiographic and ultrasonographic diagnosis of stenosing tenosynovitis of the abductor pollicis longus muscle in dogs. *Vet Radiol Ultrasound*, 53(2):135–141.

■ Johnson, K.A. (1987) Accessory carpal bone fractures in the racing greyhound. Classification and pathology. *Vet Surg*, 16(1):60–64.

■ Kirberger, R.M. (2006) The elbow joint. In: Barr, F.J., Kirberger, R.M. (eds). *BSAVA Manual of Canine and Feline Musculoskeletal Imaging*, pp. 103–118. BSAVA.

■ Kishimoto, M., Yamada, K., Pae, S.H., et al. (2009) Quantitative evaluation of hip joint laxity in 22 Border Collies using computed tomography. *J Vet Med Sci*, 71(2):247–250.

■ Marino, D.J., Matthiesen, D.T., Stefanacci, J.D., Moroff, S.D. (1995) Evaluation of dogs with digit masses: 117 cases (1981–1991). *J Am Vet Med Assoc*, 207(6):726–728.

■ Michelsen, J. (2013) Canine elbow dysplasia: aetiopathogenesis and current treatment recommendations. *Vet J*, 196(1):12–19.

■ Milton, J.L., Montgomery, R.D. (1987) Congenital elbow dislocations. *Vet Clin North Am Small Anim Pract*, 17(4):873–888.

■ Montinaro, V., Boston, S.E., Buracco, P., et al. (2013) Clinical outcome of 42 dogs with scapular tumors treated by scalpulectomy: a Veterinary Society of Surgical Oncology (VSSO) retrospective study (1995–2010). *Vet Surg*, 42(8):943–950.

■ Moores, A.P., Owen, M.R., Fews, D., et al. (2004) Slipped capital femoral epiphysis in dogs. *J Small Anim Pract*, 45(12):602–608.

■ Morgan, J.P. (1993) *Techniques of Veterinary Radiography*. 5th ed, pp. 3–272. Iowa State University Press.

■ Petazzoni, M., De Giacinto, E., Troiano, D., et al. (2018) Computed tomographic trochlear depth measurement in normal dogs. *Vet Comp Orthop Traumatol*, 31(6):431–437.

■ Pollard, R.E., Phillips, K.L. (2018) Orthopedic diseases of young and growing dogs and cats. In: Thrall DE. (ed). *Textbook of Veterinary Diagnostic Radiology*. 7th ed, pp. 348–365. Elsevier Saunders.

■ Powers, M.Y., Biery, D.N., Lawler, D., et al. (2004) Use of the caudolateral curvilinear osteophyte as an early marker for future development of osteoarthritis associated with hip dysplasia in dogs. *J Am Vet Med Assoc*, 225(2):233–237.

■ Queen, J., Bennett, D., Carmichael, S., et al. (1998) Femoral neck metaphyseal osteopathy in the cat. *Vet Rec*, 142(7):159–162.

■ Sage, J.E., Gavin, P. (2016) Musculoskeletal MRI. *Vet Clin North Am Small Anim Pract*, 46(3):421-451.

■ Samii, V., Gielen, I., Ludewig, E. et al. (2011) Joints. In: Schwarz T, Saunders J. (eds). *Veterinary Computed Tomography*; pp. 387–419 Wiley-Blackwell.

■ Schwartz, G. (2013) Spontaneous capital femoral physeal fracture in a cat. *Can Vet J*, 54(7):698–700.

■ Soler, M., Agut, A. (2014) Traumatismos y fracturas. In: Agut, A. (ed). *Diagnóstico por Imagen en Pequeños Animales*, pp. 175–186. Multimédica Ediciones Veterinarias.

■ Soler, M., Villamonte-Chevalier, A., Martínez, M., Agut, A. (2015) Diagnóstico por imagen de la displasia de codo. *Canis et Felis*, 136:110–127.

■ Spall, B.F., Fransson, B.A., Martinez, S.A., Wilkinson, T.E. (2016) Tendon volume determination on magnetic resonance imaging of supraspinatus tendinopathy. *Vet Surg*, 45(3):386–391.

■ Thrall, D.E., Robertson, I.D. (2011) *Atlas of Normal Radiographic Anatomy and Anatomic Variants in the Dog and Cat*. Elsevier Saunders.

■ Villamonte-Chevalier, A., Van Bree, H., Broeckx, B.J.G., et al. (2015) Assessment of medial coronoid disease in canine lame elbow joints: a sensitivity and specificity comparison of radiographic, computed tomographic and arthroscopic findings. *BMC Vet Res*, 11:243.

■ Zalcman, A.R., Cook, C., Mai, W. (2018) MRI of musculoskeletal diseases. In: Mai. W. (ed). *Diagnostic MRI in Dogs and Cats*., pp. 643–686. CRC Press.

Notes

Ultrasonography of the Limbs

Vicente Esteve Bernet and Patricia Laborda Vidal

Introduction

A wide variety of injuries can be diagnosed using musculoskeletal ultrasonography. The main applications of musculoskeletal ultrasonography are for imaging muscle or tendon ruptures, where there is clinical suspicion of tendinopathies, searching for foreign bodies, ultrasound-guided sampling of muscle, joint or bone masses, and monitoring the evolution of lesions.

Musculoskeletal ultrasonography is a complementary technique that is usually used alongside the acquisition of several radiographic views, complete computed tomography (CT) studies and/or magnetic resonance imaging (MRI). This is especially important in tendon injuries and injuries that may affect the appendicular skeleton. It is a cheap, fast and commonly available technique. However, the information that is obtained by musculoskeletal ultrasonography is highly dependent on the sonographer's experience and knowledge of anatomy, and the ultrasound machine that is used. The most commonly used ultrasound probe in musculoskeletal ultrasonography is the high-frequency linear probe (Fig. 1 A), as the structures to be examined are generally quite shallow and the linear probe offers the best resolution. However, the linear probe may be difficult to engage in certain anatomical regions with bony protrusions. To avoid this problem, a silicone standoff pad can be used or, alternatively, a glove filled with water or gel (avoiding the presence of gas bubbles inside). Sometimes the use of a microconvex probe (Fig. 1 B) is necessary to access deeper structures or to achieve better coupling between the probe and the anatomical region being examined. This chapter will cover the main applications of musculoskeletal ultrasonography in dogs and cats and the lesions that can be imaged by this method.

Patient Preparation

The patient should be placed in lateral recumbency. Studies should always be bilateral, looking for asymmetries and making comparisons with the contralateral anatomy. The animal may be awake, or lightly sedated if it is in pain or nervous. The area to be examined should be clipped extensively. During the ultrasound examination, two sections (longitudinal and transverse) should always be used. The same transducer position (proximal versus distal and lateral versus medial) should always be used to help the sonographer become familiar with the image, as the ultrasonographic anatomy of the musculoskeletal system can be complicated.

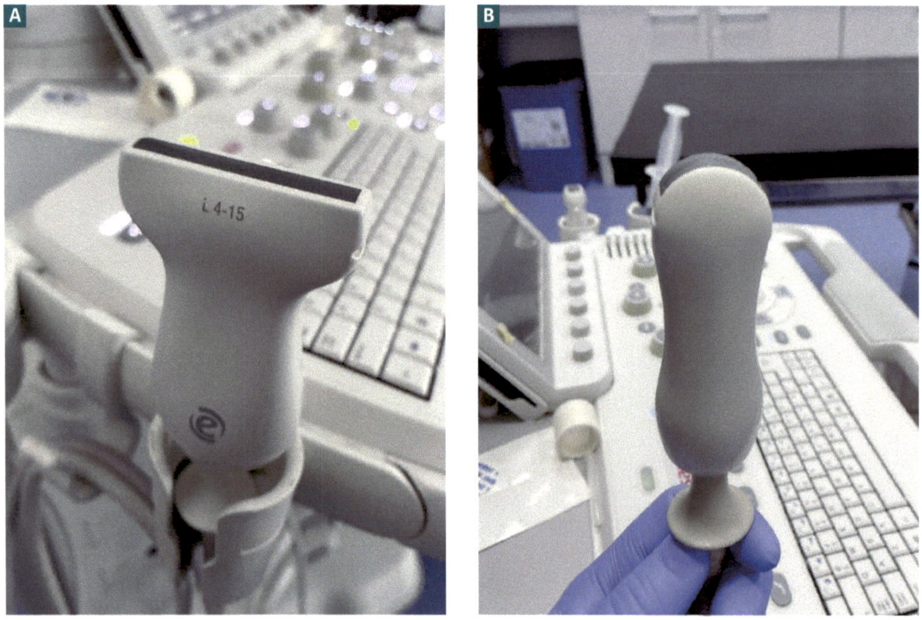

Figure 1. Ultrasound probes used in musculoskeletal ultrasonography. **A**. High-frequency linear probe. **B**. Microconvex probe.

The Shoulder

Examination Technique

Ultrasound examination of the shoulder in dogs was described by Long and Nyland (1999). Muscles in the shoulder that can be evaluated ultrasonographically are as follows:

- supraspinatus muscle
- infraspinatus muscle
- biceps brachii muscle.

The examination should be performed with the joint in external rotation (supination) in order to visualise the tendon of the biceps muscle, and in a neutral position to see the tendon insertions of the supraspinatus and infraspinatus muscles (Fig. 2 A). It is advisable, when examining all muscles, to start the examination in the muscle bellies and approach their origin or insertion in the shoulder region. To view the scapulohumeral joint, the probe is positioned on the lateral surface in a caudocranial orientation. The acromion serves as a reference point (Fig. 2 B). While holding the probe on the surface, the limb should be adducted and rotated. Access to the cranial part of the joint is hindered by the greater tubercle of the humerus, and access to the medial part is hindered by the chest wall.

Ultrasonographic Anatomy

The points of origin and insertion of the supraspinatus, infraspinatus and biceps brachii muscles are detailed in Table 1.

Table 1. Areas of origin and insertion of the supraspinatus, infraspinatus and biceps brachii muscles.

Muscle	Origin	Insertion
Supraspinatus	Supraspinous fossa	Greater tubercle of the humerus
Infraspinatus	Infraspinous fossa	Caudolateral to the greater tubercle of the humerus
Biceps brachii	Supraglenoid tubercle of scapula	Tuberosity of the ulna and tuberosity of the radius (medially)

Fig. 3 depicts the shoulder joint with the tendons of the supraspinatus, infraspinatus and biceps muscles.

The muscle belly of the **supraspinatus muscle** is hypoechoic and striated (Fig. 4 A). It crosses over to the craniomedial part of the shoulder and inserts into the greater tubercle, which appears as a convex, irregular and hyperechoic surface, with distal acoustic shadow. Owing to the orientation of the muscle fibres, the supraspinatus muscle tendon is hypoechoic with a muscle-like appearance (Fig. 4 B). The muscle belly of the **infraspinatus muscle** has a central hyperechoic fibre connecting with peripherally oriented, oblique, hyperechoic fibres and has a "fish bone" appearance (Fig. 5 A). The **deltoid muscle** is in a superficial position with respect to the infraspinatus muscle. The tendon of the infraspinatus muscle is formed of parallel hyperechoic fibres surrounded by a thin, hyperechoic peritendon (Fig. 5 B). The muscle belly of the **biceps muscle** can be scanned from the craniomedial aspect of the humeral diaphysis, moving proximally towards the tendon of origin (Fig. 6). It is hypoechoic and has the appearance of a fish skeleton due to its two muscle bellies.

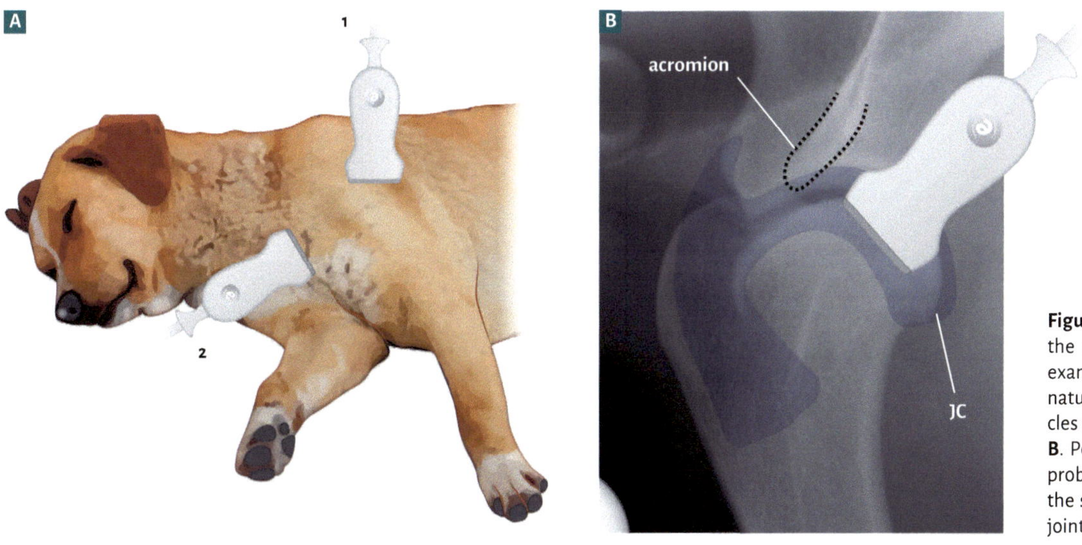

Figure 2. A. Positioning of the ultrasound probe during examination of the supraspinatus and infraspinatus muscles (1) and biceps muscle (2). **B**. Position of the ultrasound probe during examination of the scapulohumeral joint. JC: joint capsule.

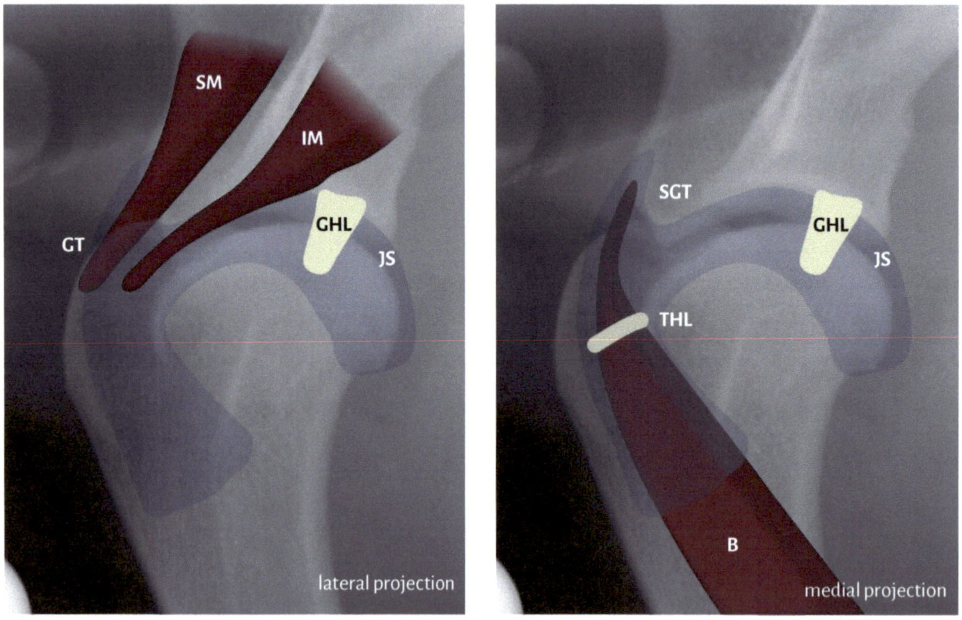

Figure 3. Shoulder joint in lateral and medial projections. SM: supraspinatus muscle; IM: infraspinatus muscle; GT: greater tubercle; GHL: glenohumeral ligament; JS: joint space; SGT: supraglenoid tuberosity; THL: transverse humeral ligament; B: biceps.

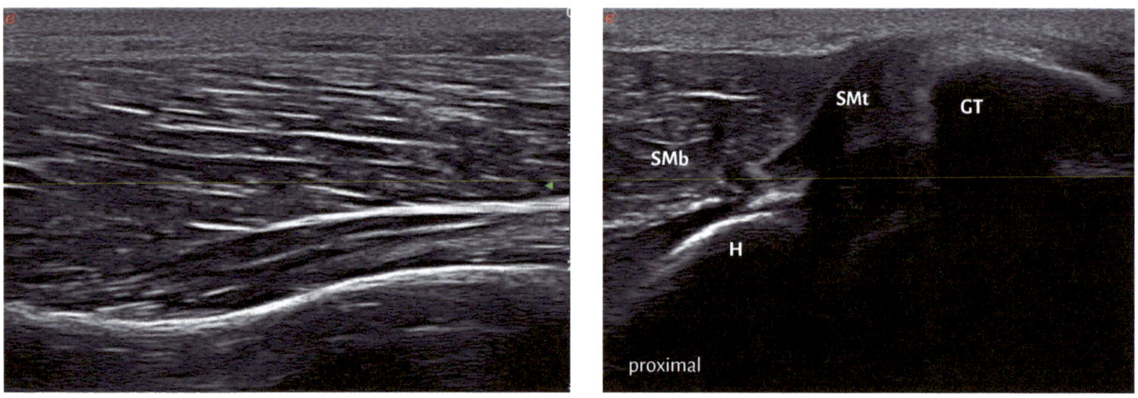

Figure 4. Supraspinatus muscle. Longitudinal ultrasound images of the muscle belly (SMb) and tendon insertion (SMt), which inserts into the greater tubercle (GT) of the humerus (H).

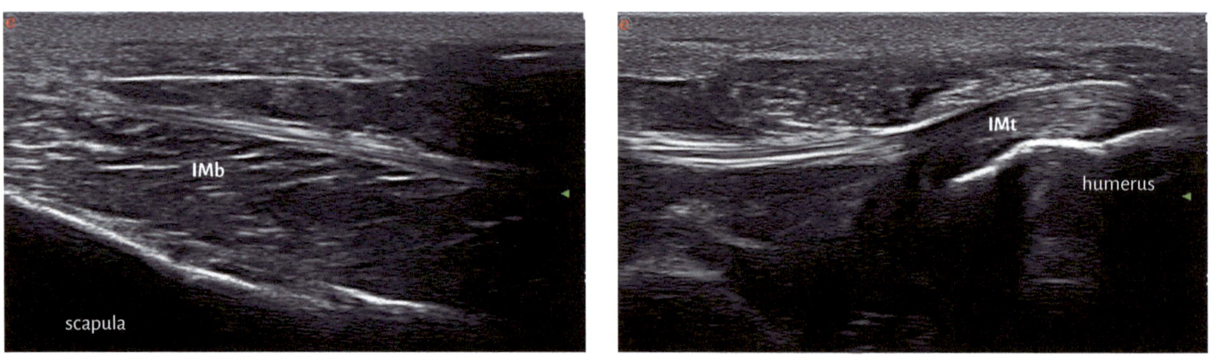

Figure 5. Infraspinatus muscle. Longitudinal ultrasound images of the muscle belly (IMb) and the tendon insertion (IMt).

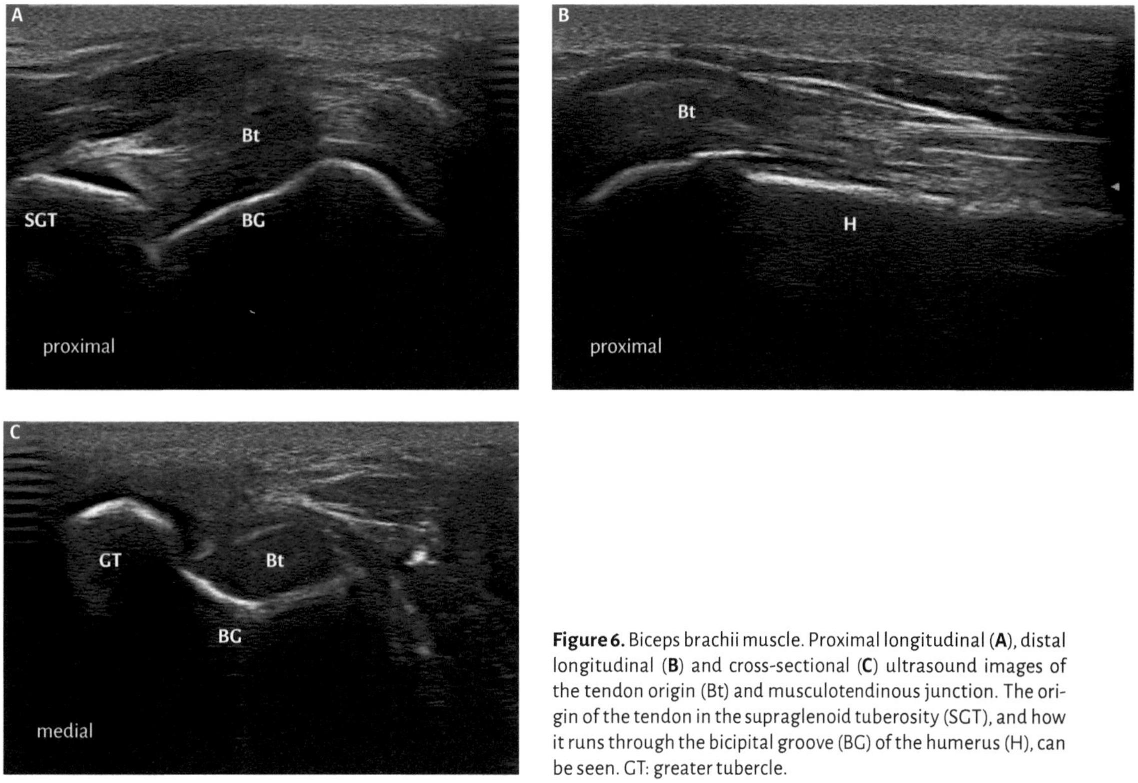

Figure 6. Biceps brachii muscle. Proximal longitudinal (**A**), distal longitudinal (**B**) and cross-sectional (**C**) ultrasound images of the tendon origin (Bt) and musculotendinous junction. The origin of the tendon in the supraglenoid tuberosity (SGT), and how it runs through the bicipital groove (BG) of the humerus (H), can be seen. GT: greater tubercle.

The tendon runs along the bicipital sulcus, medially to the greater tubercle, and is surrounded by a minimal amount of anechoic fluid within the thin hyperechoic sheath. In cross section, it is seen as an oval structure approximately 3 mm thick. It is important to place the transducer perpendicular to the tendon to avoid artefacts that could be mistaken for lesions. Proximally, it can be followed to the supraglenoid tubercle.

At the joint, the head of the humerus appears as a semicircular, convex structure, with thin, well-defined borders and a distal acoustic shadow. The hyperechoic subchondral surface is covered by anechoic articular cartilage and a thin layer of hypoechoic synovial fluid. The medial glenohumeral ligament is thin and can be seen inconsistently.

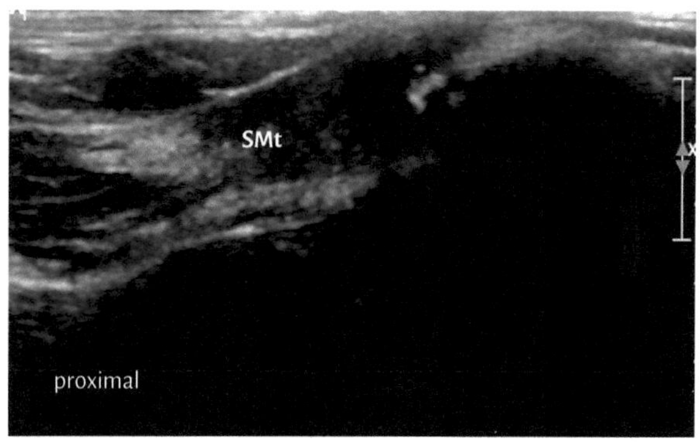

Figure 7. Longitudinal ultrasound image of the supraspinatus muscle tendon insertion (SMt) in a dog with calcifying tendinopathy.

Pathological Findings

The pathologies that are most frequently evaluated by ultrasound of the shoulder are the following:

- calcifying tendinopathy of the supraspinatus muscle
- contracture of the infraspinatus muscle
- tenosynovitis of the biceps muscle
- calcifying tendinopathy of the biceps muscle.

The general ultrasonographic appearance in acute **tendinopathies** is a thickened and hypoechoic tendon due to disruption of its fibres. In the chronic phases, echogenicity is normal or increased, presenting with reorganisation of fibres, and there is usually dystrophic mineralisation. When there is a partial breakage of fibres, hypoechoic foci can be observed in the tendon. In complete ruptures, the tendon is discontinuous, and in the area of rupture there is a cluster of hypoechoic material that corresponds with haemorrhage. The musculotendinous junction is usually retracted and has a heterogeneous echogenicity (Kramer et al., 2001b).

In **calcifying tendinopathy of the supraspinatus muscle** (Fig. 7), the tendon usually appears thickened and heterogeneous due to fibre rupture, haemorrhagic foci or fibrosis. It can displace the biceps tendon medially. Mineralised foci in tendons are observed as hyperechoic structures with an irregular area, with or without distal acoustic shadow, usually surrounded by a hypoechoic halo. Tendon mineralisation has been observed in both lame and asymptomatic animals (Lafuente et al., 2009).

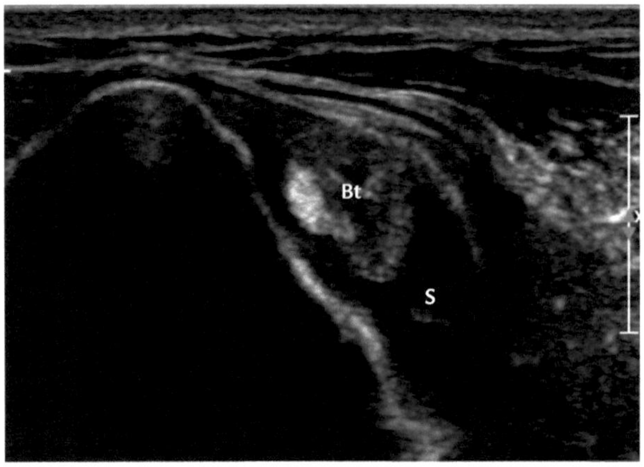

Figure 8. Cross-sectional ultrasound image of tenosynovitis of the biceps in a dog. The tendon (Bt) is thickened and irregularly shaped, and there is a large amount of anechoic fluid (S) in the tendon sheath.

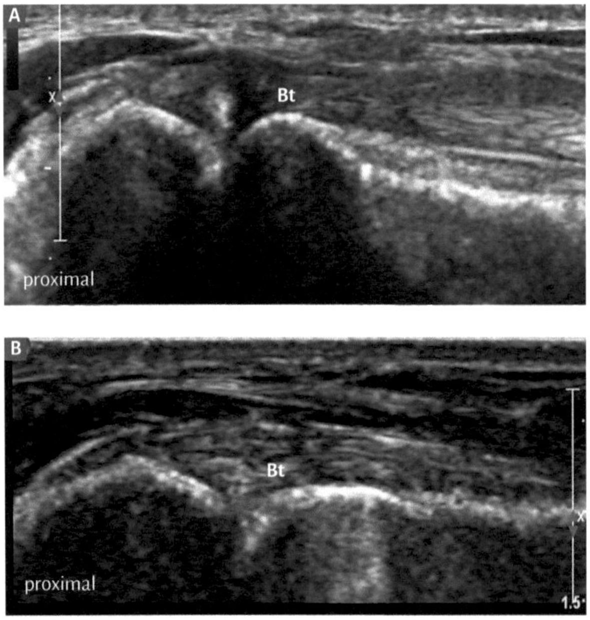

Figure 9. Longitudinal ultrasound images of (**A**) a calcifying tendinopathy of the biceps muscle and (**B**) the normal contralateral biceps tendon (Bt) in a dog. A small hyperechoic structure is observed around the tendon insertion.

Tendinopathies of the infraspinatus muscle are less common than those of the supraspinatus and have a similar appearance. **Contractures of the infraspinatus** (and supraspinatus) muscle appear as hyperechoic, heterogeneous areas with reduced muscle belly or tendon volume in chronic cases (Siems et al., 1998).

In **tenosynovitis of the biceps muscle** (Fig. 8), the tendon is usually thickened, rounded in cross section, heterogeneous, and usually presents a cluster of anechoic or hypoechoic fluid in the synovial sheath. To evaluate fibrous adhesion in the bicipital sulcus, a dynamic scan can be performed. Ultrasonographically, osteophytes can also be observed around the bicipital groove in chronic lesions, which are observed as irregular, hyperechoic structures, with or without distal acoustic shadow, and dystrophic mineralisations within the tendon sheath (calcifying tendinopathy) (Fig. 9). These mineralisations can be confused with free bone fragments, usually from osteochondritis dissecans.

In **tendon luxation**, the tendon is displaced medially, and in its place there is usually a moderate amount of effusion, which could initially be confused with a complete rupture of the tendon.

The Elbow

For the evaluation of elbow pathology, the most commonly used diagnostic techniques are radiography and CT, and occasionally MRI. Ultrasonography is primarily useful for evaluating muscles and tendons, especially the triceps tendon insertion. The ultrasonographic anatomy of the elbow has been described by Lamb and Wong (2005).

The Stifle (Knee)

Ultrasonographic Anatomy

The ultrasonographic anatomy of the stifle has been described by Kramer et al. (1999).

In the **suprapatellar approach**, the suprapatellar articular recess can be observed as a hypoechoic structure with poorly defined edges, proximal to the patella and adjacent to the femur. It should not be more than 1–2 mm thick.

In the **infrapatellar approach**, infrapatellar fat is observed ultrasonographically as a structure with poorly defined edges,

There are five different approaches to examining the stifle joint, which allow visualisation of different structures.

- **Suprapatellar: femoral quadriceps tendon, suprapatellar joint recess (Fig. 10).**
- **Infrapatellar: patellar tendon, infrapatellar fat, cruciate ligaments (Fig. 11).**
- **Lateral: lateral collateral ligament, lateral meniscus (Fig. 12 A).**
- **Medial: medial collateral ligament, medial meniscus (Fig. 12 B).**
- **Caudal: provides little information as there is poor visualisation of the joint.**

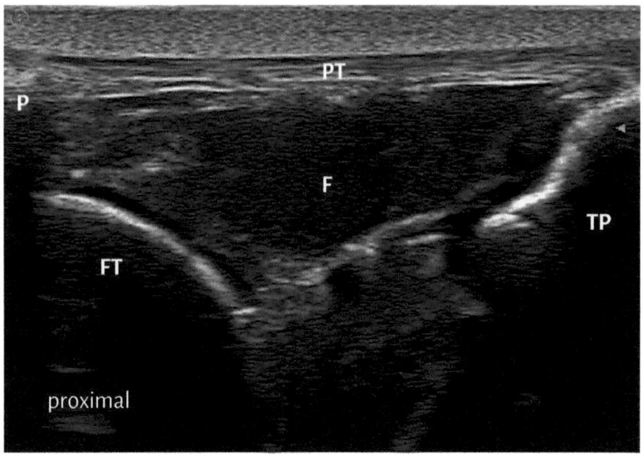

Figure 11. Ultrasonographic examination of the stifle, infrapatellar approach. The shadow produced by the patella distally (P), the patellar tendon (PT) and the infrapatellar fat (F) are observed. FT: femoral trochlea; TP: tibial plateau.

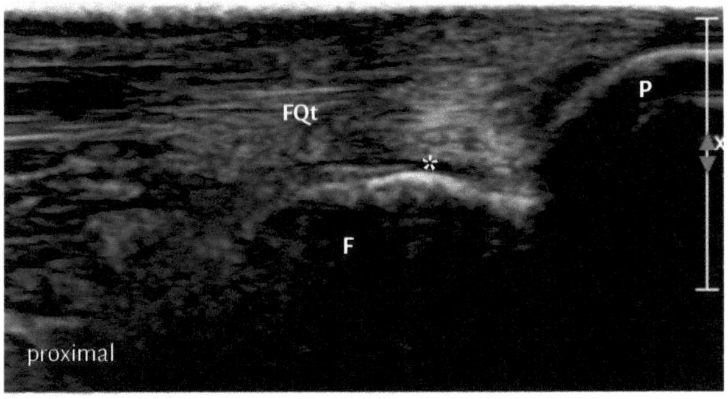

Figure 10. Ultrasonographic examination of the stifle, suprapatellar approach. The patella (P), femoral quadriceps tendon (FQt) and suprapatellar joint recess (*) are observed. F: femur.

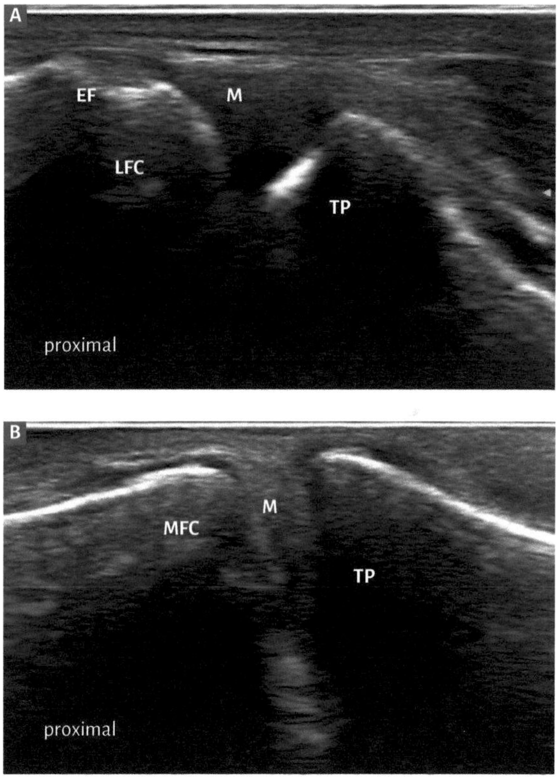

Figure 12. Ultrasonographic examination of the stifle, lateral (**A**) and medial (**B**) approaches. The lateral (in A) and medial (in B) menisci (M) and the extensor fossa (EF), where the long digital extensor muscle tendon originates (in A), are observed. MFC: medial femoral condyle; LFC: lateral femoral condyle; TP: tibial plateau.

which is hyperechoic and grainy in appearance, and which may have small vessels inside it. The cranial cruciate ligament can be observed by moving the transducer laterally by about 20°. The ligament is hypoechoic or anechoic and is located between the cranial part of the tibia and the intercondylar region of the femur. The caudal cruciate ligament is difficult to visualise.

In the **medial and lateral approaches**, the menisci are observed, which are triangular structures of moderate, homogeneous echogenicity, located between the femoral condyle and the tibial plateau. They are covered by a thin anechoic layer that corresponds to articular cartilage and synovium. The abaxial border of each meniscus should not protrude from the condylar edge and tibial plateau. The menisci can be difficult to see in small animals and in very large or obese animals. The long digital extensor muscle tendon can be seen in longitudinal section with the lateral approach (Fig. 12 A). It is located cranial to the collateral ligament, between the lateral meniscus and the joint capsule. It originates in the extensor fossa, in the craniolateral part of the lateral femoral condyle. It is thin and hypoechoic, and has a sheath that can be seen only when a certain amount of liquid accumulates inside it. In many cases, performing a dynamic stifle evaluation is important.

Pathological Findings

The most common pathologies that are evaluated by stifle ultrasonography are the following:

- cranial cruciate ligament rupture
- meniscus rupture (medial > lateral)
- ruptured patellar or quadriceps tendon
- thickening of the patellar tendon
- lateral collateral ligament rupture
- long digital extensor tendon avulsion.

The sensitivity of ultrasonography for detecting **cranial cruciate ligament rupture** is very low at around 15% (Arnault et al., 2009). However, it is possible to see the joint changes associated with cranial cruciate ligament rupture, including anechoic effusion (which can extend to both the suprapatellar recess and around the origin of the long digital extensor tendon, as well as caudally), cranial displacement of hyperechoic infrapatellar fat, osteophytes in cases of chronic joint instability, and capsular and synovial thickening. These findings are similar to those seen radiographically. To try to visualise the cranial cruciate ligament, a cranial infrapatellar approach must be used, with the knee flexed, preferably with the animal sedated. In cases of acute rupture there is usually a hypoechoic haematoma in the ligament region. In chronic ruptures, irregular hyperechoic structures representing fibrous tissue can be seen.

Meniscus rupture is most frequently observed in the medial meniscus and associated with cranial cruciate ligament rupture. The sensitivity and specificity of ultrasonography for detecting meniscus rupture have been estimated at 82% and 93%, respectively (Arnault et al., 2009). Four ultrasonographic characteristics have been described in affected menisci: these are changes in echogenicity (heterogeneous or hypoechoic), changes in shape, changes in position (usually with a bulge in the abaxial direction) and, usually, associated joint effusion.

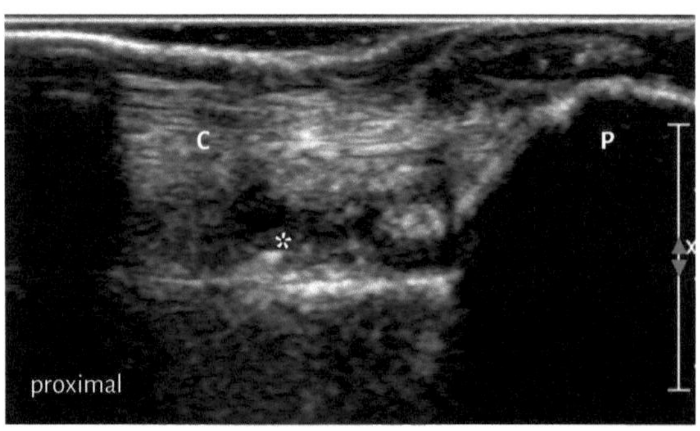

Figure 13. Ultrasonography of the stifle, suprapatellar approach. Partial rupture of the quadriceps tendon insertion (C) in a dog. The tendon appears thickened, with heterogeneous echogenicity, disruption of some fibres, hypoechoic foci (haematomas) and a small accumulation of fluid in the suprapatellar recess (*). P: patella.

Rupture of the quadriceps tendon insertion (Fig. 13) follows the same pattern of ultrasonographic findings as other tendon ruptures in the acute and repair phases. These phases are described in more detail in the following section. After tendon rupture and subsequent surgical repair, the tendon may remain thickened for many months. Postsurgical thickening of the patellar tendon may be normal after tibial plateau levelling osteotomy (up to 4 weeks; Mattern et al., 2006) and tibial tuberosity advancement surgery (up to 6 weeks; Kühn et al., 2011). This thickening may be due to hypertrophy or desmitis. In both cases it appears hypoechoic and thickened, and it is difficult to differentiate between the two causative pathologies. Hypertrophy resolves in 4–8 weeks. Desmitis is characterised by pain.

Collateral ligament rupture is observed as a discontinuity of the ligament. There may be an accumulation of hypoechoic material in the rupture area due to the formation of haematomas.

In cases of **avulsion of the long digital extensor tendon**, hyperechoic structures with distal acoustic shadows, corresponding to bone fragments, can be observed distal to the extensor fossa, in the lateral femoral condyle.

The Calcaneal Tendon

Ultrasonographic Anatomy

The ultrasonographic anatomy and pathological findings of the calcaneal tendon have been described by Kramer et al. (2001a) and Lamb and Duvernois (2005). In dogs and cats, there are five tendons that form the calcaneus:

- gastrocnemius tendon
- superficial digital flexor muscle tendon
- biceps femoris tendon
- semitendinosus muscle tendon
- gracilis muscle tendon.

The **gastrocnemius tendon** (after the two muscle bellies fuse into a single tendon) and the **superficial digital flexor tendon** are the main tendons. They are joined by the other three, which form a **common tendon**. All of them insert on to the calcaneal tuberosity in the tarsal joint. The common tendon is the deepest and is inserted into the most dorsal, proximal portion of the calcaneal tuberosity.

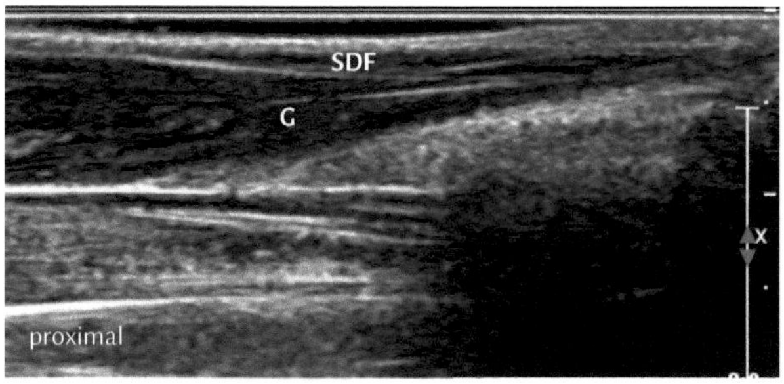

Figure 14. Ultrasound image of the normal calcaneal tendon, in which its components, the gastrocnemius (G) and the superficial digital flexor (SDF), are observed.

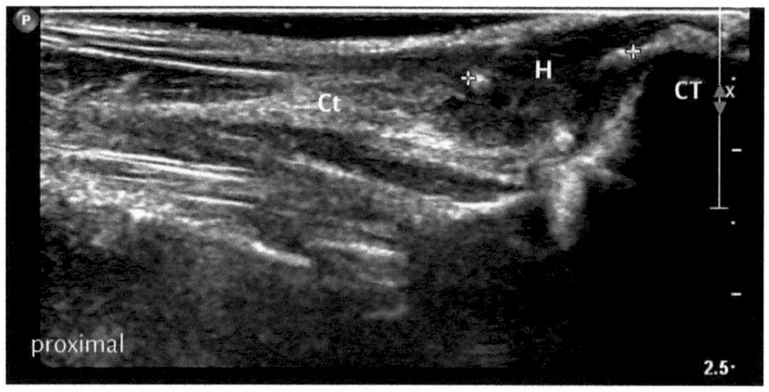

Figure 15. Ultrasound image of the calcaneal tendon (Ct), in which the almost complete acute rupture of the tendon, with chronic tendinopathy, can be seen. Separation of the tendon fibres by a hypoechoic haematoma (H) is observed, in addition to several hyperechoic foci representing dystrophic mineralisation. CT: calcaneal tuberosity.

During ultrasonographic examination, a longitudinal section should be examined first and then a cross section, examining the tendons from their musculotendinous junction to their insertion (Fig. 14). The superficial digital flexor tendon is deep to the other tendons in its proximal portion. In the middle of the diaphysis it becomes superficial. It has an insertion area in the medial and lateral part of the tuberosity of the calcaneus, and some of its fibres extend distally to the phalanges. The gastrocnemius tendon has an intermediate position between the superficial digital flexor tendon and the common tendon. The common tendon is located in the deep plane, is hyperechoic and has a fibrillar structure. In cross section, it has a rounded shape and is surrounded by a hyperechoic peritendon. The bursa of the common calcaneal tendon is normally located immediately proximal to the tuberosity of the calcaneus. It is a poorly defined, hypoechoic structure measuring approximately 5 mm in diameter.

Pathological Findings

Kramer et al. (2001a) described the **phases in the partial or complete rupture** of the calcaneal tendon.

- Day 1: hypoechoic haematoma separating the edges of the ruptured tendon.
- Weeks 1–2: haematoma organization; heterogeneous.
- Weeks 2–6: increase in the size and heterogeneity of the haematoma.
- Weeks 8–12: reduction in the size and heterogeneity of the haematoma.
- For several years: remains more heterogeneous than normal.

Enthesophytes may form on the surface of the calcaneal tuberosity; these are observed as hyperechoic structures with irregular edges. Small avulsed bone fragments and dystrophic mineralisation can also be observed in tendons. Tendon rupture may be due to trauma or may be degenerative, associated with diseases such as diabetes or hyperadrenocorticism. Fig. 15 shows an almost complete rupture of the calcaneal tendon.

Luxation of the superficial digital flexor tendon can be observed in cross section in a plantar direction to the calcaneal tuberosity (in which it is seen as an oval or semilunar-shaped tendon). The luxation may be lateral or medial. A thickened, heterogeneous tendon is observed with some hypoechoic haematoma.

The Muscles

Ultrasonographic Appearance

Normal muscles are hypoechoic and have fine hyperechoic striations running through them (Fig. 16). The fasciae are thin and hyperechoic. The fat between the intermuscular fasciae is hyperechoic.

Pathological Findings

Muscle rupture due to overexertion is more common in certain muscles, such as the iliopsoas, adductor and pectineus. In the acute phase of muscle trauma there is inflammation and oedema. Haematomas are observed as nonhomogeneous, hypoechoic or anechoic lesions and are poorly defined. There is disruption of muscle fibres. In the chronic phase, during the healing process, hyperechoic, heterogeneous lesions (representing scar formation) are seen. There may be a focal reduction in the muscle diameter.

Fibrotic myopathy of the gracilis and semitendinosus muscles has been described by several authors (Lewis et al., 1997; Vidoni et al., 2008; Gibson, 2017). German Shepherd dogs are the breed most commonly predisposed to this pathology, and it usually occurs in young animals. Ultrasonographically,

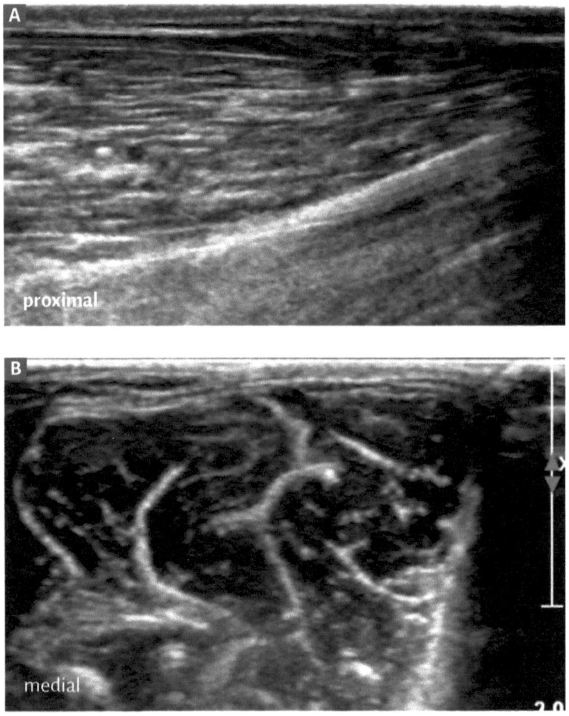

Figure 16. Ultrasound images showing the normal ultrasonographic appearance of a muscle in longitudinal section (**A**) and cross section (**B**). The muscle is hypoechoic with fine hyperechoic striations.

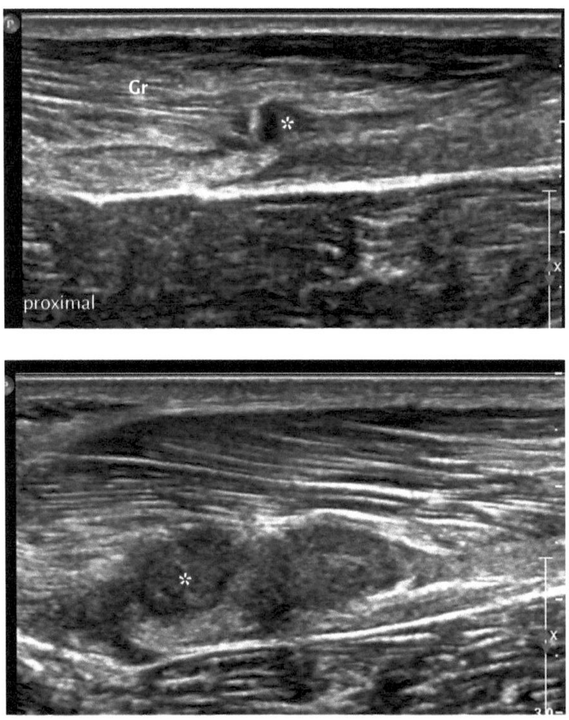

Figure 17. Muscle ultrasonography of a German Shepherd dog with bilateral fibrotic myopathy of the gracilis muscle (Gr). A heterogeneous fibrotic lesion with hypoechoic foci is observed (*).

the muscle is observed to be heterogeneous, with hypoechoic focal zones and disruption of muscle fibres (Fig. 17). On MRI, the affected muscle is shortened compared with the contralateral one, and it is also thickened in the distal portion and has a moderately thickened tendon insertion. Dystrophic mineralisation may be seen in the fibrotic lesion.

Muscular Neoplasia

Muscle neoplasms are observed as masses with variable characteristics: they can be well or poorly defined, hypoechoic, hyperechoic or heterogeneous, and of varying size (Fig. 18). They may be single or multiple, solid, cystic or mixed (and may contain hypoechoic haemorrhagic or necrotic areas). Vascularisation, even of malignant tumours, can be variable. Lipomas are usually hyperechoic.

Inflammation and Infection of Subcutaneous Tissue and Musculature

Cellulitis is inflammation of connective tissue. On ultrasonography, alternating anechoic and hyperechoic bands are seen in subcutaneous tissue or between muscle fibres (Fig. 19).

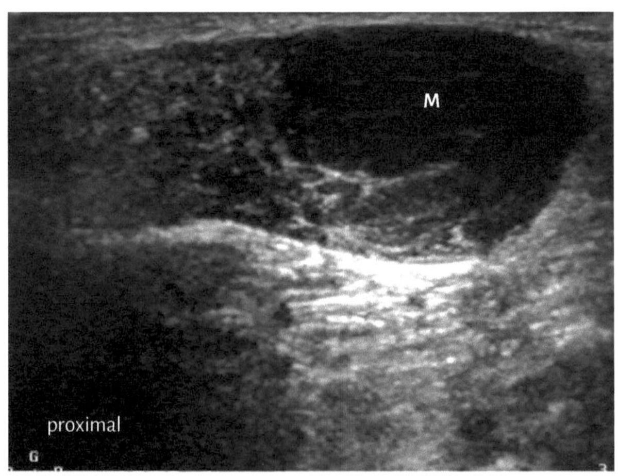

Figure 18. Muscle ultrasonography of a dog with multicentric lymphoma and hypoechoic masses (M) in the musculature. Cytology on a sample of muscle showed that the neoplasia was lymphoma.

Abscesses are usually cavitated, thick-walled, hyperechoic, well-defined lesions. **Inflammatory processes** can be caused by migrating foreign bodies, such as grass seeds, splinters or wooden sticks, thorns and other objects. Foreign bodies are usually hyperechoic, cause distal acoustic shadow, and are surrounded by a moderate amount of hypoechoic fluid (Fig. 20). In chronic processes these characteristics may change, and the foreign body may not be visible ultrasonographically. Haemorrhages change in appearance and echogenicity over time. They usually have poorly defined edges and are hypoechoic, and disappear over time.

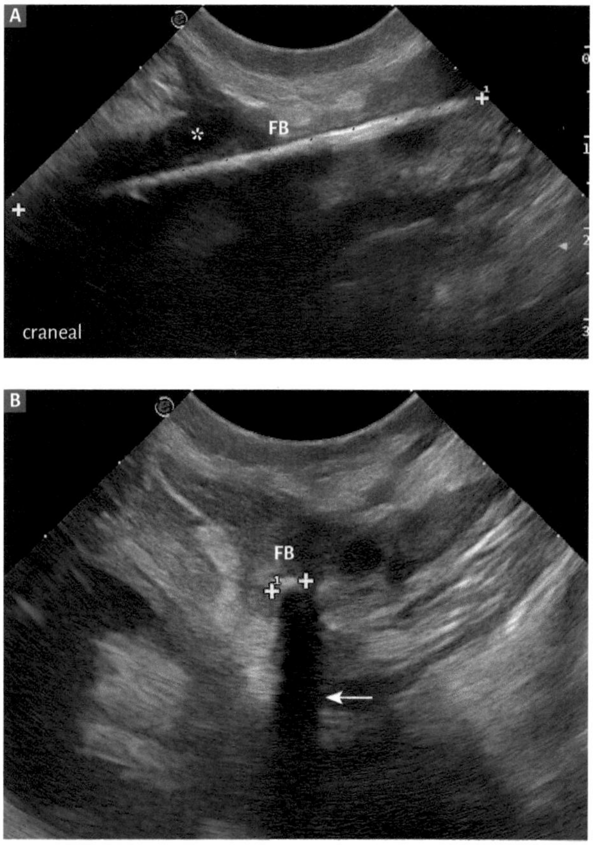

Figure 20. A. Ultrasound image of a dog with a linear foreign body (FB) located in the inguinal region. B. Cross section showing a strong distal acoustic shadow (arrow). In A, marked cellulitis and a slight amount of hypoechoic fluid (*) between the fasciae are observed.

Sampling

Ultrasonography is useful in the diagnosis of a multitude of musculoskeletal injuries, and is usually used together with other diagnostic imaging modalities such as radiography and CT. In addition, it is used for ultrasound-guided sampling in patients under light sedation (Fig. 21). Sampling can be performed by fine-needle aspiration or by using a Tru-Cut® biopsy needle. Muscle masses, masses or accumulations of fluid in soft tissue, bone lesions that occur with osteolysis and cortical destruction, and joint lesions can be sampled. With neoplastic lesions, it is recommended to perform sampling in a way that takes into account the likely surgical approach and the possibility of surgical resection of the needle tract to prevent the seeding of cancer cells.

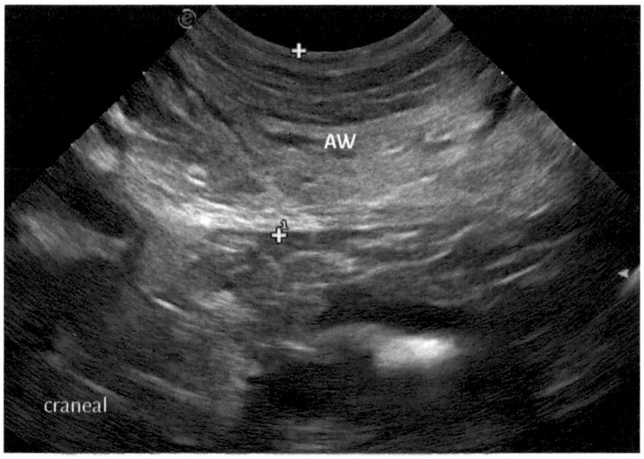

Figure 19. Ultrasound image of the abdominal wall (AW) of a dog. The wall is severely inflamed and thickened due to a traumatic rupture. The markers delimit the abdominal wall.

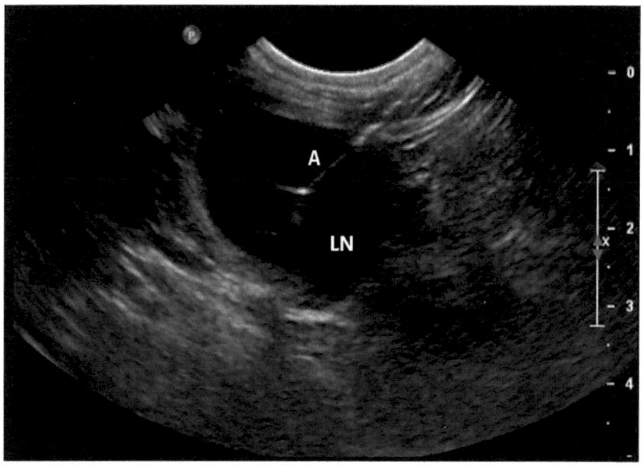

Figure 21. Ultrasound-guided fine-needle puncture (A) of an enlarged, hypoechoic, rounded lymph node (LN).

Bibliography

- Arnault, F., Cauvin, E., Viguier, E., Kraft, E., Sonet, J., Carozzo, C. (2009) Diagnostic value of ultrasonography to assess stifle lesions in dogs after cranial cruciate ligament rupture: 13 cases. *Vet Comp Orthop Traumatol*, 22(6):479–485.
- Boysen, S.R., Lisciandro, G.R. (2013) The use of ultrasound for dogs and cats in the emergency room: AFAST and TFAST. *Vet Clin North Am Small Anim Pract*, 43(4):773–797.
- Cook, C.R. (2015) Ultrasound imaging of the musculoskeletal system. *Vet Clin North Am Small Anim Pract*, 46(3):355–371.
- Doyle, A.J., Miller, M.V., French, J.G. (2000) Ultrasound of soft-tissue masses: pitfalls in interpretation. *Australas Radiol*, 44(3):275–280.
- Frances, B., Lorrie, G. (2011) *BSAVA Manual of Canine and Feline Ultrasonography*. 1st ed. BSAVA.
- Gibson, M.A., Brown, S.G., Brown, N.O. (2017) Semitendinosus myopathy and treatment with adipose-derived stem cells in working German shepherd police dogs. *Can Vet J*, 58(3):241–246.
- Mattoon, J.S., Nyland, T.G. (2015) *Small Animal Diagnostic Ultrasound*. 3rd ed. Saunders.
- Kirberger, R.M., McEvoy, F.J. (2016) *BSAVA Manual of Canine and Feline Musculoskeletal Imaging*. 2nd ed. BSAVA.
- Kramer, M., Gerwing, M., Michele, U., Schimke, E., Kindler, S. (2001a) Ultrasonographic examination of injuries to the Achilles tendon in dogs and cats. *J Small Anim Pract*, 42(11):531–535.
- Kramer, M., Gerwing, M., Sheppard, C., Schimke, E. (2001b) Ultrasonography for the diagnosis of diseases of the tendon and tendon sheath of the biceps brachii muscle. *Vet Surg*, 30(1):64–71.
- Kramer, M., Stengel, H., Gerwing, M., Schimke, E., Sheppard, C. (1999) Sonography of the canine stifle. *Vet Radiol Ultrasound*, 40(3):282–293.
- Kühn, K., Ohlerth, S., Makara, M., Hässig, M., Guerrero, T.G. (2011) Radiographic and ultrasonographic evaluation of the patellar ligament following tibial tuberosity advancement. *Vet Radiol Ultrasound*, 52(4):466–471.
- Lafuente, M.P., Fransson, B.A., Lincoln, J.D., Martinez, S.A., Gavin, P.R., Lahmers, K.K., Gay, J.M. (2009) Surgical treatment of mineralized and nonmineralized supraspinatus tendinopathy in twenty-four dogs. *Vet Surg*, 38(3):380–387.
- Lamb, C.R., Duvernois, A. (2005) Ultrasonographic anatomy of the normal canine calcaneal tendon. *Vet Radiol Ultrasound*, 46(4):326–330.
- Lewis, D.D., Shelton, G.D., Piras, A., Dee, J.F., Robins, G.M., Herron, A.J., Fries, C., Ginn, P.E., Hulse, D.A., Simpson, D.L., Allen, D.A. (1997) Gracilis or semitendinosus myopathy in 18 dogs. *J Am Anim Hosp Assoc*, 33(2):177–188.
- Long, C.D., Nyland, T.G. (1999) Ultrasonographic evaluation of the canine shoulder. *Vet Radiol Ultrasound*, 40(4):372–379.
- Mattern, K.L., Berry, C.R., Peck, J.N., De Haan, J.J. (2006) Radiographic and ultrasonographic evaluation of the patellar ligament following tibial plateau leveling osteotomy. *Vet Radiol Ultrasound*, 47(2):185–191.
- Penninck, D., d'Anjou, M.A. (2015) *Atlas of Small Animal Ultrasonography*. 2nd ed. Wiley-Blackwell.
- Siems, J.J., Breur, G.J., Blevins, W.E., Cornell, K.K. (1998) Use of two-dimensional real-time ultrasonography for diagnosing contracture and strain of the infraspinatus muscle in a dog. *J Am Vet Med Assoc*, 212(1):77–80.
- Vidoni, B., Hassan, J., Bockstahler, B., Dupré, G. (2008) Kontraktur des Musculus gracilis - Klinik, bildgebende Diagnostik und Therapie bei einer Deutschen Schäferhündin [Fibrotic gracilis myopathy - clinical signs, diagnostic imaging and therapy in a German shepherd dog]. *Wien Tierarztl Monatsschr*, 95(1):8–14.

Notes

373

Head and Spine Imaging

Radiography, Computed Tomography and Magnetic Resonance Imaging of the Head

Miriam Martínez Garrido

Introduction

The head is a complex structure, which is difficult to evaluate radiographically due to the overlap of structures (a large number of bones, soft tissues, etc.). In addition, many of the pathologies that affect the head (especially intracranially) do not present radiographic abnormalities. For these reasons, radiography of the head is often replaced by more advanced techniques such as computed tomography (CT) and magnetic resonance imaging (MRI), with which all components can be evaluated without overlapping structures and in better detail. However, head radiographs can be useful in many cases as a first approach in veterinary practices where advanced imaging techniques are not available.

Radiographic Examination of the Head

Indications

Despite their limitations, radiographs can be used to evaluate multiple structures in the head, and certain radiographic projections provide a symmetrical view that facilitates their interpretation. Therefore, a radiographic study may be indicated as a first diagnostic approach in the following cases:

- nasal pathologies, mainly chronic conditions
- mouth, periorbital or skull masses (skull deformation)
- ear disease
- fractures/trauma
- difficulty opening or closing the mouth
- dental disease.

Radiographic Technique

Radiographs of the skull of small animals should be performed with the patient under general anaesthesia or deep sedation, because good positioning of the patient is essential to achieve a symmetrical radiograph. Incorrect positioning of the patient for radiography may lead to nondiagnostic radiographs, and as a consequence certain alterations may be overlooked or pathological findings overestimated.

The radiographic technique used is the same as that used when evaluating other bone structures.

- High milliamperage (mA) and low kilovoltage (kV) should be used, since these parameters predispose to an increased photoelectric effect, causing X-rays to be absorbed by the tissues and as a result producing greater contrast.
- Focus–plate distance of 100 cm.
- Correct collimation and centring.
- A grid should be used when the thickness of the region to be radiographed is greater than 10 cm, to avoid radiation scattering.

Projections

Considering the complexity of the head, to avoid overlapping structures, multiple radiographic projections must be performed, which vary depending on the area being studied. Usually, standard projections are obtained, that is, lateral and dorsoventral (DV) or ventrodorsal (VD), and then a series of special projections depending on the area of interest.

Standard Projections

- **Lateral projection**: the patient is placed in lateral recumbency; the mid-sagittal plane of the head should be parallel to the table, ensuring that there is no rotation of the jaw and that the nasal cavity is not elevated or lowered relative to the rest of the skull. To do this, a foam wedge should be placed under the rostral portion of the head (nasal cavity and jaw). This projection provides an overview of the skull, nasal cavity, tympanic bullae, pharynx and larynx, although it should be taken into account that the structures on both sides overlap (Fig. 1).
- **DV/VD projection**: with the DV projection, more stability of the skull is achieved, and therefore it is generally used more frequently than the VD projection. For the DV projection, the patient should be placed in a sternal

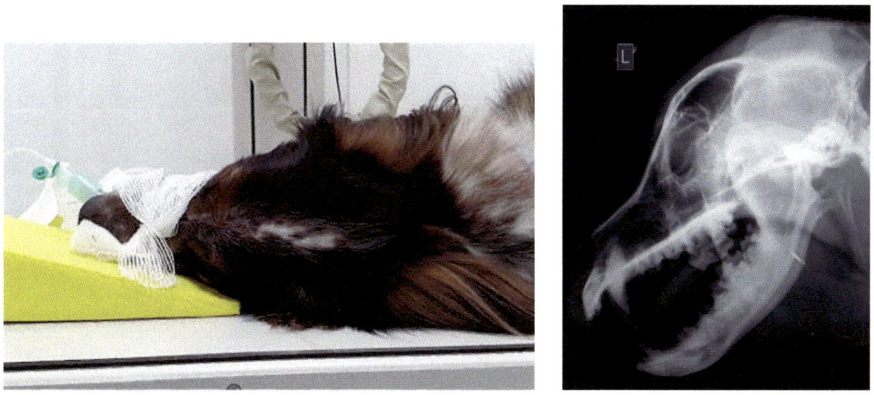

Figure 1. Positioning of the head for a lateral projection, and the resulting radiograph.

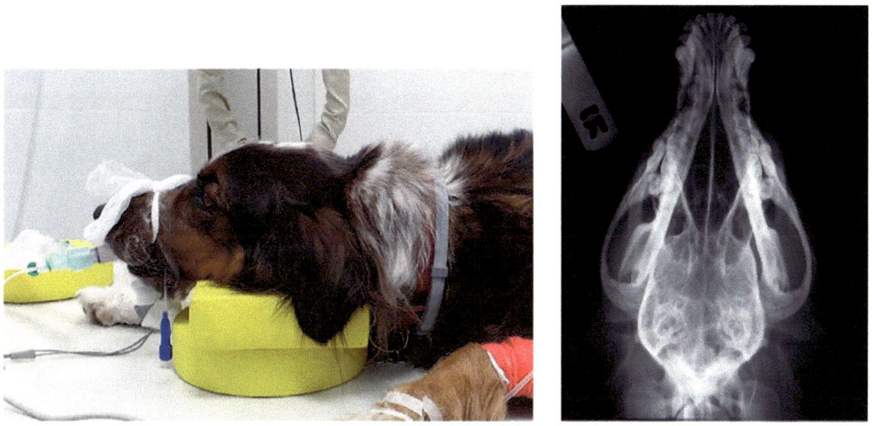

Figure 2. Positioning of the head for a DV projection, and the resulting radiograph.

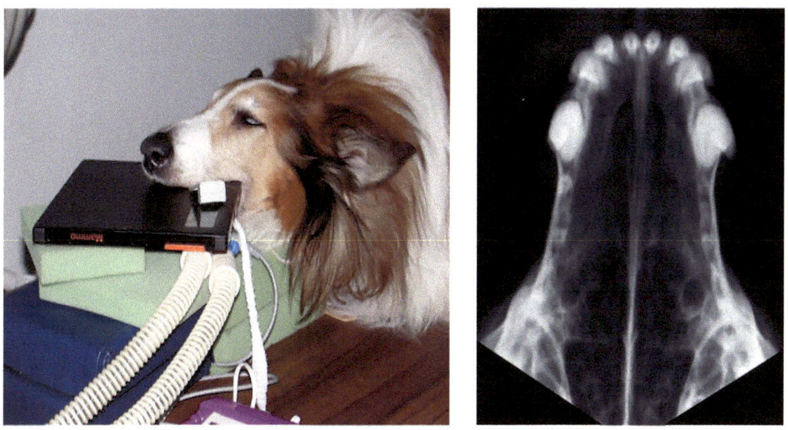

Figure 3. Positioning for an intraoral DV projection, and the resulting radiograph.

position; it is of fundamental importance that the jaw is symmetrical so that the head is not rotated. A foam wedge is placed to raise the head (to approximately the same height as the neck) and the plate, separating them from the table, to prevent rotation of the head. This projection also gives an overview of the skull and is very useful for the detection of asymmetries between different structures (Fig. 2).

Special Projections

- **Intraoral DV/oblique VD with open mouth**: with both projections, a similar radiographic image is achieved.
  - For the intraoral DV projection, the patient is positioned the same way as for a standard DV projection, with the difference that the plate is positioned inside the mouth as far as possible (Fig. 3).
  - With the oblique open-mouthed VD projection,

the patient is placed in dorsal recumbency with the hard palate parallel to the table and the jaw opened as wide as possible. The X-ray beam is then angled about 20° towards the maxillary rostral area.

With both projections, the nasal cavity and adjacent structures are visualised without overlapping with the mandible. The biggest difference between the two projections is that with the oblique VD projection, the most caudal aspect of the nasal cavity can be evaluated (Fig. 4).

- **Rostrocaudal/frontal**: the animal is positioned in dorsal recumbency; the head is flexed, forming a 90° angle with the neck, so that the hard palate is perpendicular to the plate. The X-ray beam is directed straight towards the area of the frontal sinuses. This projection is obtained to evaluate the frontal sinuses and the surface of the skull (Fig. 5).
- **Intraoral VD**: the patient is positioned in dorsal recumbency, with the hard palate parallel to the table, and the plate is placed inside the mouth. With this projection, the body of the mandible and the mandibular teeth can be evaluated (Fig. 6).
- **Oblique intraoral lateral views**: the animal is placed in lateral recumbency, the mouth is kept open, and the head is rotated on its longitudinal axis, centring the X-ray beam on the maxilla or mandible of interest. The side of interest should be the one closer to the plate. These projections are used to evaluate both the maxilla and the mandible (Fig. 7).
- **Lateral oblique (Right 20° R–LeftCd or Left 20° R–RightCd)**: the patient is placed in lateral recumbency with the area of interest near the plate and the nose is raised about 10–30°. With this projection, the temporomandibular joint and the tympanic bullae can be evaluated. The side in contact with the plate should be more rostral than the contralateral side in the radiographic image (Fig. 8).
- **Open-mouthed rostrocaudal**: the animal is positioned as for the rostrocaudal projection, but with the mouth open. In this projection, the tympanic bullae, the foramen magnum and the dens of the axis (odontoid process) can be evaluated (Fig. 9).
- **Rostro 10° ventral–caudodorsal oblique**: used to evaluate the tympanic bullae in the cat. The animal is positioned in dorsal recumbency, and a wedge-shaped piece of foam is placed behind the head so that the head is about 10° from vertical.

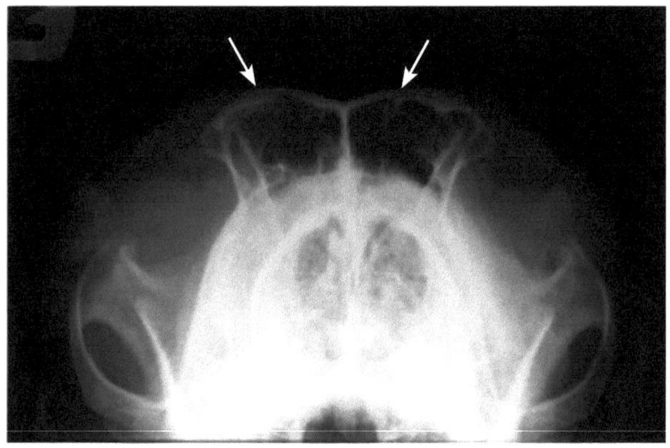

Figure 5. Rostrocaudal or frontal projection, in which the frontal sinuses are observed (arrows).

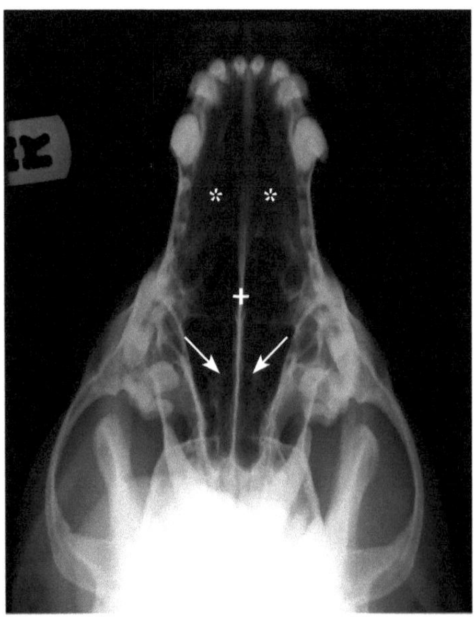

Figure 4. Oblique open-mouthed VD projection. The nasal turbinates (asterisks), the nasal septum (cross) and the cribriform plate (arrows) are observed.

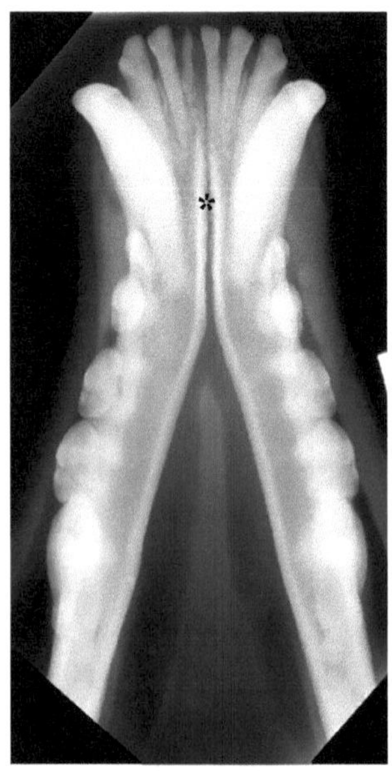

Figure 6. Intraoral VD projection of the mandible. The mandibular symphysis is observed (asterisk).

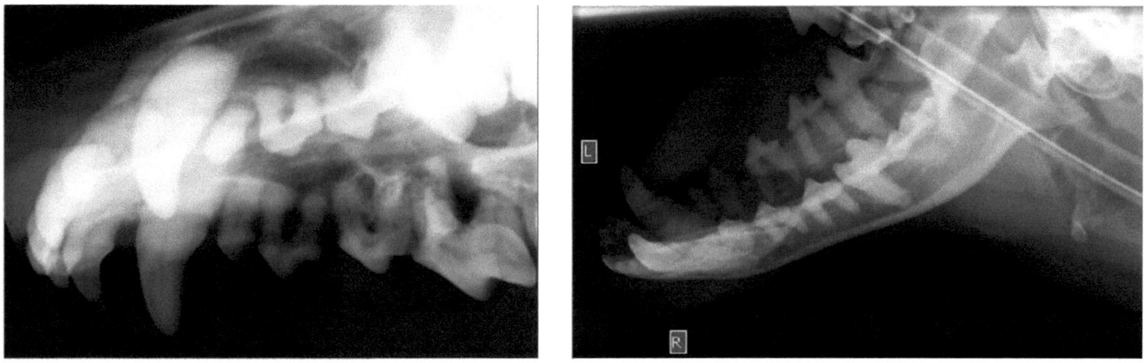

Figure 7. Oblique intraoral projections of the maxilla and mandible.

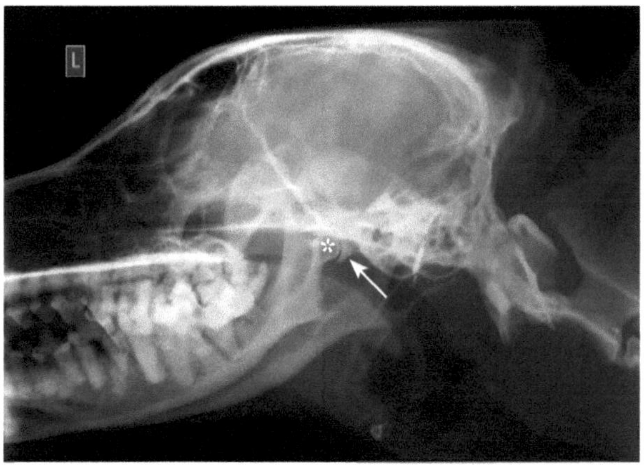

Figure 8. Oblique lateral projection (Right 20°R–LeftCd). The left temporomandibular joint is observed. The mandibular condyle (asterisk) and retroarticular process (arrow) can be seen.

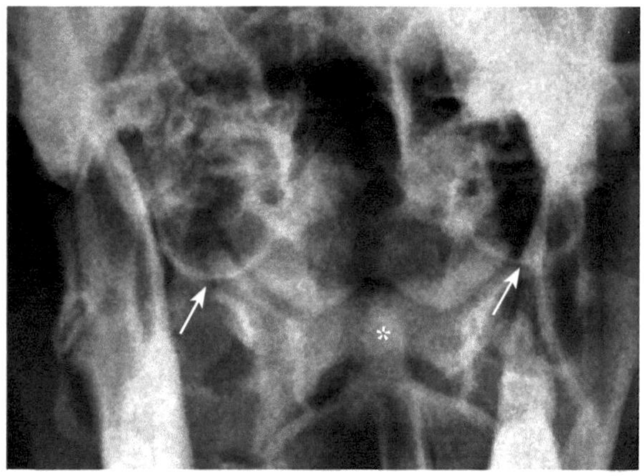

Figure 9. Rostrocaudal open-mouthed projection. The tympanic bullae with their thin, air-filled walls (arrows) and the dens of the axis (asterisk) are observed.

The Most Relevant Anatomical Structures of the Head that can be Evaluated Radiographically

The anatomical structures in the head that can be evaluated radiographically are as follows.

- The cranial cavity, especially **its boundaries and shape**.
- **The nasal cavity, frontal sinuses and maxillary recesses**. The nasal cavity (from the nostrils to the choanae and cribriform plate [lamina cribrosa]) contains the nasal turbinates, which should be clearly defined. The two nasal cavities should be symmetrical. The nasal septum consists of a cartilaginous (rostral) portion not visible on radiographs, and a caudal bony portion (formed by the vomer bone on its ventral aspect), separating the right and left nasal cavities. The cribriform plate is in the most caudal portion of the nasal cavity, and separates the nasal cavity from the intracranial region (Fig. 4).

  The frontal sinuses (Fig. 5) are defined by the frontal bone and should be filled with air. They are more prominent in large dog breeds and cats than in small dog breeds, and may be virtually absent in some brachycephalic breeds.
- **The mandible and maxilla**. The mandible is made up of two parts that come together at the mandibular symphysis (Fig. 6). Each side of the mandible is made up of the mandibular body and the ramus. Both the maxillary and mandibular regions house the teeth, which have an outer portion (crown) and a portion that is embedded in the alveolar bone (tooth root). The tooth roots are surrounded by a thin radiotransparent line that corresponds to the periodontal ligament or membrane, which in turn is delineated by a thin radiopaque layer called the lamina dura that forms part of the alveolar bone. Inside the tooth is the pulp, which decreases in size with age (Fig. 10).
- The **ear** consists of three portions: the outer ear (pinna and ear canal), the middle ear (tympanic bulla and

auditory ossicles) and the inner ear. The external auditory canal is best visualised in the VD/DV projection, as a channel of gas opacity lateral to the tympanic bulla. The tympanic bulla is visualised as a thin-walled bony structure with air inside (Fig. 9). In the cat, there is an inner bony septum that incompletely divides the bulla into two compartments, ventromedial and dorsolateral.
- **The temporomandibular joint** is formed by the condylar process of the mandible and the mandibular fossa (squamous portion of the temporal bone). In the oblique lateral projection, the mandibular condyle can be seen with a rounded shape and smooth surface, as well as the articular space separating the mandibular fossa and the retroarticular process, immediately rostral to both tympanic bullae (Fig. 8).
- **The foramen magnum** is visualised as a radiolucent oval structure at the base of the skull.

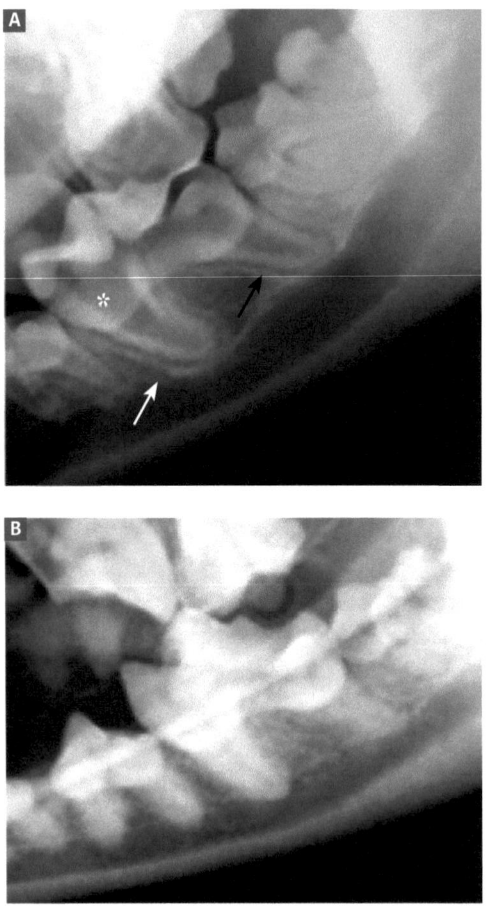

Figure 10. Detail of an oblique intraoral projection of the mandible of a young dog (**A**) and an older dog (**B**). The lamina dura (white arrow) and the periodontal ligament (black arrow) surrounding the dental root are observed. The pulp, which can be seen inside the tooth (asterisk), decreases in size with age.

CT Examination of the Head

Indications

CT allows a more detailed assessment of a wider range of structures compared with conventional radiography.

CT can be used:

- **as an alternative method on occasions when multiple radiographic projections have to be performed**
- **when radiographic studies are normal in appearance**
- **to obtain more information about abnormalities detected on radiographs**
- **to determine the extent of certain lesions.**

It is an especially useful technique for imaging the head because of the high contrast provided by bony structures and air-containing structures, and because axial imaging eliminates problems generated by overlapping structures.

Therefore, CT is useful for examining animals with exophthalmos (to evaluate the orbit and retrobulbar space), those in which otitis is suspected (to evaluate the different structures of the ear) or animals with nasal discharge (to evaluate the nasal cavity and paranasal sinuses), among others. CT shows the nasal turbinates in clear detail, and the possible invasion of bone structures, which can go unnoticed on radiographs, in addition to allowing evaluation of the regional lymph nodes.

In addition, although MRI is the technique of choice for evaluation of the nervous system, CT allows evaluation of the brain parenchyma, enabling the detection of haemorrhage (in cases of trauma), hydrocephalus and some intracranial masses. Postcontrast CT studies also allow evaluation of the extent of lesions at the intracranial level from other adjacent locations.

CT Technique: Positioning and Protocol

Positioning

To perform a head CT, the patient is placed in a sternal position, with the head elevated on a piece of foam and the limbs pulled backwards. In cases where the limbs have to be pulled

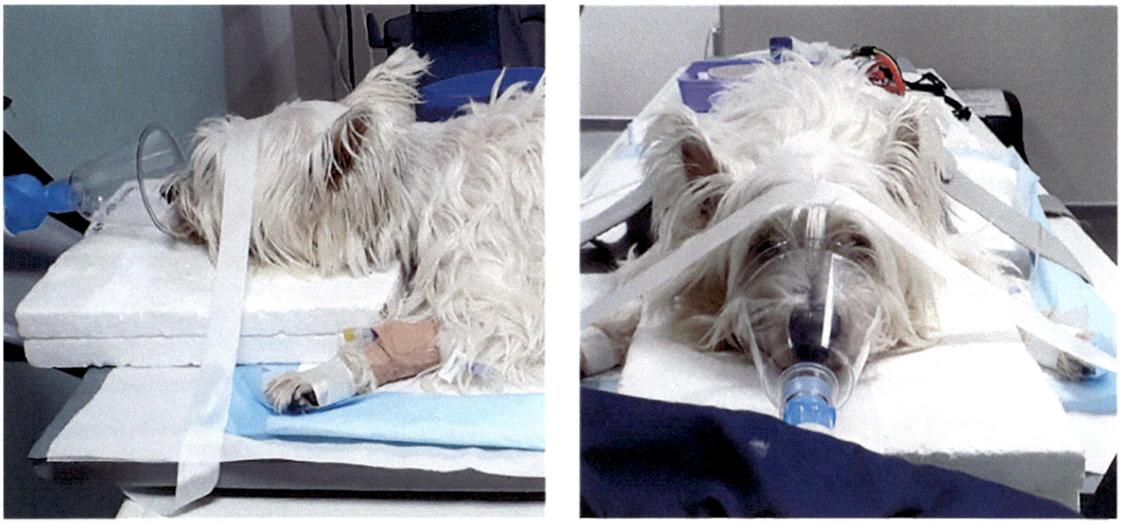

Figure 11. Patient positioning for a head CT.

forward (when the thorax is included in the scan), the head must be raised (Fig. 11).

Protocol

- The head is scanned from the nostrils to the cervical spine (C2) to ensure that the regional lymph nodes are included.
- Section thickness: 1–2 mm for bone structures but can be somewhat thicker (2–5 mm) for soft tissues, trying to maintain the smallest possible section thickness in small patients.
- Reconstruction interval: half of the section thickness used.
- Algorithms: low frequency (soft tissue) evaluated with a soft tissue window (window width [WW]: 350; window level [WL]: 40); high frequency (bone) evaluated with a bone window (WW: 2500; WL: 500). The lung window (WW: 1600; WL: –500) may also be used to evaluate the nasal turbinates.
- Pre- and postcontrast series: intravenous administration of a standard dose of contrast (600 mg I/kg).

Main Pathologies

- nasal cavity abnormalities
- ear disorders
- dental abnormalities
- abnormalities of the skull, maxilla and mandible
- abnormalities of the temporomandibular joint
- abnormalities of the orbit
- abnormalities of the salivary glands.

Nasal Cavity Abnormalities

The most common pathological processes affecting the nasal cavity are nonspecific rhinitis, fungal rhinitis, foreign bodies and neoplasms.

The main findings that can help distinguish between these pathologies are:

- the location and distribution of lesions
- changes in opacity/attenuation
- the presence of soft tissue masses or mass effect
- the destruction of nasal turbinates
- osteolysis of adjacent bones (nasal septum, cribriform plate, other skull bones)
- the extension of lesions into the paranasal sinuses.

Many of these findings can be identified by radiography, although more advanced imaging techniques (CT) are necessary to obtain a more detailed view of the lesions with the use of multiplanar images.

CT can be used to better evaluate features such as the presence of inflammation of the nasal mucosa, to differentiate fluid from soft tissue with the administration of contrast, and to more accurately determine the destruction of the nasal turbinates or the cribriform plate and the presence of intracranial involvement. In addition, regional lymph nodes can be evaluated with CT, which can help indicate an inflammatory or neoplastic process, in some cases.

However, despite CT being able to visualise all these characteristics, the different pathological processes may present common findings, and there are no pathognomonic findings for these pathologies. Therefore, rhinoscopy and sampling of the different lesions for histopathological study and culture is essential to obtain a definitive diagnosis in most cases. Aspiration of affected regional lymph nodes can also often provide important information.

Nonspecific Rhinitis

Nonspecific rhinitis is caused by bacterial, viral or parasitic infections, or allergies. It can also be secondary to dental infections. Sometimes the cause is unknown.

Radiographic changes can be minimal to severe, and normal radiographs may be obtained. In cases where there are abnormalities, the most typical pattern is an increase in opacity (soft tissue) due to the presence of mucus or a mucopurulent secretion that has been trapped, and inflammation of the nasal mucosa. This causes a loss of visualisation of the nasal turbinates (even if there is no destruction of the turbinates). Changes are usually bilateral, although they can be unilateral in some cases.

With CT, a thickening of the nasal mucosa can be seen, with marked postcontrast enhancement. The nasal turbinates can appear intact, or they may be atrophied (Fig. 12). There may also be a variable amount of secretion.

In cats, nonspecific rhinitis can cause destruction of the nasal turbinates along with increased soft tissue opacity, and it is difficult to differentiate from other more aggressive processes. Bilateral changes also often appear.

Fungal Rhinitis

Fungal rhinitis is commonly caused by *Aspergillus* species in dogs and *Cryptococcus* species in cats.

Aspergillosis causes destructive rhinitis, in which radiolucent areas are observed due to the destruction of the normal pattern of the turbinates. In addition, an increase in opacity (soft tissue) can be observed in the peripheral areas or in the caudal part of the nasal cavity, which corresponds to secretions and inflammatory and granulomatous tissue. The pathology can be either unilateral or bilateral and, in severe cases, the entire nasal cavity may be affected, although the process usually begins at the rostral level (Fig. 13).

The frontal sinuses are usually affected (sinusitis). In addition, in some cases osteolysis or bone proliferation of the frontal bone or other bones of the nasal cavity may be seen, due to osteomyelitis. It is common for there to be intracranial involvement.

With CT, bone lesions of both the nasal cavity and the frontal sinuses can be evaluated in better detail. The integrity of the cribriform plate and the presence or absence of intracranial extension can be assessed. In addition, the presence of heterogeneous attenuation and enhancement masses corresponding to fungal granulomas can be evaluated. Thickening of the mucosa, the presence of fluid or osteolysis of the frontal bone can be seen in the frontal sinuses (Fig. 13).

Foreign Bodies

Foreign bodies often cause unilateral rhinitis and are often difficult to diagnose using radiographs. Foreign bodies cannot usually be visualised on radiographs unless they present

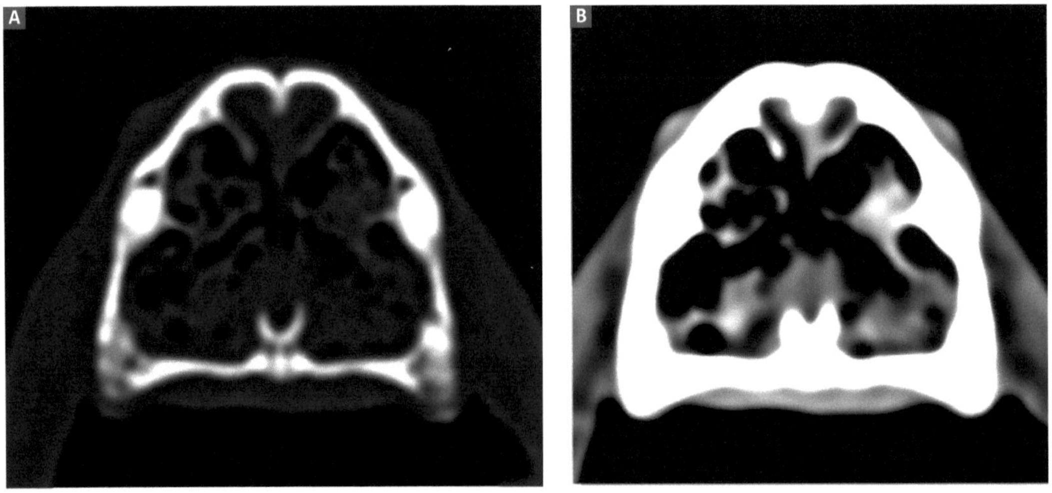

Figure 12. Transverse CT images in bone (**A**) and soft tissue (**B**) windows pre- and postcontrast respectively of the nasal cavity of a dog with nonspecific rhinitis. A moderate amount of nasal discharge is observed in both cavities, without destruction of the nasal turbinates, and with moderate enhancement of the nasal mucosa after contrast administration.

mineral or metal opacity. Therefore, only an increase in opacity of the nasal cavity where the foreign body is located is observed.

With CT, there can be a greater chance of seeing the foreign material. However, in many cases even with this modality it is still a challenge to detect foreign bodies (especially plant material, e.g. grass seeds). However, some changes can be detected associated with the presence of foreign bodies, such as a thickening of the nasal mucosa, a focal loss of the turbinates and nasal secretion.

Neoplasms

Neoplasms of the nasal cavity (carcinomas are more common in dogs and lymphoma in cats) usually appear as masses with soft tissue opacity and characteristics of aggressive bone lesions, with destruction of the nasal turbinates and osteolysis of the bones that make up the nasal cavity. Occasionally, osteolysis of the cribriform plate (assuming intracranial involvement) and invasion of other structures such as the paranasal sinuses or nasopharynx may also be observed. They are usually unilateral lesions, although if the process is advanced, with osteolysis of the nasal septum, there may be extension to the contralateral side (Fig. 14).

CT can further assess the extent of lesions, detecting subtle areas of lysis in the cribriform plate, intracranial extension or extension into the nasopharynx. In addition, the enhancement characteristics of the masses can be evaluated, and changes compatible with metastasis can be found in the regional lymph nodes (Fig. 15).

It should be taken into account that these characteristics may not be observed in all cases, and the severity of the lesions is not always the same. There are cases in which differentiation between neoplastic and nonneoplastic processes is a challenge.

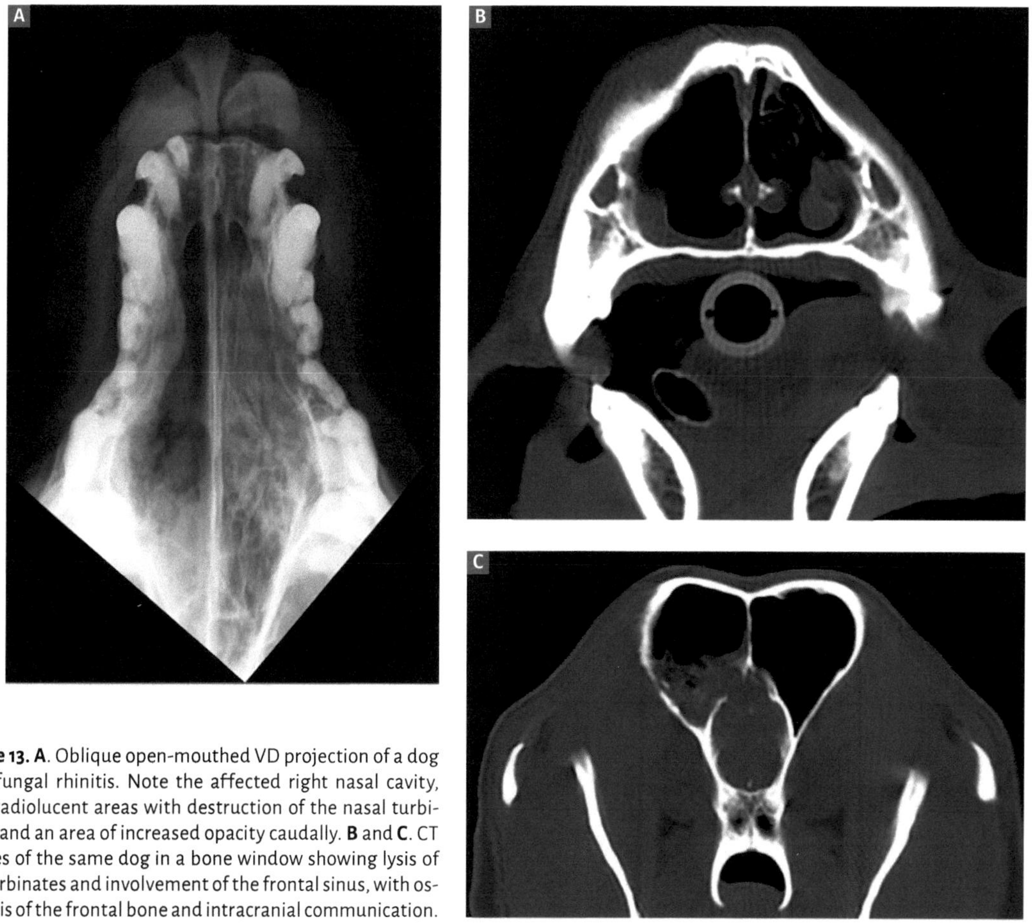

Figure 13. A. Oblique open-mouthed VD projection of a dog with fungal rhinitis. Note the affected right nasal cavity, with radiolucent areas with destruction of the nasal turbinates and an area of increased opacity caudally. **B** and **C**. CT images of the same dog in a bone window showing lysis of the turbinates and involvement of the frontal sinus, with osteolysis of the frontal bone and intracranial communication.

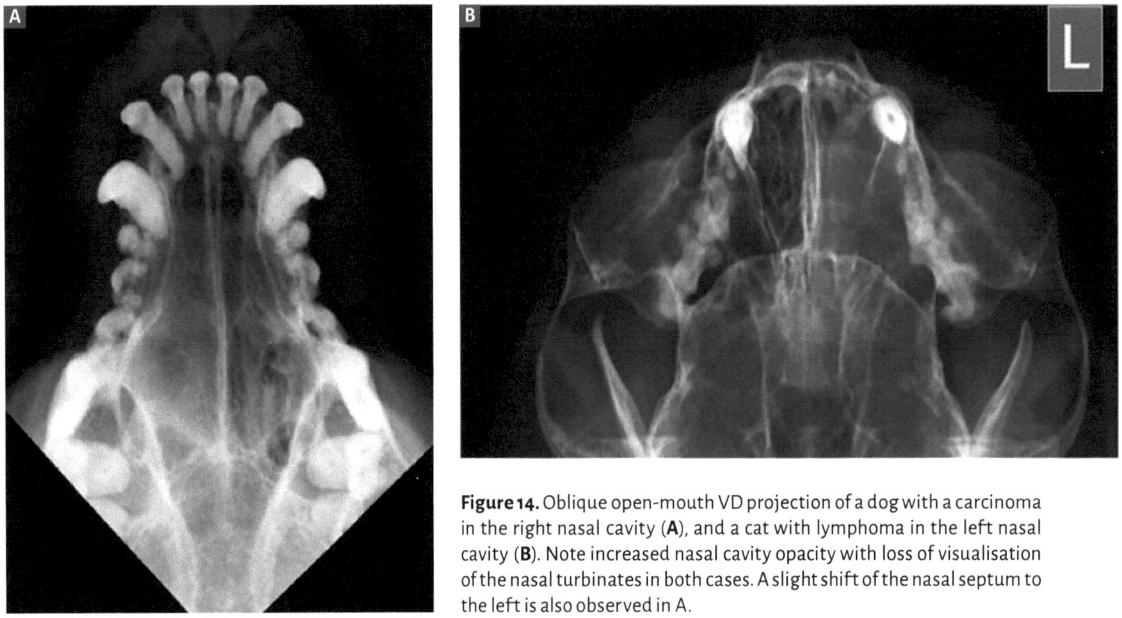

Figure 14. Oblique open-mouth VD projection of a dog with a carcinoma in the right nasal cavity (**A**), and a cat with lymphoma in the left nasal cavity (**B**). Note increased nasal cavity opacity with loss of visualisation of the nasal turbinates in both cases. A slight shift of the nasal septum to the left is also observed in A.

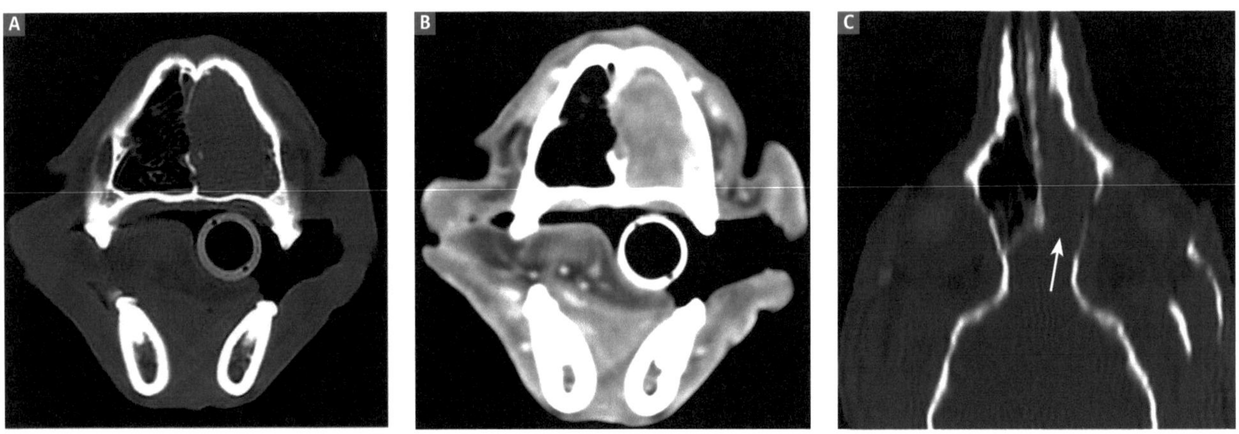

Figure 15. CT images of a dog with nasal carcinoma. In a bone window (**A**) and post-contrast soft tissue window (**B**), a soft tissue mass is observed that presents heterogeneous enhancement, causing osteolysis of the nasal turbinates and displacement of the nasal septum. **C**. Dorsal plane, in which osteolysis of the cribriform plate is observed on the left side (arrow), indicating intracranial extension.

Ear Disorders

Otitis

Inflammation affecting the ear is a fairly common process.

In cases of **otitis externa**, the radiographic findings that are observed are an increase in opacity or narrowing of the external auditory canal. This is due to an accumulation of secretions or inflammation of the external ear canal. In cases of chronic otitis, mineralisation of the cartilage of the ear canal can be seen (Fig. 16). However, this may be a finding that is observed in nonpathological cases.

Otitis media or interna is usually a consequence of the spread of infection from the external or internal auditory canal. Otitis interna cannot be diagnosed on radiographs, as the structures of the inner ear are not well defined.

Regarding otitis media, radiographs can be used to evaluate the morphology of the tympanic bullae, their wall and their content. It is possible to detect an increase in the radiopacity of the bullae, and a possible thickening of the wall. In some cases, radiographic changes may not be observed. In more serious cases, osteolysis of the wall of the tympanic bulla can be detected.

CT is an excellent modality for the diagnosis of otitis externa, media or interna, with otitis interna being the most difficult to evaluate. Inflammation and the presence of hypoattenuating material in the external auditory canal can be evaluated in otitis externa. In cases of otitis media, CT allows detection of the presence of material of liquid/soft tissue attenuation inside the bulla, and changes in the wall (thickening, irregularity or, in severe cases, areas of osteolysis) with abnormal enhancement. In some cases, some enlargement of the tympanic bulla can be observed (Fig. 17).

In otitis interna, a loss of definition of the structures of the inner ear may be observed in some cases, with sclerosis or osteolysis of the petrous portion of the temporal bone, whereas in other cases no obvious alterations may be observed. In addition, CT can help to determine the extension of lesions to other locations (intracranial or para-aural soft tissues).

Nasopharyngeal Polyps

Nasopharyngeal polyps are inflammatory polyps that develop in the middle ear or nasopharynx and can extend into the nasopharynx through the ear canal (Eustachian tube) or into the external auditory canal through the tympanic membrane. In these cases, an increase in the opacity of the tympanic bulla can be observed, with a possible increase in thickness of the bulla wall, as well as a mass with soft tissue opacity occupying the nasopharynx.

With CT, the location and extent of the polyps can be evaluated in greater detail, and their typical ring-shaped postcontrast enhancement characteristic can be observed.

Cholesteatoma

Cholesteatomas are epidermoid cysts that form expansive masses that contain keratin. They can be congenital but can also develop as a result of previous otitis. CT is the technique of choice for the diagnosis of this pathology.

Findings include expansive lesions, with osteolysis and irregular periosteal reactions of the tympanic bulla wall. The tympanic bulla is obliterated by soft tissue that usually has peripheral and heterogeneous enhancement after contrast administration. These changes usually affect only one bulla, although in some cases they are bilateral (Fig. 18).

Neoplasms

Neoplastic processes affecting the ear are usually ceruminous or squamous gland **adenomas** or **adenocarcinomas**. They are soft tissue masses that occupy the external auditory canal. In the case of adenomas, the ear canal usually retains its architecture, whereas in the case of carcinomas they are usually poorly defined masses that extend to other regions of the ear, causing osteolysis of the bulla and adjacent temporal bone.

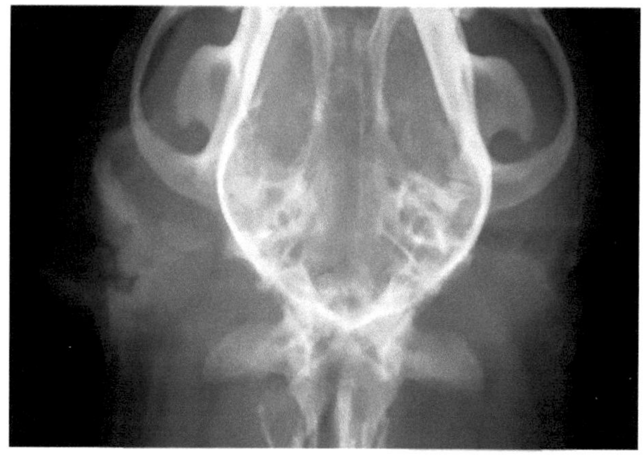

Figure 16. DV projection of the head of a dog with right-sided otitis externa and media. Note the inflammation of the soft tissue of the right temporal area; the right external auditory canal is increased in opacity, no lumen can be seen and mineralisation is present. The right tympanic bulla is of increased opacity compared with the contralateral side, which is normal in appearance.

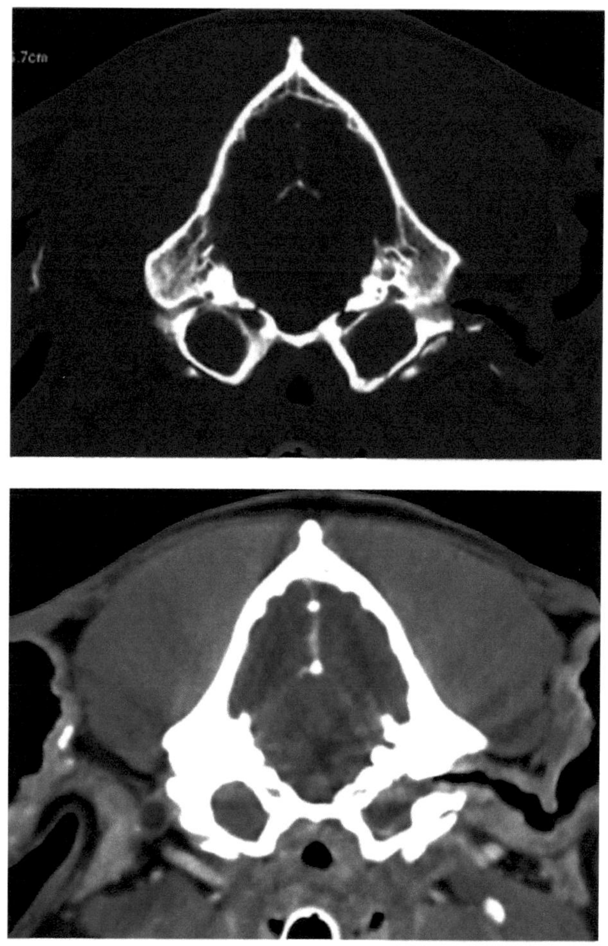

Figure 17. CT images of a dog with bilateral otitis externa and media. Thickening of the walls of the tympanic bullae is observed, and the bullae are occupied by material of soft tissue attenuation that is slightly enhanced at the periphery. The left bulla is slightly enlarged. A diffuse thickening of the wall can be seen in the external ear canal.

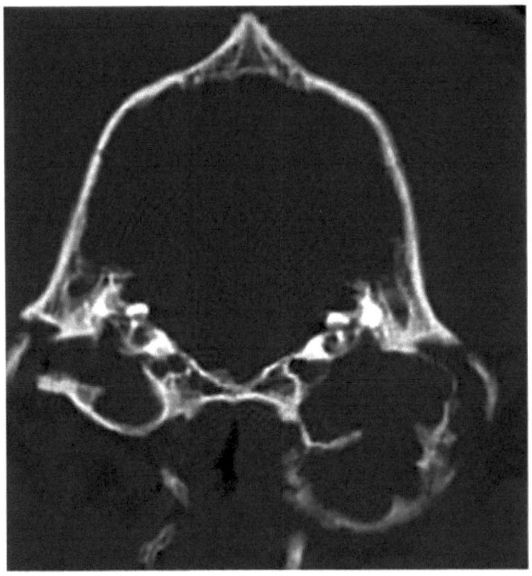

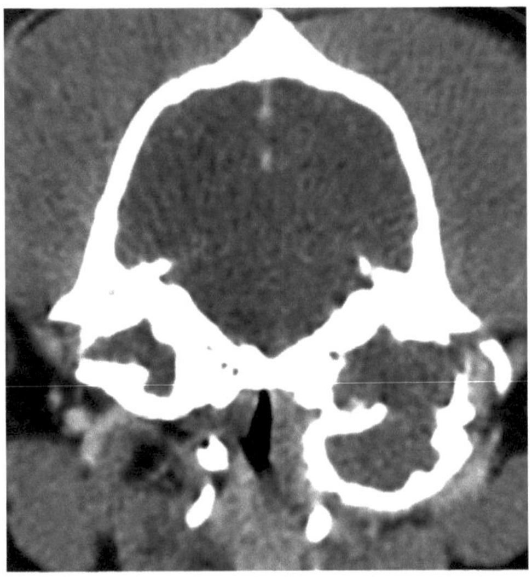

Figure 18. CT images in bone and postcontrast soft tissue windows of a dog with a cholesteatoma in the left ear. An expansive lesion is observed in the left bulla, with areas of osteolysis and bone neoformation in the wall. The bulla is occupied by material with soft tissue attenuation. The right bulla is occupied by material of soft tissue attenuation, compatible with otitis media.

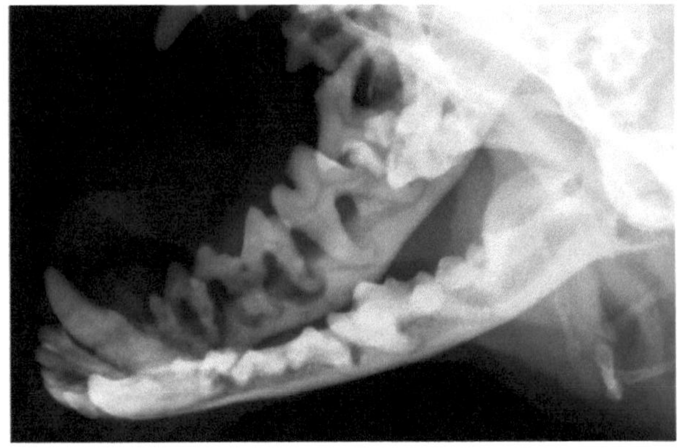

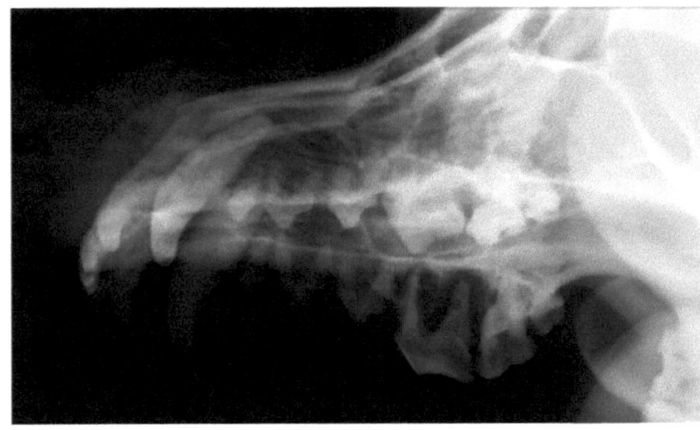

Figure 19. Oblique intraoral projections of the maxilla and mandible of a dog with periodontal disease. Widening of the periodontal ligament region is observed, with osteolysis of the adjacent alveolar bone affecting the roots of the second, third and fourth lower right premolars and the fourth upper right premolar, compatible with periapical abscesses. The roots of these teeth are slightly irregular.

Dental Abnormalities

Periodontal disease

Periodontal disease is an inflammatory/infectious disease that affects the supporting structures of the tooth and can lead to periapical abscesses.

Radiographically, a radiolucent halo is observed around the periapical region, with enlargement of the periodontal ligament, loss of visualisation of the lamina dura and osteolysis of the adjacent alveolar bone to a variable degree. Sometimes resorption of the tooth root can also be observed (Fig. 19).

CT allows all the changes described in cases of periodontal disease to be seen in great detail without the need for multiple radiographic projections.

To improve visualisation of the structures of the oral cavity, the mouth can be held open slightly using a syringe or cotton wool, facilitating the entry of air and the separation of structures.

Abnormalities of the Skull, Maxilla and Mandible

Congenital Disorders

Occipital Bone Dysplasia

Occipital bone dysplasia is a morphological variation in which the margin of the foramen magnum extends dorsally. This abnormality mainly affects miniature breeds of dog, and may be an incidental finding, although it may also be associated with neurological signs.

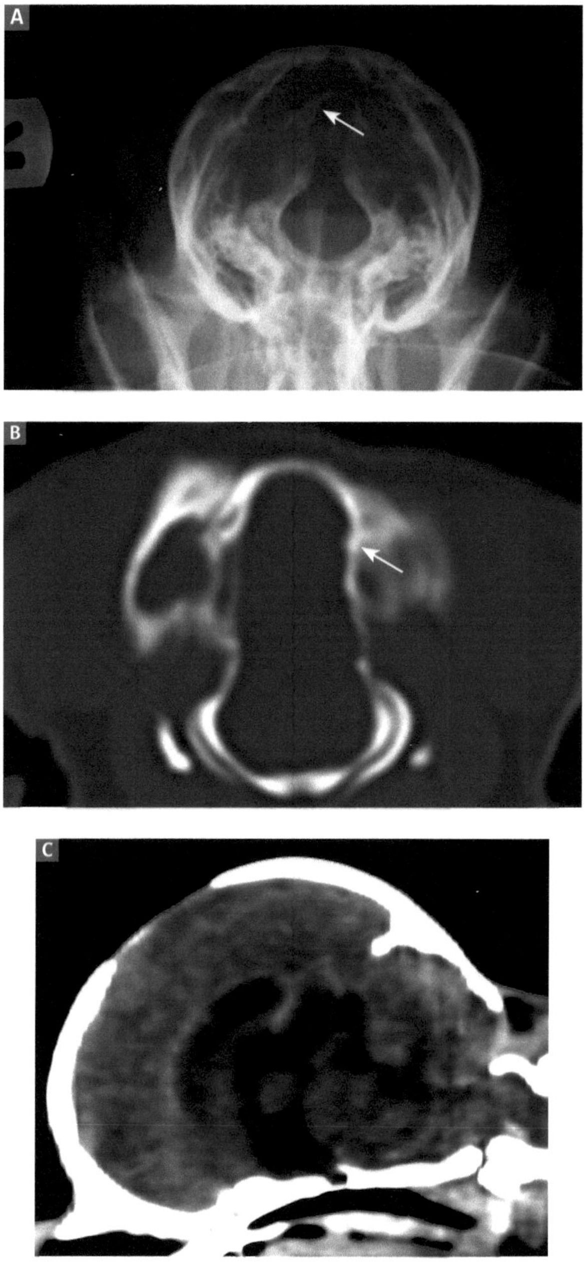

Figure 20. A. Oblique frontal projection of a dog with occipital bone dysplasia. Note the dorsal extension of the keyhole-shaped foramen magnum (arrow). **B** and **C**. CT images of another dog with the same pathology. Occipital bone dysplasia is observed in the bone window (B). In the sagittal plane with a soft tissue window (C), intracranial structures can be evaluated. The cerebellum is in a normal position and there is moderate distension of the ventricular system.

Radiographically, the foramen magnum has an abnormally elongated keyhole-like shape. The foramen magnum can also be evaluated with CT, without the need for special projections. CT is also useful to evaluate the position of the cerebellum (Fig. 20).

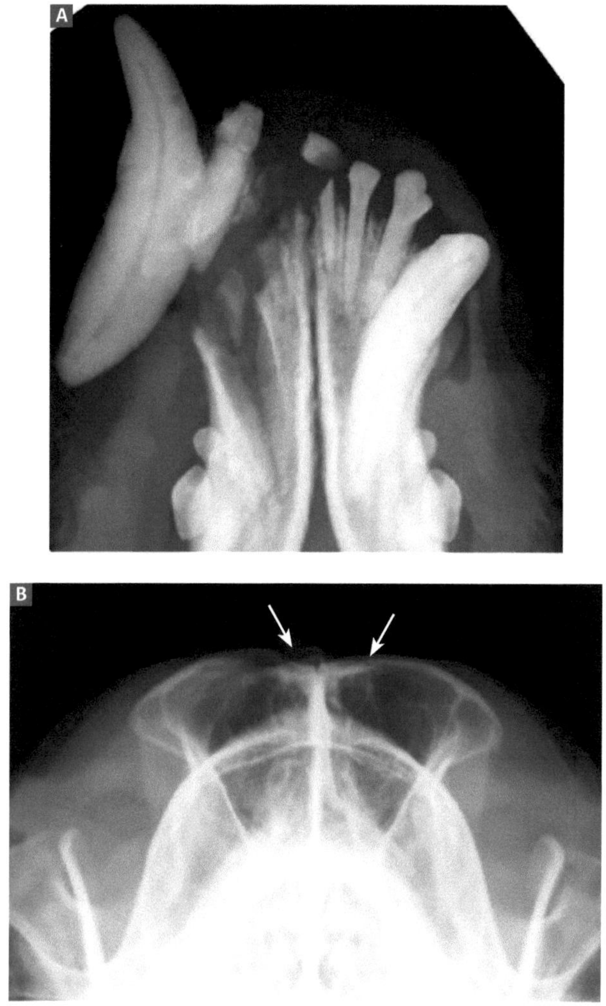

Figure 21. A. Intraoral VD projection of the mandible. A fracture of the right incisor region is observed, with fracture and displacement of the canine and right incisors and fracture of the first left incisor. The mandibular symphysis is intact. **B**. Rostrocaudal projection of the skull of a dog. Fracture lines are observed in both frontal sinuses (arrows) and there is mild depression of the right frontal sinus.

Metabolic Abnormalities

Secondary Renal Hyperparathyroidism

This pathology occurs in young dogs with renal dysplasia or, more rarely, in older dogs and cats with acquired kidney disease. It causes osteopaenia with marked changes in the bones of the skull, especially the mandible and maxilla ("rubber jaw"). Loss of visualisation of the lamina dura is observed, and osteopaenia causes the teeth to appear as if they are "floating".

Trauma

In a head injury, there may be fractures of the mandible, maxilla and other bones that make up the cranial cavity. Assessment of fractures using radiography depends on their location, extent and complexity (Fig. 21). In cases where complex fractures are suspected, performing a CT scan of the skull is preferable, as more detailed information will be provided and the need for multiple radiographic projections is avoided.

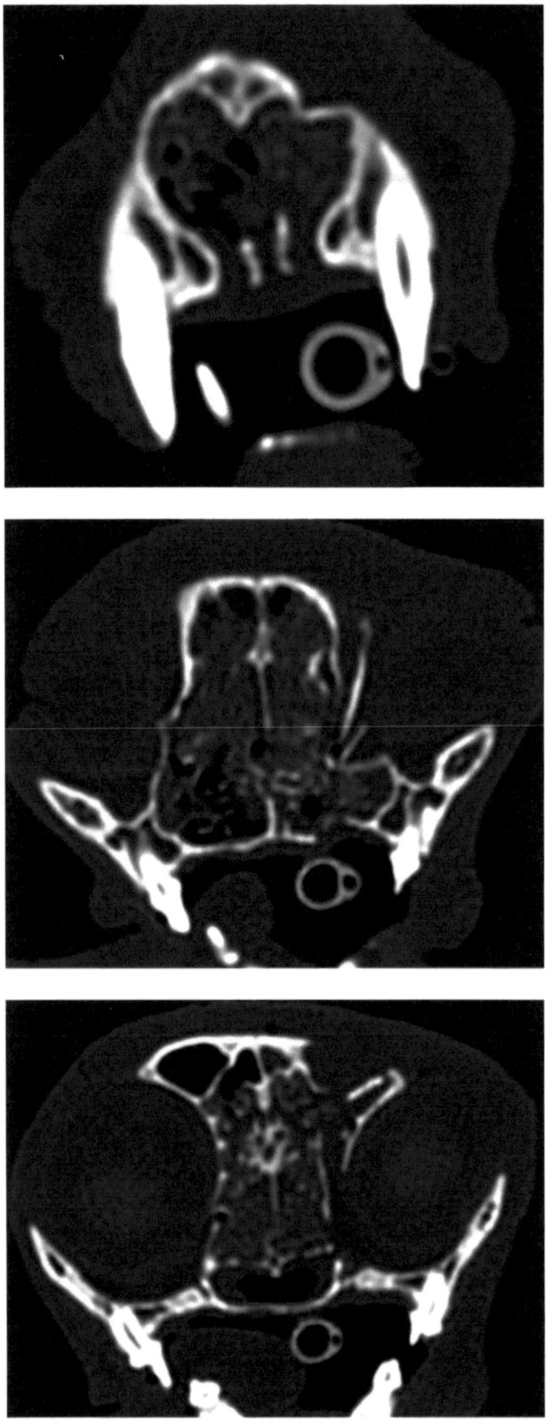

Figure 22. CT images in a bone window of a cat that was run over. Multiple fractures of the nasal, maxillary, palatal, orbital wall and left frontal bones are observed. The nasal cavity is completely occupied by material with liquid attenuation, compatible with bleeding associated with the fractures.

In addition to identifying fractured bones and detecting bone fragments and their displacement, CT allows the detection of associated haemorrhage (intracranial, nasal cavity, etc.), and the presence of gas intracranially (pneumocephalus) or in subcutaneous tissue (emphysema) (Fig. 22).

Inflammatory Disorders

Osteomyelitis

Osteomyelitis can be caused by penetrating wounds that cause abscess formation, or by trauma. In these cases, there is inflammation of the soft tissue and bone lesions are observed in one or multiple bones of the skull. These present osteolysis and aggressive periosteal reactions with poorly defined margins. In some cases, intracranial extension may occur. Some of the lesions can be so aggressive that they are difficult to distinguish from a neoplasm, so definitive diagnosis is achieved by biopsy.

CT makes it possible to evaluate bone lesions in more detail and allows their extent to be determined; adjacent soft tissues can also be evaluated and intracranial extension can be identified (Fig. 23).

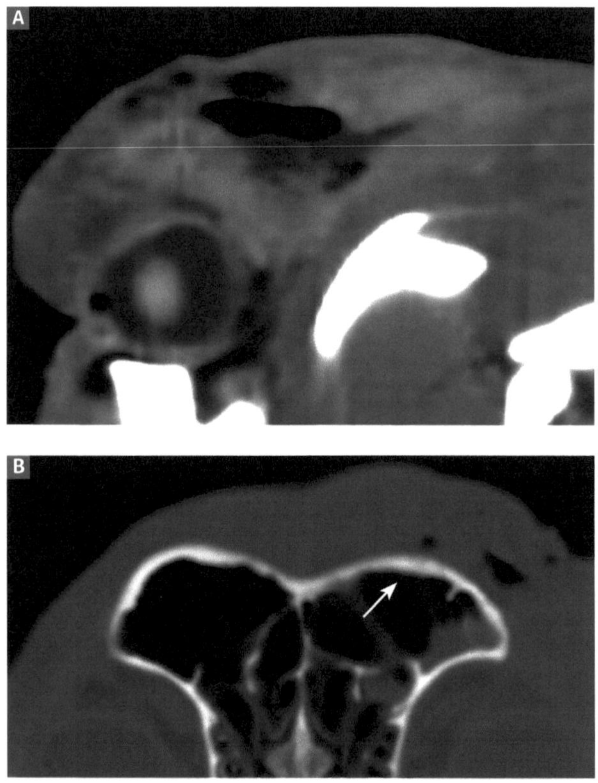

Figure 23. CT images in soft tissue and bone windows of a dog with a penetrating wound in the left frontotemporal region. **A.** A ring-enhancing lesion with irregular, well defined margins is observed, with liquid and gas inside, compatible with an abscess. **B.** Note a slight permeative osteolysis of the adjacent frontal bone (arrow), which is compatible with osteomyelitis, and the presence of fluid inside the left frontal sinus.

Neoplasms

Bones of the skull

Neoplasms affecting the bones of the skull include malignant forms of neoplasia such as osteosarcoma, chondrosarcoma and multilobular osteochondrosarcoma. These are aggressive bone processes and usually present mixed osteolysis and osteoproductive patterns (amorphous bone neoformation), as well as an associated soft tissue component/mass.

In the case of multilobular osteochondrosarcoma, it usually affects the flat bones of the skull, although it has been described in other bones of the head. The lesions are well defined, and appear as a locally invasive bone mass with a heterogeneous, granular appearance (Fig. 24). With techniques such as CT, similar characteristics are observed, and the presence of intracranial involvement can also be evaluated.

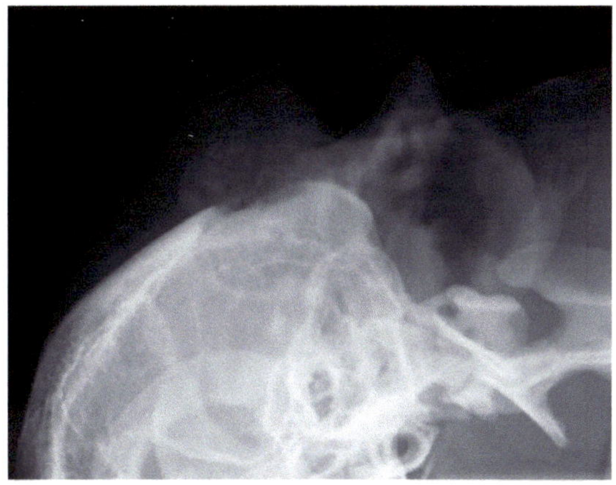

Figure 24. Lateral projection of the skull of a dog with a multilobular osteochondrosarcoma affecting the occipital bone. Note the granular-like bone mass and associated osteolysis in the occipital bone.

Oral Cavity

Neoplasms affecting the oral cavity include squamous cell carcinoma, fibrosarcoma, melanoma and odontogenic tumours.

In dogs, squamous cell carcinoma has a predilection for the rostral portion of the mandible; fibrosarcoma affects the maxilla and mandible, and has a predilection for the palate. These neoplasms have a varying radiographic appearance, with the osteolytic component predominating in some, and others being more osteoproductive. Most show both patterns, and it is not possible to determine the type of neoplasm from its radiographic characteristics.

CT allows the lesions to be evaluated in greater detail and makes it possible to establish the limits for a surgical approach (Fig. 25). In addition, other signs of aggressiveness, such as metastasis, can be evaluated, if there is alteration of the regional lymph nodes or at the pulmonary level. However, CT cannot be used to make a definitive diagnosis as most lesions have similar characteristics, but it is helpful for planning sampling (cytology, biopsy, etc.).

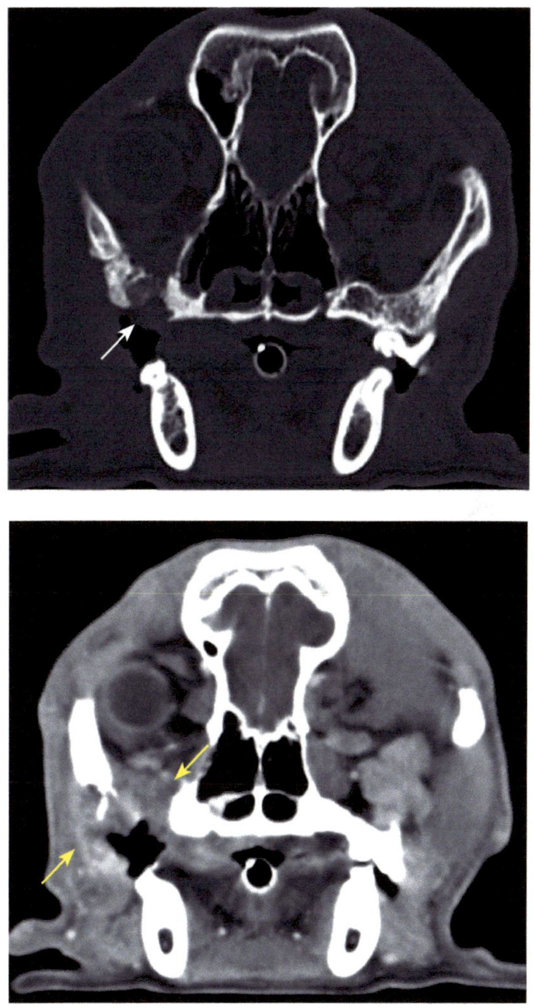

Figure 25. Transverse CT images in bone and postcontrast soft tissue windows of a dog with squamous cell carcinoma in the molar region of the right maxilla. Note the osteolysis with poorly defined margins in the maxilla, with absence of the tooth (white arrow), associated with a thickening of the soft tissue that shows homogeneous enhancement, affecting the ventral aspect of the orbit (yellow arrows).

Other Pathologies

Craniomandibular Osteopathy

Craniomandibular osteopathy is a proliferative bone disease seen primarily in young West Highland White Terriers, Scottish Terriers and Boston Terriers. It is a self-limiting disease of unknown aetiology, although in the West Highland White Terrier it has an autosomal recessive pattern of inheritance.

Radiographically, irregular bone neoformation is observed in the mandible, which can affect the temporomandibular joint, and also the tympanic bullae. Thickening of the bones of the skull (frontal, parietal, occipital) can also be observed (Fig. 26). In some cases, radiographic changes are also seen in the cortices of the metaphyses of the long bones.

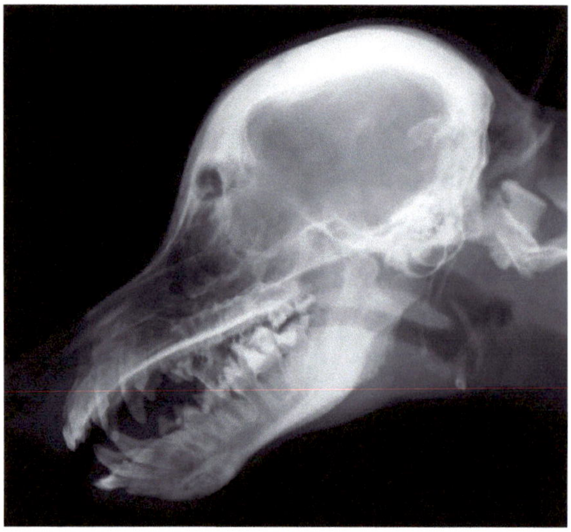

Figure 26. Lateral projection of the skull of a dog with craniomandibular osteopathy. Note the irregular bone neoformation affecting the ventral aspect of the body and the ramus of the mandible, as well as thickening and increased opacity of the skull bones.

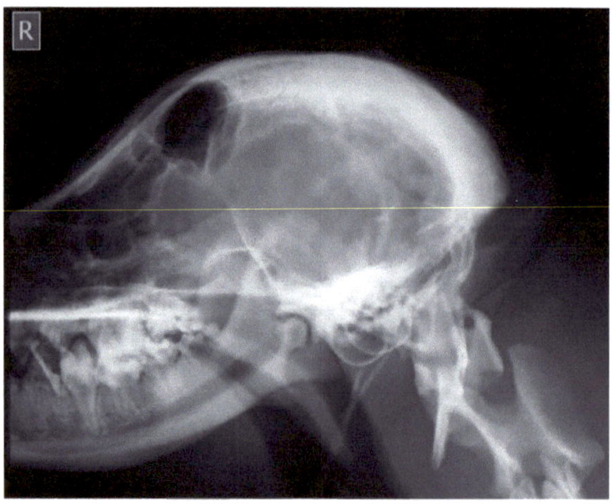

Figure 27. Lateral projection of the skull of a dog with calvarial hyperostosis. Thickening and sclerosis of the bones of the skull, with smooth margins, are observed.

Calvarial Hyperostosis

Calvarial hyperostosis is a pathology similar to craniomandibular osteopathy, but the bones of the skull are affected more. The aetiology is unknown; it affects young animals, and is mainly seen in the Bullmastiff. Radiographically, variable degrees of thickening and sclerosis of the skull bones (frontal, parietal and occipital bones) with smooth bone proliferation is observed. In these cases, no involvement of the mandible is seen (Fig. 27).

Disorders of the Temporomandibular Joint

Temporomandibular Joint Dysplasia

Temporomandibular joint dysplasia is a congenital or developmental disease that affects breeds including the Bassett Hound, Dachshund, Irish Setter and Cocker Spaniel. It is characterised by abnormalities in the morphology of the condylar process of the mandible, with flattening of the articular surfaces, and hypoplasia of the retroarticular process of the mandible (Fig. 28). Consequently, the joint space can appear wider than normal and irregular. This leads to a subluxation of the joint and can cause the coronoid process of the mandible to be trapped lateral to the zygomatic arch, leaving the patient unable to close its mouth.

Temporomandibular Luxation and Fractures

Luxation may occur secondary to trauma or as a result of joint dysplasia.

Luxation of the mandibular condyle usually occurs in the rostrodorsal direction due to the presence of the retroarticular process, which prevents it from luxating in another direction. Normally, widening of the joint space is observed, and the mandible is displaced rostrally and towards the contralateral side. Luxation can be visualised more clearly in DV or oblique lateral projections. With CT, multiplanar reconstructions facilitate the diagnosis of both luxation and subtle fractures affecting the joint (Fig. 29).

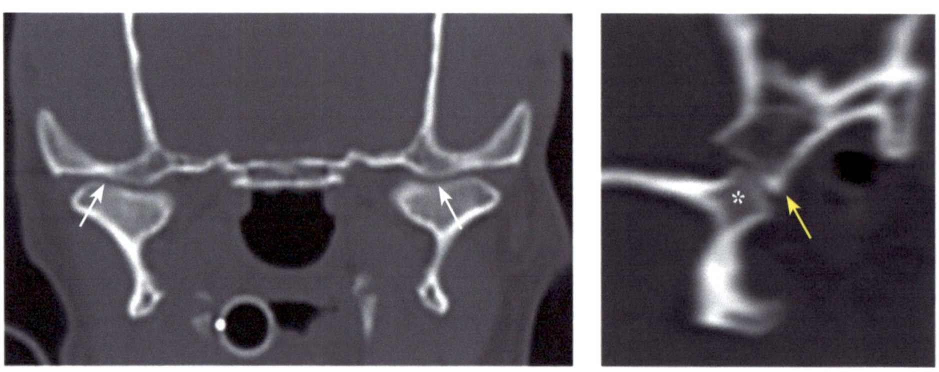

Figure 28. Transverse and sagittal CT images of a dog of a chondrodystrophic breed with temporomandibular joint dysplasia. Note that both joints have a curved shape in the transverse plane (white arrows); in the sagittal plane, an absence of the retroarticular process is observed (yellow arrow) and the condylar process is luxated slightly caudally (asterisk).

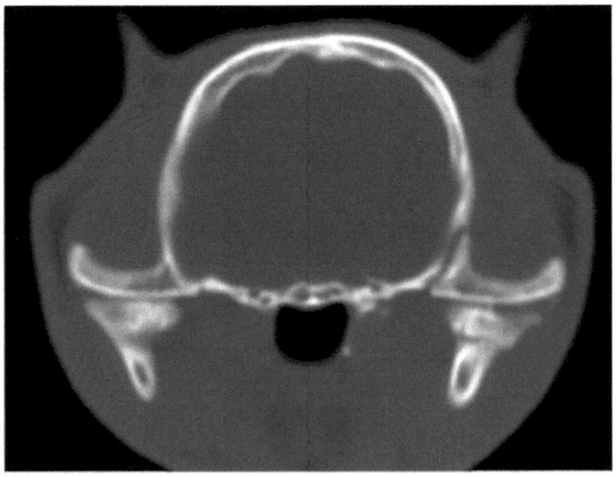

Figure 29. Transverse CT image of a cat with fracture of the left temporomandibular joint. A fracture line of the squamous portion of the temporal bone and another fracture at the base of the mandibular condylar process can be seen.

Orbit Abnormalities

CT is one of the techniques of choice for the evaluation of the orbital region, including the eyeball and all extraocular structures, due to its complex anatomy and the presence of a multitude of soft tissue structures that cannot be evaluated radiographically. The orbit contains the eyeball, extraocular muscles, optic nerve, lacrimal gland and duct, zygomatic salivary gland, medial pterygoid muscle and periorbital fat.

Cellulitis

Cellulitis is the inflammation of periorbital fat. It is usually caused by trauma, foreign bodies or infections. Among the findings that can be observed are an increase in the size of the periorbital tissue, and a loss of definition of fat and extraocular muscles.

Retrobulbar Abscess

Retrobulbar abscesses are characterised by the presence of a retrobulbar mass with liquid attenuation, with marked mass effect (causing exophthalmos), which presents marked ring or peripheral enhancement after the administration of contrast. Abscesses can invade adjacent structures that are part of the masticatory musculature (temporalis muscle). In addition, other structures in the orbit may also be affected by associated inflammatory changes (Fig. 30).

Neoplasms

Neoplasms of the orbit can originate in the soft tissues or bony structures. Soft tissue neoplasms usually have better defined margins compared with inflammatory or infectious processes. However, in many cases these pathologies are difficult to differentiate. The most common tumours include carcinoma, sarcoma and round cell neoplasia.

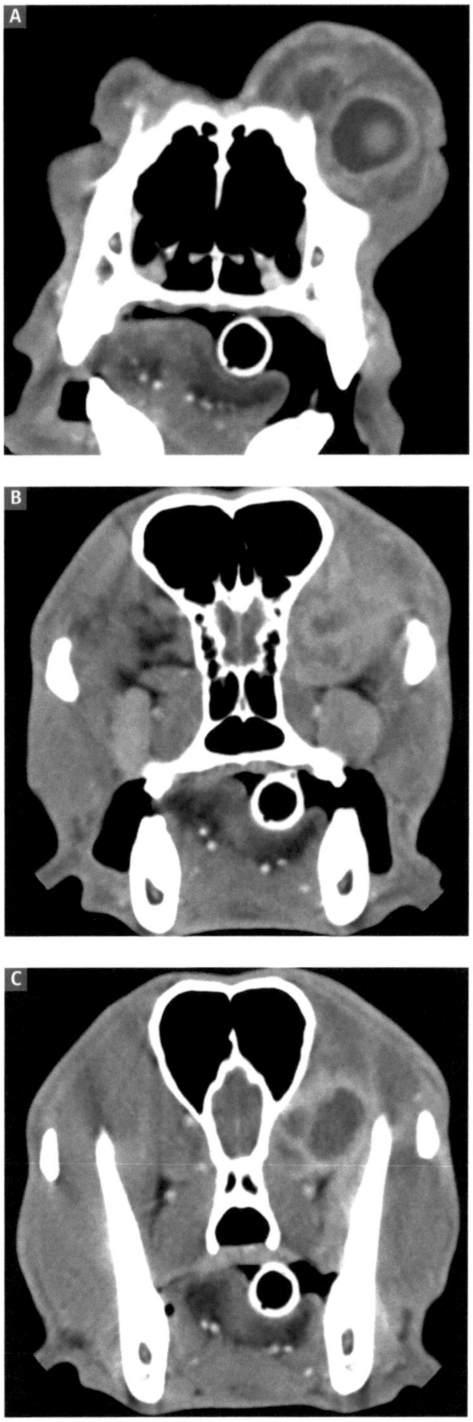

Figure 30. Transverse postcontrast CT images in a soft tissue window of a dog with periorbital cellulitis and a retrobulbar abscess in the left orbit. **A**. Note the increase in size and attenuation of periorbital fat (cellulitis) with exophthalmos. **B** and **C**. A retrobulbar mass is observed, affecting the temporalis muscle, with marked ring enhancement, compatible with an abscess.

CT helps to determine which tissues are involved in the mass, the margins and the enhancement characteristics, and also to identify the presence of osteolysis of adjacent bone structures and whether or not there is intracranial invasion.

Salivary Gland Disorders

The salivary glands comprise the zygomatic, parotid, mandibular and sublingual glands in dogs; cats have also molar salivary glands. On CT they present uniform attenuation that is greater than that of the musculature.

Sialadenitis

Sialadenitis is inflammation of the salivary glands. It can be unilateral or bilateral. The glands appear enlarged, with decreased attenuation and with marked, heterogeneous enhancement. Usually, in inflammatory processes, the glandular architecture is maintained, with loss of visualisation of periglandular fat. In these cases, enlargement of regional lymph nodes may also be detected.

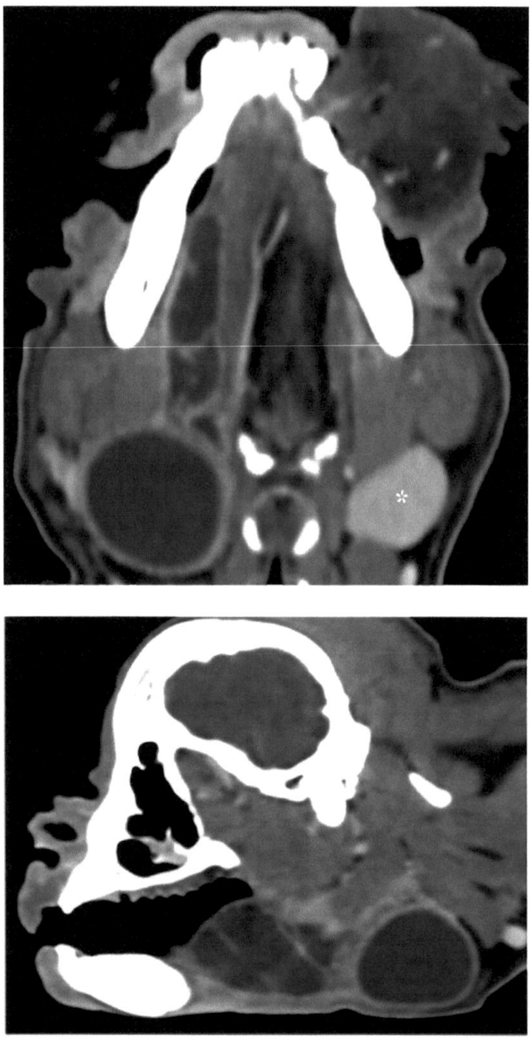

Figure 31. Dorsal and sagittal postcontrast CT images in a soft tissue window of a dog with a sialocoele in the right mandibular salivary gland. A ring-enhancing lesion is observed with liquid attenuation in the centre and with well defined margins. This lesion is rounded, affects the mandibular salivary gland and extends rostrally along the sublingual region. The contralateral mandibular salivary gland is normal (asterisk).

Sialocoele

Sialocoele is the distension of the salivary glands with an accumulation of saliva due to blockage of the salivary ducts. Imaging findings consist of well defined lesions with thin walls containing material with liquid attenuation, showing peripheral postcontrast enhancement of the wall without enhancement of the core material. These lesions affect the salivary glands and can spread to adjacent regions depending on their size. Sometimes sialoliths can be detected as the cause of the blockage, although in other cases the cause is not identified (Fig. 31).

MRI Examination of the Brain

Indications

MRI is the technique of choice for the study of the central nervous system (brain and spinal cord) as it provides greater soft tissue resolution and therefore better differentiation between white matter and grey matter. In addition, the use of different sequences allows the nature of lesions to be more accurately characterised.

Protocol

To evaluate the brain using MRI, the basic protocol consists of T2-weighted (T2W) (sagittal, transverse and dorsal planes), fluid-attenuated inversion recovery FLAIR (transverse plane), T1-weighted (T1W) (at least the transverse plane), T2* (echo gradient, transverse plane), and postcontrast T1W (at least the transverse plane) sequences.

Most Frequent Pathologies

Congenital Disorders

Hydrocephalus

Hydrocephalus is the distension of the ventricular system due to the accumulation of cerebrospinal fluid (CSF). It can be congenital or acquired.

Congenital hydrocephalus mainly affects toy and brachycephalic breeds and is caused by the obstruction of the flow of CSF, which accumulates intracranially. Acquired hydrocephalus occurs in animals of any age and is caused by any disease that secondarily causes the accumulation of CSF at the intracranial level.

Findings include distension of the ventricular system and thinning of the cerebral cortex (Fig. 32). In some cases, atrophy of the interthalamic adhesion, or the presence of associated periventricular oedema, may also be seen.

Chiari Malformation

Chiari malformation is a congenital anomaly that mainly affects Cavalier King Charles Spaniels and other small breeds. It is an abnormality in the conformation of the caudal fossa, which is reduced in size and as a consequence causes cerebellar compression. Findings that may be present include a cleft in the caudal aspect of the cerebellum caused by the occipital bone, possible cerebellar herniation through the foramen magnum and dorsal displacement of the spinal cord at the level of the atlantoaxial joint. These changes result in an irregular flow of CSF and can cause associated syringomyelia and hydrocephalus.

Some or all of these changes can be observed, with varying degrees of severity; they are more easily detected in T2W sequences in the sagittal plane (Fig. 33).

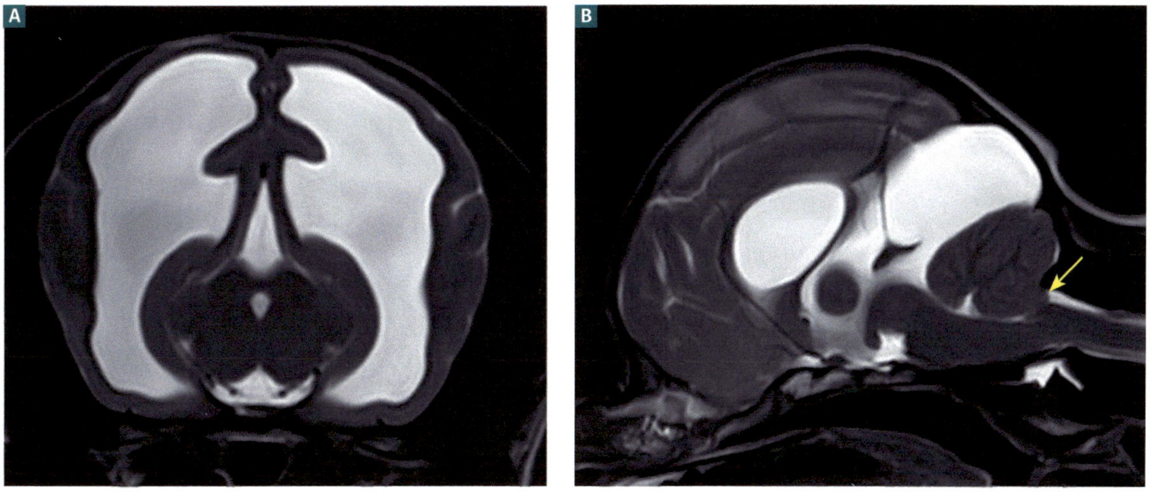

Figure 32. MRI images of a dog with congenital hydrocephalus. **A**. Transverse plane T2W. **B**. Sagittal plane T2W. Note the marked symmetrical distension of the ventricular system, with thinning of the cerebral cortex. In the sagittal plane, an accumulation of fluid is observed at the supracollicular level, with a marked mass effect on the cerebellum. The caudal aspect of the cerebellum is slightly herniated through the foramen magnum (yellow arrow).

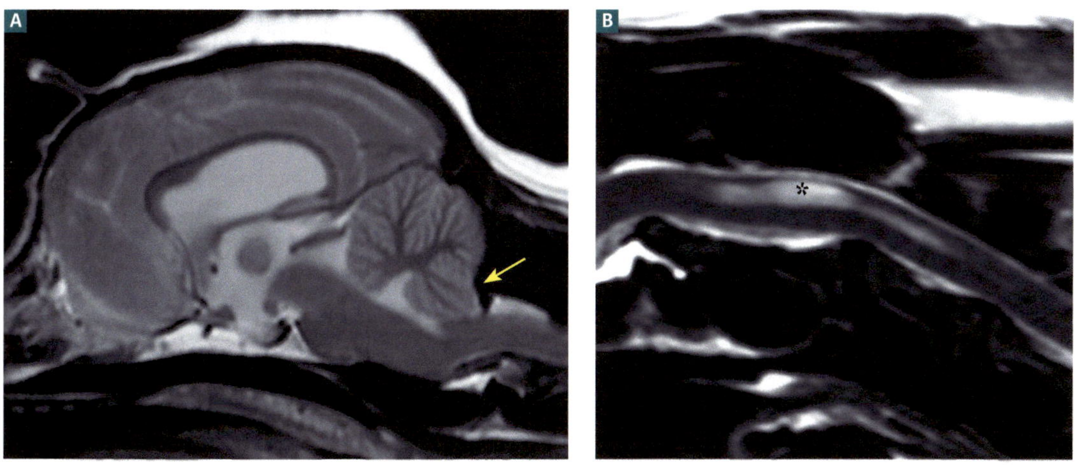

Figure 33. A. Sagittal T2W image of the skull and cervical spine of a dog with Chiari malformation or caudal occipital malformation syndrome. The following can be observed: a cleft of the occipital bone in the caudal aspect of the cerebellum (arrow), protrusion of the cerebellar vermis towards the foramen magnum, attenuation of the CSF of the cisterna magna and dorsal displacement of the spinal cord at the level of the craniocervical junction. **B**. Image of the cervical spine showing syringomyelia (asterisk).

Metabolic Diseases

Peri-ictal Changes

These changes are associated with seizures and are associated with the presence of cytotoxic and vasogenic oedema. The pathophysiology of this process is not fully known. MRI findings include diffuse lesions that are hypointense in T1W and hyperintense in T2W sequences, with no signal suppression in FLAIR. They are normally bilateral and symmetrical, but they can be unilateral. They are not usually enhanced after contrast administration, although some lesions may enhance slightly, and they can cause a slight mass effect. These lesions can affect the piriform lobe, temporal lobe and hippocampus; other locations described include the cingulate gyrus, parieto-occipital lobes, frontal lobes or olfactory bulb (Fig. 34).

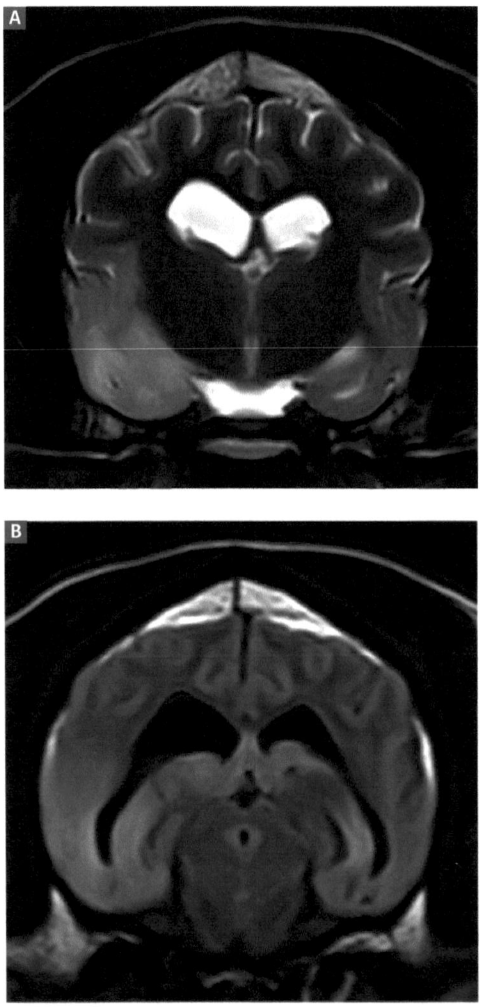

Figure 34. MRI images of a dog with seizures. **A**. Transverse T2W image showing a hyperintense diffuse zone in the piriform and temporal lobe region. **B**. FLAIR image showing symmetrical hyperintense lesions in both hippocampi, compatible with peri-ictal changes.

Inflammatory Processes

Inflammatory processes in general are characterised by multifocal, nonsymmetrical lesions of irregular morphology with poorly defined margins, which are hyperintense in T2W and FLAIR, hypo/isointense in T1W, and variably enhanced after contrast administration. These lesions may cause a mass effect, although less so than other pathologies (e.g. neoplastic processes). Sometimes these findings are associated with meningeal enhancement and thickening (pachymeninges and leptomeninges), which can be focal or diffuse.

However, inflammatory lesions can vary depending on their cause. In addition, it should be noted that inflammatory lesions have characteristics in common with vascular and neoplastic processes, so MRI findings are not pathognomonic. Based on the clinical history, examination and imaging findings (characteristics and distribution of the lesions), a list of differential diagnoses should be established from highest to lowest probability.

Noninfectious Inflammatory Processes

Meningoencephalitis of unknown origin (MUO) includes a group of idiopathic, non-infectious central nervous system diseases. MUO is subdivided into granulomatous meningoencephalitis (GME), necrotising meningoencephalitis (NME) and necrotising leukoencephalitis (NLE).

Meningoencephalitis of Unknown Origin

- **Granulomatous meningoencephalitis** (**GME**). This mainly affects toy breeds, Terriers and Poodles. Affected animals are usually young or middle aged. There are three different forms (disseminated, focal and ocular), and therefore MRI findings are variable.
  - Disseminated form: characterised by the presence of multifocal lesions that affect the white and grey matter in the forebrain, brainstem and cerebellum. The lesions have poorly defined margins, are hyperintense in T2W and FLAIR, hypo/isointense in T1W and show variable postcontrast enhancement. Lesions may be associated with perilesional oedema. Meningeal enhancement may be present (Fig. 35).
  - Focal form: characterised by a single lesion, with a mass effect displacing adjacent structures, and with variable postcontrast enhancement. It may appear similar to a neoplastic process.
- **Necrotising meningoencephalitis** (**NME**). This affects young animals. Predisposed breeds include the Pug, Maltese and Yorkshire Terrier. The lesions are multifocal, affecting grey matter and the subcortical white matter (white–grey matter demarcation) located in the cerebral hemispheres, thalamus, hippocampus, brainstem and cerebellum, with characteristics similar to those described above. In addition, there may be cystic lesions with well defined margins (hyperintense in T2W and

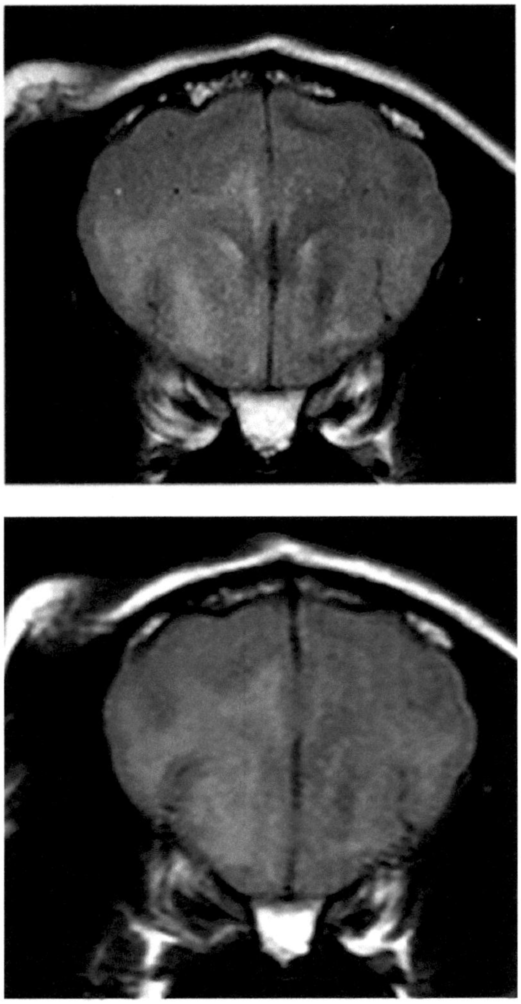

Figure 35. MRI images of a dog with granulomatous meningoencephalitis. Transverse T2W and FLAIR images showing a diffuse hyperintense lesion with poorly defined margins affecting the white and grey matter of the right hemisphere, causing slight displacement of the midline to the left.

hypointense in T1W sequences), which are characteristic of necrotic lesions (Fig. 36).

Infectious Diseases

These processes include the following: viral diseases (canine distemper, feline infectious peritonitis, etc.), bacterial (infection by extension from adjacent structures, haematogenous dissemination, trauma, etc.), protozoa (*Toxoplasma*, *Neospora*), fungal and parasitic.

Meningoencephalitis of Infectious Origin

- **Distemper**: distemper virus can affect young or adult animals, causing demyelination and grey matter necrosis in acute infections. The findings are poorly defined lesions affecting the grey matter and the grey–white

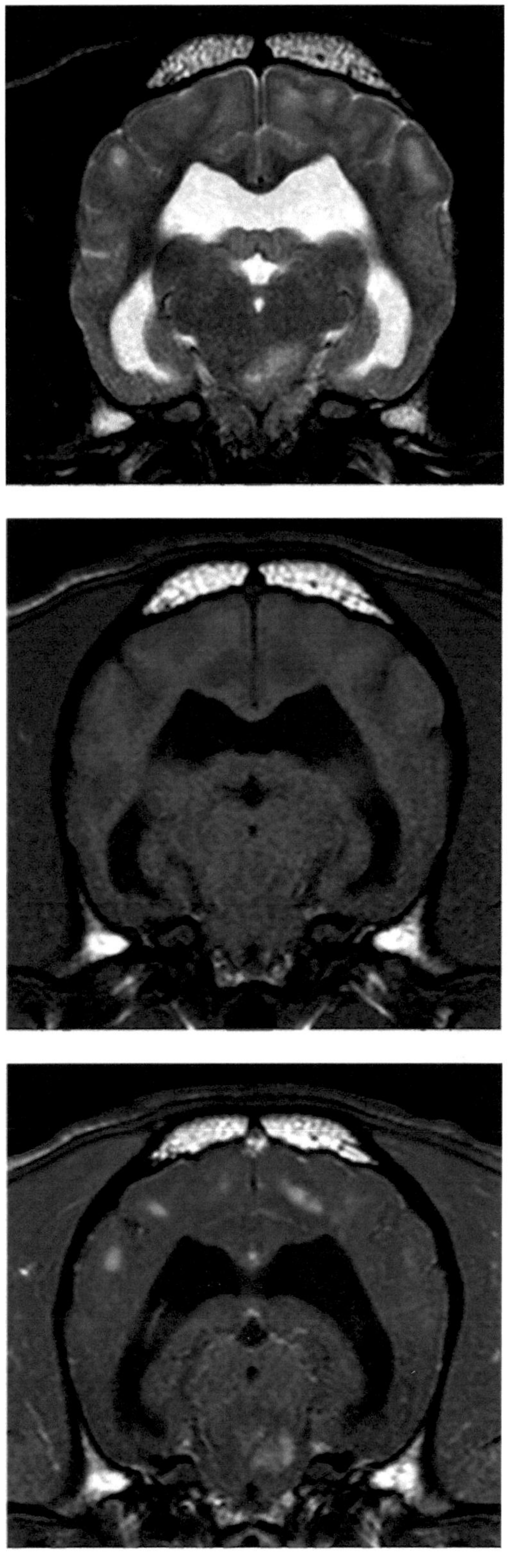

Figure 36. T2W, T1W and T1W post-contrast MRI images of a French Bulldog with necrotising meningoencephalitis. Multifocal, asymmetrical lesions are observed in the subcortical white matter, affecting both cerebral hemispheres and the brainstem. The lesions are hyperintense in T2W, isointense in T1W and show marked postcontrast enhancement.

matter interphase in the forebrain, brainstem and cerebellum. The lesions are hyperintense in T2W and hypo/isointense in T1W sequences, and show variable postcontrast enhancement (Fig. 37).

- **Feline infectious peritonitis**: this is a pyogranulomatous vasculitis that occurs in cats affected by a feline coronavirus. Lesions are characterised by distension of the ventricular system, with variable enhancement of the meninges, ependyma and periventricular area. Parenchymal lesions are focal or multifocal, hyperintense in T2W and iso/hypointense in T1W sequences, and show moderate/marked postcontrast enhancement.
- **Bacterial infections**: can be caused by haematogenous dissemination, external trauma or by the spread of infections from adjacent structures (ear, nasal cavity, etc.). Findings showing the intracranial extension of an ear infection include hyperintense, plaque-shaped T2W lesions and variable enhancement located in the brainstem, adjacent to the tympanic bulla. There is usually meningeal enhancement in the region adjacent to the tympanic bulla. In addition, material can be seen occupying the tympanic bulla, as well as postcontrast enhancement of the lining of the tympanic bulla.

Cerebrovascular Accidents: Infarctions and Haemorrhage

Cerebrovascular accidents can be divided into **ischaemic vascular accidents** due to the obstruction of a vessel and **haemorrhagic accidents** due to the rupture of a vessel. Another form of classification is based on the vasculature that is affected, such as **territorial infarctions** when they affect a large vessel or **lacunar infarctions** when they affect small vessels. There are multiple factors that predispose to the onset of infarcts, such as endocrinopathies (hyperadrenocorticism, hypothyroidism), kidney disease, sepsis, neoplasia, coagulopathies and infectious agents (e.g. *Leishmania*, *Dirofilaria*).

Ischaemic Infarcts

These are usually solitary lesions, although they can be multiple; they are more commonly located in the cerebellum, but can also be found in other locations (being limited to specific vascular territories). They are hyperintense lesions in T2W and FLAIR, normally homogeneous, with relatively well defined margins, and predominantly affect grey matter. The mass effect they usually generate is mild to moderate, depending on the severity of the infarction, and they show variable enhancement, although they do not usually present enhancement or appear in chronic stages. Diffusion sequences help to diagnose them; these show restricted water diffusion in the acute stages (hyperintense in diffusion-weighted images (DWI), and hypointense in apparent diffusion coefficient map [ADC map]) (Fig. 38).

Haemorrhages

Haemorrhages can be evaluated with MRI. It must be taken into account that changes in signal intensity are seen over time as the haemoglobin products are degraded. Thus, there are five stages (**hyperacute**, **acute**, **early subacute**, **late subacute** and **chronic**) of haemorrhage that may be seen, each of which has different characteristics on MRI (Table 1). On the other hand, the T2* echo gradient sequences are sensitive for the detection of haemorrhage, which is visualised as areas with signal void and susceptibility artefact (Fig. 39). In addition, lesions due to haemorrhage can be accompanied by variable perilesional oedema and also variable postcontrast enhancement (usually absent in acute phases, with possible appearance in later phases).

Neoplasms

Intracranial neoplasms can be classified as **extra-axial** or **intra-axial** according to their location. This classification can help in making a presumptive diagnosis. **Extra-axial** masses originate from the meninges, ventricular system, cranial nerves, etc; in short, from any structure other than the brain parenchyma.

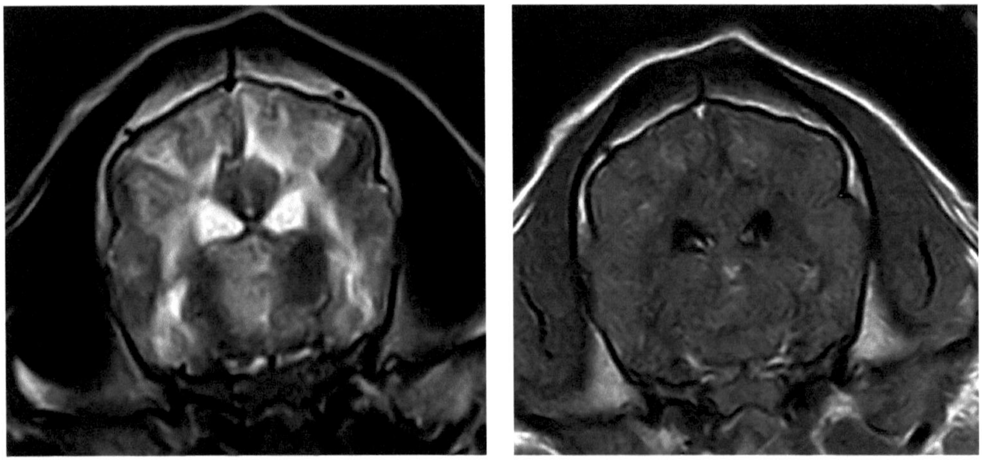

Figure 37. T2W and T1W postcontrast MRI images of a dog with infectious meningoencephalitis (distemper). Hyperintense asymmetrical multifocal lesions are observed in the T2W image, affecting the grey and white matter of both cerebral hemispheres and brainstem; the lesions present variable postcontrast enhancement.

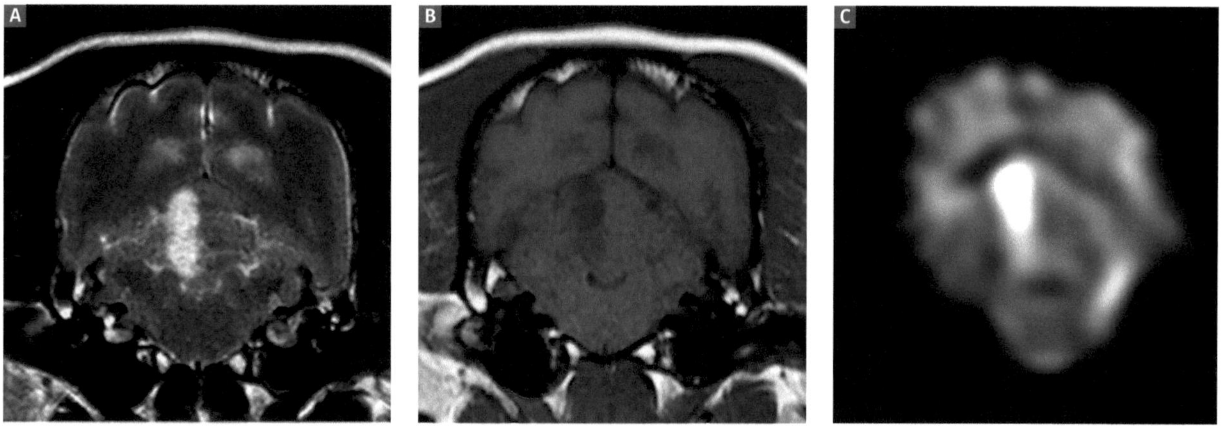

Figure 38. MRI images of a dog with an acute ischaemic cerebrovascular accident. An intra-axial lesion is observed in the rostral aspect of the cerebellum with well defined, homogeneous margins, which is hyperintense in T2W (**A**) and hypointense in T1W (**B**) sequences. In the diffusion sequence (**C**), the lesion shows restricted water diffusion, appearing markedly hyperintense. This lesion is located in the rostral cerebellar artery territory.

Table 1. MRI appearance of the stages of haemorrhage.

Stage	Time	Haemoglobin product/ distribution	T1W signal strength	T2W signal strength
Hyperacute	Immediate/within hours	Intracellular oxyhaemoglobin	Hypo/isointense	Hyperintense
Acute	Hours to days	Intracellular deoxyhaemoglobin	Hypo/isointense	Hypointense
Early subacute	>3 days	Intracellular methaemoglobin	Hyperintense	Hypointense
Late subacute	>7 days	Extracellular methaemoglobin	Hyperintense	Hyperintense
Chronic	Days to months	Extracellular haemosiderin	Hypointense	Hypointense

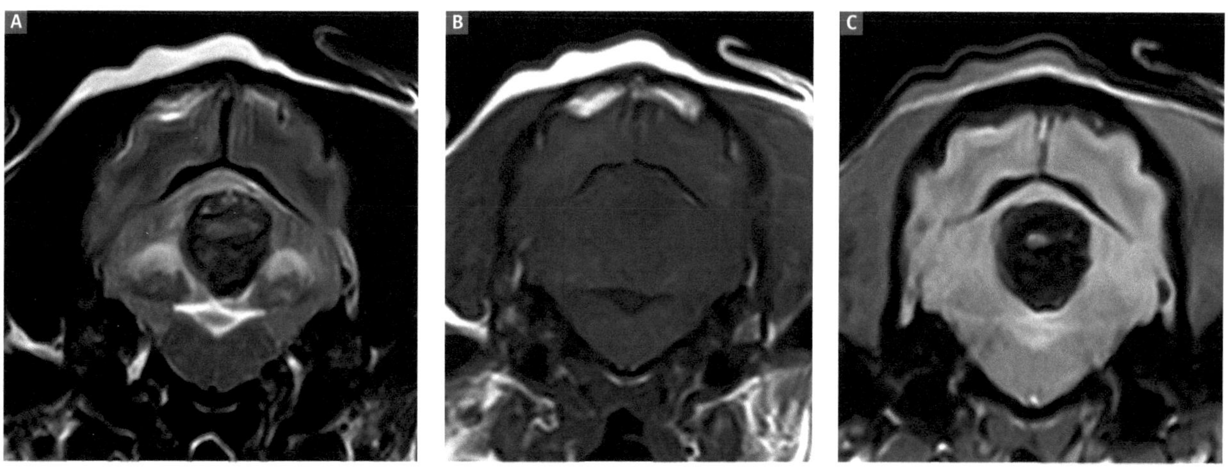

Figure 39. MRI images of a dog with a chronic cerebellar haemorrhagic lesion. **A**. T2W image, where the lesion is hypointense in the periphery and hyperintense in the central area. **B**. T1W image, where the lesion is hypointense. **C**. T2* image with associated susceptibility artefact, indicating the haemorrhagic nature of the lesion. Note the peripheral diffuse hyperintense halo surrounding the lesion in the T2W image, compatible with perilesional oedema.

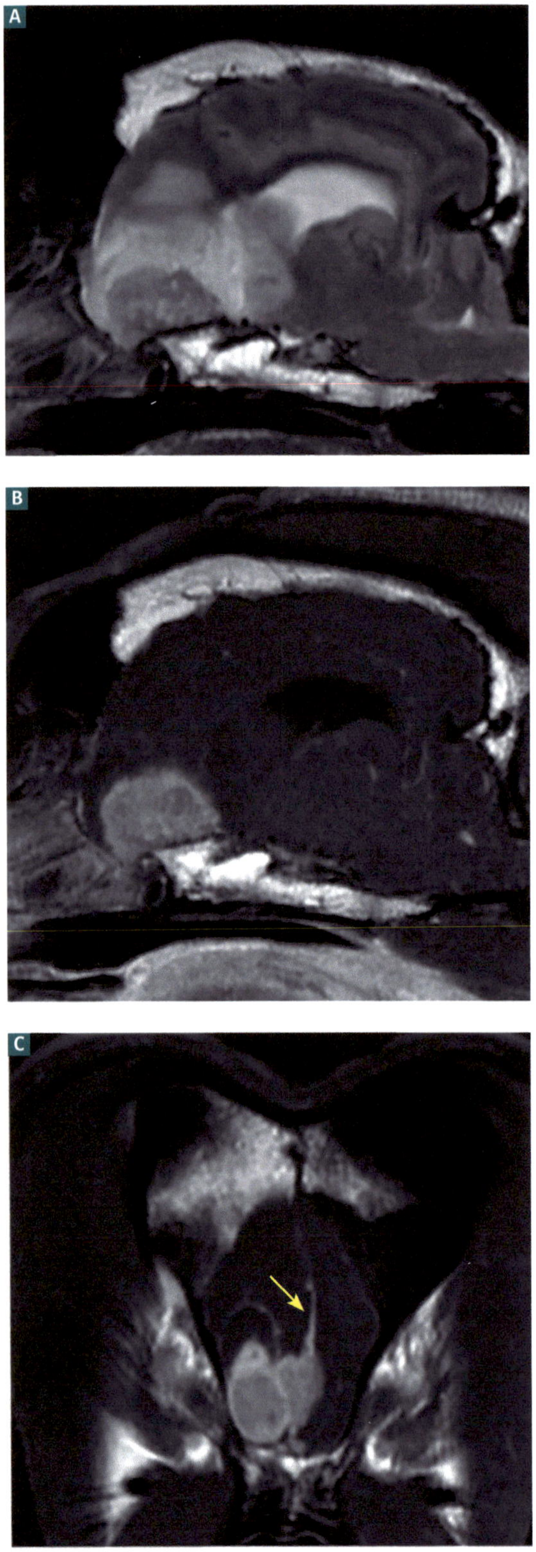

Figure 40. MRI images of a dog with a meningioma. **A**. Sagittal T2W. **B**. Sagittal T1W post-contrast. **C**. Transverse T1W post-contrast. An extra-axial mass is visualised with a wide base, well defined margins and marked postcontrast enhancement, located in the right frontal lobe in contact with the base of the skull. Note the "dural tail sign" in the transverse plane, along the midline (arrow), which is offset to the left.

Findings that may be observed in these types of lesions include the presence of a broad base in contact with the meninges/skull, bone changes in the adjacent skull, or thickening and enhancement of the meninges ("dural tail sign").

Intra-axial neoplasms are those that originate from the brain parenchyma. Among their characteristics of note, they are usually surrounded by normal brain parenchyma, which can be difficult to observe in cases of large masses or those located on the periphery. Other characteristics, such as the absence of associated meningeal enhancement or a lower postcontrast enhancement of intra-axial lesions compared with extra-axial ones, can also help differentiate them.

In general, neoplastic processes may be associated with certain features such as distension of the ventricular system due to obstruction of the flow of CSF, perilesional oedema, a moderate/marked mass effect (with midline displacement, displacement of adjacent brain parenchyma structures, etc.) and possible transtentorial, cerebellar or subfalcine herniation.

Meningeal Tumours

Meningiomas are neoplasms that originate from the meninges. They are the most common intracranial tumours in cats and dogs. They are usually single, broad-based masses, located on the periphery or associated with the midline, with variable shapes (rounded/oval or plate shaped) and well defined margins. They have a hyperintense signal intensity in T2W and are hypo/isointense in T1W, with marked postcontrast enhancement that varies from homogeneous to heterogeneous (Fig. 40). They may have the associated "dural tail sign", although it is not always present, and may cause hyperostosis of adjacent bones. In some cases, they may present mineralisation or associated haemorrhagic areas, which will be observed with a signal vacuum in T2* sequences.

Ventricular Tumours

Choroid plexus tumours are associated with the ventricular system and appear predominantly in the third and fourth ventricles. These are tumours that appear iso/hyperintense in T1W and T2W sequences, and show marked homogeneous postcontrast enhancement. Due to their location, they usually cause obstruction of the flow of CSF, with consequent distension of the ventricular system/hydrocephalus. Other findings include cyst formation, haemorrhage or associated mineralisation, and the presence of perilesional or periventricular oedema. Occasionally, associated intraventricular or subarachnoid metastases can be identified.

Glial Tumours

Glial tumours are quite common in dogs. These include astrocytomas, oligodendrogliomas and glioblastoma multiforme. Boxers and Boston Terriers are predisposed to these tumours.

Astrocytomas and **oligodendrogliomas** are usually single masses with variable morphology (from well defined to infiltrative), which are mainly located in the piriform cortex, the frontal and temporal lobes, or the thalamic region. They are usually iso/hypointense lesions in T1W and iso/hyperintense in T2W sequences. Postcontrast enhancement is variable, with enhancement being more frequent in high-grade tumours, whereas low-grade tumours tend to have less enhancement. However, histological grade cannot be determined based on MRI findings. These tumours are usually accompanied by perilesional oedema and mass effect (Fig. 41).

Other Nervous System Tumours

Round Cell Neoplasms

Lymphoma is a frequent tumour in cats; it is the second most frequent intracranial neoplasm in this species. Histiocytic sarcoma is uncommon in dogs. The lesions have a variable appearance and may be well or poorly defined, single or multifocal, and intra-axial or extra-axial in location. They have an iso/hypointense signal intensity in T1W sequences and are hyperintense in T2W, and show moderate/marked postcontrast enhancement. They usually present perilesional oedema and associated mass effect.

Tumours Associated with the Nervous System

Pituitary Gland Tumours (Adenomas and Carcinomas)

These tumours are characterised by their location in the pituitary fossa. They can be classified into **macrotumours** when they measure >10 mm (dorsoventrally) and exceed the limits of the pituitary fossa, or **microtumours** when they are small; microtumours may not be visible.

Macrotumours are usually well defined masses, with variable signal intensity (isointense in T1W, hyperintense in T2W and FLAIR, with marked postcontrast enhancement). Sometimes they can present a heterogeneous appearance by presenting cystic or haemorrhagic regions. In addition, they have an associated mass effect depending on the size of the tumour, peritumoural oedema, and can invade adjacent structures (Fig. 42).

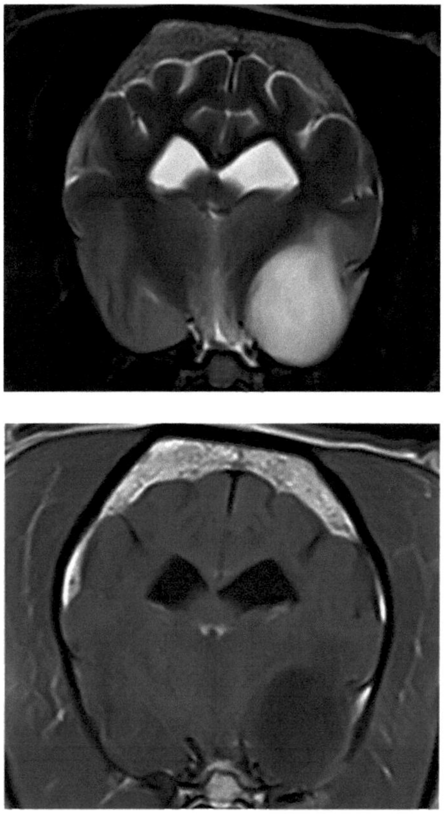

Figure 41. MRI images of a dog with a single intra-axial lesion with well defined margins located in the left piriform cortex. The lesion is hyperintense in T2W, with minimal postcontrast enhancement, compatible with a glioma. Note the moderate mass effect on the thalamus and the slight shift of the midline to the right.

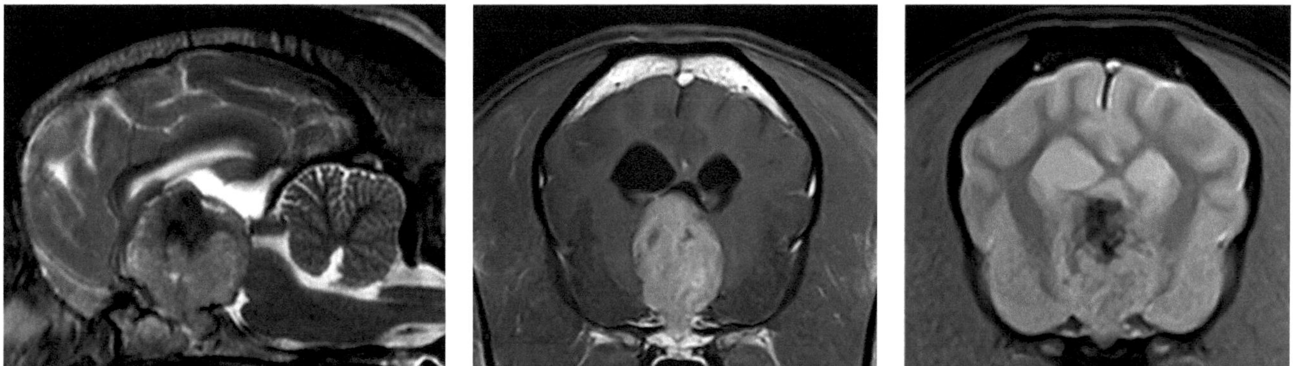

Figure 42. MRI images of a dog with a pituitary macrotumour; the animal was diagnosed with hyperadrenocorticism. Sagittal T2W, transverse T1W post-contrast and transverse T2* images. A large mass is observed at the level of the pituitary fossa, with dorsolateral extension causing a marked mass effect on the third ventricle, as well as interthalamic adhesion and mild transtentorial herniation. The mass has a mixed intensity in T2W and marked postcontrast enhancement. Note an area with signal void in the T2* image, compatible with a haemorrhagic area.

Bibliography

- Ayers, S. (2012) *Small Animal Radiographic Techniques and Positioning.* 1st ed. Wiley-Blackwell.
- Carrera, I. (2014) Cabeza (cavidad nasal y caja craneana). In: Agut, A. (ed). *Diagnóstico por Imagen en Pequeños Animales.* Multimédica Ediciones Veterinarias, pp. 197-215.
- Forrest, L. (2018) The cranial nasal cavities: canine and feline. In: Thrall, D.E. (ed). *Textbook of Veterinary Diagnostic Radiology.* 7th ed, pp. 183–203. Elsevier.
- Hecht, S., Adams, W.H. (2010) MRI of brain disease in veterinary patients part 1: basic principles and congenital brain disorders. *Vet Clin North Am Small Anim Pract,* 40(1): 21–38.
- Hecht, S., Adams, W.H. (2010) MRI of brain disease in veterinary patients part 2: acquired brain disorders. *Vet Clin North Am Small Anim Pract,* 40(1): 39–63.
- Lamb, C., Sibbing, K., Priestnall, S.L. (2016) Pathologic basis for rim enhancement observed in computed tomographic images of feline nasopharyngeal polyps. *Vet Radiol Ultrasound,* 57(2):130–136.
- Lerer, A., Chalmers, H.J., Moens, N., et al. (2014) Imaging diagnosis—Temporomandibular joint dysplasia in a Basset Hound. *Vet Radiol Ultrasound,* 55(5):547–551.
- Mai, W. (2018) *Diagnostic MRI in Dogs and Cats.* 1st ed. CRC Press.
- McConnell, J.F., Garosi, L., Platt, S.R. (2005) Magnetic resonance imaging findings of presumed cerebellar cerebrovascular accident in twelve dogs. *Vet Radiol Ultrasound,* 46(1):1–10.
- Middleton, D.L. (1993) Radiographic positioning for the spine and skull. *Vet Clin North Am Small Anim Pract,* 23(2):253–268.
- Moreno-Aguado, B., Carrera, I., Holdsworth, A. et al. (2020) CT findings in 20 dogs and six cats with confirmed nasal foreign bodies. *Vet Radiol Ultrasound,* 61(4):417–426.
- Muhlbauer, M.C., Kneller, S.K. (2013) *Radiography of the Dog and Cat: Guide to Making and Interpreting Radiographs.* 1st ed. Wiley-Blackwell.
- Nagendran, A., McConnell, J.F., De Risio, L., et al. (2021) Periictal magnetic resonance imaging characteristics in dogs with suspected idiopathic epilepsy. *J Vet Intern Med,* 35(2):1008–1017.
- Oliveira, C.R., O'Brien. R.T., Matheson. J.S., et al. (2012) Computed tomographic features of feline nasopharyngeal polyps. *Vet Radiol Ultrasound,* 53 (4):406–411.
- Palus, V., Volk, H., Lamb, C., et al. (2012) MRI features of CNS lymphoma in dogs and cats. *Vet Radiol Ultrasound,* 53 (1):44–49.
- Robertson, I.D. (2018) Magnetic resonance imaging features of brain disease in small animals. In: Thrall, D.E. (ed). *Textbook of Veterinary Diagnostic Radiology.* 7th ed, pp. 204–229. Elsevier.
- Schwarz, T., Saunders, J. (2011) *Veterinary Computed Tomography.* 1st ed. Wiley-Blackwell.
- Thrall, D.E. (2018) Basic principles of radiographic interpretation of the axial skeleton. In: Thrall, D.E. (ed). *Textbook of Veterinary Diagnostic Radiology.* 7th ed, pp. 137–152. Elsevier.
- Wisner, E., Zwingenberger, A. (2015) *Atlas of Small Animal CT and MRI.* 1st ed. Wiley-Blackwell.
- Young, B.D., Fosgate, G.T., Holmes, S.P., et al. (2014) Evaluation of standard magnetic resonance characteristics used to differentiate neoplastic, inflammatory and vascular brain lesions in dogs. *Vet Radiol Ultrasound,* 55(4):399–406.

Notes

Radiography, Computed Tomography and Magnetic Resonance Imaging of the Spine

Miriam Martínez Garrido

Introduction

Pain and spinal neuropathies are common problems in small animal practice, making the spine one of the most frequently imaged anatomical regions. Computed tomography (CT) and magnetic resonance imaging (MRI) are the modalities of choice for the complete characterisation of abnormalities of the vertebrae and spinal cord in small animals because many conditions, including intervertebral disc disease, various myelopathies, and tumours of the spinal cord, meninges and spine cannot be fully characterised using conventional radiography. However, a considerable number of pathologies can be diagnosed radiographically, and radiography can be used as a first diagnostic approach.

Radiographic Examination of the Spine and Myelography

Indications

Spinal radiographs should be performed in cases of spinal pain, neurological symptoms (ataxia, mono-, para- or tetraparesis or tetraplegia), suspected spinal malformations, masses in adjacent soft tissues, etc. Myelography is necessary for the study of lesions that affect the spinal cord because these cannot be evaluated on a plain radiograph.

The radiographic technique used is the same as that used for the rest of the skeletal system:

- **high milliamperage (mA) and low kilovoltage (kV) to increase contrast by reducing the production of scattered radiation**
- **use of a grid when the thickness of the region under study is greater than 10 cm**
- **plate–focus distance of 100 cm**
- **collimation and centring (according to the region of the spine being studied: cervical, cervicothoracic, thoracic, thoracolumbar, lumbar or lumbosacral).**

Radiographic Technique

Spinal radiographs in small animals are performed with the patient under general anaesthesia or deep sedation, because good positioning is essential to achieve a rotation-free, symmetrical radiograph. This is very important for correct interpretation taking into account the complex anatomy of the spine. To achieve optimal positioning, the use of foam, rubber, sandbags, cotton wool, and other positioning aids is advisable.

Projections

Orthogonal projections are routinely obtained, including lateral and ventrodorsal (VD) views. In trauma cases where fractures or instability of the spine (e.g. atlantoaxial luxation) is suspected, VD projections should be avoided. When performing **lateral projections**, it is important to ensure that the patient is not rotated. For this purpose, the sternum can be used as a reference; it must be in the same plane as the spine. Foam rubber wedges can be used to maintain the patient in this correct position. In addition, foam and sandbags can be used to position the limbs so they are parallel (Fig. 1).

For **VD projections**, positioning aids can be used to ensure the patient is symmetrical (Fig. 2).

Orthogonal projections should be obtained of each region of the spine to be studied (cervical, cervicothoracic, lumbosacral, etc.); lateral or VD radiographs that include the entire spine should be avoided. This is important because the divergence of the X-ray beam away from the central area of the beam affects the intervertebral spaces obliquely, which prevents correct evaluation of the areas that are furthest from the centre of the beam.

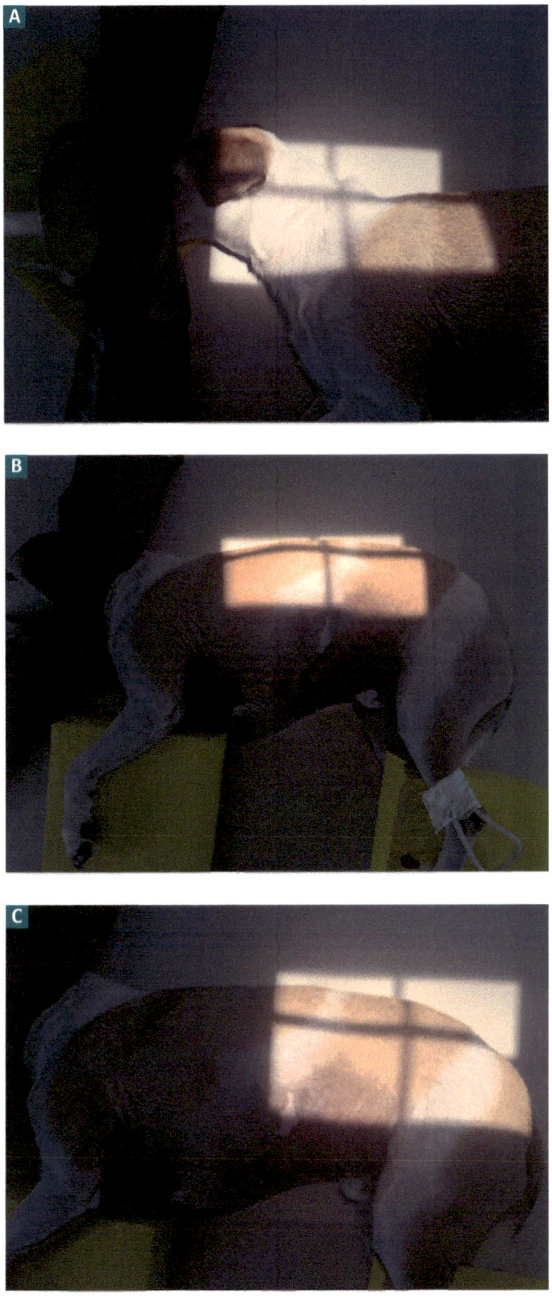

Figure 1. Lateral positioning of the patient for radiography of the cervical (**A**), thoracolumbar (**B**) and lumbosacral (**C**) spine.

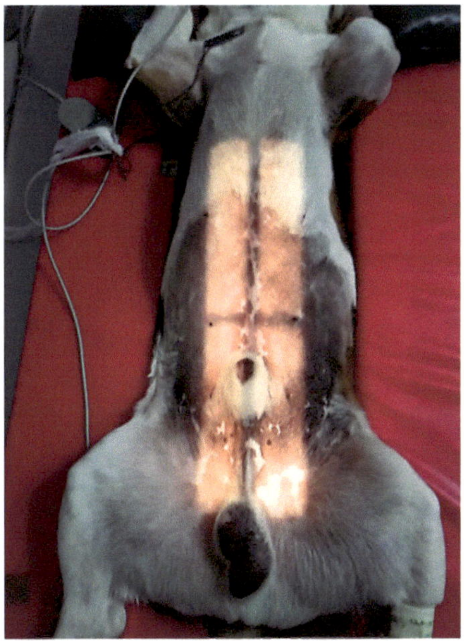

Figure 2. VD positioning of the patient for radiography of the thoracolumbar spine.

Normal Appearance and Relevant Features of the Spine

As with other regions of the body, spinal radiographs should be evaluated systematically, and it is very important that the veterinarian is familiar with the normal anatomy of the spine. The evaluation should include the following aspects.

- Evaluation of the surrounding soft tissues.
- Evaluation of the number of vertebrae in each area of the spine: in the normal spine there are 7 cervical (C1–C7), 13 thoracic (T1–T13), 7 lumbar (L1–L7), 3 sacral (S1–S3) and a variable number of caudal vertebrae.
- Assessment of whether the spine has abnormal angulations in both orthogonal projections.
- Spinal canal evaluation: diameter and opacity. The spinal canal is slightly wider in the caudal cervical region and at the level of L3–L6, due to the presence of cervical and lumbar intumescences.
- Assessment of vertebral bodies: analysis of their morphology and opacity. The body, the articular surfaces, the arch area (lamina and pedicles) and the different processes should be observed: the spinous, transverse and articular processes, the accessory and mammillary processes in the thoracic and lumbar spine, and the haemal processes in the coccygeal spine.
- Assessment of each intervertebral space: these should be radiotransparent and should be compared with the spaces cranial and caudal to it.
- Evaluation of each intervertebral foramen, which should also be radiotransparent.
- The particularities of the vertebral bodies, processes and intervertebral spaces must be taken into account:
  - C1–C2 does not have an intervertebral disc, as it is the atlantoaxial joint. The spinous processes of C1 and C2 are normally very close together, and the dorsal laminae are almost parallel in the lateral projection (Fig. 3)
  - the vertebral bodies of C7 and L7 are usually shorter than the rest

- C6 has larger transverse processes
- T1 has a pronounced spinous process compared with C7 (Fig. 4)
- T11 is the anticlinal vertebra in most dogs; however, T10 may also be referred to as the anticlinal vertebra, with its spinous process presenting in an upright position (Fig. 5)
- the ventral aspect of L3 and L4 (Fig. 6) is less well defined, because it is the area of insertion of the diaphragmatic crura; this appearance should not be confused with a lesion
- the intervertebral spaces at C7–T1, T10–T11 and in the area of L4–L6 are a little narrower
- compared with the dog, in cats the vertebral bodies (centres) are longer, the intervertebral disc spaces are narrower and the transverse processes of the lumbar vertebrae are longer (Fig. 7).

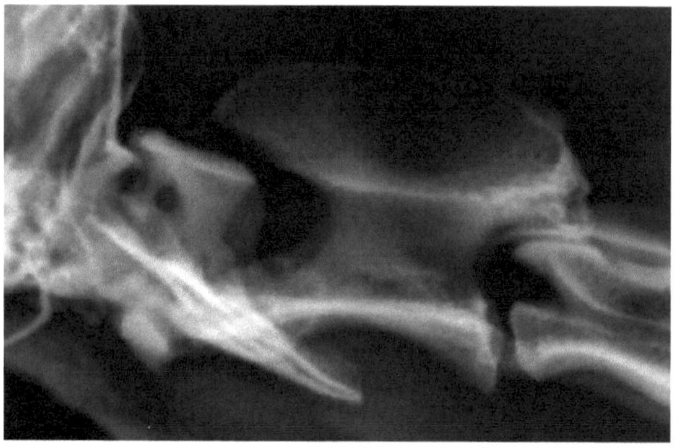

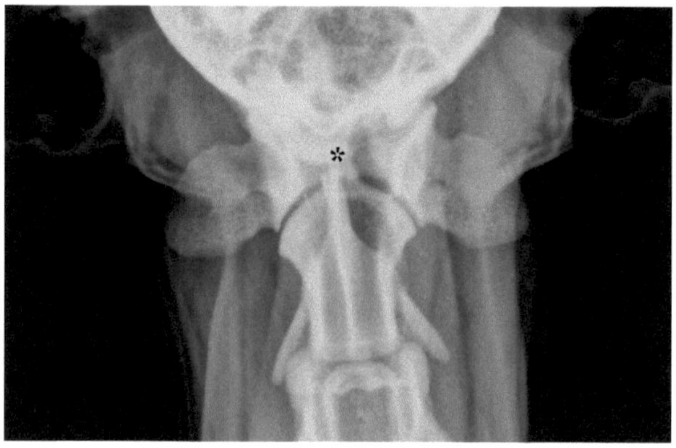

Figure 3. Lateral and VD projections of the normal atlantoaxial joint. Note the correct alignment of C1–C2 and the dens of the axis (asterisk) in the VD projection.

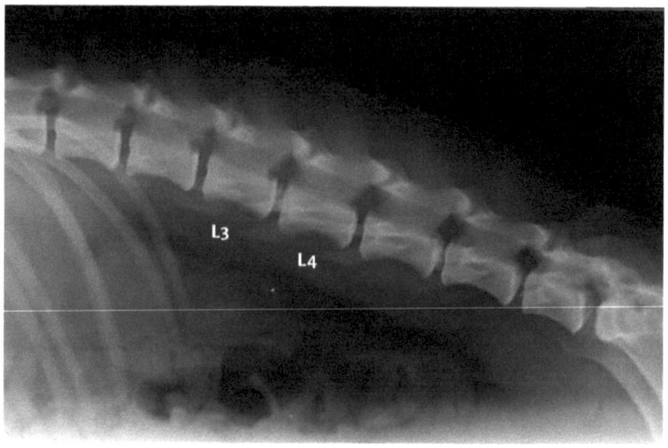

Figure 6. Lateral radiograph of the normal lumbar spine in a dog, showing the vertebral bodies of L3 and L4 with their less well defined ventral aspect due to the insertion of the diaphragmatic crura. Note that the vertebral canal is wider in the area of L3–L6 due to the presence of the lumbar intumescence.

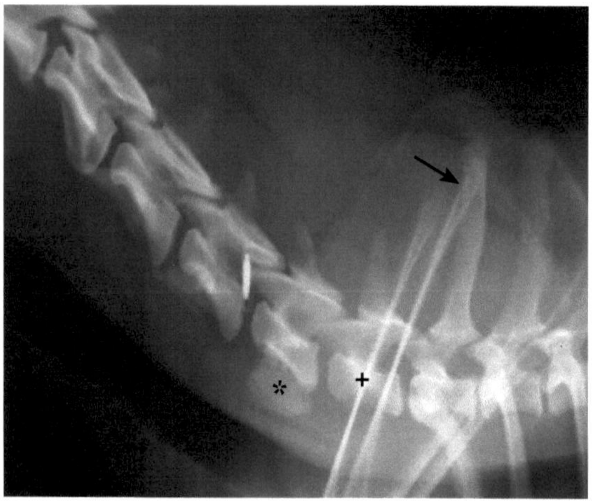

Figure 4. Lateral projection of the caudal portion of the normal cervical spine. Note the prominent transverse processes of C6 (asterisk), the vertebral body of C7, which is shorter than the rest (cross) and the more pronounced spinous process of T1 (arrow). The animal's microchip is superimposed on the spine at the level of C5.

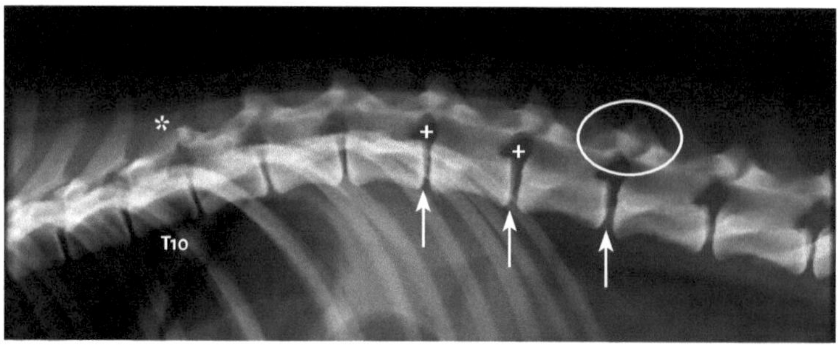

Figure 5. Lateral projection of the normal thoracolumbar spine. The spinous process of T10 is in a vertical position (anticlinal vertebra) (asterisk). The radiotransparent intervertebral spaces (arrows) and foramina (crosses) are observed, as well as the articular spaces of the articular processes (circled).

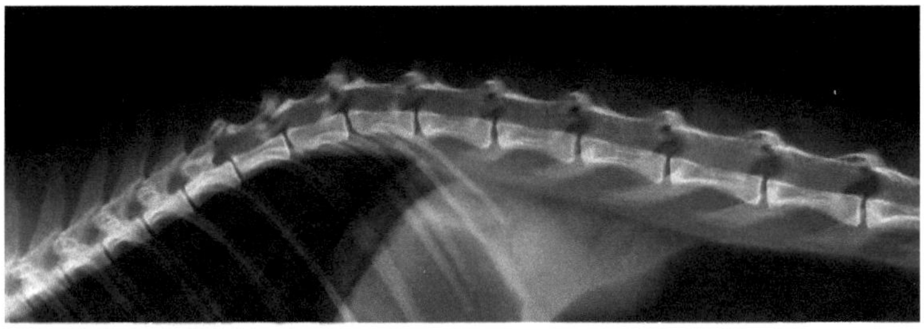

Figure 7. Lateral radiograph of the normal thoracolumbar spine of a cat, showing that the vertebral bodies are more elongated and the intervertebral spaces are narrower than in the dog.

Myelography

Myelography is a contrast technique used to evaluate the spinal cord by injecting radiopaque contrast medium into the subarachnoid space.

Indications

Myelography is indicated in cases of animals with neurological signs associated with the spinal cord in which no lesions are detected on a plain radiograph, or those in which lesions have been detected and it is necessary to assess the extent of the lesions and whether they are associated with spinal cord compression. It is usually performed in cases of suspected herniated discs, neoplasms or cervical spondylomyelopathy, and to assess the degree of spinal cord compression in cases of vertebral fractures, luxations or malformations. However, at the time of writing, with the rise of advanced imaging techniques such as CT and MRI, progressively fewer myelograms are being performed.

Contraindications

Myelography is contraindicated in cases in which meningoencephalitis is suspected, in animals with allergies to contrast medium or when the patient's condition is too unstable for it to undergo general anaesthesia.

Technique

Patient Preparation

The patient should always be under general anaesthesia and intubated to ensure a patent airway, and with a venous catheter placed. The skin where the puncture is to be performed must be clipped and prepared aseptically. It is advisable to wear sterile gloves.

Contrast Medium

The contrast medium to be used must be an iodinated, water-soluble, nonionic and low-osmolarity contrast suitable for intrathecal injection (e.g. iohexol), at a concentration of 250–300 mg I/ml. The dose varies between 0.3 ml/kg and 0.45 ml/kg patient body weight. Generally, in small animals and animals in which the lesion is distant from the injection site, a higher dose of contrast medium is administered, whereas in large animals and animals with lesions near the injection site, a lower dose is used. In large dogs, a volume of 9–10 ml of contrast medium is usually sufficient to assess the entire length of the spinal cord. The contrast medium should be warmed before injecting it, due to its viscosity; when it is warm, it will move more easily.

Types of Myelography

Depending on where the lesion is neurolocalised, puncture should be performed in the cisterna magna, when a cervical or cervicothoracic lesion is suspected, or at the lumbar level, when there is suspicion of a thoracic, thoracolumbar or lumbar lesion. There are some exceptions, for example, when the lesion is at the lumbosacral level, in which case puncture of the cisterna magna is more appropriate, to avoid the presence of contrast in the epidural space that will complicate interpretation. In cases of suspected atlantoaxial instability, manipulation of the region is not indicated and therefore puncture of the cisterna magna should be avoided.

Puncture of the Cisterna Magna

- The patient should be positioned in lateral recumbency with the neck hyperflexed, placing the nose at a 90° angle to the spine and keeping the nasal plane parallel to the table.
- Puncture is performed at the point of convergence of two imaginary perpendicular lines: one that joins the cranial edges of the wings of the atlas and one that goes from the occipital protuberance to the spinous process of the axis.
- Use of a 20–22 G 40 mm spinal needle is advisable. The needle is inserted with the bevel directed caudally until the joint capsule is crossed. Then, the guide is removed, the needle is inserted a little further, and cerebrospinal fluid (CSF) should begin to flow; a sample of CSF should be collected for analysis. CSF should never be aspirated;

instead, it should be allowed to flow out, collecting the same volume of fluid as of the contrast medium to be introduced.

- Subsequently, the contrast medium is administered slowly; if resistance is perceived, administration should be stopped.
- At the end of the contrast injection, the needle and syringe should be removed and the head and neck of the animal should immediately be raised by about 30-45° for a few minutes. After this time, lateral radiographs should be obtained and, when the lesion has been located, a VD projection should be obtained and oblique projections if necessary.

Lumbar Puncture

- The animal should be placed in lateral or sternal recumbency, with the hindlimbs pulled cranially to force maximum flexion of the lumbar spine and thus open the intervertebral space through which the contrast medium is to be injected as much as possible.
- The cranial edges of the wings of the ilium are located and between them the spinous process of L7 is palpated; using this reference, the puncture should be performed between L6 and L7 in small-breed dogs and cats, whereas in large-breed dogs it should be performed between L5 and L6.
- By palpating the spinous process of the caudal vertebra, the space where puncture is to be performed is located. The needle (in this case 90 mm in length) is inserted, directed cranially and towards the midline. When the subarachnoid space or spinal cord (cauda equina) is traversed with the needle, the animal usually contracts its hindlimbs and/or tail. The needle should be advanced until the floor of the vertebral canal is reached; the guide is then removed, and the needle is withdrawn by 1–2 mm, observing whether CSF flows out. If CSF is not obtained and there are doubts regarding the position of the needle, a small volume of contrast medium can be introduced and a radiograph then taken to check that the contrast is being administered in the correct location and not in the epidural space.
- Once the correct needle position is ensured, the entire dose of contrast medium is injected, and lateral and VD radiographs are obtained.

Normal Appearance and Evaluation of a Myelogram

On a myelogram, the contrast medium is visualised in each projection as two thin, radiopaque columns surrounding the spinal cord. When evaluating a myelogram, as for any radiograph and as mentioned above, a systematic approach should be followed.

- The depth and location of the contrast columns on both sides of the spinal cord in the two projections should be evaluated to determine whether there is any narrowing or deviation. In the lateral projection they can be called the dorsal and ventral columns, and in the VD projection they can be referred to as the right and left lateral columns.
- The diameter and position of the spinal cord should be evaluated.
- The radiopacity of the spinal cord should be evaluated.

A number of considerations that correspond to **normal myelography** should be taken into account.

- The contrast columns should be of uniform width along the vertebral canal.
- On lateral projections, the dorsal contrast column is somewhat wider than the ventral column, and is more prominent between C1 and C2 due to the presence of the cisterna magna.
- The ventral contrast column often has a slight indentation over the intervertebral disc spaces, which is more evident in the cervical spine, although this should not affect the diameter of the spinal cord.
- The spinal cord presents a slight diffuse distension in the cervical (C5–C7) and lumbar (L3–C4) intumescences, and

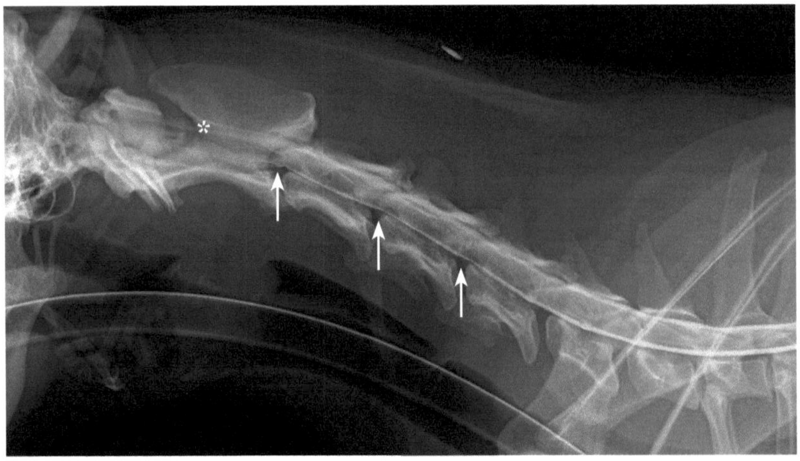

Figure 8. Lateral projection of a normal cervical myelogram in a dog. The dorsal contrast column is wider than the ventral contrast column, especially at the C1–C2 level (asterisk). The ventral contrast column presents slight normal narrowing at the level of the intervertebral discs (arrows). Note the divergence of the contrast columns at the C5–C7 level in the region of the cervical intumescence.

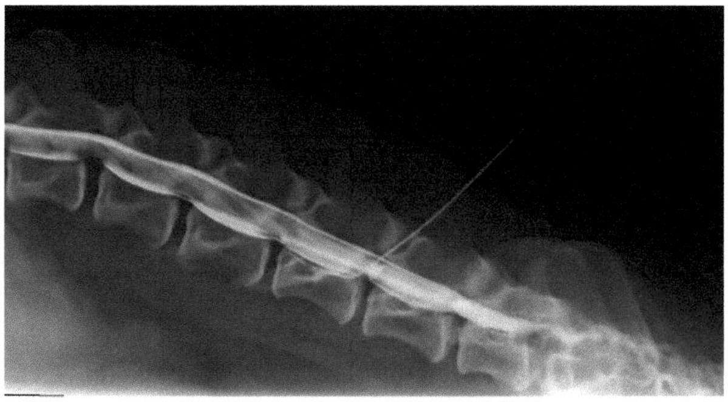

Figure 9. Lateral projection of a normal lumbar myelogram in a dog. The spinal needle is observed at the level of L5–L6 where the puncture has been performed. Note the divergence of the contrast columns in the lumbar intumescence at the L3–L4 level and convergence in the cauda equina.

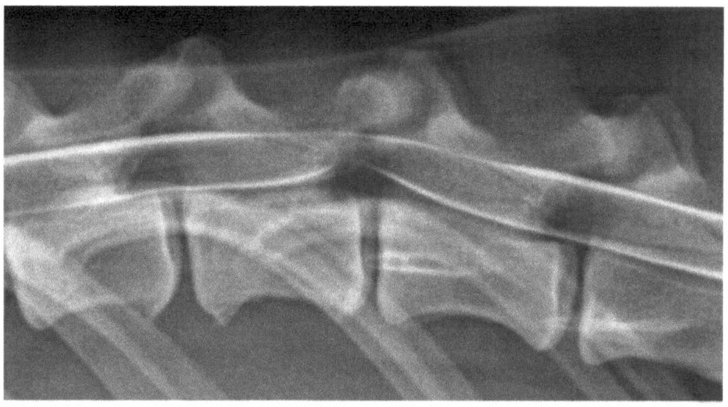

Figure 10. Lateral projection of a myelogram of a dog showing an extradural lesion in the T13–L1 intervertebral space due to a herniated disc. Note the dorsal displacement and attenuation of the ventral contrast column, and attenuation of the dorsal contrast column.

in these locations the contrast columns diverge slightly (Fig. 8).

- The spinal cord is relatively large compared with the size of the vertebral canal in small dogs and cats, and appears relatively smaller in large-breed dogs.
- In the cauda equina, the spinal cord narrows and presents a striated, convergent appearance.
- The shape of the caudal end of the dural sac is variable, and can be pointed or blunt. Its location is also variable among dogs: in most animals the dural sac enters the sacrum, but in some it ends more cranially (Fig. 9).
- In cats, the spinal cord and dural sac extend more caudally than in dogs.

Myelographic Patterns

When evaluating a myelogram, various changes in the contrast columns can be detected, including thinning, interruption, obstruction, divergence or convergence, dilation and division. Once these changes have been identified and evaluated, they must be framed in one of the three possible myelographic patterns described in the following sections.

Extradural Lesion

In the lateral projection (Fig. 10), a narrowing of the contrast column closer to the lesion and an even more marked narrowing (sometimes the continuity of the contrast is lost) in the contrast column opposite the lesion is observed, accompanied by displacement or compression of the spinal cord. In the VD projection the spinal cord will be widened, or if the lesion is lateral, an image similar to that seen in the lateral projection will be observed, but with narrowing of the corresponding left and right contrast columns. In these cases, oblique lateral projections can locate the lesion more precisely, to help determine the surgical approach. Possible causes of an extradural lesion include:

- normal variation due to very slight compression of the subarachnoid space without attenuation of the opposite contrast column. This can normally be observed at the level of the ventral contrast column in C2–C3, in the dorsal column of contrast in C3–C4–C5–C6–C7, or in the ventral column of some intervertebral spaces in large-breed dogs
- disc extrusion (Hansen type I hernia)
- disc protrusion (Hansen type II hernia)
- cervical spondylomyelopathy
- cauda equina syndrome
- spinal instability
- extradural neoplasia
- lesions in articular apophyses
- extradural haematoma or haemorrhage
- extradural infection or inflammation (granuloma, abscess or empyema).

Intradural Extramedullary Lesion

In these cases, the lesion is located in the subarachnoid space and causes widening of the contrast column on both sides of the lesion, in addition to narrowing in the opposite contrast column and variable compression of the spinal cord. Two characteristic patterns can be observed, one in which the contrast column divides surrounding the lesion ("golf tee"), and another in which it widens with an abrupt ("teardrop-shaped") termination (Fig. 11). Possible causes of an intradural extramedullary lesion include:

- subarachnoid cysts/diverticula
- neoplasms (meningioma, nerve sheath tumour, nephroblastoma)
- herniated disc material with ruptured dural membrane
- haematoma or intradural haemorrhage.

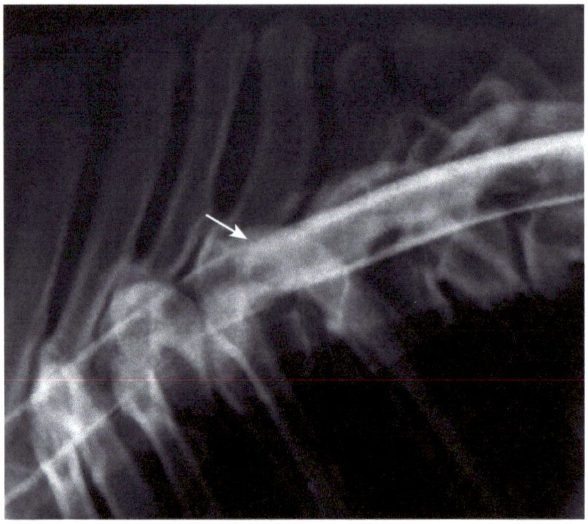

Figure 11. Lateral projection of a myelogram in which an intradural extramedullary lesion is observed with a "teardrop-shaped" pattern in the dorsal contrast column (arrow).

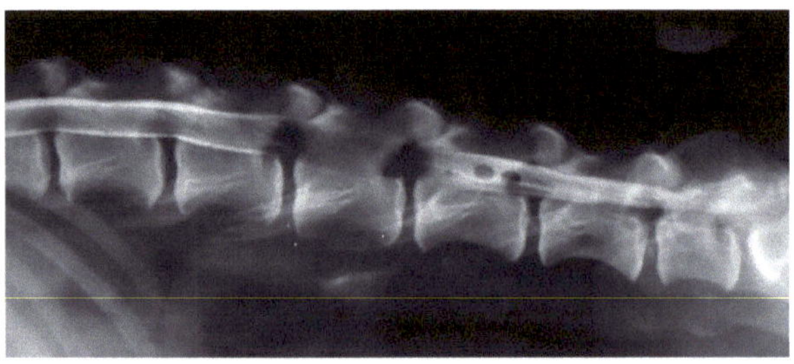

Figure 12. Lateral projection of a lumbar myelogram in which an intramedullary pattern is observed. There is divergence and attenuation of the ventral and dorsal columns of contrast at the L4 level, with an increase in the size of the spinal cord. Note the two radiolucent circular structures, compatible with iatrogenic gas bubbles introduced when contrast medium was injected.

Intramedullary Lesion

In these cases, the lesion originates in the spinal cord, so it will appear widened, with narrowing and divergence of the contrast columns in both projections (Fig. 12).

Possible causes of an intramedullary lesion include:

- physiological (at the level of the cervical or lumbar intumescences)
- primary neoplasm, metastasis or intradural neoplasm invading the spinal cord
- haemorrhage or oedema
- ischaemic myelopathy
- granulomatous meningoencephalitis
- syringohydromyelia
- dermoid or epidermoid cysts
- myelomalacia, where contrast can be seen inside the spinal cord.

CT Examination of the Spine

Indications and Anatomy

Indications

Spinal CT is indicated in cases of trauma or neurological deficits in which the lesion is located in the spine. With this technique, complex spinal fractures, lytic lesions (neoplasms, infection) and cases of degenerative disc diseases can be evaluated. Although CT does not provide much detail of the spinal cord, meaning that MRI is usually the technique of choice

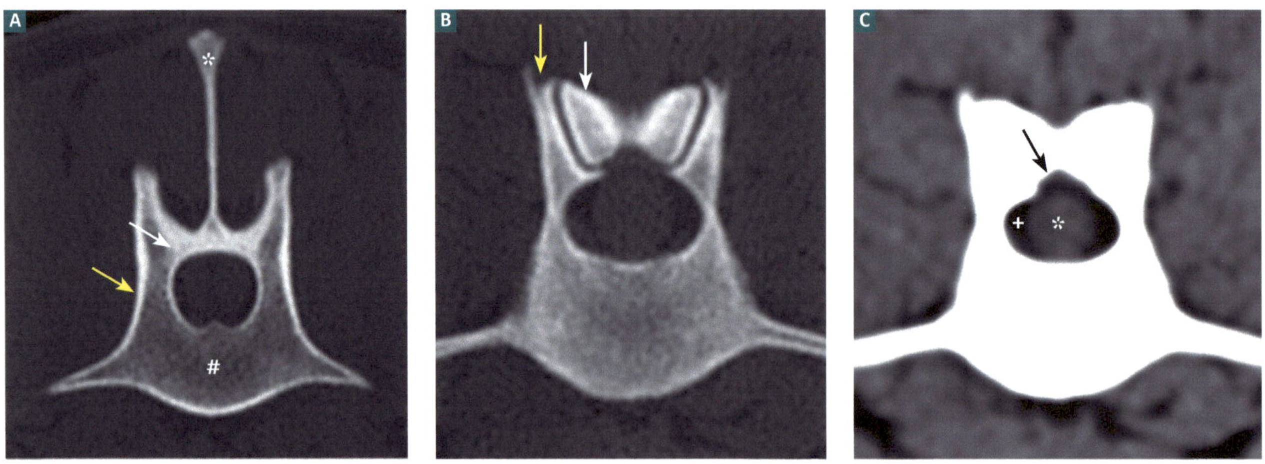

Figure 13. Cross-sectional CT images of the normal lumbar spine. **A** and **B**. Bone algorithm, in which the spinous process (asterisk), dorsal lamina (white arrow), pedicle (yellow arrow), vertebral body (hash), cranial articular process (yellow arrow) and caudal (white arrow) can be seen. **C**. Soft tissue algorithm, in which the spinal cord (asterisk), epidural fat (cross), and yellow ligament (black arrow) can be seen.

to evaluate the spine, it does allow the evaluation of lesions that cause compression of the spinal cord when performing myelography (myeloCT).

Anatomy

In CT images, the cortical bone is thin and of uniformly high attenuation, with smooth margins, allowing accurate assessment of the trabeculation of the cancellous bone. All components of the vertebra (lamina, pedicles, body, orifices, basivertebral venous canal, bony apophyses) are visualised in detail on CT. Occasionally, the ligamentum flavum (yellow ligament) can be seen. The ventral, dorsal, interspinous and intertransverse ligaments are usually indistinguishable from the surrounding structures. Epidural fat is hypoattenuating with respect to the soft tissue structures of the vertebral canal. The combination of the spinal cord, blood vessels, subarachnoid space with the CSF and meninges form a structure with soft tissue attenuation and round/oval morphology in the middle of the vertebral canal that is surrounded by a border of hypoattenuating epidural fat. Nerve roots can be seen as structures that are isoattenuating with respect to soft tissue and circular or linear in shape, depending on their plane of orientation (Fig. 13).

When a CT scan is performed after myelography, the thecal sac is hyperattenuated, which allows more accurate differentiation between intramedullary, intradural and extradural lesions. CT myelography can be achieved by injecting nonionic iodinated contrast medium into the subarachnoid space at 25% of the regular myelographic dose; this provides excellent definition of the spinal cord and is useful for characterising extradural lesions in cases of disc herniations with noncalcified disc material, intradural extramedullary lesions (subarachnoid diverticula, meningiomas, etc.) or intramedullary lesions (inflammation or neoplasms).

CT Technique

Positioning

For a spinal CT, the patient must be under general anaesthesia and placed in dorsal recumbency, with the limbs as far away as possible from the region to be imaged.

Protocol

The protocol that should be followed when performing a spinal CT scan is as follows:

- the different regions of the spine are scanned depending on the neurological location of the lesion
- a section thickness of about 1–2 mm is used
- the reconstruction interval is half the section thickness
- the algorithms used are low frequency (soft tissue) evaluated in a soft tissue window (window width [WW]: 300; window level [WL]: 50–100) and high frequency (bone) evaluated in a bone window (WW: 2500–3500; WL: 500)
- pre- and postcontrast (intravenous) series are obtained when performing a myeloCT as a complementary technique in cases where this is deemed necessary.

MRI Examination of the Spine

Indications and Anatomy

Indications

MRI is the technique indicated to confirm or rule out injuries affecting the spinal cord, spine or paravertebral soft tissues. MRI and the different sequences that can be performed enable the spinal cord and subarachnoid space to be evaluated in great detail, without the need for intrathecal contrast administration.

Anatomy

On MRI, the cortical bone appears as a hypointense layer around the vertebrae in all sequences. On T1-weighted (T1W) images, the bone marrow is isointense or slightly hypointense compared with the intervertebral discs. The epidural and paraspinal fat is hyperintense. The intervertebral discs have a medium signal strength. The spinal cord and nerve roots are isointense to the intervertebral discs, and are surrounded by a hypointense halo that represents the CSF in the subarachnoid space and the meninges. In some cases, the hyperintense grey matter in the central region of the spinal cord can be differentiated from the white matter surrounding it. The dorsal and ventral longitudinal ligaments, as well as the ligamentum flavum, are visible only in the intervertebral areas, and are hypointense.

On T2-weighted (T2W) images, the bone marrow is hypointense compared with the intervertebral discs. The epidural and paraspinal fat is hyperintense, and the spinal cord and nerve roots are hypointense. As in T1W sequences, in some cases the grey matter at the centre of the spinal cord can be seen with a hyperintense signal compared with the peripheral white matter. The spinal cord is surrounded by the CSF, which forms a hyperintense halo with a signal intensity similar to epidural fat and can be difficult to differentiate in some cases. Sequences such as SSFSE (single shot fast spin echo) or HASTE (half Fourier acquisition single shot turbo spin echo) enhance the CSF signal while suppressing the tissue signal, giving a myelogram-like appearance. Normal intervertebral discs have a hyperintense signal due to the high water content in the nucleus pulposus and the inner portion of the annulus fibrosus (Fig. 14). Fat suppression techniques make it possible to differentiate normal fat (in the vertebral bone marrow, epidural space and paraspinal musculature) from other hyperintense tissues, which can be pathological.

Protocol

The patient is positioned in dorsal recumbency, and sagittal, dorsal and transverse planes of the different sequences are obtained. The minimum protocol includes the sagittal plane in T2W, dorsal plane in T2W, and transverse planes in T2W and T1W of the areas of interest or where pathologies are detected. T1W imaging after contrast administration is optional depending on the abnormalities present. Fat suppression sequences (short tau inversion recovery; STIR) can also be used in the dorsal plane, especially to evaluate soft tissues.

Main Pathologies

The main pathologies of the spine are:

- congenital or developmental abnormalities
- fracture, luxation or subluxation
- inflammatory or infectious processes
- degenerative disease
- intervertebral disc disease
- vascular diseases (ischaemic myelopathy)
- myelomalacia
- neoplasia.

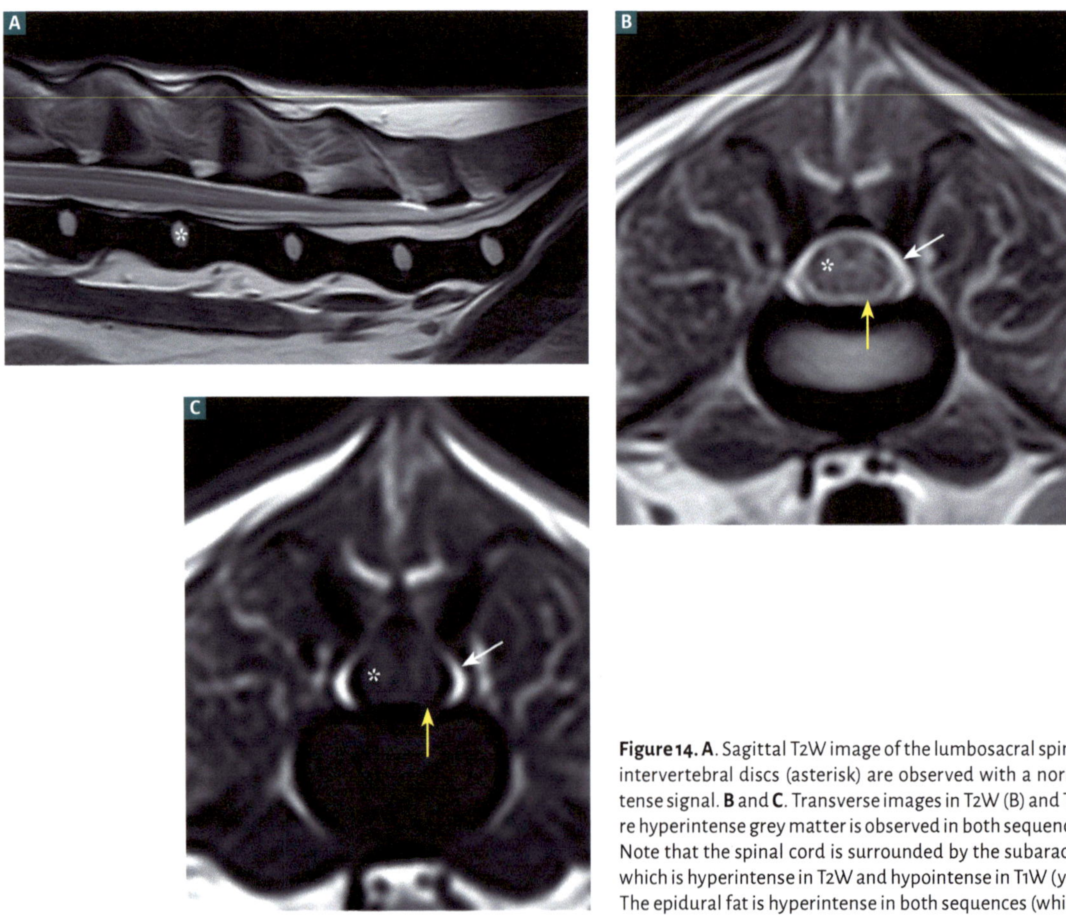

Figure 14. A. Sagittal T2W image of the lumbosacral spine, where the intervertebral discs (asterisk) are observed with a normal hyperintense signal. **B** and **C**. Transverse images in T2W (B) and T1W (C), where hyperintense grey matter is observed in both sequences (asterisk). Note that the spinal cord is surrounded by the subarachnoid space, which is hyperintense in T2W and hypointense in T1W (yellow arrow). The epidural fat is hyperintense in both sequences (white arrows).

Congenital or Developmental Disorders

Atlantoaxial Subluxation

Atlantoaxial subluxation is a pathology that mainly affects small-breed and toy dogs, such as the Yorkshire Terrier, Toy Poodle or Chihuahua. Normally, atlantoaxial instability and subluxation is associated with hypoplasia or aplasia of the dens of the axis (odontoid process), nonunion of the dens or abnormalities of the ligaments. However, this pathology can also be traumatic due to fracture of the dens or rupture of the ligaments. Among the radiographic findings (Fig. 15), separation of the spinous process of the axis from the dorsal lamina of the atlas, dorsal displacement of the body of the axis and misalignment of the vertebral canal can be observed. To evaluate these changes more easily, a lateral projection with the neck slightly flexed can be performed, although it must be performed with care, as flexing the neck in patients with atlantoaxial joint instability carries high risk. In addition, in a slightly oblique lateral projection, the morphology of the dens of the axis can be evaluated, and malformations can be detected in cases of aplasia or hypoplasia of the dens. In cases of atlantoaxial instability that are of traumatic origin, the presence of dens fractures may also be evaluated.

CT provides a more thorough assessment of bone structures with the use of multiplanar reconstructions. In cases of congenital atlantoaxial luxation, the dens of the axis is observed to be missing or hypoplastic, and this may be accompanied by an occipital atlantoaxial malformation. In cases of ligament abnormalities, the dens tends to protrude dorsally and into the spinal cord. When the abnormality is of traumatic origin, fracture of the odontoid process can be observed.

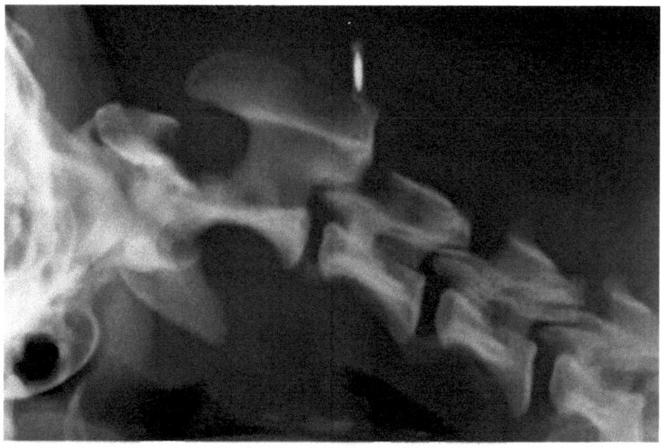

Figure 15. Lateral radiograph of the atlantoaxial joint of a dog with atlantoaxial subluxation, in which the dorsal lamina of the atlas is not parallel to that of the axis, the axis (including the dens) is displaced dorsally and there is misalignment of the vertebral canal.

Abnormalities or fractures of the dens of the axis can be more clearly identified in sagittal or dorsal planes. Subluxation causes a narrowing of the diameter of the vertebral canal and spinal cord compression, which can be more easily identified when multiplanar reconstructions are available.

MRI is useful in determining the extent of soft tissue lesions associated with atlantoaxial instability. Narrowing of the dorsal or ventral subarachnoid space at the level of the dens, dorsal deviation of the spinal cord and possible associated intramedullary lesions that may represent oedema, haemorrhage, gliosis or degeneration, as well as syringomyelia, can be seen. Abnormalities in the ligaments can also be detected, such as lack of visualisation of the transverse ligament, or thickening of the apical and alar ligaments.

Vertebral Anomalies

Anomalies of the vertebral bodies are common, especially in brachycephalic breeds such as Bulldogs and Pugs. Although many are incidental findings without clinical significance, others can cause clinical signs by causing spinal cord compression due to narrowing of the vertebral canal. These anomalies can occur in a single vertebra or in multiple vertebrae and are more common in the thoracic vertebrae.

Several types of vertebral abnormalities can be distinguished.

- **Block vertebrae** result from a failure in vertebral segmentation, in which part of the adjacent vertebral elements are not divided. These typically do not cause spinal deformity.
- **Hemivertebrae**, wedge-shaped vertebrae and butterfly vertebrae are the result of the abnormal development of a portion of a vertebral element (Fig. 16).
- **Transitional vertebrae** are those that show characteristics of two different anatomical divisions. These abnormalities occur at the cervicothoracic, thoracolumbar and lumbosacral junctions and usually affect the vertebral arch rather than the body (Fig. 17). The main clinical significance of transitional vertebral abnormalities relates to the use of the more caudal ribs as a reference point to identify the site of access for spinal decompression surgery. They have been reported in various breeds of dog, such as Dachshunds and German Shepherd Dogs, in the lumbosacral junction.

These abnormalities most commonly cause no clinical signs and are incidental findings, but they may result in clinical signs associated with progressive spinal canal stenosis and spinal instability (Fig. 18). In cases of vertebral anomalies, vertebral alterations and misalignment of the vertebral canal can be seen in more detail with CT. In addition, myeloCT can be used to determine whether there is associated spinal cord compression.

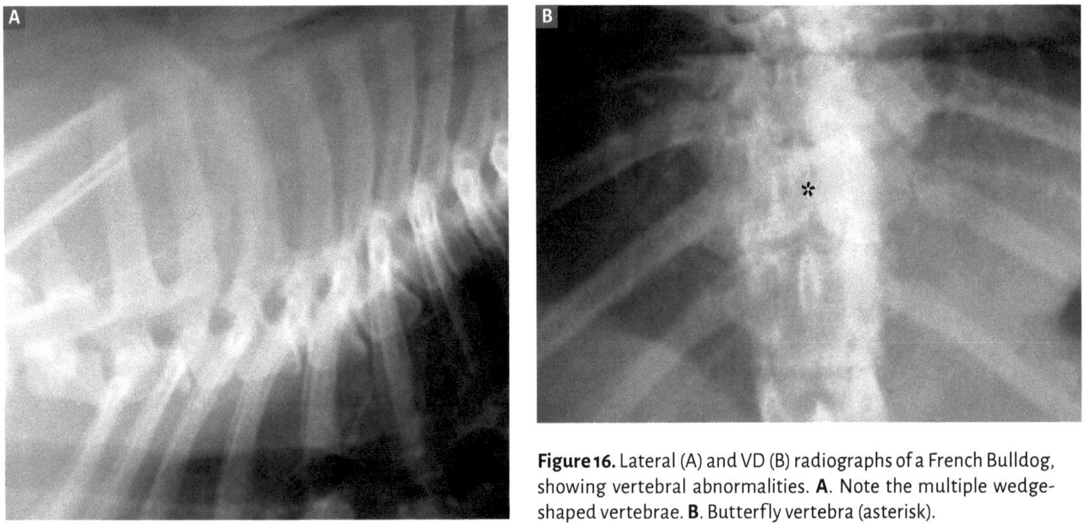

Figure 16. Lateral (A) and VD (B) radiographs of a French Bulldog, showing vertebral abnormalities. **A**. Note the multiple wedge-shaped vertebrae. **B**. Butterfly vertebra (asterisk).

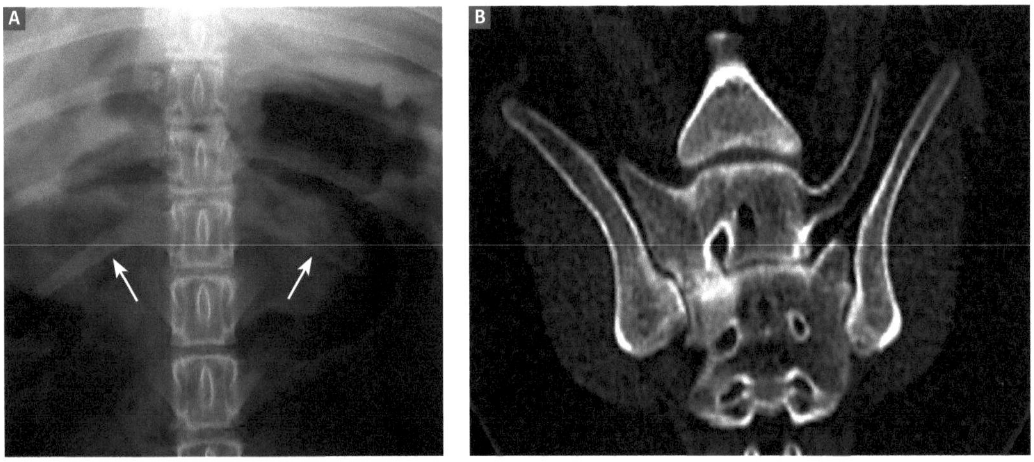

Figure 17. A. VD projection of a thoracolumbar spine showing thoracoisation of L1, which has two vestigial ribs replacing the transverse processes (arrows). **B**. Dorsal CT image of a dog with lumbarisation of S1, which is not completely fused to the rest of the sacrum and has a transverse process on the left side.

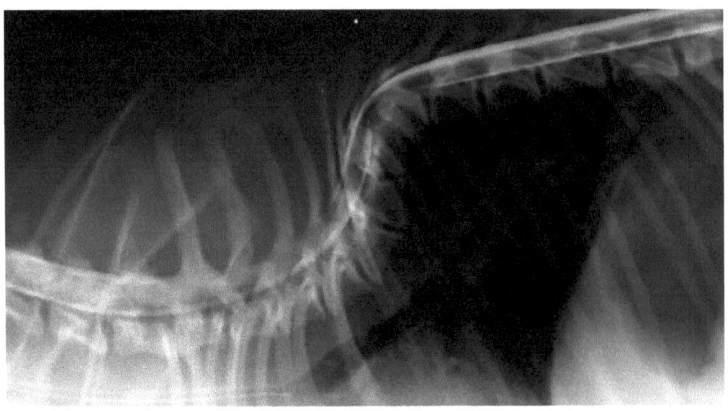

Figure 18. Lateral radiograph with myelography of the thoracic spine of a dog with kyphosis due to wedge- and butterfly-shaped vertebrae. Note the attenuation of the ventral contrast column at the point of greatest angulation of the column.

Depending on the type of vertebral anomaly, different types of spinal deformities are observed.

- **Kyphotic abnormalities cause excessive focal convex dorsal curvature of the spine, which is best seen in lateral projections or sagittal planes (Fig. 18).**
- **Kyphoscoliotic abnormalities cause excessive focal convex dorsal curvature along with exaggerated focal lateral curvature of the spine; the latter is best seen on VD projections or dorsal planes.**

The main advantage of MRI over CT in imaging these anomalies is that, in addition to evaluating bone structures (albeit in somewhat less detail than with CT), MRI enables evaluation of the spinal cord to determine whether there is a spinal contusion/compression or other alterations associated with the abnormalies. T1W imaging is preferred for providing bone detail, while T2W and myelographic imaging allow secondary changes such as arachnoid diverticula, syringomyelia and intramedullary hyperintensity, associated with oedema or gliosis secondary to compression, to be evaluated.

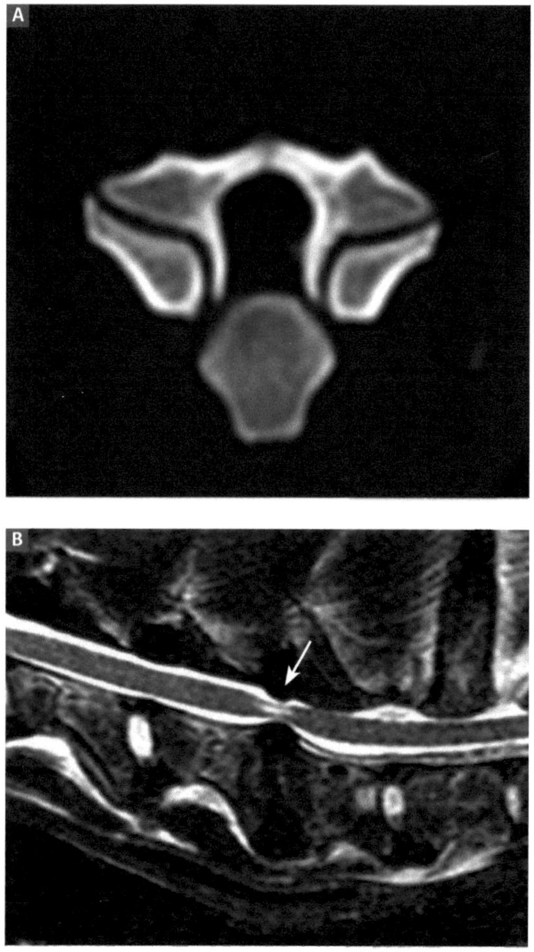

Figure 19. Images of two dogs with cervical spondylomyelopathy. **A**. Cross-sectional CT image in a bone window of a young dog. Note the thickening/hypertrophy of the articular processes of the cervical vertebrae causing laterolateral stenosis of the vertebral canal. **B**. Sagittal T2W MRI image of an adult Dobermann. Note the protrusion of the C6–C7 intervertebral disc and associated spondylosis, together with hypertrophy of the ligamentum flavum (arrow), causing dorsoventral compression of the spinal cord. An intramedullary focal hyperintense area can be seen.

Cervical Spondylomyelopathy

Cervical spondylomyelopathy or "wobbler syndrome" is a pathology that affects the cervical spine of large- or giant-breed dogs, resulting in progressive, chronic compression of the spinal cord. This spinal cord compression may be associated with abnormalities of the bone structures or abnormalities of the intervertebral discs. Bone abnormalities are more frequent in young and giant-breed patients (Great Dane), whereas abnormalities associated with intervertebral discs are more typical in adult and large-breed animals (Dobermann).

This syndrome is characterised by several abnormalities: vertebral bodies of abnormal or misaligned morphology, hypertrophy and osteoarthrosis of the articular processes, disc protrusions that are sometimes associated with hypertrophy of the dorsal longitudinal ligament, and hypertrophy of the ligamentum flavum. All of them lead to stenosis of the spinal canal, resulting in static or dynamic compression of the cervical spinal cord. Among the radiographic changes, "funnel-shaped" stenosis of the vertebral canal can be observed, with narrowing of the cranial aspect of the canal in the affected vertebrae, as well as misalignment or subluxation of some vertebrae, with dorsal displacement of the cranial aspect of the vertebrae forming small steps along the vertebral canal. Affected vertebrae sometimes have cranioventral flattening due to abnormal formation or remodelling, with the vertebral body being narrower at its cranial aspect. Osteoarthritic changes can be detected in the articular processes, as well as changes compatible with disc disease (narrowing of the intervertebral space or mineralisation of the intervertebral disc).

The use of myeloCT or MRI is required to evaluate disc degeneration or protrusion and the extradural compression of the associated spinal cord, with the latter technique used only to evaluate hypertrophy of the joint capsule and alteration in the flavum or interarcual ligament (Fig. 19).

Spina Bifida

Spina bifida is the result of a failure in the fusion of the vertebral arch dorsally during its development, causing the absence or incomplete development of the spinous process. It may be associated with neural tube defects, with the presence of meningocoele or myelomeningocoele. Spina bifida is most common in brachycephalic breeds of dog such as Bulldogs, Pugs and Boston Terriers, and in Manx cats. It can occur at any location in the spine but is frequently described at the lumbar or sacral level. There are several types, which range from abnormalities of no clinical importance, with small defects in the affected vertebra without abnormalities in the spinal cord (occult spina bifida), to significant defects associated with meningocoele or myelomeningocoele that lead to neurological problems (manifest spina bifida). Radiographs will show the divided or absent spinous process. The vertebral canal may also be widened at the level of the affected vertebra.

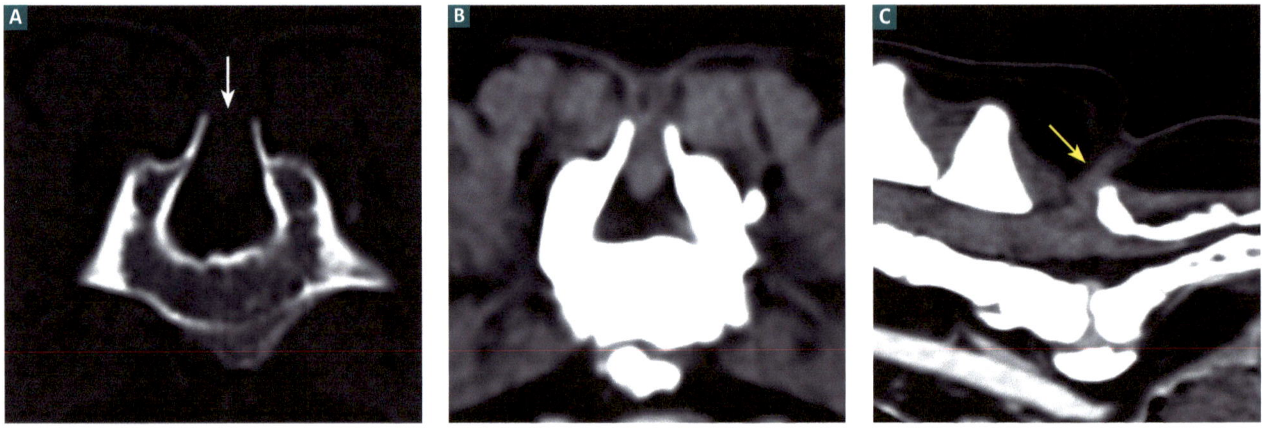

Figure 20. CT images of an English Bulldog with spina bifida with the presence of myelomeningocoele and associated dermoid sinus. **A**. Image obtained in a bone window at the level of L7 showing a bone defect in the dorsal lamina with absence of the spinous process (arrow). **B**. Image obtained in a soft tissue window, in which the medullary cone is displaced dorsally and protrudes through the bone defect, compatible with a myelomeningocoele. **C**. Image in the sagittal plane, in which a defect in the skin and subcutaneous tissue is observed, as well as a soft tissue band that connects this defect with the medullary canal (yellow arrow), compatible with a dermoid sinus.

Advanced imaging techniques are necessary for a more thorough evaluation (Fig. 20). MRI is preferred to characterise the presence and extent of any neural tube defects. In T1W sequences, incomplete fusion of the dorsal lamina of the affected vertebra is observed. In T2W in cases of meningocoele or myelomeningocoele, the subarachnoid space or spinal cord extends dorsally through the bone defect.

Aplasia and Hypoplasia of the Caudal Articular Processes

Aplasia and hypoplasia of the caudal articular processes consists of the absence or malformation of these processes. Pugs are predisposed to this anomaly, although many other breeds may be affected. The most common location is in the caudal thoracic spine and cranial lumbar spine. They are usually incidental lesions with no clinical significance, although a small proportion of cases may be associated with progressive signs of spinal cord dysfunction.

Radiographically, the absence of the caudal articular processes or abnormal morphology is observed. These anomalies can be better visualised with CT. However, as with radiography, it is not possible to visualise other associated abnormalities that are the cause of the clinical signs (spinal cord compression or subarachnoid diverticula). To visualise these associated abnormalities, a myeloCT scan is necessary. The absence or partial loss of the structure of the articular processes can be observed on MRI (visualised in T1W), as well as the production of fibrocartilage and bone proliferation. Dorsolateral or dorsal compression of the spinal cord is also observed at the level of the affected joints.

Arachnoid Diverticula

Arachnoid diverticula are focal enlargements of the subarachnoid space. They are not true cysts, as they lack an epithelial lining. They are usually congenital abnormalities that develop and expand over time; however, they can also be acquired. They are mainly located in the cervical spine (in large breeds) or in the thoracolumbar spine (in small breeds). MyeloCT or MRI findings include distension of the teardrop-shaped subarachnoid space, usually located dorsal to the spinal cord, producing a variable degree of spinal cord compression (Fig. 21).

Fracture, Luxation and Subluxation

Vertebral fractures and luxations typically occur at regional junctions, for example, atlanto-occipital, atlantoaxial, cervicothoracic or thoracolumbar, as these junctions are subject to greater flexion extension, torsion and axial loading. Most traumatic spinal fractures and luxations occur in the thoracolumbar region (T10–L3). In cases where this type of lesion is suspected, a lateral projection must be obtained, which is usually sufficient to be able to observe fracture lines or a poor alignment of the vertebrae (Fig. 22). Other features observed include asymmetry of the articular processes and vertebral articular faces, narrowing of the vertebral canal and, in compression fractures, shortening of the vertebral body.

Evaluating each vertebral compartment to determine the severity and instability of vertebral fractures and luxations is recommended, dividing each vertebra into three

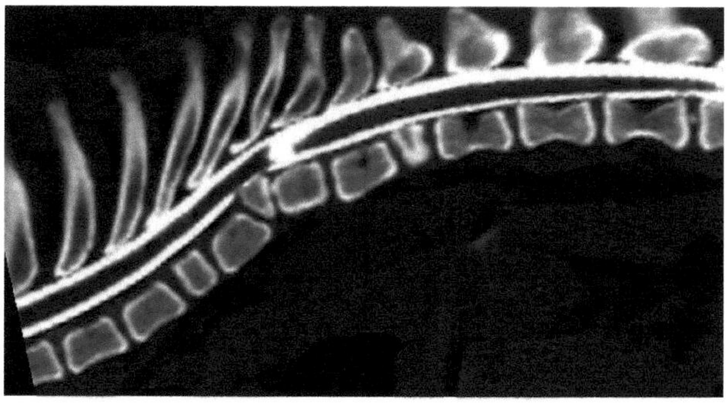

Figure 21. Sagittal plane of a myeloCT of the thoracic spine of a dog with a subarachnoid diverticulum. A teardrop-shaped focal distension of the dorsal subarachnoid space resulting in severe spinal cord compression is observed. These findings are associated with kyphosis due to a wedge-shaped vertebra.

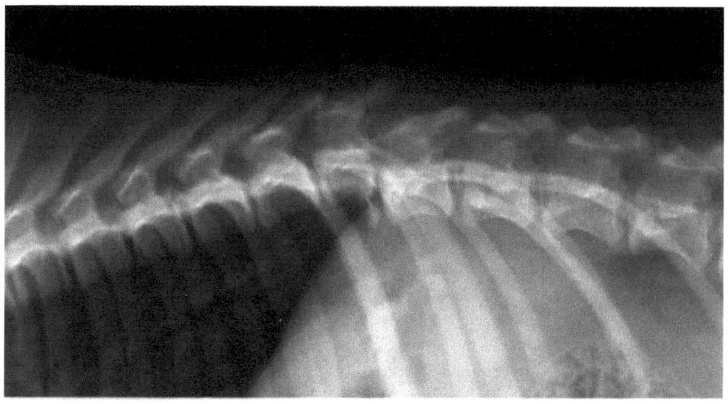

Figure 22. Lateral projection of a dog that had been run over. A fracture of the caudal physis of T11 is observed, with subluxation of the spine at the level of T11–T12, ventral displacement of the caudal portion of the spine and an increase in the movement of the articular processes.

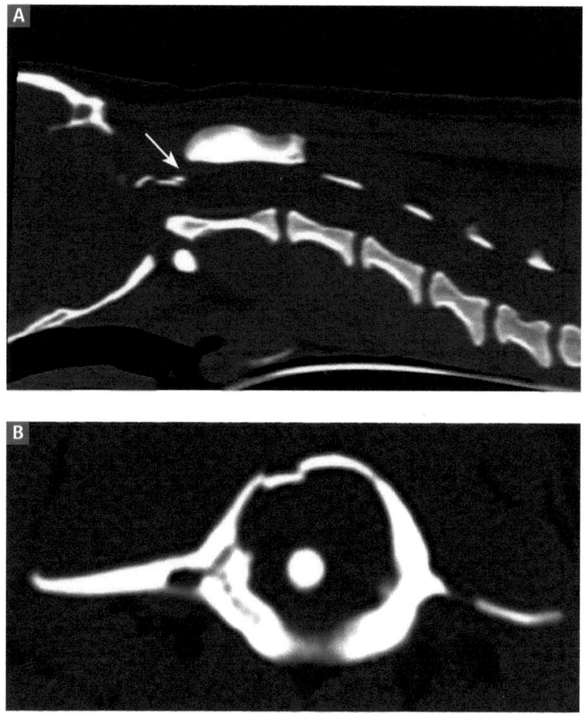

Figure 23. Sagittal plane (**A**) and transverse plane (**B**) in a bone algorithm of a CT scan of a dog with a traumatic atlantoaxial subluxation, showing that the lamina of the atlas is not parallel to that of the axis (arrow). In (B), a fracture of the dorsal arch of the atlas with multiple bone fragments is visible.

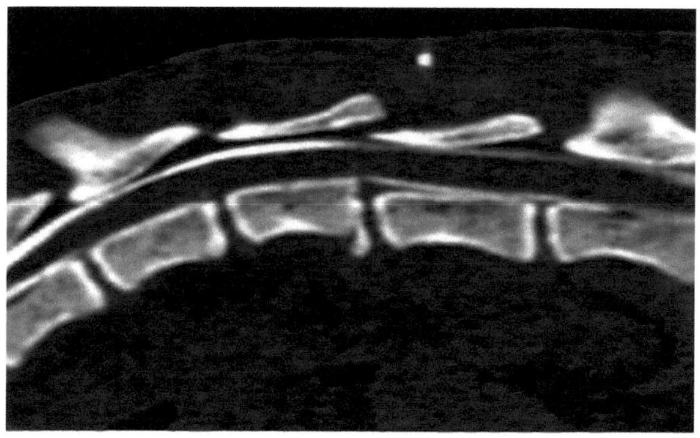

Figure 24. Sagittal plane in a bone algorithm of a myeloCT of a cat with fracture of the caudal epiphysis of L1, with a slight subluxation of the spine, showing slight attenuation of both contrast columns at the level of L1–L2.

compartments: dorsal, middle and ventral. The **dorsal compartment** contains the spinous process, the vertebral dorsal lamina, the articular processes, the vertebral pedicles and the dorsal ligaments (supraspinous ligaments, interspinous ligaments and ligamentum flavum); the **middle compartment** contains the dorsal longitudinal ligament, the dorsal portion of the annulus fibrosus and the dorsal aspect of the vertebral body (the floor of the vertebral canal); the **ventral compartment** includes the rest of the vertebral body, the lateral and ventral aspects of the annulus fibrosus, the nucleus pulposus and the ventral longitudinal ligament. If two or more compartments of a vertebra are affected, the fracture or luxation is likely to be unstable and require stabilisation.

With vertebral fractures and luxations, soft tissue injuries involving the spinal cord, intervertebral discs and other connective tissues may be found; therefore, CT or MRI should be considered in all animals with vertebral injury, especially if a lesion affecting the spinal cord is suspected. **CT** (Fig. 23) provides excellent detail of bone structures, and is very useful for identifying subtle, nondisplaced fractures or fissures that are not visible on radiographs and in cases of complex fractures; multiplanar reconstructions can help in planning the surgical approach. In addition, CT allows rapid assessment of the spine (compared with MRI). Spinal cord compression can be assessed by performing a myeloCT scan (Fig. 24).

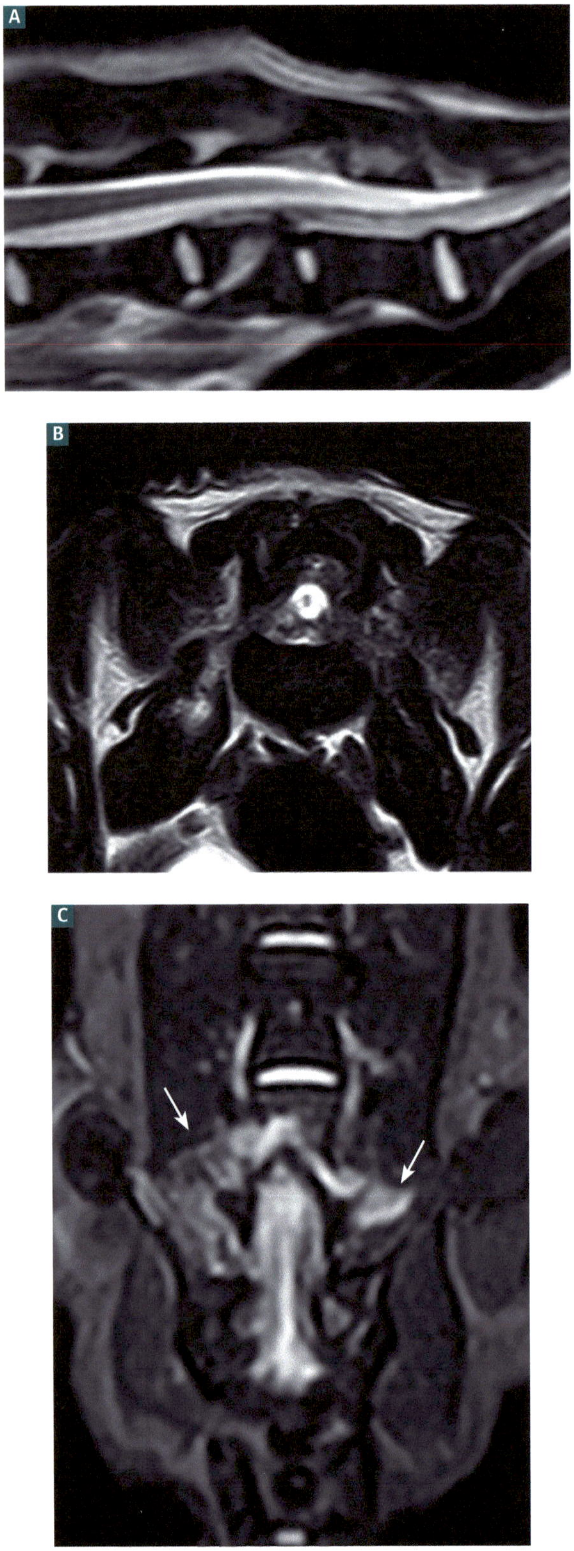

Figure 25. MRI of the spine of a dog following trauma. **A**. Sagittal plane T2W image, in which an oblique fracture of the vertebral body of L6 is observed. **B**. Transverse plane T2W image, in which thickening of the right nerve root of L6, compatible with neuritis, is observed. **C**. Dorsal plane STIR image showing diffuse hyperintensity of the paravertebral musculature (arrows) compatible with inflammation secondary to trauma.

The main advantage of **MRI** in these cases is that it can be used to evaluate spinal cord compression or contusion without the need for administration of intrathecal contrast medium. In addition, it allows the presence of changes in the epidural space (haemorrhage etc.) and changes in the paravertebral soft tissues to be evaluated in more detail (Fig. 25).

Haemorrhage

Paravertebral, extradural or intramedullary haemorrhage may occur as a consequence of traumatic spinal injuries in dogs and cats. The method of choice for its diagnosis is MRI, in which areas of focal hyperintense medullary contusion in T2W with variable postcontrast enhancement can be seen. T2* echo gradient sequences are very useful as they show areas of signal void when haemorrhage is present in either the epidural or the intramedullary space (Fig. 26).

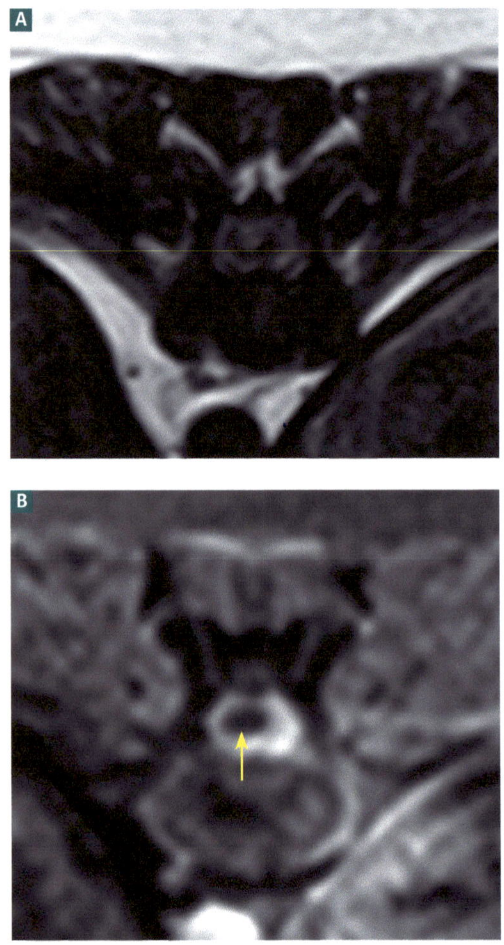

Figure 26. MRI of the spine of a dog with intramedullary haemorrhage secondary to a traumatic hernia. **A**. T2W transverse plane image, in which the spinal cord can be seen with a focal lesion of mixed intensity. **B**. Transverse plane T2* image, where the same lesion is observed with signal void (arrow).

Dural Tears

Trauma can cause tearing of the dura, leading to the loss of CSF from the subarachnoid space. A CT scan may show an associated vertebral fracture or subluxation; myeloCT is required to visualise the leakage of contrast medium from the subarachnoid space at the site of the lesion to the extradural or intramedullary spaces (Fig. 27).

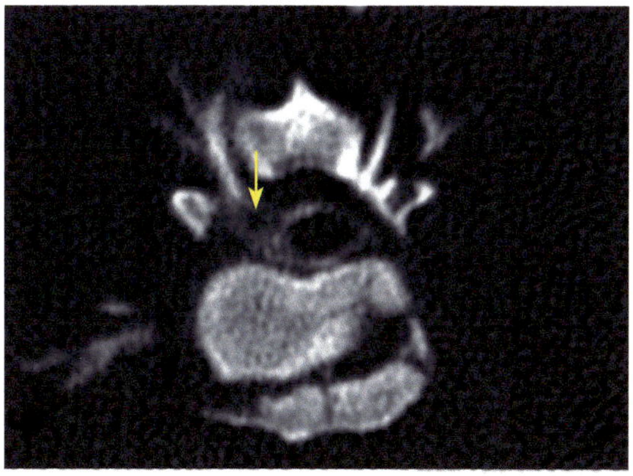

Figure 27. Transverse plane of a myeloCT in a bone algorithm of a dog with a fracture of the vertebral body of L1. Attenuation of the dorsal and ventral contrast columns is observed, as well as leakage of contrast into the right epidural space (arrow) due to a dural tear.

Inflammatory and Infectious Processes

Discospondylitis

Discospondylitis is the infection of an intervertebral disc, which affects the articular surfaces of the vertebral bodies adjacent to the disc. It usually occurs as a result of haematogenous dissemination, and is frequently associated with urogenital infections, paraspinal abscesses or the migration of a foreign body. It generally affects middle-aged and large-breed dogs, and is less common in cats, although it has a similar aetiopathogenesis in this species. The radiographic findings (Fig. 28 A) vary depending on the time point at which the radiograph is performed because discospondylitis is a process that evolves over time. In an initial or early phase, the articular surfaces adjacent to the affected disc are observed with irregular and poorly defined edges due to the osteolysis they are undergoing, and the intervertebral space is visualised as somewhat wider than the contiguous spaces, although in some cases there is collapse or narrowing of the latter spaces. In later phases, bone neoformation of the bony surfaces occurs, the articular surfaces become better defined again, the intervertebral space narrows because it is remodelled over time, and fusion between two vertebrae can occur in the presence of spondylosis. In some cases, areas of secondary subluxation may be detected. In cases of discospondylitis, CT allows bone lesions to be visualised in greater detail. In addition, it allows evaluation of the adjacent soft tissues for a cause or secondary abnormalities (foreign bodies, abscesses, etc.); here, the intravenous administration of contrast medium plays a fundamental role (Fig. 28 B).

MRI is superior to CT and radiography for the detection of discospondylitis. It is very useful in cases where this pathology is suspected but the changes are subtle or atypical on radiographs, as it is more sensitive to early changes. Fat suppression sequences are very useful for the visualisation of areas of hyperintensity around the articular surfaces, and postcontrast sequences are also useful because they show areas of enhancement. Among the MRI findings, irregular articular surfaces of vertebral bodies can be visualised, with loss of the normal appearance of the nucleus pulposus, and marked enhancement

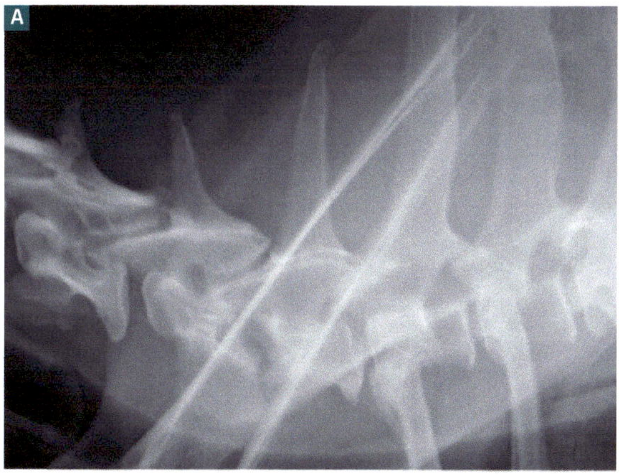

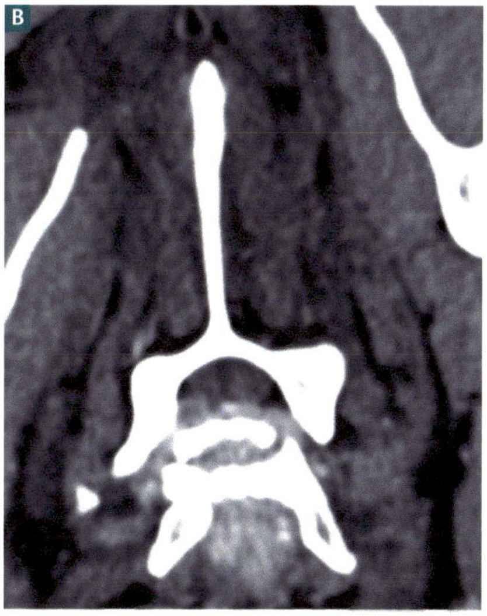

Figure 28. Images of the cervical spine of a dog with acute discospondylitis at C6–C7. **A.** Lateral radiograph, in which an increase in the intervertebral space is observed, with lysis of the caudal vertebral articular surface of C6 and the cranial surface of C7, surrounded by areas of sclerosis. **B.** Transverse plane CT image post intravenous contrast in a soft tissue window, in which marked contrast uptake by the soft tissues surrounding the intervertebral disc is observed.

of the articular surfaces and the intervertebral disc. In addition, if the process extends into the epidural space, or if there is compression of the spinal cord associated with the alteration of the intervertebral disc (protrusion/extrusion) or vertebral subluxation is present, these can also be detected.

Spondylitis

Vertebral **spondylitis** or osteomyelitis is the process that takes place if infection is focused on a vertebral body without affecting the adjacent intervertebral disc. Common causes of spondylitis include microbial infection, foreign body migration, *Spirocerca lupi* infection, and paraspinal abscesses that can spread to the spine and cause spondylitis. Radiographic changes are an irregular periosteal reaction at the ventral border of the affected vertebral body, so a differential diagnosis with bone metastases should be made. Parasite-induced spondylitis results in bone neoformation in the ventral aspect of the vertebral bodies of T8–T11.

Vertebral **physitis** occurs in young dogs due to septic processes. Initial radiographic signs include osteolysis of the physes of the affected vertebrae with preservation of the endplates. As physitis progresses, there is collapse of the cranial or caudal aspect of the vertebral body and endplate sclerosis.

Meningomyelitis

Inflammation of the meninges and spinal cord occurs rarely in dogs and cats. As in cases of meningoencephalitis, the causes are infectious or noninfectious. Viral, bacterial, fungal and parasitic organisms are found among the causes of infectious meningomyelitis. Among the noninfectious causes are granulomatous meningoencephalitis and steroid-responsive meningitis–arteritis.

On CT, the use of intravenous contrast medium is necessary to visualise lesions. However, meningomyelitis is difficult to diagnose and, even with contrast use, lesions may not be observed, or heterogeneous contrast uptake in the spinal cord may be observed, as well as meningeal enhancement. On MRI, poorly defined multifocal intramedullary lesions can be observed, which are hyperintense in T2W, hypo- or isointense in T1W, and show heterogeneous and variable enhancement after contrast administration (Fig. 29).

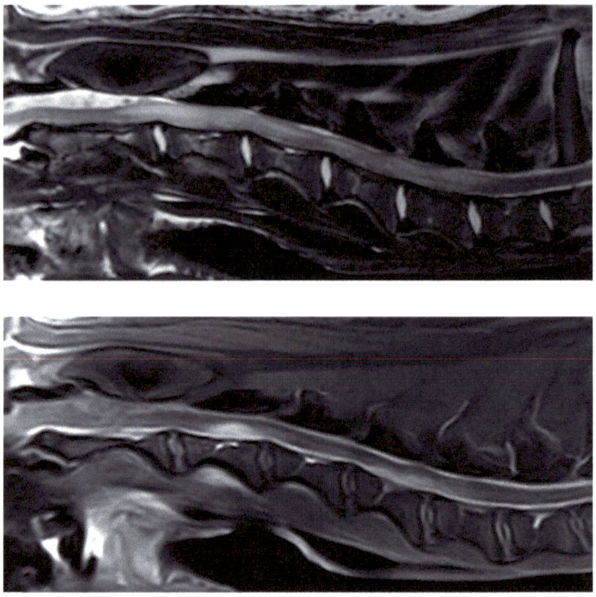

Figure 29. Sagittal plane MRI images in T2W and T1 with postcontrast fat saturation of a dog with meningomyelitis of unknown origin. Multiple hyperintense diffuse intramedullary lesions are observed in T2W, with marked enhancement showing poorly defined margins. Note the marked postcontrast meningeal enhancement.

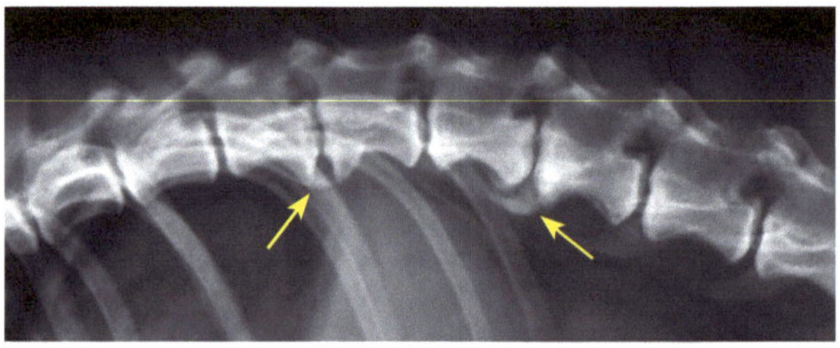

Figure 30. Lateral projection of the thoracolumbar spine of a dog with spondylosis at the level of T13–L1 and L2–L3 (arrows).

Degenerative Disease

Spondylosis

Spondylosis is a degenerative disease of the vertebral bodies. It is common in dogs, especially Boxers and large breeds, and is usually seen in the thoracolumbar and lumbosacral regions in middle-aged and elderly animals. The exact cause is unknown, but the aetiopathogenesis includes repetitive trauma, instability and ageing, as well as hereditary predisposition. It is unclear whether intervertebral disc degeneration is a factor influencing the development of deforming spondylosis, but it is common for disc protrusions to be associated with areas of spondylosis. In most patients, spondylosis is an incidental finding except in those in which it may be associated with disc protrusions. Compression of nerve roots due to spondylosis is rare, except in cases with lumbosacral instability.

On radiography, the presence of bone neoformations (osteophytes) with different degrees of development on the ventral articular surfaces of the vertebral bodies is seen (Fig. 30).

These changes seen on radiography are not usually associated with clinical signs, although sometimes the bone neoformations can join together, form bridges, and cause stiffness and decreased mobility of the affected area.

Diffuse Idiopathic Skeletal Hyperostosis

This pathology is characterised by bone neoformation along multiple vertebral bodies. The aetiology is unknown, but it is believed to be a form of degenerative disease. It is described in young dogs of large or giant breeds (Boxers, Great Danes, etc.). It may be associated with hyperthyroidism, hyperthyrocalcitonism or hyperparathyroidism.

The radiographic findings consist of smooth bone neoformation linking the ventral and lateral aspects of multiple consecutive vertebral bodies (three or more) while the intervertebral discs remain intact, as well as bone neoformation in the articular processes, pseudoarthrosis between the spinous processes, and mineralisation of the insertions of soft tissue structures on the long bones (enthesopathies) (Fig. 31).

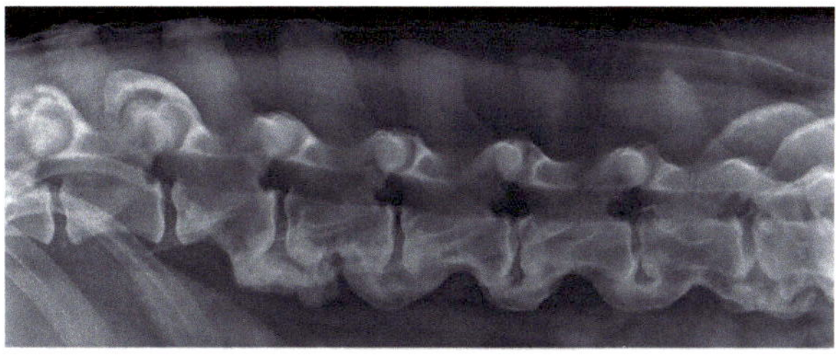

Figure 31. Lateral radiograph of the thoracolumbar spine of a dog with diffuse idiopathic skeletal hyperostosis. Ventral bone neoformation is observed along the vertebral bodies of the lumbar spine, and bone neoformation is observed in the articular processes of T13–L1 and L1–L2.

Degenerative Lumbosacral Disease

Degenerative lumbosacral disease is commonly known as "cauda equina syndrome" and mainly affects large-breed dogs (German Shepherd Dogs especially), middle-aged or old dogs, and males. There are multiple aetiopathological factors that can contribute to this condition, such as degeneration and herniation of the intervertebral disc (most commonly protrusion), lumbosacral instability or subluxation with ventral displacement of the lamina sacralis, misalignment of the articular processes, foraminal stenosis, or hypertrophy of the ligamentum flavum and joint capsule of the articular processes. CT and MRI are excellent modalities for diagnosing this disease.

CT (Fig. 32) allows evaluation of the protrusion of the intervertebral disc. There is a loss of visualisation of the epidural fat ventrally, and the presence of bone neoformation (spondylosis) on the articular surfaces, causing narrowing of the intervertebral foramina, or at the level of the articular processes. In addition, after intravenous administration of contrast medium, enhancement or thickening of the nerve roots (indicating neuritis) secondary to the compression can be seen. In these cases, studies can be done with the spine extended or flexed at the level of the affected disc(s), since there are cases in which the compression is dynamic and can be observed in greater detail when studies are performed in different positions.

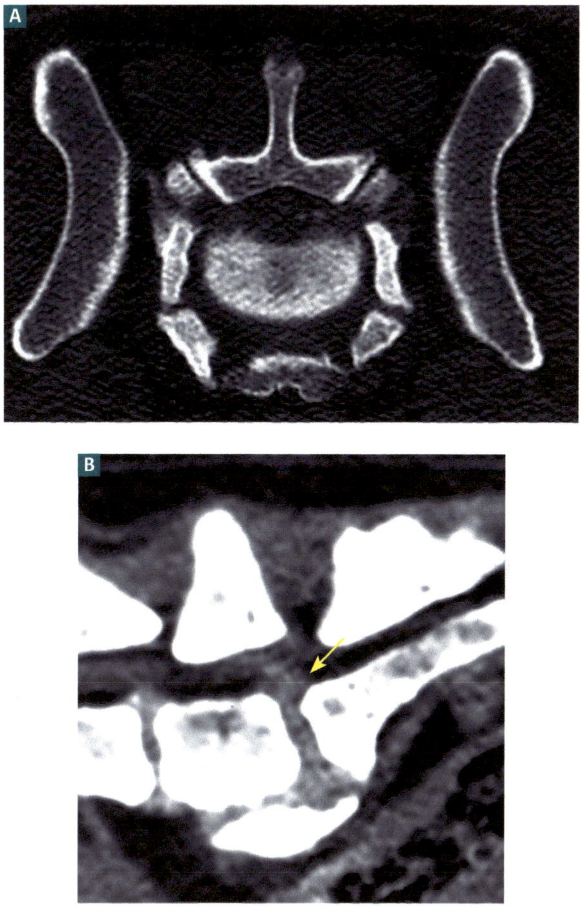

Figure 32. Transverse plane in a bone window (A) and sagittal plane in a soft tissue window (B) CT images of a dog with lumbosacral degenerative disease. **A.** Ventrolateral bone neoformation is observed causing stenosis of both intervertebral foramina. **B.** Note the L7–S1 disc protrusion (arrow), with loss of visualisation of ventral epidural fat.

On MRI, degeneration of the disc (evident as a decrease in the intensity of the normal signal of the nucleus pulposus on T2W images) and protrusion of the lumbosacral intervertebral disc (a protuberance of the annulus fibrosus) towards the vertebral canal or intervertebral foramina, with loss of visualisation of the epidural fat signal within the vertebral canal, are observed. Spondylosis, a vertebral misalignment between L7 and S1, and ventral displacement of the dorsal lamina of the sacrum, the presence of transitional vertebrae (most commonly lumbarisation of S1) and hypertrophy of the interarcual and dorsal longitudinal ligaments can also be seen.

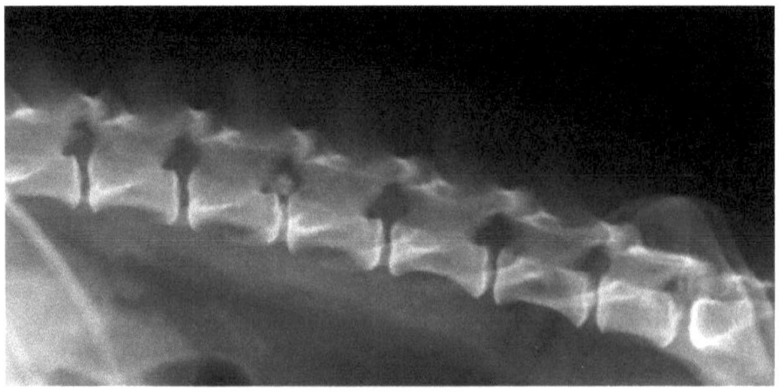

Figure 33. Lateral radiographic projection of the lumbar spine of a dog with disc disease (disc extrusion), in which a narrowing of the L3–L4 intervertebral space is observed, with the presence of mineralised disc material occupying the vertebral canal superimposed at the level of the intervertebral foramen.

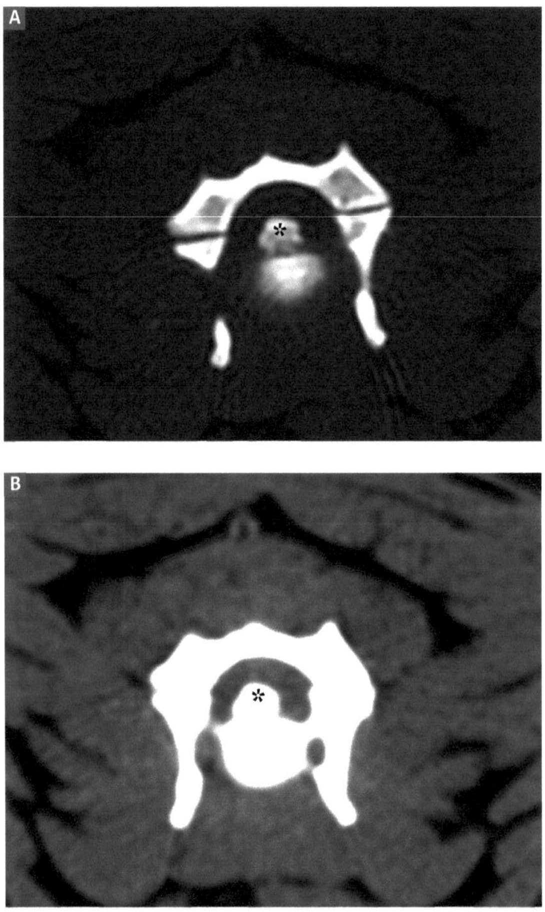

Figure 34. Transverse CT planes of the spine in a bone window (**A**) and a soft tissue window (**B**) of a dog with a disc extrusion. The presence of mineralised disc material (asterisk) located in the ventral aspect of the vertebral canal is observed, causing displacement and compression of the spinal cord dorsally.

These changes cause displacement or compression of the dural sac or nerve roots, and narrowing or stenosis of the intervertebral foramen (uni- or bilateral) with compression of the nerve roots, which can appear thickened and inflamed. In addition, associated changes in the paraspinal musculature (a symmetrical or asymmetrical decrease in muscle mass) can be observed.

The limitations of both CT and MRI include, but are not limited to, the poor correlation between imaging findings and clinical signs.

Intervertebral Disc Disease

The term "disc disease" is a very broad description that encompasses all the changes that can occur in the intervertebral discs, whether they are clinically relevant or not. This pathology can be better characterised through the use of MRI, which allows the characteristic changes of the different types of disc disease that are described in the literature to be classified and observed in a more precise way. The radiographic signs that can be detected in some cases of disc disease are narrowing of the intervertebral space, an increase in opacity, narrowing or change in the shape of the intervertebral foramen, the presence of mineralised disc material in the vertebral canal and the presence of associated spondylosis (Fig. 33). In most cases, no radiographic changes are visualised and the presence of lesions should always be confirmed by myelography, CT or MRI.

CT is very useful in cases of degenerative disc disease. Findings that can be observed are a decrease in the intervertebral space, sclerosis of the articular surfaces of the vertebral bodies and even the presence of gas (vacuum sign) in the intervertebral space. In cases of disc extrusions where the disc material is mineralised, the presence of hyperattenuating material can be observed occupying the vertebral canal (Fig. 34). In these cases, the exact location and extent of the extradural material and whether it is lateralised or not can be assessed. In some cases, associated bleeding may be observed, with the presence of hyperattenuating material extending cranially or caudally from the site of compression and diffuse intramedullary contrast acquisition zones related to medullary contusion or slightly hypoattenuating areas of oedema. In cases where the disc material is not mineralised, myeloCT is useful to identify the site of disc herniation, whether there is lateralisation and the degree of extradural compression of the spinal cord, but rarely provides significant information on the state of the spinal cord, so it is performed as an alternative method to study disc disease when MRI is not available (Fig. 35).

With the use of MRI, disc disease can be classified into several categories, because a more exhaustive interpretation of the different patterns can be made, and the spinal cord can be studied in more detail due to the greater resolution provided by this technique.

Intervertebral Disc Extrusion (Hansen Type I Hernia)

Hansen type I hernia is a chondroid degeneration of the disc, with subsequent herniation of the degenerated nucleus pulposus through the annulus fibrosus extending along the vertebral canal. It usually affects young dogs and chondrodystrophic breeds. Among the findings, degenerative changes can be seen at the level of the intervertebral disc, with loss of the normal hyperintense signal in T2W sequences of the nucleus pulposus. In cases of extrusion, the changes usually affect a single intervertebral disc, and the disc material extruded into the vertebral canal extends along the vertebral body beyond the intervertebral space and may be lateralised on many occasions. This extradural material has a variable signal intensity (although it is generally hypointense in T1W and T2W) and causes a variable mass effect, with loss of visualisation of the epidural fat and subarachnoid space, and compression and displacement of the spinal cord.

Sequences in T2* help to detect the presence of epidural or spinal cord haemorrhage as a result of disc extrusion, and show lesions with a signal vacuum. In addition, MRI allows the presence of contusion and inflammation of the spinal cord secondary to compression to be detected (Fig. 36).

Foraminal disc extrusions are more common at the C6–C7 and C5–C6 intervertebral spaces, with hypointense extruded material being observed in T2W sequence images within the intervertebral foramen, causing impingement of the nerve roots.

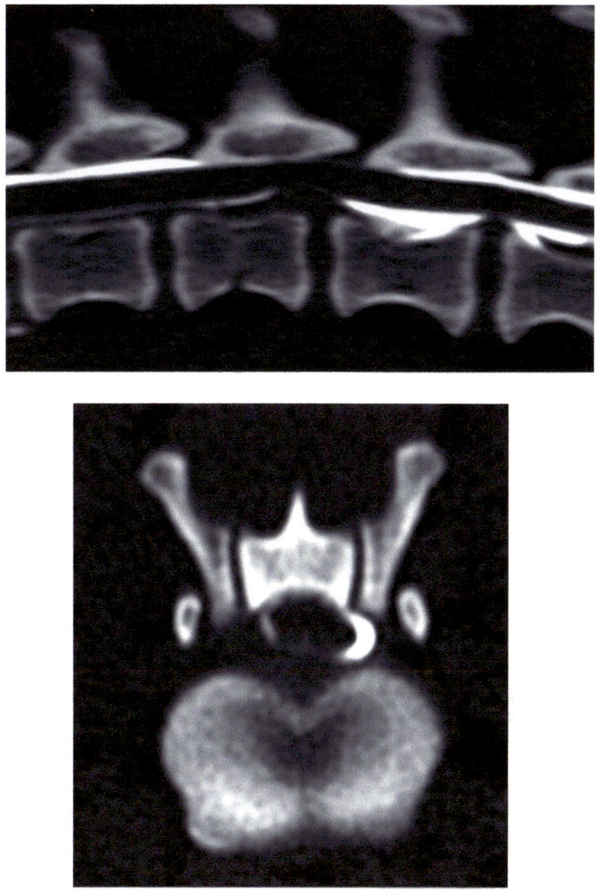

Figure 35. Sagittal and transverse planes of a myeloCT of a dog with a disc extrusion with nonmineralised disc material. An extradural lesion lateralised to the right is observed, causing displacement and narrowing of the ventral contrast column and narrowing of the dorsal contrast column in the T13–L1 intervertebral space, and extending cranially along T13.

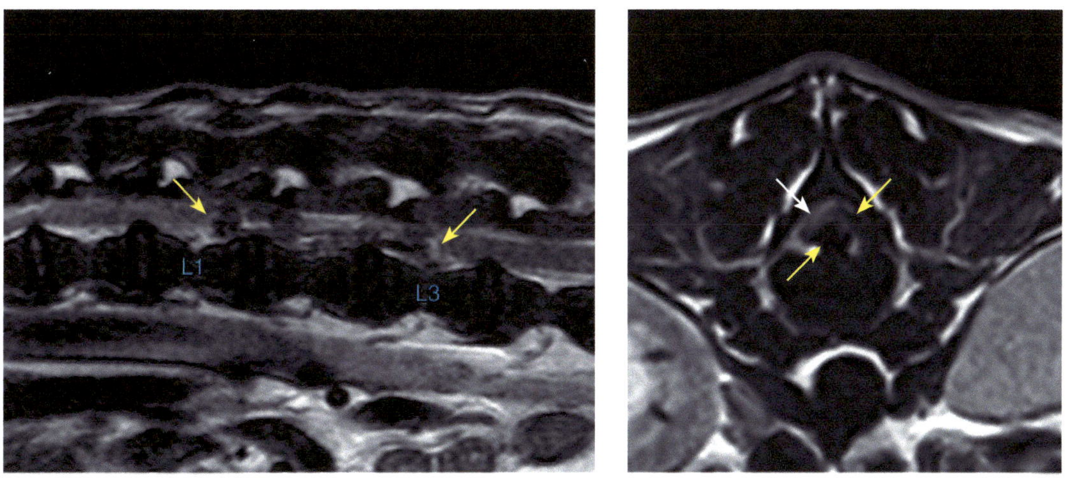

Figure 36. Sagittal and transverse planes in T2W sequences of an MRI of the lumbar spine of a dog with a disc extrusion. Note the presence of extradural material of mixed intensity, lateralised to the left, that extends from the caudal aspect of L1 to the middle aspect of L3 (yellow arrows). The material occupies 70% of the diameter of the vertebral canal and compresses the spinal cord markedly. The spinal cord is diffusely hyperintense, compatible with oedema, contusion or gliosis (white arrow).

Protrusion of the Intervertebral Disc (Hansen Type II Hernia)

Hansen type II hernia is a fibrinoid degeneration in which degeneration of the annulus fibrosus is observed, with rupture of the inner layers and hypertrophy of the annulus fibrosus and a displacement (protrusion) of the nucleus pulposus. It usually affects older dogs and nonchondrodystrophic breeds. The presence of intervertebral discs with a diminished signal is observed in T2W (hypointense), protruding towards the vertebral canal to a variable degree, leaving the extradural disc material confined in the intervertebral space. Normally, loss of visualisation of the subarachnoid space occurs at the ventral level and can cause alterations to the rounded morphology of the spinal cord, depending on its severity (Fig. 37).

There are cases in which it can be difficult to differentiate between a protrusion and a disc extrusion, although, regardless of the type of hernia, with MRI it will always be possible to evaluate the degree of compression and the state of the spinal cord at the site of the lesion.

Acute Noncompressive Disc Extrusion (High Velocity, Low Volume Hernia or Traumatic Hernia)

In acute noncompressive disc extrusion, the nondegenerated nucleus pulposus becomes extruded during exercise or trauma, causing rupture of the annulus fibrosus and resulting in a contusion of the spinal cord immediately dorsal to the intervertebral disc. The segment of the spine where it most often occurs is T13–L3. Among the imaging findings, a decrease in intervertebral space is observed, with decreased volume and intensity of the nucleus pulposus of the intervertebral disc, and with an associated intramedullary lesion dorsal to the disc. The intramedullary lesion is characterised by a diffuse zone that is hyperintense in T2W and isointense in T1W without contrast uptake, although it may be enhanced if the MRI is performed several days after the onset of the clinical signs. In T2*, zones with signal void, compatible with haemorrhage, can be detected. In some cases, changes in signal intensity can be seen in the epidural space or the presence of a very small amount of disc material that does not cause spinal cord compression (Fig. 38).

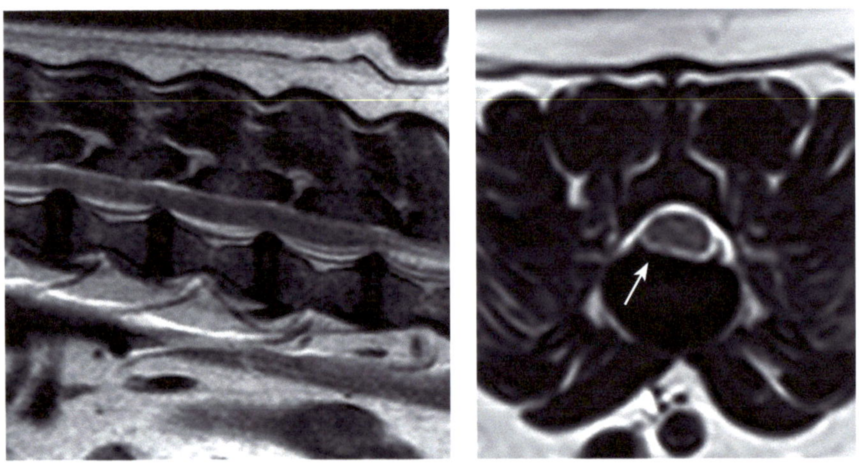

Figure 37. Sagittal and transverse planes of an MRI of the lumbar spine of a dog with multiple disc protrusions. Hypointense intervertebral discs (degenerated/dehydrated) that protrude slightly into the vertebral canal are observed. In the transverse plane, this protrusion (arrow) causes a thinning of the ventral subarachnoid space and flattening of the spinal cord.

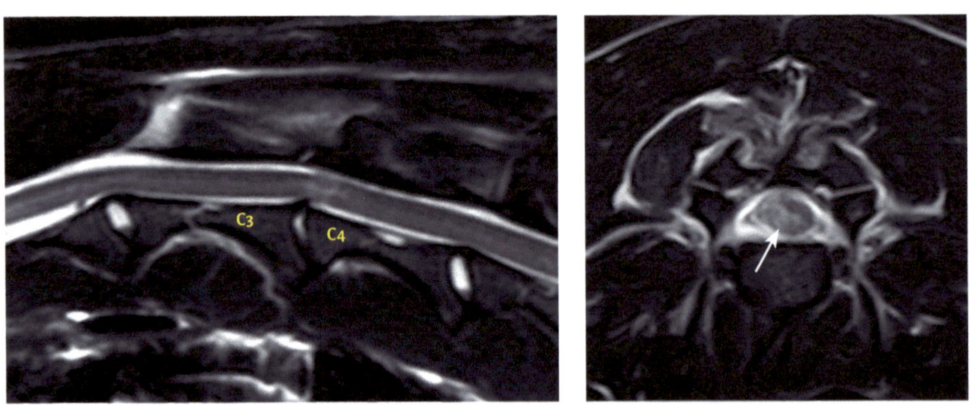

Figure 38. Sagittal and transverse planes of MRI of a dog with an acute noncompressive disc extrusion at the level of C3–C4. Note the decrease in volume of the intervertebral disc, and a focal area of lateralised hyperintensity on the right affecting the spinal cord (grey and white matter) dorsal to the intervertebral space (arrow). Diffuse hyperintensity of the associated paravertebral musculature is also visualised.

Regarding prognosis, it has been suggested that when the intramedullary hyperintense lesion exceeds 90% of the area of the spinal cord in a T2W transverse plane, there is an association with a poor prognosis in 92% of cases. The imaging findings are most useful for predicting the prognosis.

Compressive Hydrated Nucleus Pulposus Extrusion

Compressive hydrated nucleus pulposus extrusion consists of the hydrated and nondegenerated disc material being extruded into the vertebral canal, causing spinal cord compression. This type of extrusion occurs more frequently in the cervical region.

Findings include hyperintense material in T2W, which is isointense to the nucleus pulposus (nondegenerate nucleus pulposus), from a dorsal extradural location to the intervertebral space. In addition, there is an associated decrease in the volume of the nucleus pulposus. Variable spinal cord compression is also observed.

Intramedullary Disc Extrusion

This acute extrusion causes a tear of the dura mater, and the extruded disc material ends up at the intramedullary level. This type of hernia is poorly described. In these cases, a focal intramedullary lesion is observed at the dorsal level of the intervertebral disc. This lesion usually has a mixed intensity on MRI due to the presence of disc material, spinal contusion and haemorrhage. In addition, a line/pathway can be observed that is hyperintense in T2W and hypointense in T1W, with peripheral enhancement, extending along the spinal cord from the intervertebral space. The affected disc shows a decrease in signal strength.

Herniated Intravertebral Disc (Schmorl's Node)

Intravertebral disc herniation is usually diagnosed radiographically or with CT but can be seen in more detail on MRI.

This type of hernia causes a defect in the articular aspect of the vertebral body adjacent to the intervertebral disc, through which disc material is herniated. The lesion on the vertebral articular surface presents a hyperintense signal in T2W and STIR images, and is hypointense in T1W with or without endplate enhancement. Sclerosis of the joint surfaces is also observed in some cases (hypointense foci in T1W and T2W without enhancement).

Vascular Disorders

The most common cause of ischaemic myelopathy in dogs and cats is fibrocartilaginous embolism. Other causes include thrombi of parasitic, septic or neoplastic origin, or pathologies that predispose to thrombus formation.

Ischaemic myelopathy primarily affects the grey matter and can occur in all segments of the spinal cord, but predisposed sites in dogs are L4–S3, C6–T2 and T3–L3, whereas in cats cervical spinal cord involvement is more frequent. MRI is useful to recognise the changes associated with ischaemic myelopathy and differentiate it from other conditions with similar clinical presentations, such as spinal trauma or intervertebral disc herniation. Generally, in T2W images, a hyperintense intramedullary lesion with fairly well defined margins affecting the grey matter, which is usually asymmetrical and lateralised, is observed. These lesions are hypo- or isointense in T1W, with variable postcontrast enhancement during the first week (Fig. 39).

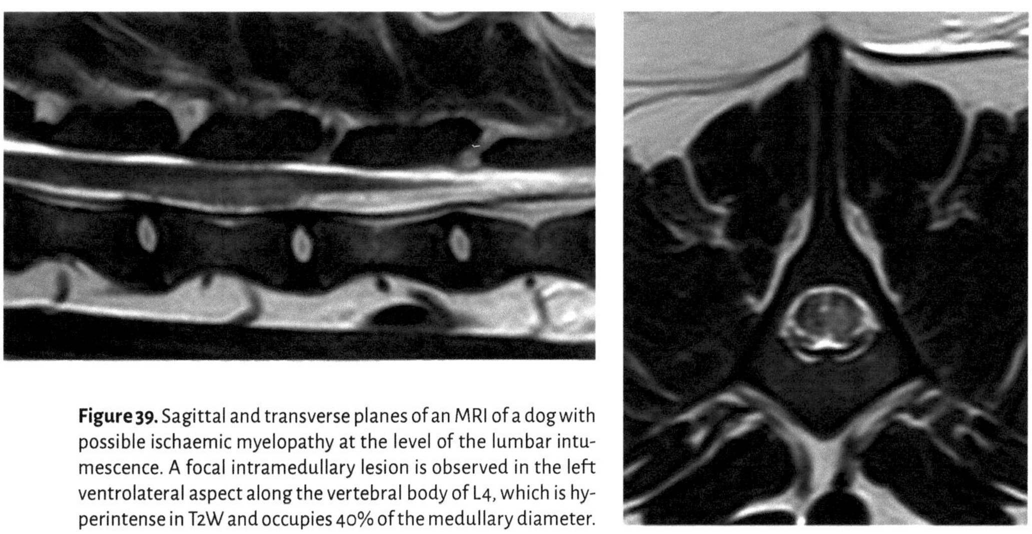

Figure 39. Sagittal and transverse planes of an MRI of a dog with possible ischaemic myelopathy at the level of the lumbar intumescence. A focal intramedullary lesion is observed in the left ventrolateral aspect along the vertebral body of L4, which is hyperintense in T2W and occupies 40% of the medullary diameter.

Myelomalacia

Myelomalacia is necrosis of the parenchyma of the spinal cord. It can occur secondary to any acute damage to the spinal cord; after the initial damage, secondary damage is caused by vascular compromise. Myelomalacia can be focal or diffuse, extending cranially or caudally (ascending or descending myelomalacia). Between 1% and 9% of dogs with acute spinal cord damage at the thoracolumbar level will have diffuse myelomalacia. The prognosis is guarded.

With CT, hyperattenuating areas can be observed in the spinal cord, and after performing myeloCT, contrast can be seen in the spinal cord parenchyma, as well as inflammation of the spinal cord.

MRI is useful in determining the degree of involvement. Hyperintense areas are observed in T2W, and iso-/hypointense areas in T1W. There may be inflammation of the spinal cord resulting in a loss of visualisation of the CSF hyperintense signal on T2W sequences.

Neoplasia

Neoplastic processes of the spine can be classified according to their location as extradural, intradural extramedullary or intramedullary.

Extradural Tumours

Extradural tumours are those that affect the vertebral bodies, paraspinal soft tissues and epidural space. They are the most common category of neoplasms affecting the spine. These tumours can invade the spinal canal and cause spinal cord compression. Among extradural tumours, neoplasms that affect bone structures, such as osteosarcoma, chondrosarcoma, haemangiosarcoma, lymphoma, multiple myeloma, metastases and histiocytic sarcoma, are found, as well as others that affect the paraspinal soft tissues, such as soft tissue sarcoma and infiltrative lipoma.

Primary Bone Tumours

Primary bone neoplasms affecting the vertebrae can produce osteolytic foci, bone neoformations (periosteal reaction) or mixed lesions. The most common tumour types are osteosarcoma, chondrosarcoma, fibrosarcoma and multiple myeloma. Except for multiple myeloma, these neoplasms usually affect a single vertebra (monostotic), with the lesion being localised to the vertebral body, the dorsal lamina and the processes. The radiographic signs of vertebral neoplasia are nonspecific and typical of an aggressive bone response, and include bone lysis and bone production; pathological fractures can be associated with these changes. In the case of **multiple myeloma**, its presentation is characteristic because it produces multiple, more or less rounded osteolytic foci, with sharp but not sclerotic edges, affecting several vertebrae (polyostotic) and present in any part of the vertebra. In these cases, a differential diagnosis should be made with lymphoma and other round cell neoplasms (Fig. 40). CT allows bone lesions to be evaluated in more detail, which is of great importance where the lesions are subtle. In addition, CT enables evaluation of whether the lesions affect and invade the vertebral canal, and with myeloCT the degree of spinal cord compression can be studied (Fig. 41).

On MRI, the signal intensity of the neoplastic lesion itself is highly variable, ranging from iso- to hyperintense or hypointense in T1W and T2W sequences, with contrast enhancement also being variable, although it is often heterogeneous. However, it is possible to evaluate in great detail whether the lesion causes invasion of the vertebral canal, and the degree of spinal cord involvement.

Bone Metastases

Bone metastases usually affect more than one vertebral body and even other bones. They can be osteolytic, osteoproductive or mixed lesions. In the case of metastases of prostate, bladder, and urethral carcinomas, they usually cause periosteal reactions in the ventral aspects of the vertebral bodies of the lumbar and sacral spine, whereas metastases of mammary carcinomas usually have a variable location depending on the location of the primary tumour (Fig. 42).

Paraspinal Soft Tissue Neoplasms

Several types of neoplasms that originate in the paraspinal soft tissues can invade the vertebral canal and cause spinal cord compression. Examples include fibrosarcoma and other soft tissue sarcomas. The techniques of choice for the evaluation

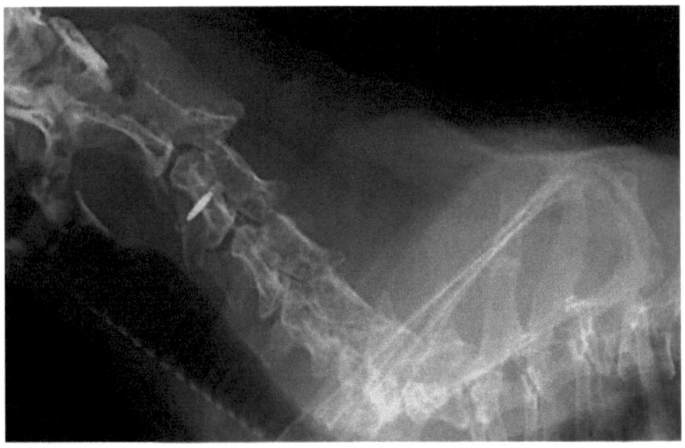

Figure 40. Lateral radiographic projection of the cervical spine of a dog with multiple myeloma. Multiple osteolytic foci are observed affecting all cervical vertebrae.

of these pathologies are CT and MRI; both enable the extent and characteristics of the lesions to be assessed, and help in planning a surgical approach, if indicated. With both techniques, the administration of contrast is very useful to evaluate the enhancement characteristics of the lesions.

Extramedullary Intradural Tumours

Extramedullary intradural tumours are located between the dura mater and the spinal cord. This group includes neoplasms such as meningioma, nerve sheath tumours and nephroblastoma, among others. Most of these neoplasms affect adult geriatric dogs and cats, but nephroblastomas are typically found in young dogs. The techniques of choice to evaluate this type of neoplasm are CT and MRI. When a myeloCT scan is performed, a widened subarachnoid space with the appearance of a "golf tee" is observed in the contrast column that is affected by the lesion in sagittal and dorsal reconstructions, in some cases extending to the spinal cord and appearing to be intramedullary.

Meningiomas

Meningiomas are usually single, well defined masses with a broad base, which cause a variable degree of spinal cord compression. The cranial cervical spine (cranial to C3) is the most commonly affected region (Fig. 43). On MRI, meningiomas are usually hyperintense in T2W and T1W compared with the spinal cord, with strong contrast uptake. Sometimes, they are accompanied by a "dural tail sign".

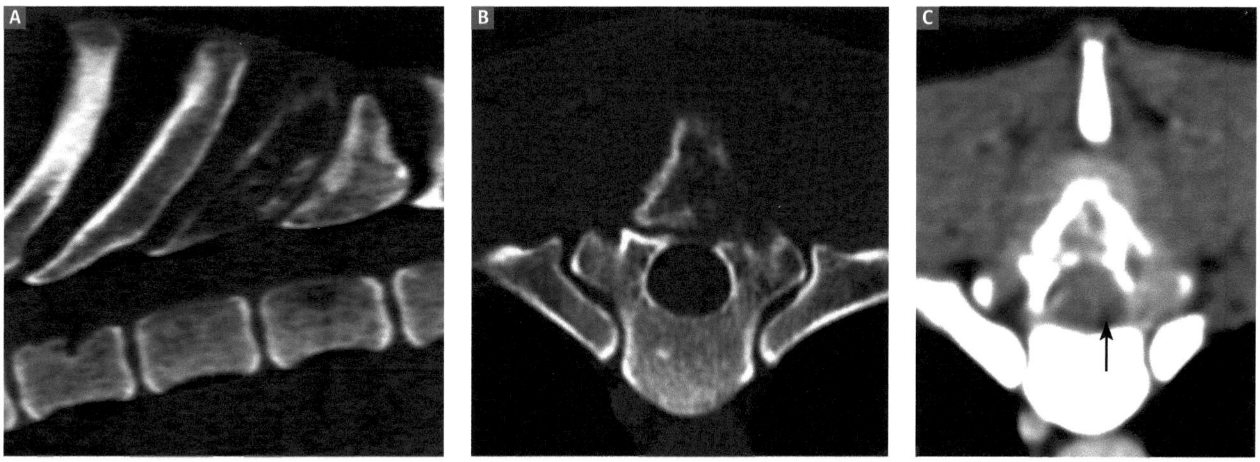

Figure 41. CT images of a dog with a bone neoplasm: sagittal (A) and transverse (B) planes in a bone window, and transverse plane in a soft tissue window after intravenous contrast administration (C). **A** and **B**. Note the aggressive expansive monostotic bone lesion with osteolysis and mild irregular periosteal reaction affecting T9 (spinous process, dorsal lamina and left vertebral pedicle). **C**. A soft tissue component with marked enhancement is observed that extends into the dorsolateral aspect of the vertebral canal (arrow) and compresses the spinal cord slightly.

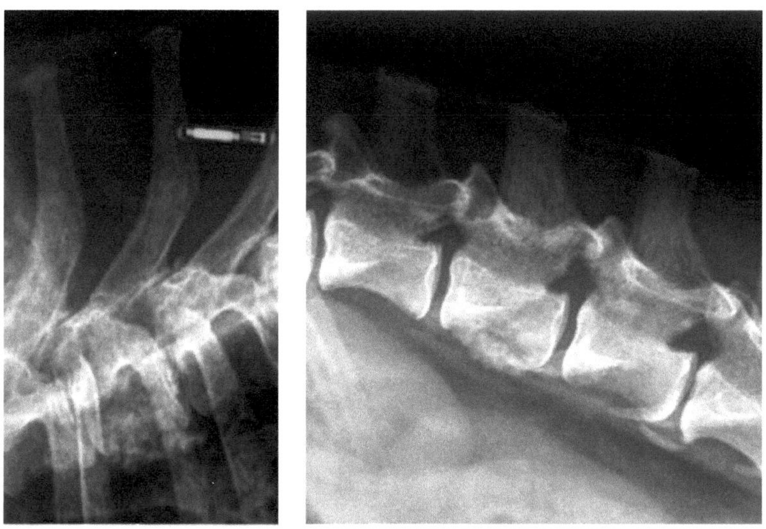

Figure 42. Lateral radiographic projections of the thoracic and lumbar spine of a dog with polyostotic bone lesions, with the presence of a solid and irregular periosteal reaction in the ventral aspect of several vertebral bodies. These lesions are compatible with bone metastases.

Nerve Sheath Tumours

Nerve sheath tumours usually cause widening of the intervertebral foramen and the presence of a hypercaptive tubular structure due to the enlargement of the nerve root, which may be visible in detail on CT (Fig. 44). On MRI, the appearance is usually a well defined tubular mass, which is iso- or hypointense to the spinal cord in T1W images and hyperintense in T2W images, with moderate postcontrast enhancement, extending from the intradural compartment through the intervertebral foramen and into the paravertebral soft tissues.

Intramedullary Spinal Tumours

Intramedullary tumours are rare; glial tumours are the most common in dogs, whereas lymphosarcoma is more common in cats. Intramedullary metastases are rare, but they can occur. General MRI features of intramedullary neoplasia include thinning or attenuation of the epidural space at the level of the lesion, which is best seen on T2W images, and widening of the spinal cord with lesions that are isointense in T1W and hyperintense in T2W, with variable enhancement after contrast administration.

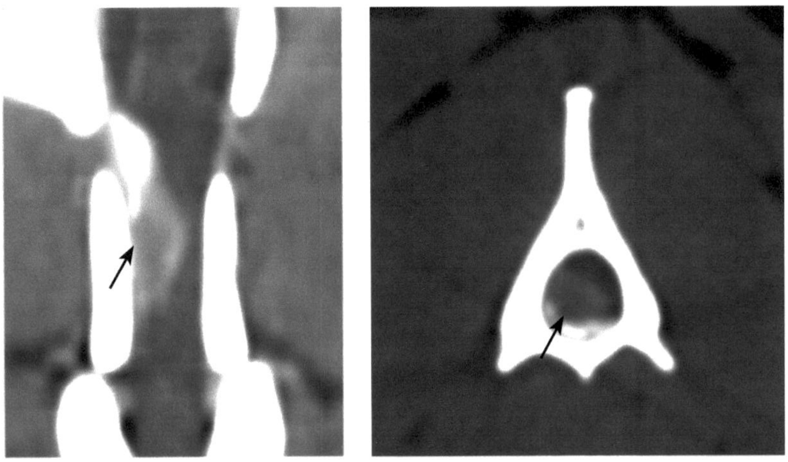

Figure 43. Dorsal and transverse planes CT images with intravenous postcontrast, with soft tissue algorithms, of a dog with a lesion compatible with a meningioma. A broad-based mass with homogeneous marked enhancement and well defined margins is observed at the ventral level and lateralised to the right, at the level of the C1–C2 space (arrows). The lesion causes marked spinal cord compression.

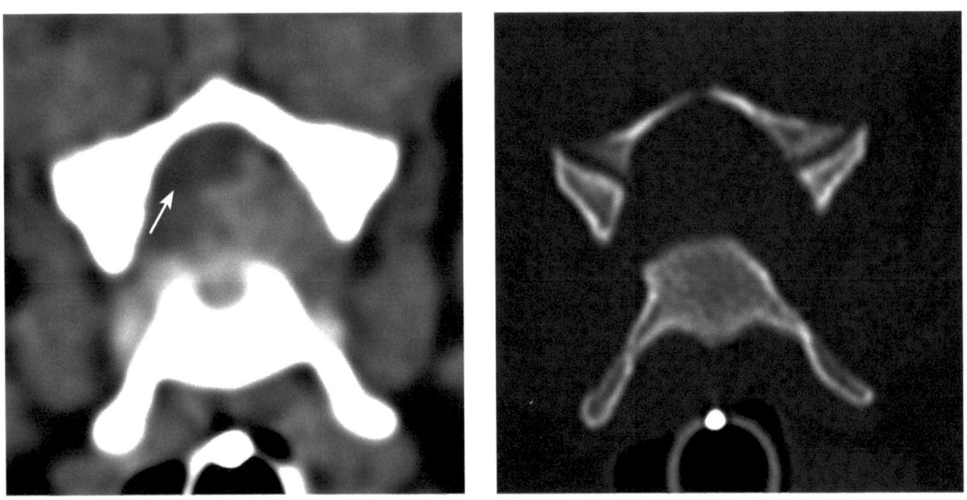

Figure 44. Transverse CT planes in a postcontrast soft tissue window and a bone window of a dog with a nerve sheath tumour. A mass is observed affecting the left C7 nerve root, with marked homogeneous enhancement, which extends into the spinal canal, causing marked compression of the spinal cord (arrow). Note the widening of the left intervertebral foramen.

Bibliography

- Ayers, S. (2012) *Small Animal Radiographic Techniques and Positioning*. 1st ed. Wiley-Blackwell.
- Bertram, S., Haar, G.T., De Decker, S. (2018) Caudal articular process dysplasia of thoracic vertebrae in neurologically normal French bulldogs, English bulldogs, and Pugs: prevalence and characteristics. *Vet Radiol Ultrasound*, 59(4):396–404.
- Da Costa, R.C. (2018) Cervical spondylomyelopathy. In: Mai, W. (ed). *Diagnostic MRI in Dogs and Cats*. 1st ed, pp. 447–471. CRC Press.
- Dennis, R., Kirberger, R.M., Wrigley, R.H., et al. (2010) *Handbook of Small Animal Radiology and Ultrasound. Techniques and Differential Diagnoses*. 2nd ed. Elsevier.
- Fenn, J., Drees, R., Volk, H.A., et al. (2015) Inter- and intraobserver agreement for diagnosing presumptive ischemic myelopathy and acute noncompressive nucleus pulposus extrusion in dogs using magnetic resonance imaging. *Vet Radiol Ultrasound*, 57(1):33–40.
- Gomes, S.A., Volk, H.A., Packer, R.M., et al. (2016) Clinical and magnetic resonance imaging characteristics of thoracolumbar intervertebral disk extrusions and protrusions in large breed dogs. *Vet Radiol Ultrasound*, 57(4):417–426.
- Gutierrez-Quintana, R., Guevar, J., Stalin, C., et al. (2014) A proposed radiographic classification scheme for congenital thoracic vertebral malformations in brachycephalic "screw-tailed" dog breeds. *Vet Radiol Ultrasound*, 55(6):585–591.
- Johnson, P., Beltran, E., Dennis, R., et al, O. (2012) Magnetic resonance imaging characteristics of suspected vertebral instability associated with fracture or subluxation in eleven dogs. *Vet Radiol Ultrasound*, 53(5):552–559.
- Lim, C., Kweon, O.K., Choi, M.C., et al. (2010) Computed tomographic characteristics of acute thoracolumbar intervertebral disc disease in dogs. *J Vet Sci*. 11(1):73–79.
- Llabrés, F. (2014) Columna vertebral y mielografía. In: Agut, A. *Diagnóstico por Imagen en Pequeños Animales*. 1st ed. Multimédica Ediciones Veterinarias.
- Mai, W. (2018) Normal MRI spinal anatomy, degenerative disc disease, and disc herniation. In: Mai, W. (ed). *Diagnostic MRI in Dogs and Cats*. 1st ed, pp. 413–446. CRC Press.
- Mai, W. (2018) Magnetic resonance imaging and computed tomography features of canine and feline spinal cord disease. In: Thrall, D.E. (ed). *Textbook of Veterinary Diagnostic Radiology*. 7th ed, pp. 271–304. Elsevier.
- Mai, W. (2018) Spinal neoplasia. In: Mai, W. (ed). *Diagnostic MRI in Dogs and Cats*. 1st ed, pp. 527–564. CRC Press.
- Mauler, D.A., De Decker, S., De Risio, L., et al. (2014) Signalment, clinical presentation, and diagnostic findings in 122 dogs with spinal arachnoid diverticula. *J Vet Intern Med*, 28(1):175–181.
- Muhlbauer, M.C., Kneller, S.K. (2013) *Radiography of the Dog and Cat: Guide to Making and Interpreting Radiographs*. 1st ed. Wiley-Blackwell.
- Sande, R.D. (1992) Radiography, myelography, computed tomography and magnetic resonance imaging of the spine. *Veterinary Clinics of North America: Small Animal Practice*. 22 (4):811-31.
- Seiler, G., Kinns, J., Dennison, S., et al. (2011) Vertebral column and spinal cord. In: Schwarz T, Saunders J. (eds). *Veterinary Computed Tomography*. 1st ed, pp. 209–228. Wiley-Blackwell.
- Seim, H.B., Withrow, S.J. (1982) Pathophysiology and diagnosis of caudal cervical spondylomyelopathy with emphasis on the Doberman Pinscher. *J Am Anim Hosp Assoc*, 18:241–251.
- Widmer, W.R., Thrall, D.E. (2018) Canine and feline vertebrae. In: Thrall, D.E. (ed). *Textbook of Veterinary Diagnostic Radiology*. 7th ed, pp. 249–270. Elsevier.
- Wisner, E., Zwingenberger, A. (2015) *Atlas of Small Animal CT and MRI*. 1st ed. Wiley-Blackwell.

Ultrasonography of the Neck and Head

Vicente Esteve Bernet and Patricia Laborda Vidal

Introduction

Ultrasonography of the neck and head is not performed very often. The most frequent reasons for its use are:

- examination of masses in the cervical or head region
- assessment of regional lymph nodes for metastasis
- assessment of the thyroid and parathyroid glands
- ultrasound-guided sampling
- investigation of laryngeal paralysis.

Patient Preparation and Technique

The sedated patient is usually placed in dorsal recumbency, with the neck extended. It is important that the patient is positioned straight and symmetrically because the head and neck together constitute an anatomically complex region. As most anatomical structures in the head and neck are bilateral, it is important to examine both sides and look for symmetry between the right and left sides. The area should be clipped extensively. A high-frequency linear probe is usually used because superficial structures will be evaluated. The location of the structures to be evaluated on ultrasonographic examination of the neck is shown in Fig. 1.

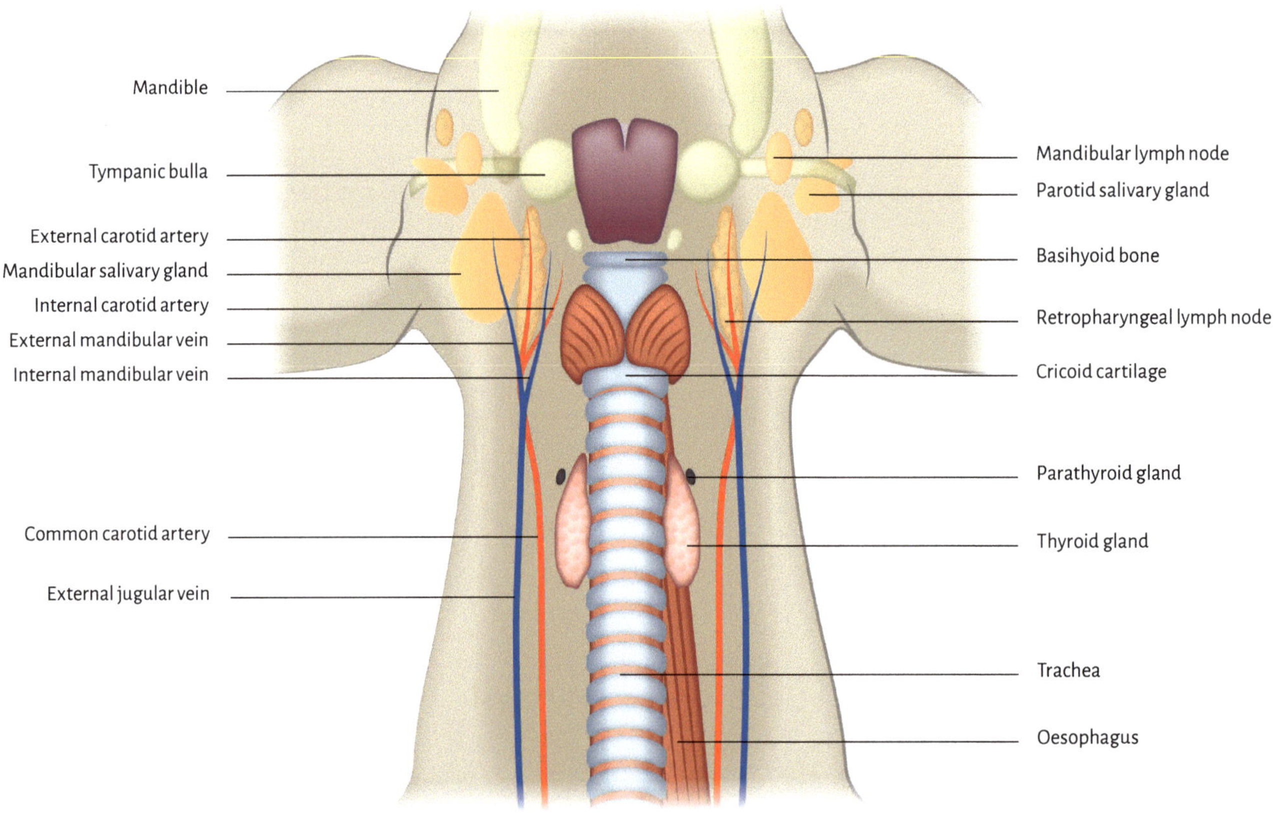

Figure 1. Representative diagram of the location of the cervical structures that can be evaluated using ultrasonography.

Lymph Nodes

Ultrasonographic Anatomy

The retropharyngeal and mandibular lymph nodes are normally evaluated. Both groups of lymph nodes are usually approximately 5 mm thick. The **retropharyngeal lymph nodes** (Fig. 2) are quite elongated (4–5 cm in length in dogs, 3–4 cm in cats) and are located caudomedial to the mandibular salivary gland. The **mandibular lymph nodes** (Fig. 3) are very superficial and are located around the linguofacial vein. There are usually two or three of these lymph nodes on each side. **Deep cervical lymph nodes** are usually poorly developed and are not usually visible ultrasonographically. **Superficial cervical lymph nodes** are located lateroventrally in the caudal part of the neck, cranial to the supraspinatus muscle. They are usually larger and their size correlates with the animal's body weight. Lymph nodes are usually isoechoic or slightly hypoechoic relative to the surrounding fat.

Pathological Findings

The pathologies that affect the lymph nodes are of inflammatory, infiltrative neoplastic or regional metastatic origin. Inflamed or neoplastic lymph nodes are usually enlarged, and their margins may appear poorly defined or irregular if the fat around them is inflamed. They are rounded and hypoechoic (Fig. 4). Occasionally, especially in cases of multicentric lymphoma in dogs, they can be anechoic and show posterior enhancement, so they can be confused with cysts or cystic lymph nodes. In inflammatory processes, lymph nodes may be cavitated due to abscess formation or, in the case of neoplastic nodules, due to necrosis or haemorrhage.

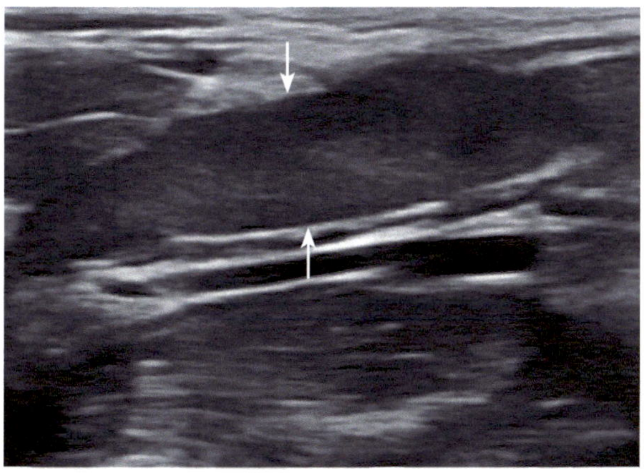

Figure 2. Ultrasound image of a retropharyngeal lymph node in a dog.

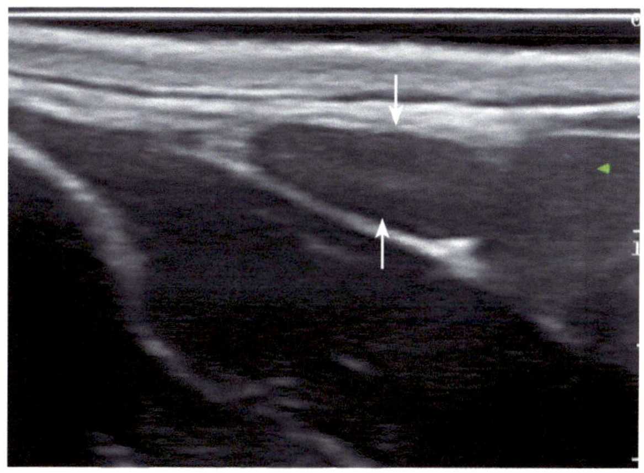

Figure 3. Ultrasound image of a mandibular lymph node in a dog.

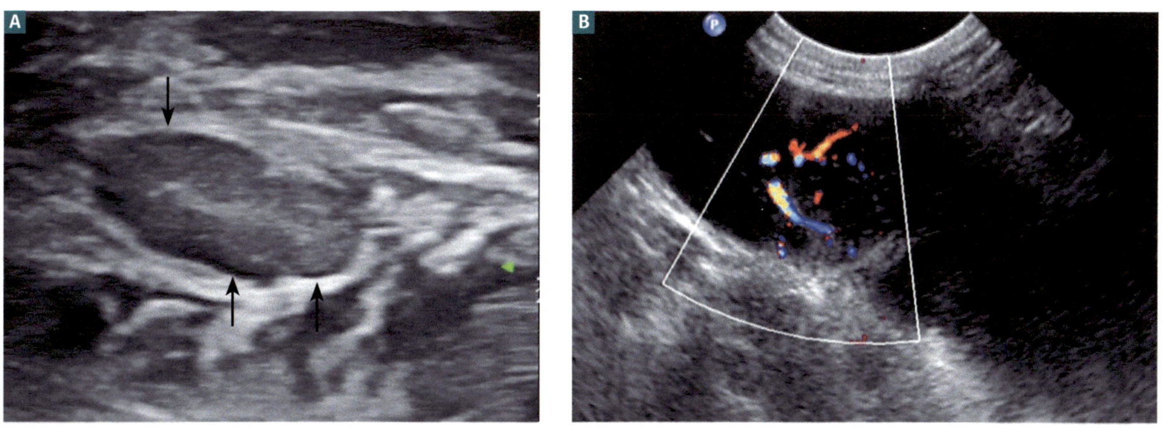

Figure 4. Ultrasound images of two lymph nodes in a dog. **A**. Reactive mandibular lymph node, which has irregular borders and a thin subcapsular hypoechoic halo (arrows); the surrounding fat is strongly hyperechoic. **B**. Neoplastic superficial cervical lymph node, which is enlarged, rounded and anechoic. Colour Doppler shows that it is vascularised and has no cystic content.

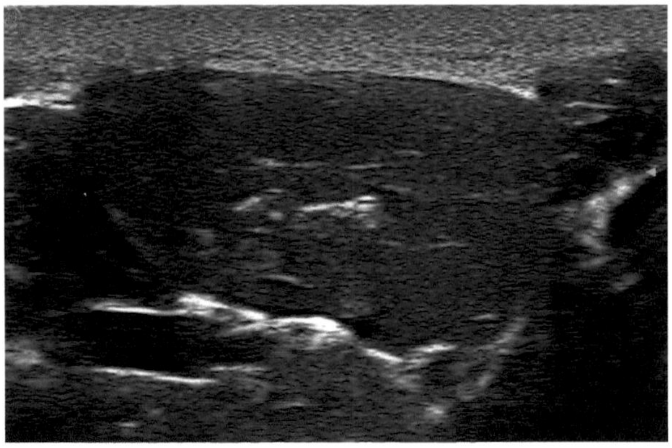

Figure 5. Ultrasound image of the mandibular salivary gland of a dog.

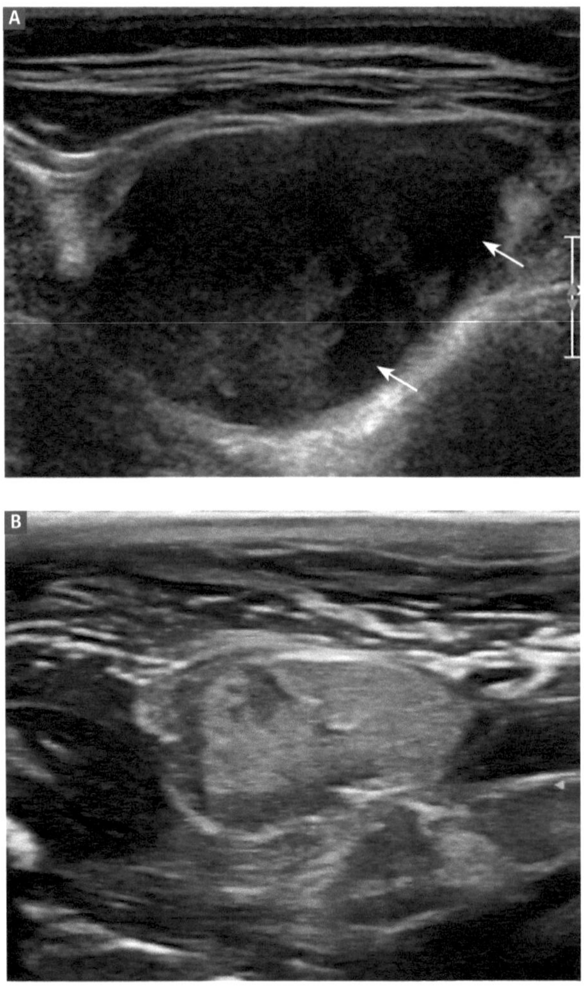

Figure 6. Ultrasound images of mandibular salivary glands from two dogs with sialadenitis and cellulitis/oedema in the neck. **A**. The salivary gland is increased in size and shows heterogeneous echogenicity and irregular anechoic foci (arrows). **B**. The salivary gland has a small, irregularly shaped hypoechoic focus.

Metastatic lymph nodes occasionally have a normal size and reduced or normal echogenicity. It is not possible to differentiate ultrasonographically between inflammatory and neoplastic processes. Performing a fine-needle aspiration is necessary to obtain a sample for cytology.

Salivary Glands

Ultrasonographic Anatomy

The **mandibular salivary gland** is located caudal to the mandibular ramus and lateral to the medial retropharyngeal lymph node. It is surrounded by the internal and external maxillary veins cranial to the junction where the jugular vein is formed. It is large, oval and hypoechoic, with hyperechoic striations in its interior. It has a hyperechoic central hilum and is surrounded by a thin hyperechoic capsule (Fig. 5). The **parotid salivary gland** is located ventral and lateral to the external auditory canal, and superficial and dorsal to the mandibular salivary gland. It is small and heterogeneous, with poorly defined edges, and distinguishing it ultrasonographically may not be possible.

Pathological Findings

Pathologies affecting the salivary glands include cysts, sialoliths, sialadenitis, sialocoele/mucocoele, salivary duct cysts and neoplasms. They are rare.

In **sialadenitis**, the salivary glands are enlarged and hypoechoic (Fig. 6). If there is obstruction of the duct, they may appear to be filled with liquid, and the duct may be visible. Sometimes a sialolith is observed inside. **Sialocoeles** can be associated with sialadenitis. If there is inflammation or oedema of the surrounding tissue, it may appear hyperechoic or striated. Sialocoeles have a thin wall and content ranging from anechoic to moderately hyperechoic. If the zygomatic salivary gland is affected, a mass effect may appear from the retrobulbar region. **Neoplasms** usually alter the normal shape and structure of the salivary gland and cause disruption of the capsule.

Thyroid Gland

Ultrasonographic Anatomy

The thyroid gland is composed of two lobes, the right and the left. The lobes are located caudal to the larynx and dorsolateral to the trachea, between the trachea and the common carotid artery, in an asymmetrical position. The oesophagus is located dorsal to the left lobe. The parenchyma of the thyroid gland is homogeneous and thin, and slightly hyperechoic.

The lobes are elongated and fusiform, with a rounded cranial rim and a pointed caudal rim. The size of each lobe is proportional to the size of the animal. In cats they measure approximately 2 × 0.2 × 0.3 cm (length × thickness × height). It is recommended to begin searching for the thyroid gland in a cross section; once it has been located, a sagittal section can be visualised to see both lobes individually.

Pathological Findings

Hyperthyroidism

Hyperthyroidism is common in older cats and is frecuently caused by an adenoma or adenomatous hyperplasia. A discrete nodule or diffuse enlargement of the thyroid gland may be observed. In 70% of cases both lobes are affected (Mooney, 2002) (Fig. 7).

- **Adenomatous hyperplasia**: the thyroid gland is isoechoic or hypoechoic to the surrounding tissue and is hypoechoic compared with a normal thyroid gland.
- **Benign neoplasm (adenoma)**: the thyroid gland may have a nodule or be generally enlarged. Hyperplasia cannot be differentiated from an adenoma ultrasonographically.
- **Incidental cysts**: these present posterior reinforcement, and should not be confused with parathyroid glands, which are also hypoechoic or anechoic but do not show posterior enhancement.

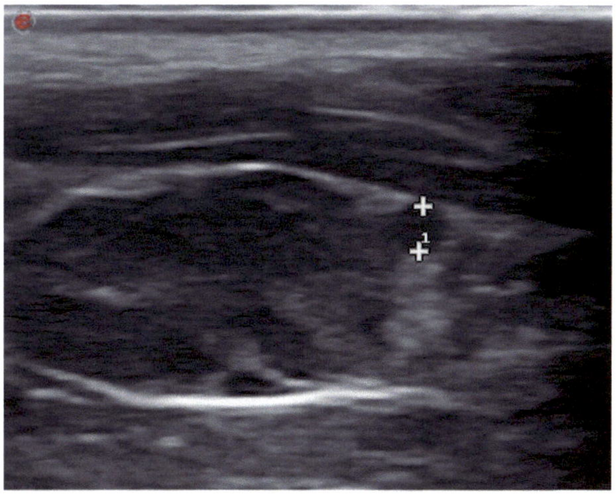

Figure 7. Ultrasound image of the thyroid gland of a cat, in which both lobes were enlarged and had heterogeneous echogenicity. The parathyroid gland is seen between the crosses, embedded in the parenchyma of the caudal pole of the thyroid gland.

Hypothyroidism

In hypothyroidism (in dogs), the thyroid gland is generally small, irregular and hypoechoic; however, it may be heterogeneous and have a capsule with irregular margins.

Thyroid carcinomas

Thyroid carcinomas (more common in dogs than in cats) are rare neoplasms and are usually very locally aggressive and metastatic. Retropharyngeal lymph nodes are usually affected. In approximately 50% of cases, mineralisation of the masses occurs, which can be observed as hyperechoic foci with a distal acoustic shadow. When the masses are very large, their origin may be difficult to determine by ultrasonography, so computed tomography or magnetic resonance imaging may be indicated. They can displace or invade other structures in the neck, especially blood vessels. **Ectopic thyroid carcinomas** can be located from the base of the tongue to the mediastinum.

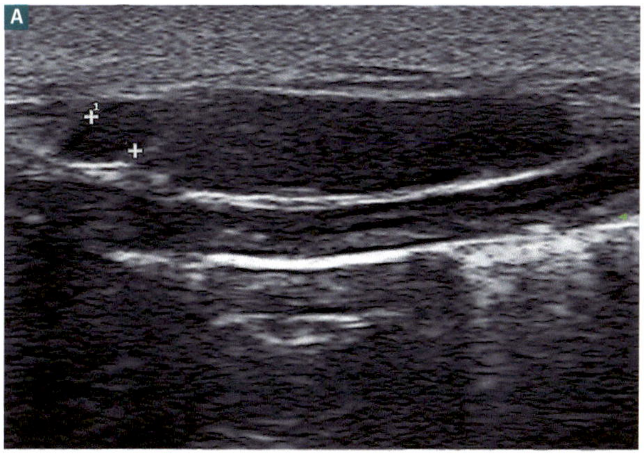

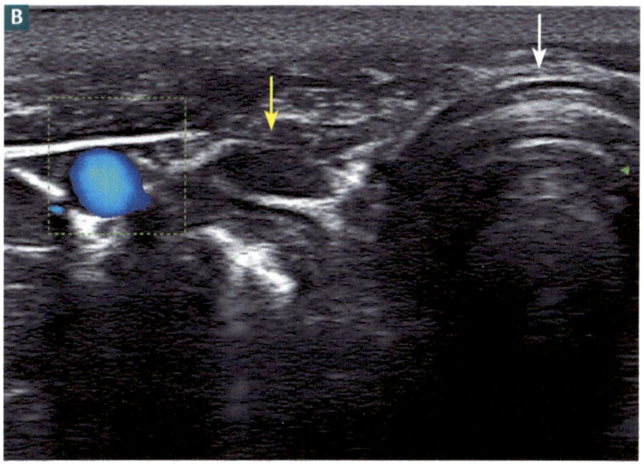

Figure 8. Sagittal (A) and transverse (B) ultrasound images of the thyroid gland in a dog. **A**. One of the parathyroid glands is located at the cranial pole of the thyroid lobe (between the crosses). **B**. Medial to the thyroid gland (yellow arrow) is the trachea (white arrow) and laterally is the carotid artery, indicated with colour Doppler.

Parathyroid Glands

Ultrasonographic Anatomy

There are usually two parathyroid glands associated with each thyroid lobe. One is adjacent to each cranial thyroid lobe (Fig. 8) and the other is embedded in the caudal part of the thyroid parenchyma (Fig. 7). They may vary in number and location between individuals. They are anechoic. They measure 2 × 3.3 mm (Reusch et al., 2000; Wisner et al., 1997). They can be difficult to visualise, especially in cats.

Pathological Findings

Pathologies affecting the parathyroid glands include **diffuse hyperplasia**, **adenomatous hyperplasia**, **adenomas** and, less frequently, **carcinomas**. All of them are characterised by enlargement of one or more of the parathyroid glands. In dogs with hypercalcaemia, it is important to differentiate between primary and secondary hyperparathyroidism (Reusch et al., 2000). In primary hyperparathyroidism, a single gland is enlarged. In secondary hyperparathyroidism (renal, nutritional or malignant hypercalcaemia), all the parathyroid glands are increased in size. They are usually more hyperechoic than normal parathyroid glands but remain hypoechoic relative to the thyroid gland. Regarding their size, nodules measuring more than 4 mm in diameter are usually of neoplastic origin (adenoma, carcinoma) and cause primary hyperparathyroidism. Nodules that are less than 4 mm in diameter are usually due to primary hyperplasia or have a secondary origin (renal, nutritional or malignant hypercalcaemia).

Vascular Structures

The vascular structures that can be evaluated ultrasonographically in the head and neck region are:

- common carotid artery:
  - external carotid artery
  - internal carotid artery
- external jugular vein:
  - linguofacial vein
  - maxillary vein.

Differentiation Between Arteries and Veins

Generally, arteries and veins can be differentiated by their location, wall echogenicity, pulsatility, flow direction on colour Doppler and firmness when pressure is exerted on them.

Pathologies

The pathologies that can be detected ultrasonographically are the following:

- thrombosis (Cushing's disease, protein-losing nephropathy, secondary to placement of an intravenous catheter, etc.) (Fig. 9)
  - anechoic: acute thrombosis
  - hyperechoic: chronic thrombosis
- stenosis
- aneurysm
- neoplasm: carotid body tumour (in brachycephalic breeds): hypoechoic, highly vascularised
- invasion by nearby neoplasia: carcinoma.

Larynx

Laryngeal Paralysis

Laryngeal paralysis is a neuropathy of the recurrent laryngeal nerve. It causes unilateral or bilateral paralysis of the vocal cords. Ultrasonography can be used to observe a reduction or asymmetry in the movement of the vocal cords or cuneiform cartilages; this is observed in approximately 50% of dogs with suspected laryngeal paralysis. Other associated signs are laryngeal collapse during inspiration and caudal displacement of the larynx.

Other Pathologies

Other pathologies that can be identified by ultrasonography are:

- laryngeal neoplasms (hypoechoic masses)
- laryngeal/retropharyngeal abscesses.

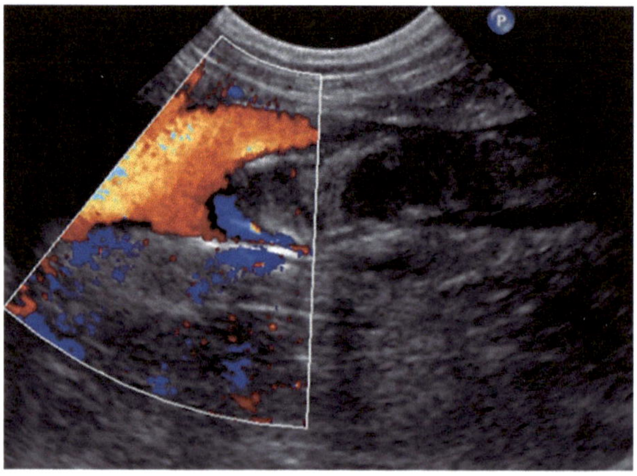

Figure 9. Ultrasonographic appearance of a thrombus. The blood vessel appears in a longitudinal position, and a hyperechoic thrombus can be seen inside it. Doppler helps to identify the lack of blood flow in the vessel caused by the thrombus.

Other Cervical Masses

Cervical masses with origins other than the lymph nodes, or the thyroid and parathyroid glands, can be haematomas, abscesses or neoplasms (mainly sarcomas and lipomas). **Neoplasms** are usually solid and have variable or mixed echogenicity. **Haematomas** are usually hypoechoic in their acute phase. Over time their echogenicity increases, septa may appear, and they reduce in size and eventually disappear. **Abscesses** usually have a thick wall and hypoechoic contents; they may be associated with penetrating wounds or migrating foreign bodies. **Foreign bodies** are usually observed as hyperechoic structures with distal acoustic shadowing. They are usually associated with **oedema**, which is observed ultrasonographically as hypoechoic or anechoic areas separated by thin hyperechoic septa. The inflamed fatty tissue appears thickened and hyperechoic.

Retrobulbar Space

The retrobulbar space should be explored with a high-frequency linear probe. It can be accessed through the cornea or eyelid, using the eyeball as an acoustic window.

Under normal conditions it is possible to observe a cone-shaped area; the edges of the cone are the extraocular muscles, which appear as two hypoechoic lines. The muscles are surrounded by fat that appears hyperechoic. In the centre of the image the optic nerve can be observed as a central hypoechoic line. The main pathologies that are seen in this location are haemorrhages, abscesses, neoplasms and inflammation (myositis or cellulitis) (Fig. 10).

Bibliography

- Barr, F., Gaschen, L. (2011) *BSAVA Manual of Canine and Feline Ultrasonography*. 1st ed. BSAVA.
- Boysen, SR., Lisciandro, GR. (2013) The use of ultrasound for dogs and cats in the emergency room: AFAST and TFAST. *Vet Clin North Am Small Anim Pract*, 43(4):773–797.
- Doyle, A.J., Miller, M.V., French, J.G. (2000) Ultrasound of soft-tissue masses: pitfalls in interpretation. *Australas Radiol*, 44(3):275–280.
- Mattoon, J.S., Nyland, T.G. (2015) *Small Animal Diagnostic Ultrasound*. 3rd ed. Elsevier Saunders.
- Mooney, C.T. (2002) Pathogenesis of feline hyperthyroidism. *J Feline Med Surg*, 4(3):167–179.
- Penninck, D., d'Anjou, M-A. (2015) *Atlas of Small Animal Ultrasonography*, 2nd ed. Wiley-Blackwell.
- Reusch, C.E., Tomsa, K., Zimmer, C., et al. (2000) Ultrasonography of the parathyroid glands as an aid in differentiation of acute and chronic renal failure in dogs. *J Am Vet Med Assoc*, 217(12):1849–1852.
- Rudorf, H., Barr, F.J., Lane, J.G. (2001) The role of ultrasound in the assessment of laryngeal paralysis in the dog. *Vet Radiol Ultrasound*, 42(4):338–343.
- Wisner, E.R., Penninck, D., Biller, D.S., et al. (1997) High-resolution parathyroid sonography. *Vet Radiol Ultrasound*, 38(6):462–466.

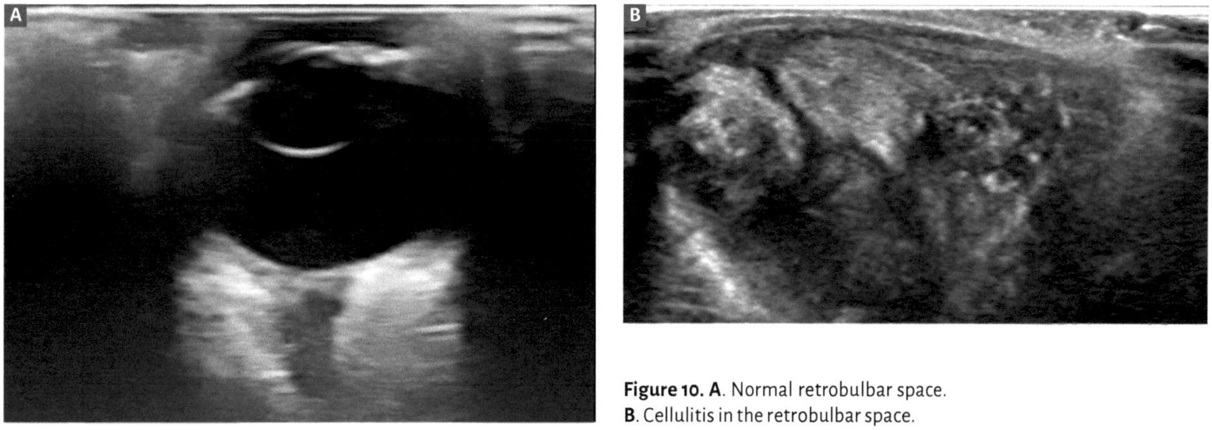

Figure 10. A. Normal retrobulbar space.
B. Cellulitis in the retrobulbar space.

Self-assessment

(Answers on page 458)

COMPUTED TOMOGRAPHY

Xavier Sánchez Salguero

1. Which of the following combinations of window width (WW) and window level (WL) should be selected to assess lung parenchyma?
   a. WW 300/WL 1500.
   b. WW 1500 / WL -500.
   c. WW 400/WL 60.
   d. None of the above are correct.

2. Which of the following combinations of parameters should be used for a CT study where the intention is to rule out the presence of lung metastases?
   a. 5 mm sections, 80 kV, 50 mA.
   b. 3 mm sections, 140 kV, 150 mA.
   c. 4 mm sections, 100 kV, 100 mA.
   d. 1.25 mm sections, 120 kV, 300 mA.

3. Which of the following combinations, for the interpretation windows in images A and B, is correct?
   a. A: bone window, B: lung window.
   b. A: lung window, B: bone window.
   c. A: soft tissue window, B: bone window.
   d. A: lung window, B: mediastinal window.

4. Which of the following combinations in image C is correct?
   a. Sagittal reconstruction, MinIP projection.
   b. Dorsal reconstruction, MIP projection.
   c. Transverse section, MIP projection.
   d. Dorsal reconstruction, MinIP projection.

5. Which of the following combinations, related to the planes of the reconstructions in images D, E and F, is correct?
   a. D: dorsal, E: transverse, F: sagittal.
   b. D: sagittal, E: dorsal, F: transverse.
   c. D: sagittal, E: transverse, F: dorsal.
   d. D: transverse, E: dorsal, F: sagittal.

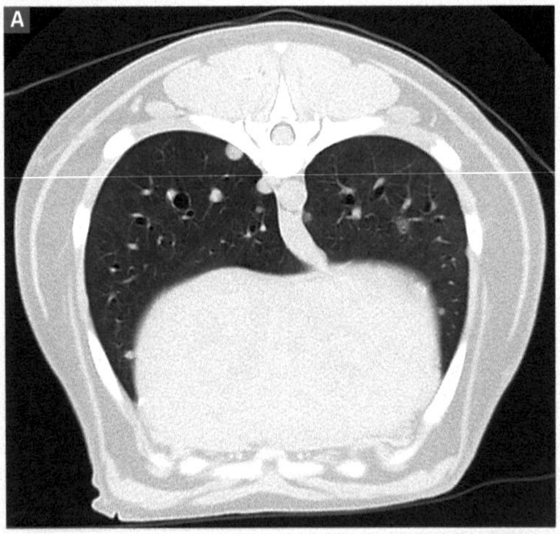

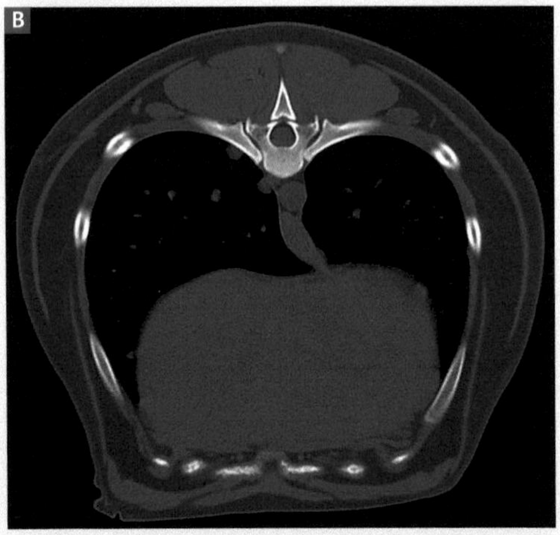

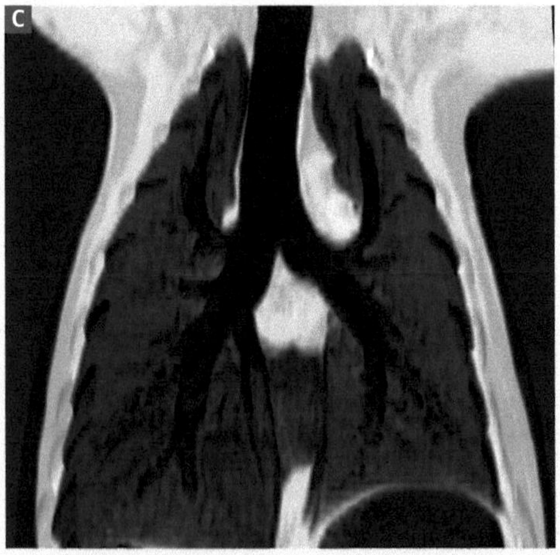

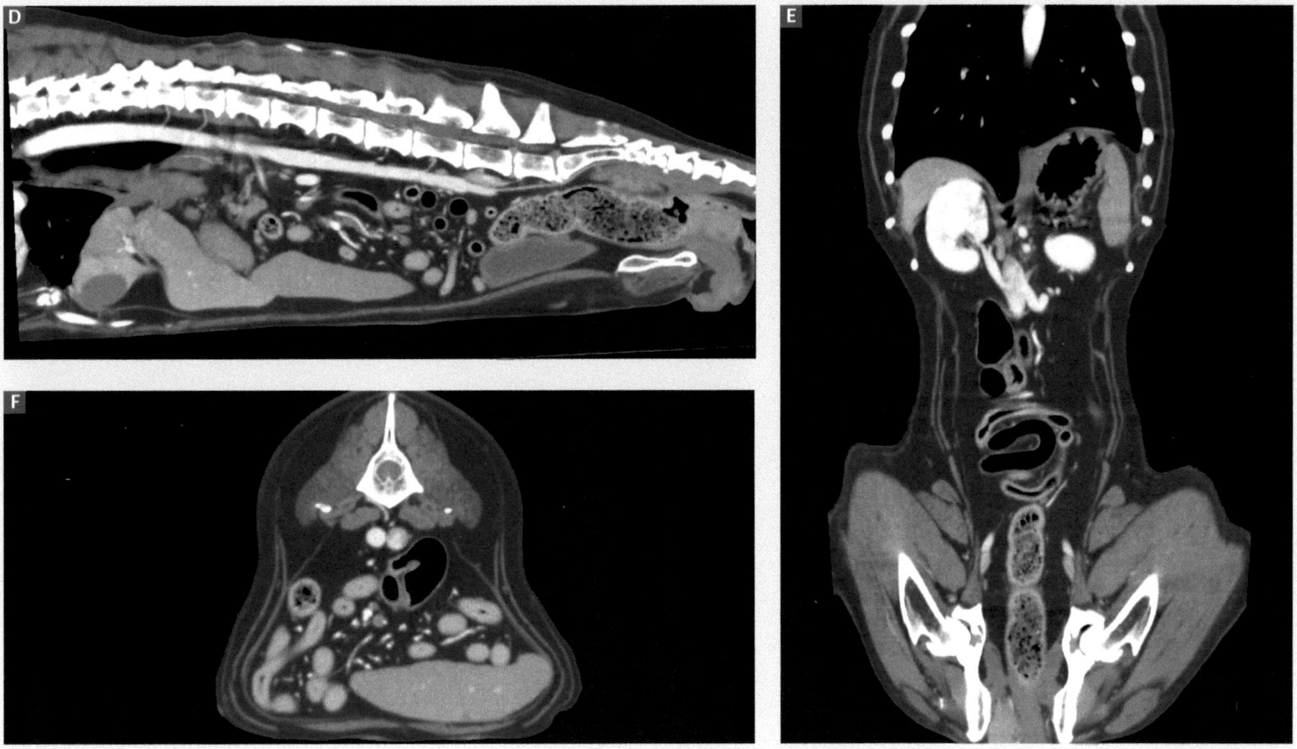
D
E
F

Magnetic Resonance Imaging

Pablo Amengual Batle

Test

1. **Which of the following statements is true regarding protons?**
   a. Only protons exposed to a powerful external magnetic field rotate on their axis.
   b. In the presence of an external magnetic field, all protons are parallel to it.
   c. Precession movement is defined as the movement that a proton makes when rotating around its axis, like a spinning top losing speed.
   d. The Larmor equation shows that the stronger the external magnetic field, the lower the precession speed.

2. **Which of the following statements is true regarding magnetisation vectors?**
   a. The longitudinal magnetisation created by protons can be detected by magnetic resonance.
   b. The transverse magnetisation created by protons can be detected by magnetic resonance.
   c. Sending a radiofrequency pulse allows protons to maintain their longitudinal magnetisation.
   d. When capturing energy using the radiofrequency pulse, the precession movement of the protons loses coordination, which is known as phase shift.

3. **Which of the following statements is true about relaxation times?**
   a. T1 relaxation is caused by phase loss between the different protons in the precession motion.
   b. T1 relaxation can be described as the time in which 37% of the transverse magnetisation is lost.
   c. T2 relaxation occurs when protons realign with the external magnetic field, increasing their longitudinal magnetisation.
   d. T2 relaxation can be described as the time in which 37% of the transverse magnetisation is lost.

4. **Which of the following statements is true regarding MRI sequences?**
   a. Spin echo sequences are characterised by a 90° radiofrequency pulse followed by a second 180° pulse.
   b. The 90° pulse is of utmost importance, as it allows the effects caused by external interference to be eliminated.
   c. Inversion recovery sequences, such as T2*, suppress the signal of certain tissues, such as free fluid or fat.
   d. In reversal recovery sequences, reversal time is defined as the time between 90° pulses.

5. **Which of the following statements is true regarding T1-enhanced sequences?**
   a. In this case, long repetition times are used, to enhance the T1 relaxation effect.
   b. The use of short echo times allows the T2 relaxation effect to be minimised.
   c. In this sequence, fluid and soft tissue have a similar intensity, whereas fat is hypointense.
   d. They are mainly used to detect pathological processes.

6. **Which of the following structures physiologically captures contrast?**
   a. Caudate nuclei.
   b. Facial nerve.
   c. Pituitary gland.
   d. Olfactory recesses.

7. **Which of the following statements is true regarding T2-enhanced sequences?**
   a. Long repetition times are used to minimise the T1 relaxation effect.
   b. In conventional T2-enhanced sequences, fluid appears hyperintense whereas fat is hypointense.
   c. The main use of this sequence is anatomical, especially when compared with FLAIR.
   d. The use of fast and turbo spin echo T2W sequences allows fluid to appear hypointense.

8. **Which of the following statements is true about inversion recovery sequences?**
   a. An initial pulse of 180° is used.
   b. In the case of FLAIR, the inversion time is short.
   c. In the case of STIR, the inversion time is long.
   d. After the 180° pulse, a second pulse of between 50° and 70° is performed, unlike in spin echo sequences, in which it is 90°.

Clinical Case

- 13-year-old male neutered Golden Retriever, with a chronic history (1 month) of head tilt to the left side, dragging the left side of the body and right-sided facial paralysis.
- The physical examination was normal.
- Neurological examination shows the mental state to be mildly affected, with a marked head tilt to the left and vestibular ataxia with a tendency to fall to the left. In addition, some proprioceptive ataxia is observed, especially on the left side of the body. Postural responses are decreased on the left side and normal on the right. Spinal reflexes are normal. Absence of the threat response is observed on the left side, as well as absence of the left eyelid reflex and horizontal spontaneous pathological nystagmus with the rapid phase on the right. No pain is observed on palpation of the spine or manipulation of the neck.

1. **Where is the lesion located?**

2. **Which tests should be performed on this animal?**
   An MRI of the head is performed, which reveals the following (Fig. 1).

3. **From these images, identify the following:**
   A. Region shown/structures present.
   B. Type of sequences.
   C. Plane of these sequences.

4. **Describe the lesion based on the parameters previously described.**

5. **List four differential diagnoses for this lesion.**

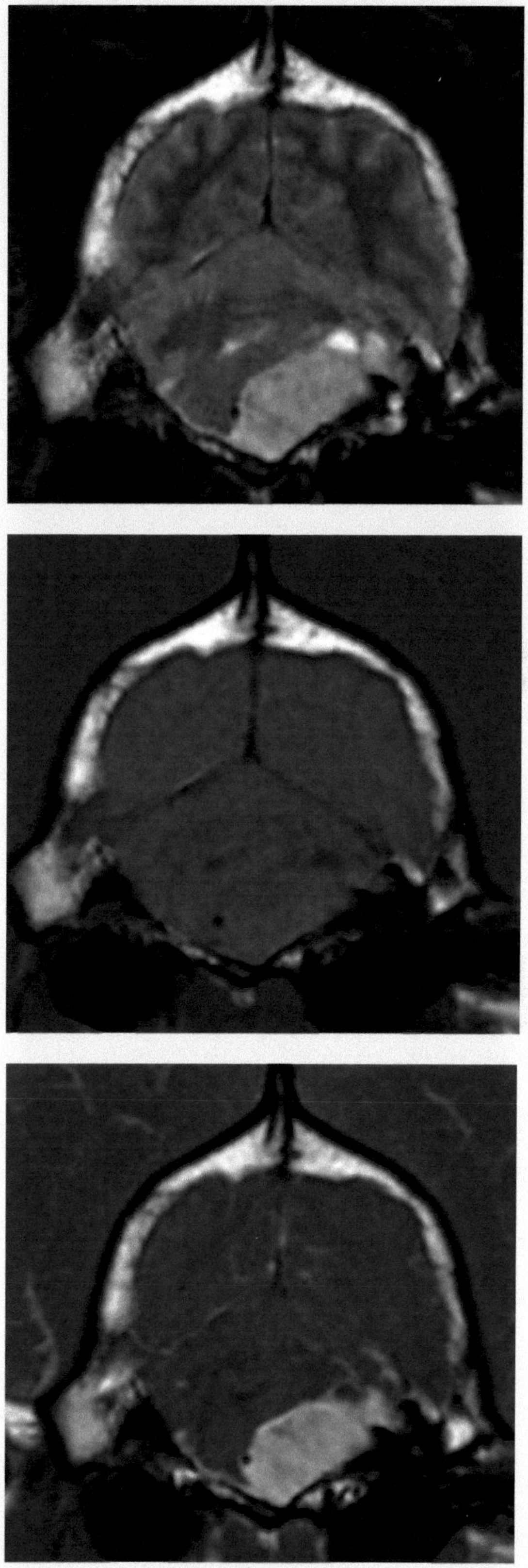

Figure 1. MRI of the head.

Abdominal Lymph Node Ultrasonography

Raquel Salgüero Fernández

Test

1. **What is the technique of choice for the evaluation of abdominal lymph nodes in first opinion practice?**
   a. Radiography.
   b. Ultrasonography.
   c. Computed tomography.
   d. Magnetic resonance.

2. **What probes should be used to get a better picture of the iliac lymph nodes in a kitten?**
   a. Convex.
   b. Microconvex.
   c. Linear.
   d. The choice of probe is not important.

3. **The medial iliac lymph nodes are part of which lymph centre?**
   a. Aortic lymph centre.
   b. Iliosacral lymph centre.
   c. Mesenteric lymph centre.
   d. They do not belong to any lymph centre.

4. **Which of the following statements is false?**
   a. Puppies have larger iliac lymph nodes than adult dogs.
   b. Puppies have iliac lymph nodes similar in size to those of adults.
   c. Mesenteric lymph nodes are larger in puppies than in adults.
   d. The lymph nodes in puppies may have a different ultrasonographic appearance.

5. **The lymph nodes in normal patients are usually:**
   a. Hyperechoic relative to fat.
   b. Isoechoic to hypoechoic relative to fat.
   c. Heterogeneous in echogenicity.
   d. Hypoechoic with a perinodal reaction.

6. **Which of the following statements is true?**
   a. Most normal lymph nodes do not present vascularisation when examined using Doppler.
   b. In normal situations, vascularisation can be identified in all lymph nodes.
   c. Normal vascularisation of the lymph nodes is peripheral.
   d. Colour Doppler is not required to assess lymphatic vascularisation.

7. **When can mineralisation be found in lymph nodes?**
   a. In normal patients.
   b. In reactive lymph nodes.
   c. In cases of metastasis of prostate carcinomas.
   d. Mineralisation is never found in lymph nodes.

8. **What is the normal ratio between the short axis and the long axis (S/L) of a lymph node?**
   a. >0.7.
   b. <0.7.
   c. 1.
   d. >2.

9. **How are areas of necrosis in lymph nodes visualised ultrasonographically?**
   a. Anechoic lesions with posterior reinforcement or enhancement.
   b. Hyperechoic lesions with posterior reinforcement or enhancement.
   c. No areas of necrosis can be identified ultrasonographically.
   d. Hypoechoic lesions.

10. **In cases of feline infectious peritonitis (FIP), the lymph nodes are:**
   a. Always enlarged.
   b. Always normal in size and echogenicity.
   c. Variable, from normal to greatly enlarged in size.
   d. Lymph nodes are not usually evaluated in cases of FIP.

Clinical Case

- 8-month-old unneutered female cat, weighing 2.5 kg, with a history of decline, hyporexia and weight loss. Leukaemia positive.
- Clinical examination showed poor body condition, fever (40 °C) and abdominal pain. Cardiac and pulmonary auscultation was normal.
- Complete blood count showed marked anaemia (haematocrit 11%) and biochemistry showed a slight increase in amylase (1670 U/L, reference range: 410–1100).
- Abdominal ultrasonographic examination demonstrated the presence of a moderate amount of hyperechoic abdominal free fluid (Fig. 1 A), as well as thickening and a hyperechoic appearance to the peritoneum. In addition, there was generalised thickening of the intestinal loops (3.8–5 mm). Cranial ileocolic and mesenteric lymph nodes appeared moderately enlarged (7.3 mm thick) with rounded edges, and were slightly heterogeneous but mainly hypoechoic in appearance (Figs. 1 B and 1 C).
- Abdominocentesis was performed, as well as fine-needle aspiration of the abnormal lymph nodes. The abdominal fluid was compatible with an inflammatory exudate that was positive on the Rivalta test, and cytology was compatible with a granulomatous process.
- Clinical, analytical, ultrasonographic, and fluid and lymph node findings confirmed the presence of feline infectious peritonitis.

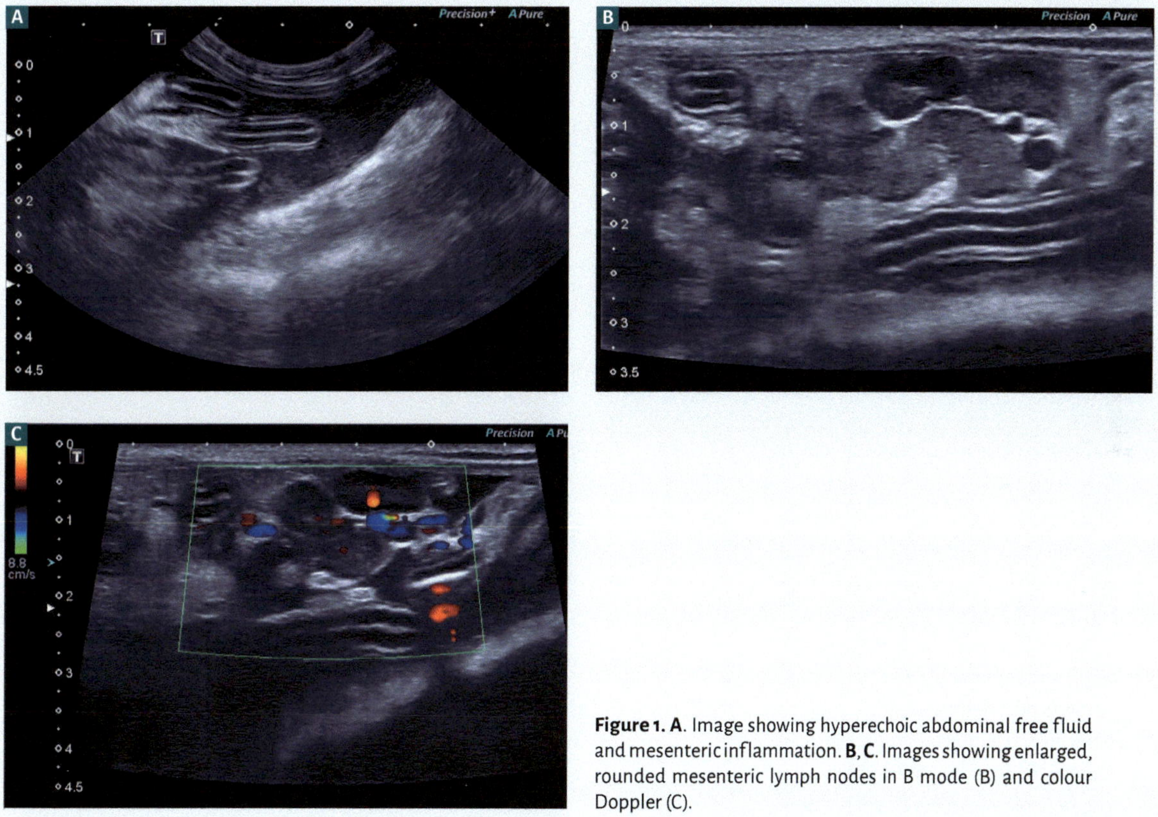

Figure 1. A. Image showing hyperechoic abdominal free fluid and mesenteric inflammation. **B, C**. Images showing enlarged, rounded mesenteric lymph nodes in B mode (B) and colour Doppler (C).

Application of Doppler

Abby Caine

Test

1. **Which is the most cranial vessel entering the portal vein, immediately cranial to the hepatic hilum (porta hepatis)?**
    a. Cranial mesenteric vein.
    b. Caudal mesenteric vein.
    c. Splenic vein.
    d. Gastroduodenal vein.

2. **Which of the following presentations would not be considered a possible cause of thromboembolism, according to Virchow's triad?**
    a. A cat with hypertrophic cardiomyopathy.
    b. A dog with a right adrenal tumour.
    c. A cat with a right circumcaval ureter.
    d. A dog that had undergone splenectomy the previous day.

3. **Adrenal tumours can invade:**
    a. The aorta.
    b. The caudal vena cava.
    c. The internal thoracic vein.
    d. The portal vein.

4. **A duplicate caudal vena cava:**
    a. Is a congenital anomaly discovered by chance.
    b. Is always associated with congenital portal anomalies.
    c. Is due to the presence of a common coeliacomesenteric trunk.
    d. Increases the incidence of renal vein thrombosis.

5. **A mean hepatopetal portal velocity of 28 cm/s in a dog measured in the hepatic hilum can be seen in:**
    a. Hepatic carcinoma.
    b. Portal vein thrombus.
    c. Arterioportal fistula.
    d. An intrahepatic portocaval shunt.

Clinical Case

An 11-year-old female neutered Border Terrier was presented as an emergency with pyrexia, neutrophilia with left shift, and abdominal pain. On clinical examination the dog was cardiovascularly stable, and on examination with point-of-care ultrasound (POCUS) there was no abdominal free fluid.

During the abdominal ultrasound examination, a left adrenal mass was identified (see Fig. 1, obtained from a right dorsolateral approach, in which the mass can be seen in the left adrenal gland *); the mass was located deep to the cranial mesenteric artery and the coeliac trunk (white arrows). The caudal vena cava was dilated, and completely full at this level with material of heterogeneous echogenicity (between the yellow arrowheads). In Video 1 (which can be viewed at: publication.improveinternational.com) the ultrasound scan can be seen, using a right lateral approach to the caudal vena cava, from cranial to caudal; material can be seen filling the caudal vena cava and extending along the entire abdominal portion of the vessel, and can be seen extending as far as the paired renal veins and the external iliac veins.

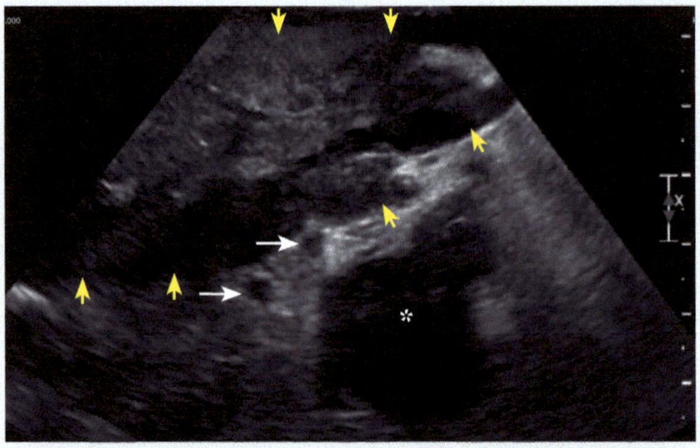

Figure 1. Right dorsolateral approach in which a mass is observed in the left adrenal gland (*), deep to the coeliac trunk and the cranial mesenteric artery (white arrows). The caudal vena cava (CVC) was dilated and filled with a material with heterogeneous echogenicity (between the yellow arrowheads). The CVC can be seen in detail in Video 1.

Portal vein flow was normal (Fig. 2), with an average hepatopetal portal velocity of 16 cm/s.

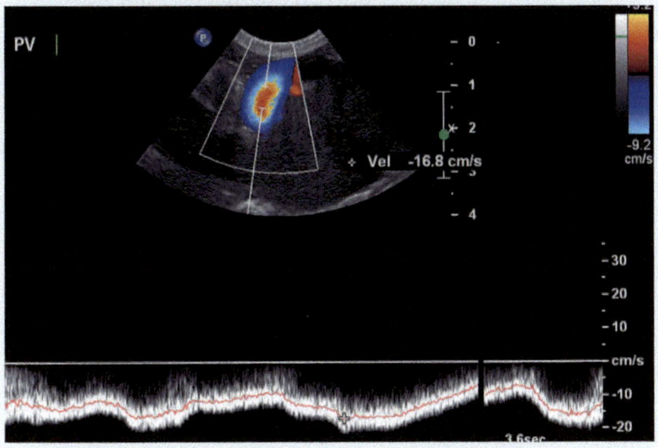

Figure 2. Image showing normal flow in the portal vein.

The retroperitoneal fat was hyperechoic compared with what was expected. Among the fat, several fine, branch-shaped, anechoic structures presenting blood flow were visualised (Fig. 3, and also in Video 2 (which can be viewed at: publication.improveinternational.com), in which the retroperitoneal space is scanned caudally from the caudal pole of the kidney). These vessels were in a location where there are normally no vessels.

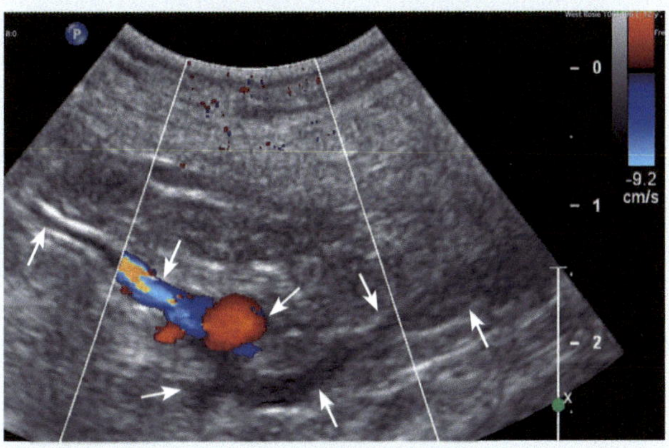

Figure 3. Several vessels were observed in the retroperitoneal fat, in locations where they are not usually present (see Video 2).

The conclusion after the ultrasound examination was that a malignant neoplasm of the left adrenal gland had caused a thromboembolism that completely filled the caudal vena cava and some of the veins draining into it. This completely obstructed the caudal vena cava and consequently collateral vessels had developed to maintain venous return to the heart. These vessels differ from an acquired portosystemic shunt that develops due to portal hypertension (in this case there was no portal hypertension), because these shunts go from the systemic venous circulation to the systemic venous circulation. An article written by Specchi et al. (2014) describes the patterns of collateral circulation identified by CT that develop as a result of a caudal vena cava obstruction in the dog. This location represents an intermediate pathway between the ureters and the uterus (if present); however, other pathways have been identified, including superficial (subcutaneous) vessels and a deep pathway through the lumbar veins and within the vertebral venous plexus, as well as systemic venous circulation to a portal collateral pathway. Many of these pathways could not be identified on ultrasonography due to their location; however, if detected, they must be confirmed to be a consequence of caudal vena cava obstruction and not the result of a separate pathology.

Liver, Spleen, Gastrointestinal, Urinary, Reproductive and Adrenal Glands

Amalia Agut

1. **How are lymphangiectasias visualised on ultrasound in cases of protein-losing enteropathies?**
   a. Hyperechoic lines in the mucosal layer.
   b. Thickened muscular layer.
   c. Thickened mucosal layer.
   d. Hyperechoic lines in the muscular layer.

2. **In an ultrasound of a normal dog's liver, how would you identify the hepatic artery?**
   a. By its hyperechoic walls.
   b. It is not visualised.
   c. By its hypoechoic walls.
   d. As an anechoic structure.

3. **Which of these statements is true regarding ultrasound?**
   a. The spleen is isoechoic compared to the liver.
   b. The spleen is hypoechoic compared to the renal sinus.
   c. The spleen is hypoechoic compared to the renal cortex.
   d. All are true.

4. **Indicate the correct answer:**
   a. The intestinal serosa layer is hypoechoic.
   b. The intestinal mucosa layer is hyperechoic.
   c. The intestinal muscular layer is hypoechoic.
   d. The intestinal submucosa layer is hypoechoic.

5. **In the case of a generalised decrease in liver echogenicity, which of the following could be the cause?**
   a. Hepatitis.
   b. Lipidosis.
   c. Steroid hepatopathy.
   d. Fibrosis.

6. **Indicate the correct answer regarding biliary mucocele:**
   a. It produces acoustic shadowing.
   b. It is more frequently observed in cats than in dogs.
   c. The characteristic image is usually that of a "kiwi image."
   d. It is a mobile echogenic material inside the gallbladder.

7. **What ultrasound measurement is recommended to estimate the age of the foetus in the first half of gestation?**
   a. Outer diameter of the embryonic sac.
   b. Inner diameter of the embryonic sac.
   c. Outer biparietal diameter.
   d. Inner biparietal diameter.

8. **What is the most sensitive measure of changes in the size of the adrenal glands?**
   a. The thickness of the cranial pole in the longitudinal plane.
   b. The thickness of the caudal pole in the longitudinal plane.
   c. The thickness of the cranial pole in the transverse plane.
   d. The thickness of the caudal pole in the transverse plane.

9. **The size of the kidney in dogs, evaluated by ultrasound, can be estimated by the ratio of the length of the kidney to the diameter of the aorta, which is considered normal if:**
   a. It is less than 5.5.
   b. It is greater than 5.5 and less than 9.1.
   c. It is greater than 9.1.
   d. It is greater than 3.5 and less than 7.3.

10. **The hyperechoic line at the corticomedullary junction can be observed in:**
    a. Healthy dogs.
    b. Dogs with renal lymphoma.
    c. Dogs with ethylene glycol poisoning.
    d. All are true.

Thoracic Radiography

Vicente Esteve Bernet

Test

1. **Select the correct answer regarding alveolar patterns:**
   a. In pulmonary oedema due to heart failure, a cranioventral distribution can be expected.
   b. A vesicular pattern is characteristic of pulmonary torsion.
   c. It is possible to visualise the blood vessels.
   d. In patients with aspiration pneumonia, a perihilar distribution is seen most often.

2. **Select the correct answer regarding interstitial patterns:**
   a. This pattern indicates the most serious type of pulmonary pathologies.
   b. The silhouette sign is characteristic of this type of pattern.
   c. An increase in pulmonary radiopacity is observed, but visualisation of the blood vessels is possible.
   d. The unstructured interstitial pattern is characteristic of lung metastases.

3. **Select the correct answer regarding bronchial patterns:**
   a. Finding an increase in the radiopacity of the bronchial walls in chondrodystrophic patients is always secondary to a pathological process.
   b. Bronchiectasis is typical of acute processes.
   c. Aerial bronchograms are pathognomonic for this type of pattern.
   d. They are characterised by an increase in the thickness or radiopacity of the bronchial walls.

4. **Select the correct answer regarding pulmonary pathologies:**
   a. Primary pulmonary neoplasms, such as bronchoalveolar carcinomas, typically produce small-sized pulmonary nodules with a multifocal distribution.
   b. Bronchopneumonia mainly has a caudodorsal distribution.
   c. Pulmonary fibrosis characteristically presents with an alveolar pattern of multifocal distribution.
   d. All the above are incorrect.

5. **Select the correct answer regarding thoracic radiographs:**
   a. Thoracic radiographs are performed on expiration, to decrease kinetic blurring produced by movement during the respiratory cycle.
   b. Normally only one projection is performed, either a lateral or a ventrodorsal (VD) view.
   c. The imaging technique of choice to search for lung metastases is radiography.
   d. Lateral views with the X-ray beam horizontal help in the detection of pneumothorax, mainly when there is a small amount of air in the pleural space.

6. **Select the correct answer regarding pulmonary vessels:**
   a. On a lateral radiograph the pulmonary vessels of the caudal lobes can be assessed.
   b. On a lateral radiograph the arteries are ventral to the bronchus and the veins are dorsal.
   c. On a VD/DV radiograph the pulmonary vessels of the caudal lobes can be assessed.
   d. On a VD/DV radiograph the arteries are medial to the main bronchus and the veins are lateral.

7. **Select the incorrect answer regarding vascular patterns:**
   a. An increase in the size of the pulmonary arteries may be compatible with dirofilariasis.
   b. An increase in the size of the pulmonary veins may be compatible with left-sided heart failure.
   c. A decrease in the size of the pulmonary vessels may be compatible with dehydration.
   d. An increase in the size of both the pulmonary arteries and pulmonary veins may be associated with mild cases of left-sided heart failure.

8. **Select the correct answer regarding the pleural space:**
   a. On a lateral thoracic radiograph, dorsal displacement of the cardiac silhouette is pathognomonic for pneumothorax.
   b. In a tension pneumothorax, ipsilateral displacement of the mediastinal structures can be seen.
   c. In a tension pneumothorax, contralateral displacement of the mediastinal structures can be seen.
   d. The primary neoplasm found in the pleura is haemangiosarcoma.

9. Select the correct answer regarding the pleural space:

a. In patients with pleural effusion, a VD radiograph must be performed to visualise the cardiac silhouette.

b. In patients with pleural effusion, a DV radiograph must be performed order to visualise the cardiac silhouette.

c. In patients with pleural effusion, a right lateral radiograph must be performed to visualise the cardiac silhouette.

d. In patients with pleural effusion a DV radiograph with the X-ray beam horizontal must be performed to visualise the cardiac silhouette.

Clinical Case

A domestic shorthair cat was brought into the practice presenting with tachypnoea and a chronic cough.

Radiographic description

- Skeletally mature cat.
- Radiographs show a severe bronchial pattern, diffusely distributed throughout the pulmonary parenchyma (Fig. 1, red arrows), with thickening of the bronchial wall possibly due to a peribronchial infiltrate.
- There is excessive distance from the heart to the diaphragm and slight flattening of the diaphragmatic crura; this may be indicative of inspiratory effort secondary to bronchial disease.
- Old rib fractures with bone callus formation (Fig. 1, yellow arrows), possibly secondary to old trauma or pathological fractures due to inspiratory effort.
- In the left cranial lobe in the ventral area (Fig. 1, black circle) there is an area with increased radiopacity and loss of visualisation of blood vessels, a focal alveolar pattern, possibly due to mucous exudate or obstruction of the main bronchus.

Differential diagnoses

The most likely diagnoses to be considered should be severe feline asthma, neoplasia (bronchoalveolar carcinoma) or haematogenous bacterial infection.

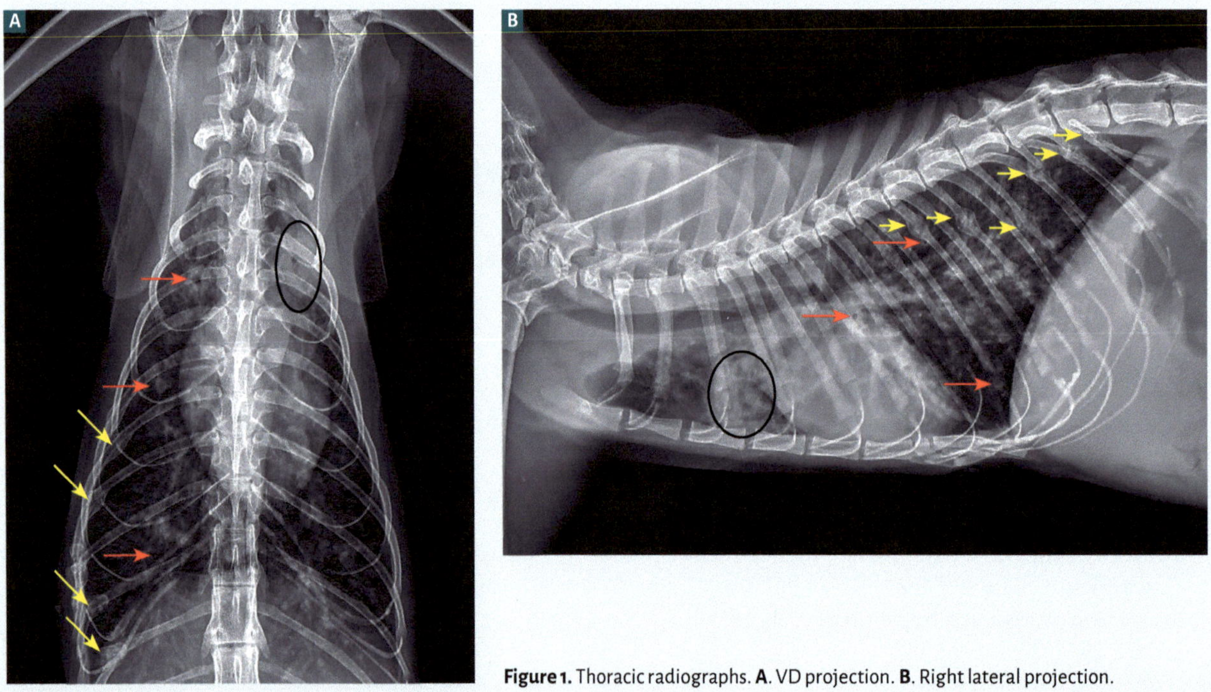

Figure 1. Thoracic radiographs. **A.** VD projection. **B.** Right lateral projection.

Cardiac and Mediastinal Thorax

Patricia Laborda Vidal

Test

1. **On the following thoracic radiographs of a 3-year-old English Bulldog, the most likely diagnosis is:**

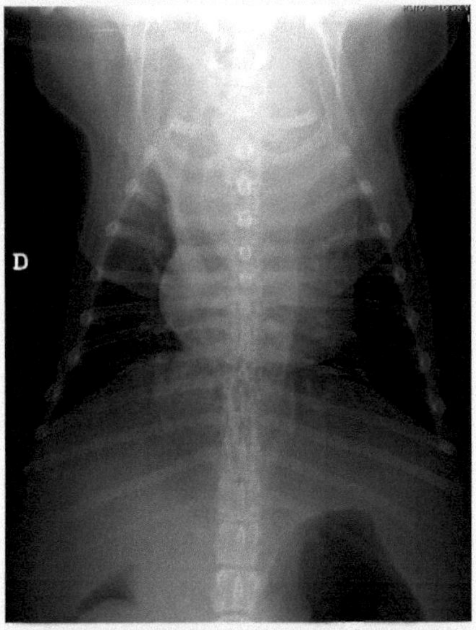

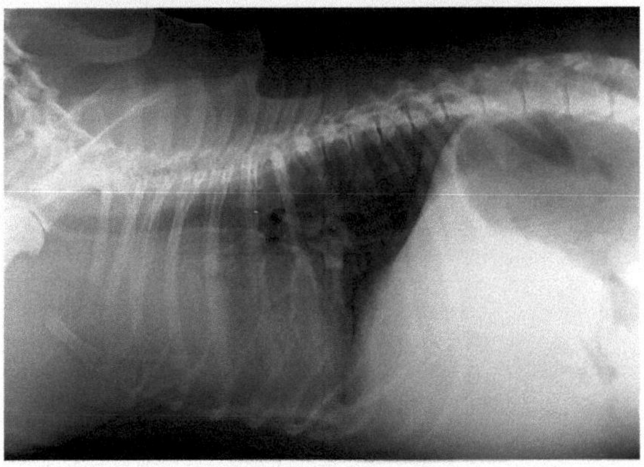

   a. Normal thoracic radiograph, taking the breed into account.
   b. Lymphoma, with cranial mediastinal lymphadenopathy.
   c. Left cranial lung lobe torsion.
   d. Persistence of the fourth right aortic arch.

2. **Which of the following options is false according to the clock analogy, in the dorsoventral view?**
   a. The aorta is located at 12–1 o'clock.
   b. The pulmonary trunk is located at 1–2 o'clock.
   c. The left atrium is located at 2–3 o'clock.
   d. The left ventricle is located at 3–5 o'clock.

3. **According to the clock analogy, in the lateral view:**
   a. The left atrium is located at 12–2 o'clock.
   b. The left ventricle is located at 5–9 o'clock.
   c. The right ventricle is located at 3–5 o'clock.
   d. The main pulmonary artery is located at 2–3 o'clock.

4. **Which of the following options is false regarding the size of the cardiac silhouette?**
   a. Its width in the lateral view should measure 2.5–3.5 intercostal spaces (in dogs).
   b. Its width in the lateral view should measure 2.0–2.5 intercostal spaces (in cats).
   c. Its width in the dorsoventral view should not exceed 65% of the width of the thorax.
   d. Its height in the lateral view should not exceed 60% of the thoracic height.

5. **Cardiac size in dogs, according to the vertebral cardiac index, is:**
   a. 8.7–10.
   b. 9.7–10.
   c. 9.2–10.
   d. 8.1–10.

6. **What radiographic features can be observed in a dog with a patent ductus arteriosus?**
   a. Bulging at 11–1, 1–2 and 2–3 o'clock according to the clock analogy in the lateral view.
   b. Bulging at 11–1, 1–2 and 2–3 o'clock according to the clock analogy in the dorsoventral view.
   c. Bulging at 1–2, 2–3 and 3–4 o'clock according to the clock analogy in the lateral view.
   d. Bulging at 1–2, 2–3 and 3–4 o'clock according to the clock analogy in the dorsoventral view.

7. **The bulges observed in a dog with a patent ductus arteriosus correspond to which cardiovascular structures?**
   a. Right atrium, aortic arch, pulmonary trunk.
   b. Right auricular appendage, aortic arch, pulmonary trunk.
   c. Aortic arch, pulmonary trunk, left atrium.
   d. Aortic arch, pulmonary trunk, left auricular appendage.

8. Indicate which of the following options is false. What radiographic features can be observed in a dog with pulmonary stenosis?

a. Right cardiomegaly, reverse D shape in the dorsoventral view.
b. Bulging at 1–2 o'clock according to the clock analogy in the dorsoventral view.
c. Hypervascular pattern (both arteries and veins).
d. Hat sign in the lateral view.

9. What are the radiographic features in a dog with a persistent fourth right aortic arch?

a. Oesophageal dilation caudal to the cardiac base.
b. Focal curvature of the trachea to the right in the dorsoventral view.
c. Ventral displacement of the trachea at the height of the cardiac base.
d. Presence of an abnormal duct of soft tissue opacity at the height of the cardiac base.

10. In cats with advanced hypertrophic cardiomyopathy, which of the following may be observed?

a. An increase in the size of the left atrium due to dilation.
b. The typical "Valentine's heart".
c. Pleural effusion and pulmonary oedema.
d. All of the above are correct.

11. Indicate which of the following options is false. The radiographic characteristics that can be observed in the case of megaoesophagus are:

a. Aspiration pneumonia.
b. Tracheo-oesophageal band sign.
c. Displacement of the trachea ventrally and to the left.
d. Ventral displacement of the cardiac silhouette.

12. Which of the following radiographic characteristics may be observed in the case of cranial mediastinal masses in a German Shepherd dog?

a. Displacement of the carina caudal to the sixth intercostal space.
b. Displacement of the carina caudal to the fifth intercostal space.
c. Thickening of the cranial mediastinum (>2.5–3 times the width of the thoracic vertebral body in the dorsoventral view).
d. Thickening of the cranial mediastinum (>1 times the width of the thoracic vertebral body in the dorsoventral view).

Clinical Case

- 2-year-old English Springer Spaniel.
- Grade III/VI murmur.

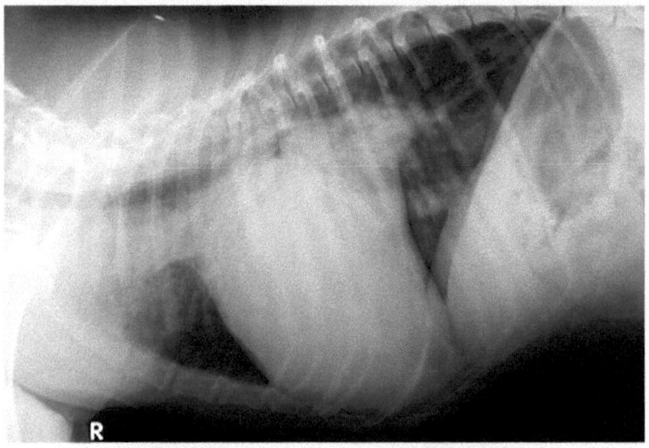

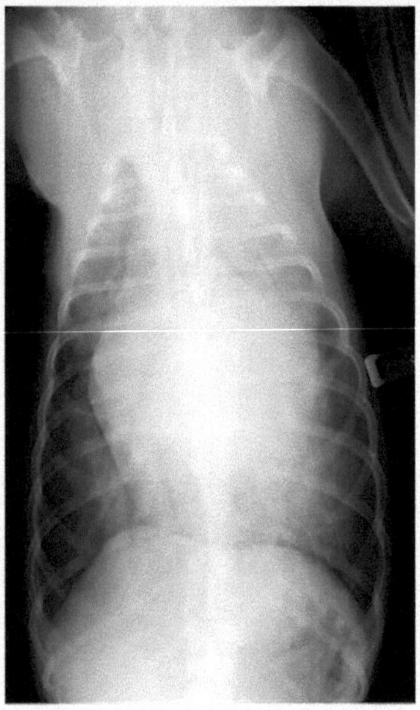

Radiographic description

- Moderately to severely enlarged cardiac silhouette with dorsal deviation of the trachea.
- Straightening and increased high of the caudal edge of the cardiac silhouette.
- Bulging at 1–3 o'clock in the lateral view, with compression of the caudal main stem bronchi. In the dorsoventral view, there is an abaxial deviation of the caudal main stem bronchi and a double wall sign.

- Moderate increase in the opacity of the pulmonary parenchyma, which is more marked in the perihilar area and in the left cranial pulmonary lung lobe, where there are several aerial bronchograms and a mild border effacement of the left part of the cardiac silhouette.
- Pulmonary vessels are moderately enlarged (arteries and veins) but poorly defined by the border effacement.
- Visible parts of the abdomen and musculoskeletal system appear normal.

Summary and differential diagnoses

- Left-sided cardiomegaly with congestive heart failure (differential diagnosis: consider congenital disease given the age of the animal, mitral dysplasia or patent ductus arteriosus. Other pathologies such as degenerative mitral valve disease or dilated cardiomyopathy cannot be ruled out).
- Interstitial alveolar pattern (differential diagnosis: cardiogenic pulmonary oedema).

Comments

An echocardiography and cardiology consultation is recommended.

Echocardiography I

M. Josefa Fernández del Palacio

1. Indicate which of the following is false regarding two-dimensional (2D) echocardiography:

a. The image that is observed in 2D does not appear in real time but is formed by an M-mode image reconstruction.
b. 2D mode was the second mode to be used in cardiology.
c. It allows visualisation of the movement of the cardiac structures, as well as measurement of the size of the chambers.
d. It is the base mode for obtaining the M, Doppler, and 3D modes.

2. Indicate which of the following is false regarding M mode echocardiography:

a. When using M mode, the heart is scanned according to a combination of linear images.
b. It is mainly used for the measurement of cardiac structures.
c. M mode is obtained from 2D images.
d. M mode is obtained from right short-axis parasternal images.

3. State which of the following is correct regarding Doppler echocardiography:

a. Pulsed Doppler allows blood flow velocities greater than 5 m/s to be measured.
b. Continuous Doppler allows the exact point of measurement of blood flow velocity to be selected.
c. Colour Doppler is a type of continuous Doppler.
d. Tissue Doppler allows measurement of myocardial velocities.

4. Indicate which of the following is false regarding a right four-chamber parasternal image:

a. In this image, the right-sided chambers are smaller than the left-sided ones.
b. The coronary sinus appears as a rounded structure approximately 1 cm in diameter in normal dogs and cats.
c. The right pulmonary vein and artery appear of similar size in healthy dogs.
d. The fossa ovalis is observed as an area where there are few echoes.

5. Indicate which of the following is correct regarding a right short-axis transventricular parasternal projection:

a. The left ventricle is observed as an oval shape in normal animals.
b. The tricuspid valve leaflets are clearly visible in the right ventricle.
c. Three papillary muscles in the left ventricle are seen protruding into the ventricular cavity.
d. This image is always the ideal for guiding M mode and for measuring the walls and chamber of the left ventricle.

6. Indicate which of the following is correct regarding measurements in M mode:

a. Measurements of cardiac structures should be obtained only in systole.
b. The use of a synchronous electrocardiogram is recommended to achieve greater precision in the measurements.
c. Measurements of cardiac structures in cats depend on their age.
d. Measurements of cardiac structures in dogs are calculated by dividing weight by age.

7. Indicate what is correct regarding echocardiographic projections:

a. Right parasternal and subcostal access windows are used for the entire examination.
b. Through the right parasternal access, only long-axis sections of the heart are obtained.
c. Subcostal access is used to obtain pulmonary flow velocities.
d. Left parasternal access is best suited to assess atrioventricular valve flows using spectral Doppler.

8. Indicate which of the following is false regarding the left parasternal projection:

a. The transducer is placed both in an apical and a cranial position.
b. Using the apical position, four- and five-chamber sections are obtained.
c. Long- and short-axis sections are obtained using the cranial position.
d. Aortic flow velocity can be easily measured using the cranial position.

9. Indicate which of the following is false regarding transvalvular flow:

a. Transmitral flow is observed during left ventricular diastole.
b. Atrial fibrillation affects the number of flow velocity peaks for the atrioventricular valves.
c. Pulmonary flow can be obtained by both right and left parasternal access.
d. Aortic flow velocity can be obtained only using subcostal access.

ECHOCARDIOGRAPHY II

M. Josefa Fernández del Palacio

1. **Which of the following echocardiographic findings is not characteristic in a dog with subaortic stenosis?**
   a. Aortic flow velocities of 1.8 m/s obtained using a subcostal access.
   b. Left ventricular concentric hypertrophy.
   c. Poststenotic dilation of the ascending aorta.
   d. A mitral flow pattern of abnormal relaxation.

2. **Indicate which is correct regarding pulmonary stenosis:**
   a. It is diagnosed when the pulmonary flow velocity is greater than 2.6 m/s.
   b. Type A presents a dome shape of the sigmoid valves during systole.
   c. The diagnosis can be made using colour Doppler.
   d. Right ventricular hypertrophy is pathognomonic of pulmonary stenosis.

3. **Indicate which of the following is false regarding tetralogy of Fallot:**
   a. Echocardiography allows the visualisation of all defects.
   b. Contrast echocardiography makes it possible to diagnose this heart disease.
   c. Dextroposition of the aorta is observed using a right long-axis parasternal access.
   d. The pulmonary artery may appear hypoplastic.

4. **Which of the following statements is false?**
   a. Ventricular septal defects are best visualised using a left apical four-chamber parasternal access.
   b. Restrictive defects are characterised by blood flow velocities exceeding 4.5 m/s through them.
   c. Atrial septal defects can be visualised using a right long-axis four-chamber parasternal access.
   d. In ostium primum-type atrial septal defects, the septal leaflet of the tricuspid valve and the anterior leaflet of the mitral valve have a common origin in the ventricular septum.

5. **Which of the following is correct regarding chronic mitral degenerative disease in dogs?**
   a. In early stages, mitral valve prolapse can be observed using M-mode echocardiography.
   b. Fractional shortening is a reliable parameter for determining the severity of mitral regurgitation.
   c. In advanced stages of the disease, there is a characteristic pattern of abnormal relaxation.
   d. Mitral regurgitation volume can be assessed semiquantitatively by colour Doppler.

6. **Which of the following is false regarding dilated cardiomyopathy (DCM) in dogs?**
   a. 2D echocardiography reveals a dilation of the left-sided chambers.
   b. A fractional shortening of less than 30% suggests systolic dysfunction in DCM.
   c. Doppler echocardiography may reveal diastolic dysfunction when considering the E/A ratio.
   d. Systolic and diastolic dysfunction coexist in DCM.

7. **Which of the following is true regarding feline cardiomyopathies?**
   a. Hypertrophic cardiomyopathy in cats is characterised by eccentric hypertrophy.
   b. In restrictive cardiomyopathy, the fractional shortening may be normal.
   c. Pulsed Doppler makes it possible to differentiate between the different types of cardiomyopathy.
   d. Dynamic obstruction of the left ventricular outflow tract is assessed by evaluating transmitral flow.

8. **Which of the following is correct regarding cardiac neoplasms?**
   a. Only those measuring more than 2 cm in diameter are observed by echocardiography.
   b. Cardiac base tumours are best seen using transoesophageal echocardiography.
   c. Mesotheliomas can be easily diagnosed using the 2D mode.
   d. M mode allows evaluation of the echogenicity of tumours.

9. **In a dog with severe abdominal distension secondary to pericardial tamponade, what is the most characteristic echocardiographic sign?**
   a. Tricuspid regurgitation with a velocity greater than 2.8 m/s.
   b. Increased size of the left-sided chambers.
   c. Compression of the right atrial wall caused by elevated intrapericardial pressure.
   d. Paradoxical movement of the interatrial septum.

10. **Which of the following is false regarding pulmonary hypertension?**
   a. Tricuspid regurgitation velocities greater than 3.0 m/s suggest pulmonary hypertension.
   b. Pulmonary regurgitation velocities higher than 2.2 m/s suggest pulmonary hypertension.
   c. The right-sided cavities may appear generally dilated.
   d. The left-sided cavities are seen to be reduced in size in severe cases.

Radiographic Diagnosis of the Musculoskeletal System

Marta Soler Laguía

Test

1. Indicate which of the following statements is true:

a. The epiphysis is located between the diaphysis and the metaphysis.
b. The physis, epiphyseal line or growth plate is located between the epiphysis and the metaphysis.
c. The nutrient artery is located in the metaphysis.
d. The metaphysis in young animals is radiotransparent.

2. Which statement is true?

a. Osteolytic changes are radiographically evident about 10–14 days after the onset of bone injury.
b. Changes in osteogenesis are radiographically evident at least 5–7 days after the onset of bone injury.
c. Changes in osteogenesis are radiographically evident at least 10–14 days after the onset of bone injury.
d. Osteolytic changes are radiographically evident on the second day after the onset of bone injury.

3. Which statement is true?

a. The solid model for osteogenesis can be palisade, spiculated or amorphous.
b. In a bone lesion, the "Codman's triangle" is not pathognomonic of osteosarcoma.
c. In a bone lesion, if the transition zone is narrow, it indicates malignancy.
d. In a joint, visualisation of intracapsular gas is a sign of synovial effusion.

4. Which statement is true?

a. In degenerative joint diseases, increased opacity of the subchondral bone is called sclerosis.
b. The primary bone healing of a fracture occurs by the process of endochondral ossification.
c. Salter–Harris type fractures occur in radiographically mature animals.
d. In a fracture, bone callus should be seen radiographically after 5 days.

5. Which terminology would be most adequate when taking a radiograph of a cat's metacarpals with the X-ray beam centred on the third metacarpal and the cassette behind it?

a. Anteroposterior projection.
b. Craniocaudal projection.
c. Dorsopalmar projection.
d. Dorsoplantar projection.

6. Indicate which is the correct answer:

a. Metastatic bone tumours usually have monostotic distribution.
b. Haematogenous osteomyelitis usually has a polyostotic distribution.
c. Primary bone tumours usually have polyostotic distribution.
d. Bone marrow tumours usually have a monostotic distribution.

7. Which is the correct answer:

a. In cases of multiple epiphyseal dysplasia, a radiopaque stipple is visualised on the epiphyses of the long bones.
b. In secondary renal hyperparathyroidism, generalised osteopaenia occurs, especially in the long bones.
c. In cases of rickets, osteopaenia occurs that affects the bones of the skull.
d. In cases of hypertrophic osteopathy, an amorphous pattern of periosteal reaction is visualised in the cortices of the distal long bones of the extremities.

8. If osteolytic foci are observed on a radiograph along with significant inflammation of the soft tissues of the stifle joint in a large-breed dog, the first suspected differential diagnosis should be:

a. Leishmaniasis.
b. Synovial cell sarcoma.
c. Lupus erythematosus.
d. Rheumatoid arthritis.

9. If a large-breed adult/geriatric dog presents with pain and inflammation in the carpus and tarsus, what pathology should be considered first?

a. Metaphyseal osteopathy.
b. Haematogenous osteomyelitis.
c. Hypertrophic osteopathy.
d. Osseous cysts.

10. Regarding fracture resolution, indicate the correct answer:

a. Check-ups should be every 6 weeks.
b. Intramembranous repair is also known as secondary repair.
c. Endochondral repair occurs by perfect apposition of the fragments and there is no formation of bone callus.
d. During intramembranous repair, bone attachment occurs through the prior formation of a haematoma and granulation tissue.

Clinical Case

Producing a radiographic report

1. Identify the patient: species, sex, body condition and type of breed (when known); indicate whether the animal is adult or radiographically immature.

2. Identify the projections taken.

3. Evaluate the radiographic technique used to obtain the images: mention whether there are any characteristics that could have been improved to improve the radiographic quality (if there is rotation, if the right/left side/extremity is labelled, if the image is overexposed or underexposed, if it is properly collimated and centred, or if the presence of an artefact is observed). If nothing is observed that could have been improved, the radiographic technique is noted as being correct.

4. Describe the radiographic findings: the radiographic image should be described so that someone reading the report without seeing the radiographs could visualise it with all the information provided.

5. Provide a radiographic diagnosis (this will not always be the definitive diagnosis, as a radiographic diagnosis may coincide with several possible diagnoses).

6. Prepare a list of differential diagnoses: when a radiographic diagnosis is compatible with more than one possible definitive diagnosis, the differential diagnoses should be indicated on a list, ordered from highest to lowest probability of occurrence.

7. Comments/recommendations/other means of diagnosis: what is the next step to be taken to reach the definitive diagnosis (other radiographic projections, an ultrasound examination, a blood test, a fine-needle aspiration/biopsy, a CT or MRI study, etc).

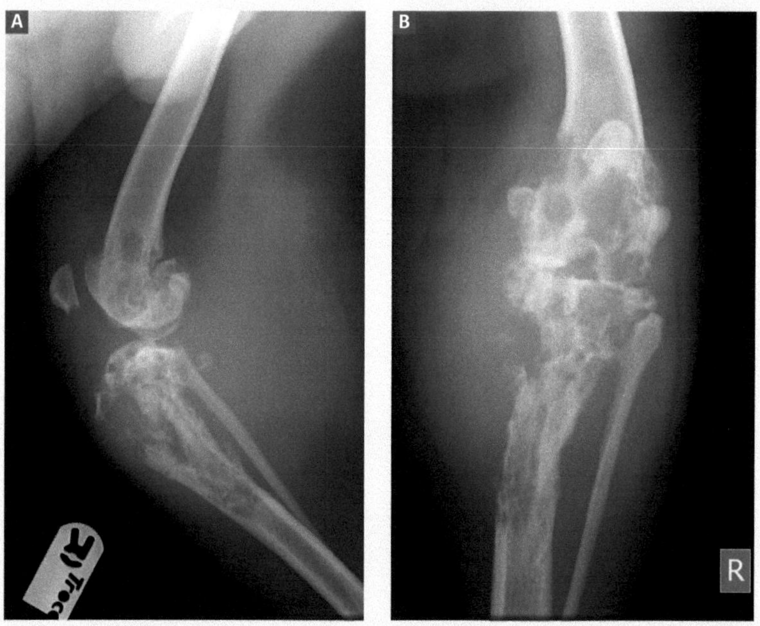

Diagnostic Imaging of the Limbs

Marta Soler Laguía

Test

1. **Indicate the correct answer regarding osteochondrosis:**
   a. In the shoulder, it usually affects the greater tubercle of the humerus.
   b. In the elbow, it usually affects the lateral epicondyle of the humerus.
   c. In the shoulder, it usually affects the caudal portion of the head of the humerus.
   d. In the tarsus, it usually affects the lateral edge of the trochlea of the talus.

2. **Which statement is true?**
   a. Nonunion of the anconeal process can be diagnosed from 5 months of age.
   b. Fragmentation of the medial coronoid process is diagnosed with a lateral elbow projection in forced flexion.
   c. Fragmentation of the medial coronoid process is diagnosed with a craniocaudal projection of the elbow.
   d. Diagnosis of fragmentation of the medial coronoid process is achieved using computed tomography.

3. **To diagnose hip dysplasia:**
   a. It is not necessary to sedate the animal.
   b. Radiography is performed in a dorsoventral projection.
   c. The entire wing of the ilium up to the tibial tuberosities should be included.
   d. It is not necessary for the stifle to be centred on the femoral condyles.

4. **Regarding avascular necrosis of the head of the femur, which is the correct answer?**
   a. It is best diagnosed by performing a lateral radiograph of the affected femur.
   b. It is diagnosed when osteolytic foci are visualised in the femoral head and neck, among other radiographic signs.
   c. In most cases, there is bilateral involvement.
   d. It usually affects medium- and large-breed dogs.

5. **Which is the correct answer?**
   a. Supraglenoid scapular tubercle avulsions are characteristic of adult animals.
   b. The best projection for visualisation of fractures of the scapula is the forced lateral or "swimmer's" view.
   c. Scapula fractures are common and usually bilateral.
   d. The best projection for visualisation of fractures of the scapula is the skyline projection of the shoulder.

6. **Which is the correct answer:**
   a. The lateral coronoid process of the ulna is fragmented more frequently than the medial one.
   b. To diagnose elbow dysplasia, performing a lateral radiograph in oblique flexion is necessary.
   c. If there is an alteration of the medial coronoid process of the ulna, it can be diagnosed with a lateral radiograph of the elbow in flexion.
   d. When there is a fragmentation of the medial coronoid process of the ulna, other radiographic signs, such as sclerosis of the subtrochlear notch of the ulna, among others, are usually observed.

7. **Which is the correct answer:**
   a. Incomplete ossification of the humeral condyle can be diagnosed from 2 months of age.
   b. Incomplete ossification of the humeral condyle is diagnosed by lateral radiographs of the elbow in forced flexion.
   c. A craniocaudal elbow radiograph is needed to diagnose incomplete ossification of the humeral condyle.
   d. Incomplete ossification of the humeral condyle is usually unilateral.

8. **Which is the correct answer:**
   a. To diagnose hip dysplasia, the Norberg angle must be less than 90°.
   b. Morgan's line is a radiopaque line that appears on the femoral head in cases of hip dysplasia.
   c. Morgan's line is a radiopaque line that appears on the femoral neck in cases of hip dysplasia.
   d. In cases of hip dysplasia, the femoral neck is usually affected, showing osteolytic foci in the area of insertion of the joint capsule.

9. Which is the correct answer:

a. If a lateral stifle radiograph shows cranial displacement of the tibia with respect to the femur, a rupture of the caudal cruciate ligament can be suspected.
b. Feline metaphyseal osteopathy usually occurs in young cats.
c. Medial patella luxation usually occurs in large-breed dogs.
d. Lateral patella luxation usually occurs in miniature-breed dogs.

10. Which is the correct answer:

a. Squamous cell carcinoma of the nail matrix always presents a palisade reaction model.
b. Squamous cell carcinoma of the nail matrix usually exhibits a marked pattern of osteogenesis.
c. Squamous cell carcinoma of the nail matrix is often accompanied by inflammation of the soft tissues of the distal phalanx.
d. Answers b and c are correct.

Clinical Case

- 6.5-month-old, 12 kg mixed-breed dog.

Producing a radiographic report

1. Identify the patient: species, sex, body condition and type of breed (when known); indicate whether the animal is adult or radiographically immature.

2. Identify the projections taken.

3. Evaluate of the radiographic technique used to obtain the images: mention whether there are any characteristics that could have been altered to improve the radiographic quality (if there is rotation, if the right/left side/extremity is labelled, if the image is overexposed or underexposed, if it is properly collimated and centred, or if the presence of an artefact is observed). If nothing is observed that could have been improved, the radiographic technique is noted as being correct.

4. Describe the radiographic findings: the radiographic image should be described so that someone reading the report without seeing the radiographs could visualise it with all the information provided.

5. Provide a radiographic diagnosis (this will not always be the definitive diagnosis, as a radiographic diagnosis may coincide with several possible diagnoses).

6. Prepare a list of differential diagnoses: when a radiographic diagnosis is compatible with more than one possible definitive diagnosis, the differential diagnoses should be indicated on a list, ordered from highest to lowest probability of occurrence.

7. Comments/recommendations/other means of diagnosis: what is the next step to be taken to reach the definitive diagnosis (other radiographic projections, an ultrasound examination, a blood test, a fine-needle aspiration/biopsy, a CT or MRI study etc)?

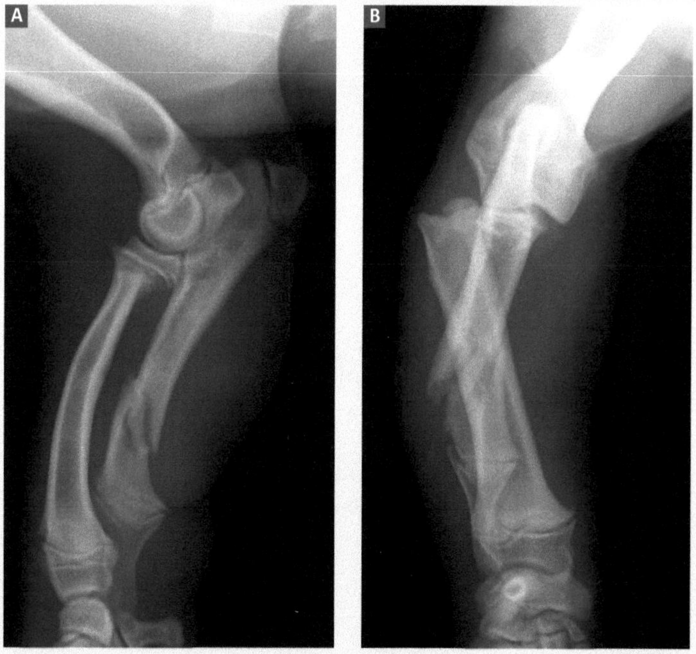

Head and Neck, Limbs and Noncardiac Thorax

Patricia Laborda Vidal

Test

1. The most likely diagnosis for these ultrasound images of the neck (thyroid gland) of a cat with polyphagia is:

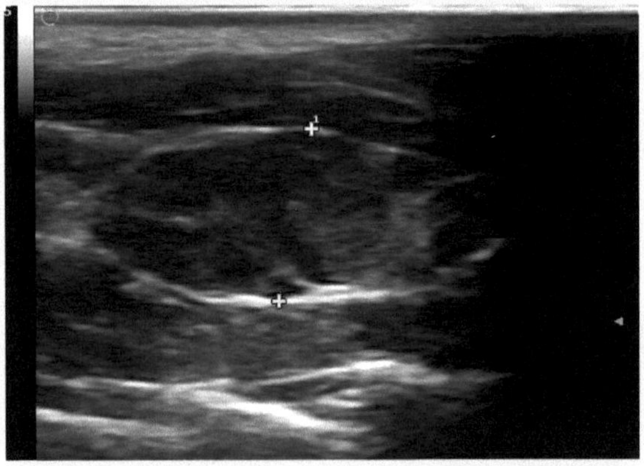

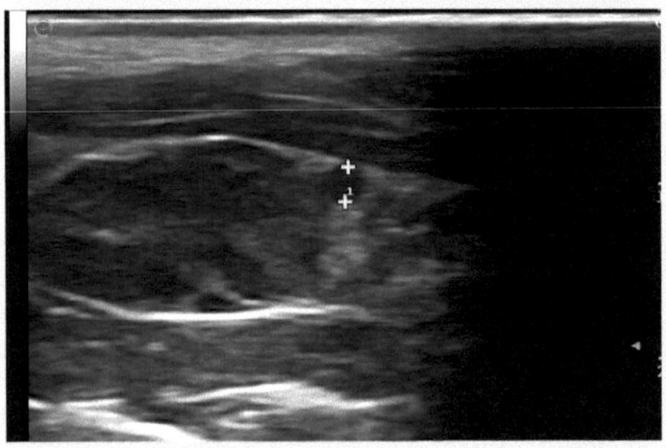

a. Thyroid adenoma or adenomatous hyperplasia.
b. Thyroid carcinoma
c. Cysts in the thyroid gland.
d. Hyperparathyroidism.

2. Indicate whether the following statement is true or false:
In the above ultrasound images of the thyroid gland, the small, rounded, hypoechoic structure (indicated with markers) probably represents the caudal parathyroid gland, which is embedded in the thyroid parenchyma.

3. Regarding ultrasonographic visualisation of the mandibular salivary gland:
a. It is located ventrally and laterally to the external auditory canal.
b. It is located superficially and dorsally to the parotid salivary gland.
c. It is the largest salivary gland.
d. It is located medial to the retropharyngeal lymph node.

4. An 8-year-old, male Flat-Coated Retriever is presented with a history of cough, apathy and anorexia for the past week. In the following thoracic mediastinal ultrasound images, what are the anechoic structures likely to be?

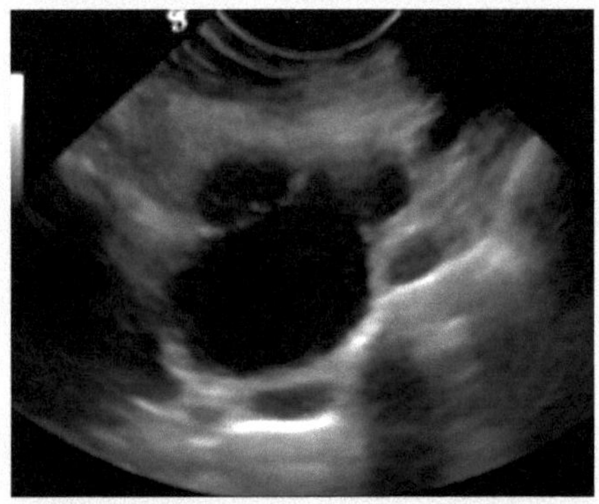

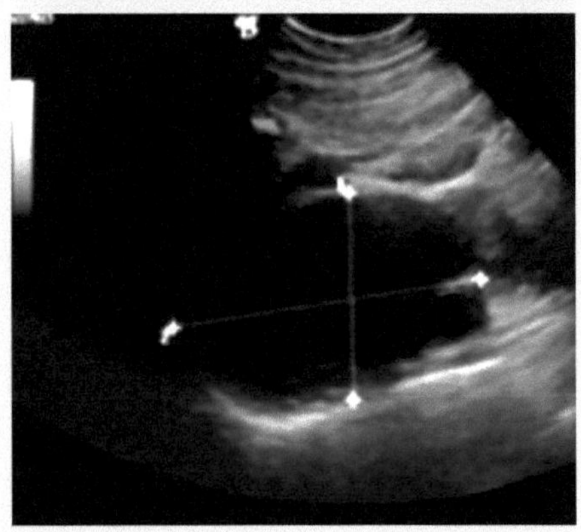

a. Mediastinal cysts.
b. Mediastinal vessels in cross section.
c. Cranial mediastinal lymph nodes.
d. Fat necrosis.

5. What is the most likely diagnosis in the above images of the mediastinum of a Flat-Coated Retriever?
a. Fungal infection (probably aspergillosis).
b. Neoplasia (probably histiocytic sarcoma).
c. Mediastinitis (probably due to a foreign body).
d. Parasitic infection (probably associated with *Spirocerca* migration).

6. **Indicate which is the right answer regarding lung ultrasonography:**
   a. A lines occur in normal lung.
   b. A lines can occur in cases of alveolar oedema.
   c. A lines can occur in cases of pleural effusion.
   d. A lines do not occur in cases of pneumothorax.

7. **Indicate which is the right answer regarding lung ultrasonography:**
   a. B lines occur in normal lung.
   b. B lines can occur in cases of alveolar oedema.
   c. B lines can occur in cases of pleural effusion.
   d. B lines can occur in cases of pneumothorax.

8. **Which are among the most common muscle pathologies of the shoulder that can be examined ultrasonographically?**
   a. Calcifying deltoid tendinopathy.
   b. Calcifying tendinopathy of the biceps femoris.
   c. Supraspinatus tenosynovitis.
   d. Biceps tenosynovitis.

9. **Indicate which of the following options is true regarding ultrasonography of the stifle:**
   a. The medial meniscus cannot be seen using ultrasound.
   b. The lateral meniscus is seen as a hyperechoic triangle.
   c. It is the method of choice for examining cruciate ligaments.
   d. Collateral ligaments cannot be observed because they are very superficial.

10. **Indicate which of the following options is false regarding ultrasound examination of tendon ruptures:**
   a. In the acute phase (1 day), the presence of hypoechoic foci that represent a haematoma can be observed.
   b. In the initial chronic phase (4–6 weeks) heterogeneous foci that represent haematoma organisation can be observed.
   c. In the late chronic phase (>3 months), they appear completely normal.
   d. Normal tendons appear as structures with hyperechoic fibres.

11. **Which of the following options is correct regarding muscle ultrasonography:**
   a. Muscles are more hypoechoic than tendons.
   b. The fat in the intermuscular fascia is hyperechoic in comparison to muscle.
   c. The echogenicity of muscle is heterogeneous, with fine hyperechoic strips.
   d. All of the above are correct.

Clinical Case

- 7-year-old, female Greyhound.
- Acute lameness in the right hindlimb after running through a field.
- Ultrasonographic examination of the stifle is performed (Fig. 1).

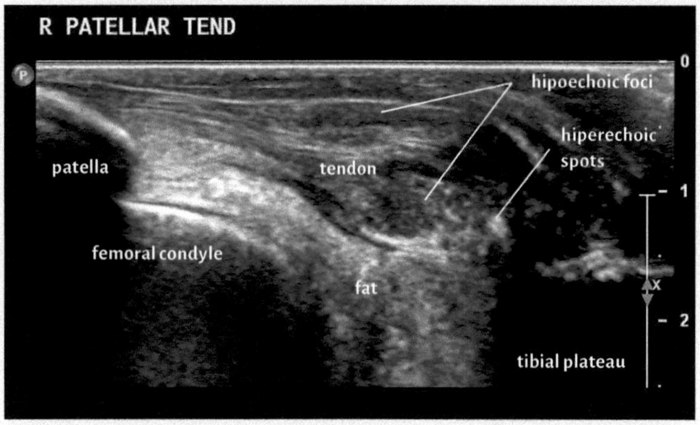

Figure 1. Ultrasound image of the stifle of an adult dog.

Description

- Ultrasound examination of the stifle, via an infrapatellar approach.
- There is thickening of the distal half of the right patellar tendon. Its fibres lose their linear structure, and it acquires a heterogeneous echogenicity. There are some hypoechoic foci (haematomas) with small hyperechoic spots (mineralisation) in the distal part of the tendon, where no normal fibres are seen.
- The visible surface of the patella and femoral condyle are smooth. The surface of the tibial plateau has a rough appearance. Infrapatellar fat is compressed/ displaced caudally.

Interpretation and differential diagnoses

Acute rupture of the right patellar tendon with possible avulsion of small bone fragments from the tibial plateau.

Comments

- The stifle must be evaluated both clinically and ultrasonographically to assess whether the rupture is complete (in this image it appears to be).
- An ultrasound examination of the contralateral stifle should be performed to evaluate possible chronic injuries, and radiographs of both stifles should be performed before the ultrasound examination.

Correct Answers

Computed Tomography

Test: **1.**b; **2.**d; **3.**b; **4.**d; **5.**b

Magnetic Resonance Imaging

Test: **1.**c; **2.**b; **3.**d; **4.**a; **5.**b; **6.**c; **7.**b; **8.**a

Clinical Case

1. Left central vestibular system (brainstem).
2. a. Complete blood tests with complete blood count and biochemistry.
   b. MRI of the head.
   c. Cerebrospinal fluid sampling and analysis.
3. A. Region shown/structures present: caudal fossa, occipital cortex, cerebellum, medulla oblongata.
   B. Sequence type: T2W, T1W precontrast, T1W postcontrast.
   C. Plane of these sequences: transverse.
4. **Presence of a focal, extensive, broad-based, extra-axial lesion located ventrolateral to the medulla oblongata, causing compression of the medulla oblongata on the left side.** The lesion is markedly hyperintense in T2W and isointense in T1W compared with the cortical grey matter, and shows homogeneous enhancement and marked contrast enhancement. The lesion causes a marked mass effect with midline displacement and distortion of the fourth ventricle.
5. a. Meningioma.
   b. Histiocytic sarcoma.
   c. Lymphoma.
   d. Fungal granuloma.

Abdominal Lymph Node Ultrasonography

Test: **1.**b; **2.**c; **3.**b; **4.**a; **5.**b; **6.**a; **7.**c; **8.**b; **9.**a; **10.**c

Application of Doppler

Test: **1.**d; **2.**c; **3.**b; **4.**a; **5.**d

Liver, Spleen, Gastrointestinal, Urinary, Reproductive and Adrenal Glands

Test: **1.**a; **2.**b; **3.**b; **4.**c; **5.**a; **6.**c; **7.**b; **8.**b; **9.**b; **10.**d

Thoracic Radiography

Test: **1.**b; **2.**c; **3.**d; **4.**d; **5.**d; **6.**c; **7.**d; **8.**c; **9.**a

Cardiac and Mediastinal Thorax

Test: **1.**b; **2.**c; **3.**a; **4.**d; **5.**a; **6.**b; **7.**d; **8.**c; **9.**c; **10.**d; **11.**c; **12.**a

Echocardiography I

Test: **1.**a; **2.**a; **3.**b; **4.**b; **5.**d; **6.**b; **7.**d; **8.**d; **9.**d

Echocardiography II

Test: **1.**a; **2.**b; **3.**b; **4.**a; **5.**d; **6.**b; **7.**b; **8.**b; **9.**c; **10.**a

Radiographic Diagnosis of the Musculoskeletal System

Test: **1.**b; **2.**c; **3.**b; **4.**a; **5.**c ; **6.**b; **7.**a; **8.**b; **9.**c; **10.**a

Clinical Case

1. These are two radiographic images of the right stifle of a radiologically mature canine patient.
2. There is a mediolateral projection (ML) and a craniocaudal projection (CrCd).
3. Radiographic technique is adequate.
4. Multiple osteolytic foci are visualised affecting the distal metaphysis and femoral condyles, as well as the tibial condyles and the proximal tibial metaphysis; osteolytic lesions also extend caudally, affecting the proximal third of the tibia. These osteolytic foci affect both the medullary and cortical cavities of the bones (femur and tibia). These are foci with poorly defined margins, of variable size, that seem to converge and form more extensive areas of osteolysis. At the level of the cortices, there is thinning and loss of continuity in all of them, but this is more intense in the medial and cranial cortex of the proximal tibial metaphysis. The distal pole of the patella presents an osteolytic focus. The sesamoid bones of the gastrocnemius cannot be clearly assessed due to overlapping of structures, and in the ML projection, the sesamoid bone of the popliteus appears to be distally displaced, with an irregular surface and decreased opacity. The soft tissues show marked increases in opacity and volume both intra-articularly and extra-articularly, especially at the medial and caudal levels of the joint. The transition zone of the lesions is wide, and there is little definition of the margins of these lesions.
5. The radiographic diagnosis consists of an aggressive bone lesion with a marked osteolytic component that affects all the bones of the stifle joint, with involvement of the cortical and medullary cavity and intense inflammation of the adjacent soft tissues.
6. The differential diagnoses for an aggressive bone lesion are neoplasia and infection (osteomyelitis/erosive arthritis). Among the possible differentials for neoplasia, given that this is a large joint in an adult large-breed dog, the first would be synovial cell sarcoma; however, other neoplasms of bone origin, such as haemangiosarcoma, fibrosarcoma or even osteosarcoma cannot be ruled out despite the lesion not being in their most common form.
7. A radiographic study of the thoracic cavity (since the animal is already in the X-ray room) and biopsy of the lesion should be recommended first to reach a definitive diagnosis.

Diagnostic Imaging of the Limbs

Test: 1.c; **2.**d; **3.**c; **4.**b; **5.**b; **6.**d; **7.**c; **8.**c; **9.**b; **10.**c

Clinical Case

1. Two radiographic images of the ulna and radius of a radiographically immature canine patient. Observing the morphology of the bones, the animal presents characteristics of a chondrodystrophic breed.
2. There is a mediolateral projection (ML) and a craniocaudal projection (CrCd).
3. Radiographic technique is adequate.
4. An oblique fracture is visualised at the level of the middle shaft of the ulna, with slight cranial and medial displacement of the distal fragment with respect to the proximal fragment. In the radius, a fracture is observed at the level of the proximal physis (growth line), with lateral displacement of the shaft. The proximal epiphysis (head of the radius) remains in its anatomical position articulating with the humerus. The adjacent soft tissues are increased in thickness and opacity, especially at the caudal and medial level of the forelimb. There are no other alterations in the area of the elbow and carpal joints.
5. The radiographic diagnosis consists of a mid-distal diaphyseal oblique fracture of the ulna with slight craniomedial displacement of the distal fragment and a type I Salter–Harris fracture at the level of the proximal physis of the radius, with lateral displacement of the diaphysis of the radius.
6. In this case there are no differential diagnoses because the radiographic diagnosis coincides with the definitive diagnosis.
7. No other diagnostic tests are necessary because a definitive diagnosis is reached through the radiographic study.

Head and Neck, Limbs and Noncardiac Thorax

Test: 1.a; **2.**True; **3.**c; **4.**c; **5.**b; **6.**a; **7.**b; **8.**d; **9.**b; **10.**c; **11.**d

List of Abbreviations

Abbreviations

APM: anterior papillary muscle
ASD: atrial septal defect
BPH: benign prostatic hyperplasia
CC: congenital cardiopathy
CCT: carcinoma de células transicionales
CdCr: caudocranial
CdVC: caudal vena cava
CR: computed radiography
CrCd: craniocaudal
CrVC: cranial vena cava
CSF: cerebrospinal fluid
CT: computed tomography
CVC: caudal vena cava
CW spectral Doppler: continuous-wave spectral Doppler
DCM: dilated cardiomyopathy
DDR: direct digital radiography
DFOV: display field of view
DJD: degenerative joint disease
DP: dorsopalmar
DPt: dorsoplantar
DPG: Doppler pressure gradient
DV: dorsoventral
ECG: electrocardiogram
FFD: film-focus distance
FIP: feline infectious peritonitis
FMCP: fragmentation of the medial coronoid process
GDV: gastric dilatation-volvulus
GME: granulomatous meningoencephalitis
HU: Hounsfield units
HV: hepatic vein
IBD: inflammatory bowel disease
IOHC: incomplete ossification of the humeral condyle
IR: inversion recovery
kV: kilovoltaje
LA: left atrium
LV: left ventricle
LVFW: left ventricular free wall
LVOT: left ventricular outflow tract
LVS: left ventricular septum
mAs: milliamperage
MED: multiple epiphyseal dysplasia
MinIP: minimum intensity projection
MIP: maximum intensity projection
ML: mediolateral
MRI: magnetic resonance imaging
MUO: meningoencephalitis of unknown origin
NLE: necrotising leukoencephalitis
NME: necrotising meningoencephalitis
OC: osteochondrosis
OCD: osteochondritis dissecans
OFD: object-to-fil distance
PA: pulmonary artery
PDA: patent ductus arteriosus
PI: pulsatility index
PPM: posterior papillary muscle
PSS: portosystemic shunt
PW Doppler: pulsed-wave Doppler
RA: right atrium
RI: resistive index
RP: radiofrequency pulse
RV: right ventricle
RVOT: right ventricular outflow tract
S/L ratio: ratio of the short axis and the long axis of a lymph node
SE: spin echo
SFOV: scan field of view
STIR: short tau inversion recovery
VD: ventrodorsal
VHS: vertebral heart score
V_{max}: maximum velocity
VSD: ventricular septal defect
WL: window level
WW: window width

Notes